Image-based Questions in

Obstetrics and Gynecology

Image-based Questions in

Obstetrics and Gynecology

MRCOG, NEET SS/NEET PG Aspirants and OBGYN Residents (MD & DNB)

Richa Saxena
MBBS MD (OBGYN)
PG Diploma in Clinical Research, RCOG Associate
Obstetrician Gynecologist (Let's talk woman's health)
Course Mentor and Director (Cracking MRCOG-DigiNerve)
New Delhi, India

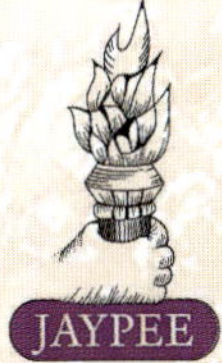

JAYPEE BROTHERS MEDICAL PUBLISHERS
The Health Sciences Publisher
New Delhi | London

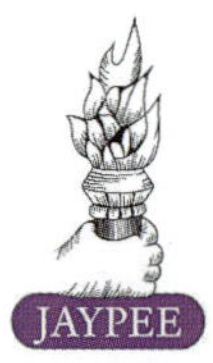

JAYPEE **Jaypee Brothers Medical Publishers (P) Ltd**

Headquarters
EMCA House, 23/23-B
Ansari Road, Daryaganj
New Delhi 110 002, India
Landline: +91-11-23272143, +91-11-23272703
+91-11-23282021, +91-11-23245672
e-mail: jaypee@jaypeebrothers.com

Corporate Office
4838/24, Ansari Road, Daryaganj
New Delhi 110 002, India
Phone: +91-11-43574357
Fax: +91-11-43574314
e-mail: jaypee@jaypeebrothers.com

Overseas Office
JP Medical Ltd.
83, Victoria Street, London
SW1H 0HW (UK)
Phone: +44-20 3170 8910
e-mail: info@jpmedpub.com

EU GPSR Authorised Representative
Logos Europe, 9 rue Nicolas Poussin
17000, La Rochelle, France
Phone: +33 (0) 6 67 93 73 78
e-mail: contact@logoseurope.eu

Website: www.jaypeebrothers.com
Website: www.jaypeedigital.com

© 2026, Jaypee Brothers Medical Publishers

The views and opinions expressed in this book are solely those of the original contributor(s)/author(s) and do not necessarily represent those of editor(s) or publisher of the book.

All rights reserved. No part of this publication may be reproduced, stored or transmitted in any form or by any means, electronic, mechanical, photocopying, recording or otherwise, without the prior permission in writing of the publishers.

All brand names and product names used in this book are trade names, service marks, trademarks or registered trademarks of their respective owners. The publisher is not associated with any product or vendor mentioned in this book.

Medical knowledge and practice change constantly. This book is designed to provide accurate, authoritative information about the subject matter in question. However, readers are advised to check the most current information available on procedures included and check information from the manufacturer of each product to be administered, to verify the recommended dose, formula, method and duration of administration, adverse effects and contraindications. It is the responsibility of the practitioner to take all appropriate safety precautions. Neither the publisher nor the author(s)/editor(s) assume any liability for any injury and/or damage to persons or property arising from or related to use of material in this book.

This book is sold on the understanding that the publisher is not engaged in providing professional medical services. If such advice or services are required, the services of a competent medical professional should be sought.

Every effort has been made where necessary to contact holders of copyright to obtain permission to reproduce copyright material. If any have been inadvertently overlooked, the publisher will be pleased to make the necessary arrangements at the first opportunity.

Inquiries for bulk sales may be solicited at: jaypee@jaypeebrothers.com

Image-based Questions in Obstetrics and Gynecology

First Edition: **2026**

ISBN: 978-93-6616-436-6

Printed at: Samrat Offset Pvt. Ltd.

Dedication

Dedicated to my mother, Mrs Bharati Saxena

For always being there....

"My mother is the most beautiful woman I have ever seen. All I am I owe to my mother.

I attribute all my success in life to the moral, intellectual and physical education I have received from her."

—George Washington

Preface

In an era of visually driven learning and rapid advancements in obstetrics and gynecology, *Image-based Questions in Obstetrics and Gynecology* is designed to bridge the gap between theoretical knowledge and clinical application through an interactive and visually engaging format. This book brings together over 500 image-based questions, each rooted in clinical scenarios commonly encountered in everyday practice.

"In the vivid clarity of images lies the power to transform knowledge into understanding,"

—Anonymous

This quote captures the essence of this book, emphasizing how the visual learning deepens comprehension, making complex medical concepts clearer and more memorable.

The unique, three-column layout of this book is its defining feature and a powerful tool for learners and practitioners alike. Column 1 presents clinical scenarios structured as multiple-choice questions (MCQs), encouraging readers to think critically about diagnoses and management strategies. Column 2 provides concise and accurate answers, allowing for quick assessment and reinforcement of knowledge. Finally, Column 3 dives into evidence-based explanations, offering readers an in-depth understanding of each answer's rationale and linking clinical decisions to current guidelines and research.

This book is intended to be a comprehensive resource for students preparing for exams, as well as a reliable reference for clinicians seeking a practical review. Through vibrant, high-quality images and clear, structured answers, this atlas aims to foster a deeper, more practical understanding of obstetrics and gynecology.

This book is particularly beneficial for candidates preparing for the MRCOG Part 1 and NEET SS/NEET PG exams, where image-based questions play a critical role in testing applied clinical knowledge. With an emphasis on real-world scenarios and high-quality visuals, the format closely mirrors the style and rigor of these examinations. Furthermore, the structured approach of this book aligns well with the Objective Structured Clinical Examinations (OSCEs), now a core component of the residency, particularly the DNB exam. By combining practice with precise, evidence-based explanations, this atlas serves as a comprehensive tool to support success in a range of certification and postgraduate exams in obstetrics and gynecology.

The multiple-choice questions (MCQs) in this book follow the Single Best Answer (SBA) format, consistent with the MRCOG exam structure. While there may be several closely related options, each question has been carefully crafted to highlight the single best answer.

I hope that this image-based color atlas not only serves as a valuable resource in your learning journey but also inspires a passion for lifelong learning and clinical excellence in our field.

Writing a book is a colossal task. It can never be completed without divine intervention and approval. Therefore, I have decided to end this preface with a small prayer of thanks to the Almighty, which I was taught in my childhood.

"Father, lead me day by day, ever in thy own sweet way,
Teach me to be pure and good and tell me what I ought to do."

—Amen

I would like to extend my thanks and appreciation to all the related authors and publishers whose references have been used in this book. Book creation is teamwork, and I acknowledge the way the entire staff of M/s Jaypee Brothers Medical Publishers (P) Ltd., New Delhi, India, worked hard on this manuscript to give it a final shape. I would especially like to thank Mr Jitender P Vij (Group Chairman), Mr Ankit Vij (Managing Director), Mr MS Mani (Group President), Mr Sabyasachi Hazra (Director, PG and PNR Content), Ms Pooja Bhandari (Director Production), Mr Ashwani Kumar (Senior Manager), Ms Aarti Kushwah (Development Editor), and Mr Sunil Rawat (Typesetter).

I believe that writing a book involves a continuous learning process. Though extreme care has been taken to maintain accuracy while writing this book, inadvertent errors can sometimes creep in. Therefore, constructive criticism would be greatly appreciated. Please e-mail me your comments at richa@drrichasaxena.com. Also, please feel free to visit my website www.drrichasaxena.com for obtaining information related to various other books written by me and to make use of the free resources available for the doctors.

As always, I wish the readers every success in their studies and their future careers in obstetrics and gynecology.

Richa Saxena
(richa@drrichasaxena.com)
(www.drrichasaxena.com)

Contents

List of Abbreviations

A & E	Accident and Emergency
A-A	Artery-to-Artery
AC	Abdominal Circumference
ACOG	American College of Obstetricians and Gynecologists
AFI	Amniotic Fluid Index
AFP	Alpha Fetoprotein
AFS	American Fertility Society
ANC	Antenatal Care
APAS	Antiphospholipid Antibody Syndrome
APGAR	Activity, Pulse, Grimace, Appearance and Respiration
APH	Antepartum Hemorrhage
APLA	Antiphospholipid Antibody
APTT	Activated Partial Thromboplastin Time
ART	Assisted Reproductive Technology
ASRM	American Society of Reproductive Medicine
AUB	Abnormal Uterine Bleeding
BBT	Basal Body Temperature
BMI	Body Mass Index
BPD	Biparietal Diameter
BPP	Biophysical Profile
BSO	Bilateral Salpingo-Oophorectomy
CA MRSA	Community acquired Methicillin resistant staphylococcus aureus
CC	Clomiphene Citrate
CCT	Controlled cord traction
CDC	Centers for Disease Control and Prevention
CHM	Complete Hydatidiform Mole
CL	Corpus Luteum
CNS	Central Nervous System
COCP	Combined Oral Contraceptive Pills
CPD	Cephalopelvic Disproportion
CPP	Central Precocious Puberty
CRL	Crown-Rump Length
CST	Contraction Stress Test
CT	Computerized Tomography
CTG	Cardiotocography
D&C	Dilatation and Curettage
DFMC	Daily Fetal Movement Count
DHEA	Dehydroepiandrosterone
DHEAS	Dehydroepiandrosterone Sulfate
DIC	Disseminated Intravascular Coagulation
DMPA	Depot Medroxyprogesterone Acetate
DUB	Dysfunctional Uterine Bleeding
DV	Ductus Venosus
DVT	Deep Vein Thrombosis
EB	Endometrial Biopsy
ECV	External Cephalic Version
EDD	Expected Date of Delivery
EFW	Expected Fetal Weight
ER	Extended Release
ESHRE	European Society of Human Reproduction and Embryology
ETT	Endotracheal Tube
FBS	Fasting Blood Sugar
FDA	Fetal Descending Aorta
FDP	Fibrinogen Degradation Product
FGM	Female Genital Mutilation
FHR	Fetal Heart Rate
FHS	Fetal Heart Sound
FL	Femur Length
FNAC	Fine Needle Aspiration Cytology
FSH	Follicle Stimulating Hormone
GA	General Anesthesia
GCT	Glucose Challenge Test
GDM	Gestational Diabetes Mellitus
GFR	Glomerular Filtration Rate
GnRH	Gonadotropin-Releasing Hormone
GTD	Gestational Trophoblastic Disease
GTN	Gestational Trophoblastic Neoplasia
GTT	Glucose Tolerance Test
H. mole	Hydatidiform mole
HbS	Hemoglobin S
HC	Head Circumference
hCG	Human Chorionic Gonadotropin
HELLP	Hemolysis, Elevated Liver Enzymes, Low Platelets
HIE	Hypoxic-Ischemic Encephalopathy
HIV	Human Immunodeficiency Virus
HPE	Histopathology Examination
HPV	Human Papillomavirus

HRT	Hormone Replacement Therapy
HSG	Hysterosalpingogram
ICSI	Intracytoplasmic Sperm Injection
ICU	Intensive Care Unit
IUCD	Intrauterine Contraceptive Device
IUD	Intrauterine Death
IUGR	Intrauterine Growth Retardation
IUI	Intrauterine Insemination
IVF	In Vitro Fertilization
IVH	Intraventricular Hemorrhage
IVIG	Intravenous Immunoglobulin
KFT	Kidney Function Test
LA	Local Anesthesia
LCG	Labor Care Guide
LAVH	Laparoscopic-Assisted Vaginal Hysterectomy
LGA	Large for Gestational Age
LH	Luteinizing Hormone
LHRH	Luteinizing Hormone-Releasing Hormone
LMA	Left Mentoanterior
LMP	Left Mentoposterior
LMT	Left Mentotransverse
LMWH	Low-Molecular-Weight Heparin
LNG-IUS	Levonorgestrel-Intrauterine System
LOA	Left Occiput Anterior
LOD	Laparoscopic Ovarian Drilling
LOP	Left Occiput Posterior
LOT	Left Occiput Transverse
LSA	Left Sacroanterior
LSCS	Lower Segment Cesarean Section
LSH	Laparoscopic Supracervical Hysterectomy
MCA	Middle Cerebral Artery
MCH	Mean Corpuscular Hemoglobin
MCHC	Mean Corpuscular Hemoglobin Concentration
MCV	Mean Corpuscular Volume
MRI	Magnetic Resonance Imaging
MSAFP	Maternal Serum Alpha Fetoprotein
MTP	Medical Termination of Pregnancy
MVA	Manual Vacuum Aspiration
NAAT	Nucleic Acid Amplification Test
NICU	Neonatal Intensive Care Unit
NSAID	Nonsteroidal Anti-Inflammatory Drug
NST	Nonstress Test
OCP	Oral Contraceptive Pill
OFD	Occipitofrontal Diameter
OGTT	Oral Glucose Tolerance Test
OHSS	Ovarian Hyperstimulation Syndrome
OPD	Out-patient Department
PCOD	Polycystic Ovarian Disease
PCOS	Polycystic Ovarian Syndrome
PEFR	Peak Expiratory Flow Rate
PHM	Partial Hydatidiform Mole
PID	Pelvic Inflammatory Disease
PHM	Partial Hydatidiform Mole
PMS	Premenstrual Syndrome
PNDT	Prenatal Diagnostic Techniques
POC	Products of Conception
POG	Period of Gestation
POI	Progestogen Only Injectable
POP	Progestogen Only Pill
PP	Postprandial
PPH	Postpartum Hemorrhage
PROM	Premature Rupture of Membranes
PSTT	Placental Site Trophoblastic Tumor
PUBS	Percutaneous Umbilical Cord Blood Sampling
RCOG	Royal College of Obstetricians and Gynaecologists
RDW	Red Cell Distribution Width
RMA	Right Mentoanterior
RMI	Risk of Malignancy Index
RMP	Right Mentoposterior
RMT	Right Mentotransverse
ROA	Right Occiput Anterior
ROM	Rupture of Membranes
ROP	Right Occiput Posterior
ROT	Right Occiput Transverse
RSA	Right Sacroanterior
RSP	Right Sacroposterior
RST	Right Sacrotransverse
SFH	Symphysis-Fundal Height
SGA	Small for Gestational Age
SHBG	Serum Hormone Binding Globulin
SIS	Saline Infusion Sonography
STD	Sexually Transmitted Disease
STI	Sexually Transmitted Infection
SUI	Stress Urinary Incontinence
TAH	Total Abdominal Hysterectomy
TAS	Transabdominal Sonography
TB	Tuberculosis
TBG	Thyroid Binding Globulin
TCD	Transverse Cerebellar Diameter
TCRE	Transcervical Resection of Endometrium
TNF	Tumor Necrosis Factor

TOA	Tubo-ovarian Abscess
TORCH	Toxoplasma, Other viruses, Rubella, Cytomegalovirus, Herpes virus
TRAP	Twin Reversed Arterial Perfusion
TRH	Thyroid Releasing Hormone
TSH	Thyroid Stimulating Hormone
TTTS	Twin-to-Twin Transfusion Syndrome
TVS	Transvaginal Sonography
UGF	Urogenital Fistula
USG	Ultrasound
UTI	Urinary Tract Infection
V-V	Vein-to-Vein
VBAC	Vaginal Birth after Cesarean (Section)
VVC	Vulvovaginal Candidiasis
VVF	Vesicovaginal Fistula
β-hCG	Beta Human Chorionic Gonadotropin

SECTION 1

Obstetrics

CHAPTER 1

Reproductive Anatomy and Physiology

REPRODUCTIVE AND GENERALIZED ANATOMY

Question	Answer	Comment
Q1. A 30-year-old woman presents to the gynecology clinic with complaints of heavy menstrual bleeding. During the evaluation, the clinician considers the vascular supply to the uterus as a potential factor contributing to her symptoms. Based on the image provided, identify the primary arterial supply to the uterus, labeled as A. 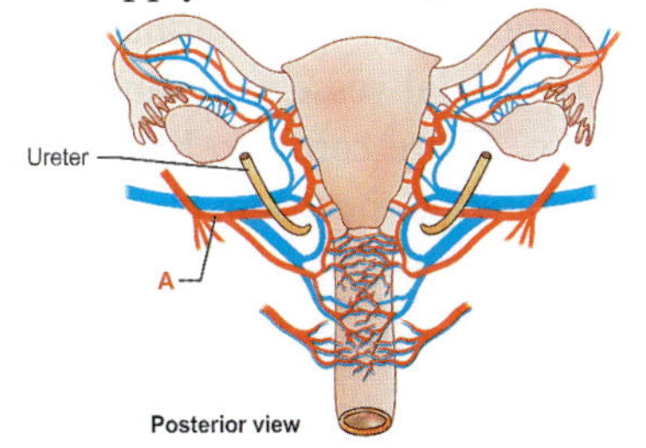 A. Ovarian artery B. Uterine artery C. Vaginal artery D. Internal iliac artery E. External iliac artery	**Ans: B (Uterine artery)** Blood supply to the uterus is mainly by the uterine arteries with the collateral supply from the ovarian arteries **(Fig. 1)**. Uterine arteries are main branches of the internal iliac arteries. 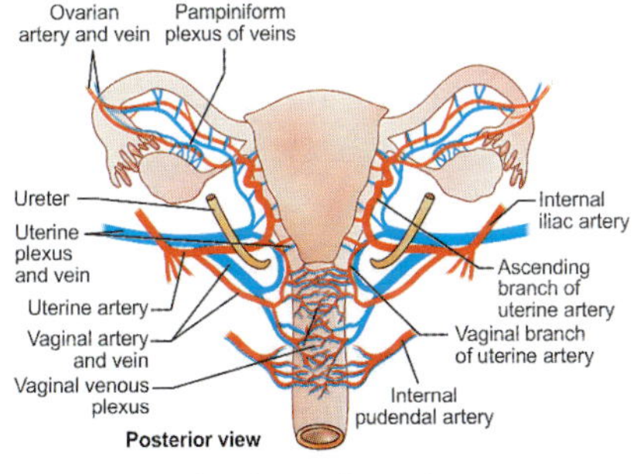 **Fig. 1:** Blood supply to the uterus.	**Explanation:** The uterine artery passes inferiorly from its origin into the pelvic fascia. It runs medially in the base of broad ligament to reach the uterus. After reaching the internal os, it then ascends along the lateral margin of the uterus within the broad ligament. It continues to move along the lower border of the fallopian tubes where it ends by anastomosing with the ovarian artery. **Potential questions:** There can be questions related to the blood vessels, supplying vagina, cervix, or ovary. There can also be questions related to the origin of these blood vessels.
Q2. Identify X in the image below. 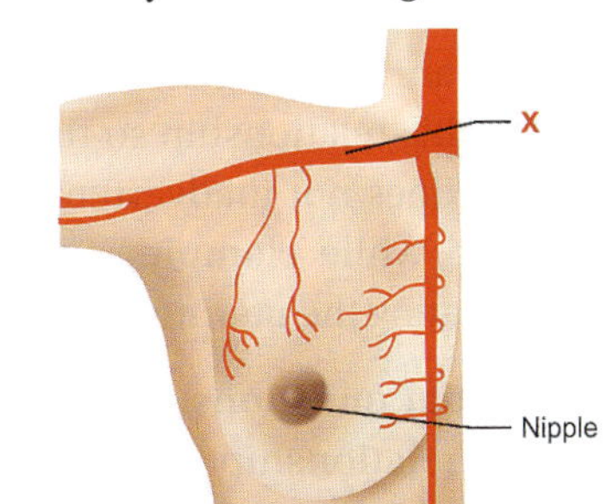 A. External thoracic artery B. Internal thoracic artery C. Lateral thoracic artery D. Thoracoacromial artery E. Posterior intercostal artery	**Ans: D (Thoracoacromial artery)** **Figure 2** shows arterial supply to the breasts. 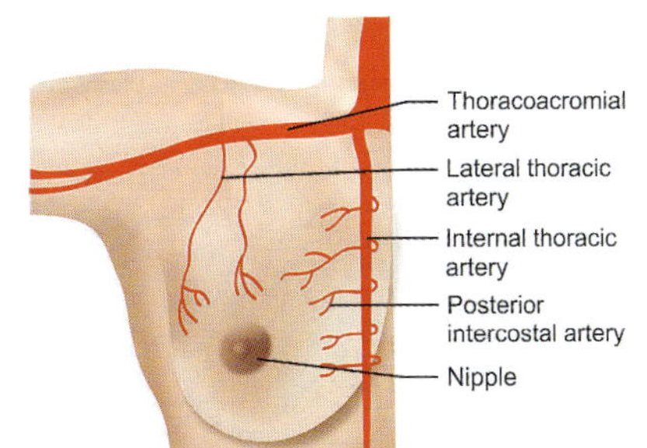 **Fig. 2:** Arterial supply to the breasts.	**Explanation:** Blood supply to the breasts is mainly derived from the perforating branches (second to fifth perforators) of internal mammary arteries derived from internal thoracic arteries. Other blood vessels which supply the breast tissues include thoracoacromial artery and lateral thoracic artery. **Potential questions:** There can be questions regarding the identification of other important vessels supplying the breast, e.g., lateral thoracic or internal thoracic, and questions related to origin of these vessels.

<table>
<tr><th>Question</th><th>Answer</th><th>Comment</th></tr>
<tr>
<td>

Q3. Identify the artery labeled X in the image.

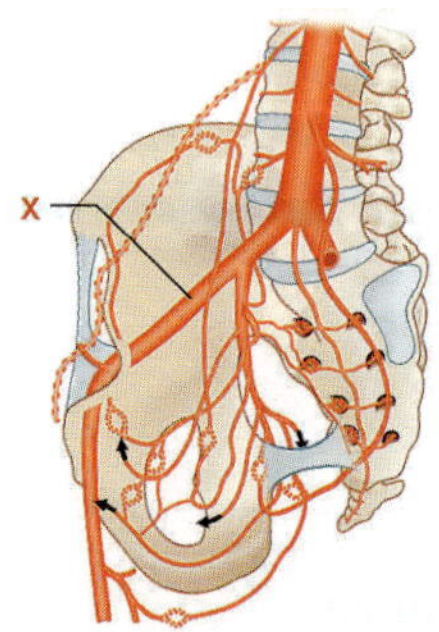

A. External iliac artery
B. Uterine artery
C. Internal iliac artery
D. Superior mesenteric artery
E. Pudendal artery

</td>
<td>

Ans: C (Internal iliac artery)

The artery labeled X in the adjacent image is the internal iliac artery. As shown in **Figure 3**, blood supply to the pelvis is mainly by the internal iliac artery.

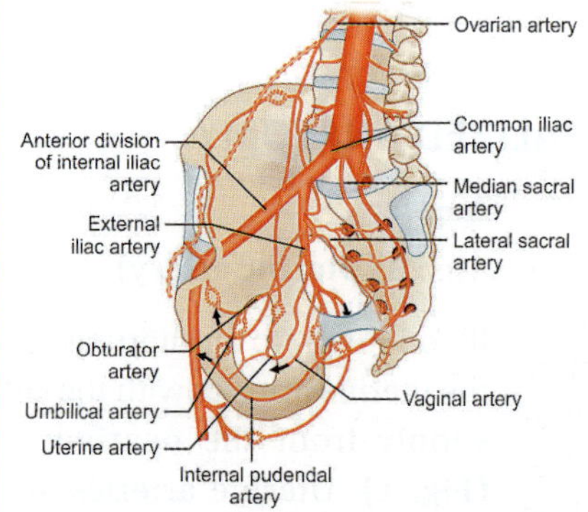

Fig. 3: Blood supply to the pelvic structures.

</td>
<td>

Explanation: Internal iliac artery, also known as the hypogastric artery, is a branch of the common iliac artery at the level of sacroiliac joint. This artery is important as it supplies the majority of the pelvic organs, including the reproductive organs, urinary bladder, and rectum. The other arteries mentioned do not play a significant role in supplying the pelvic organs, with the external iliac artery primarily serving the lower limbs and the renal artery supplying the kidneys.

Potential questions: Besides the internal iliac vessels, there can be questions related to other blood vessels traveling through the pelvic region, e.g., external iliac vessels, pudendal vessels, uterine vessels, etc. There can also be questions related to the origin and branches of these vessels.

</td>
</tr>
<tr>
<td>

Q4. In the image below, identify the structure labeled X and describe its relationship to the adjacent structures.

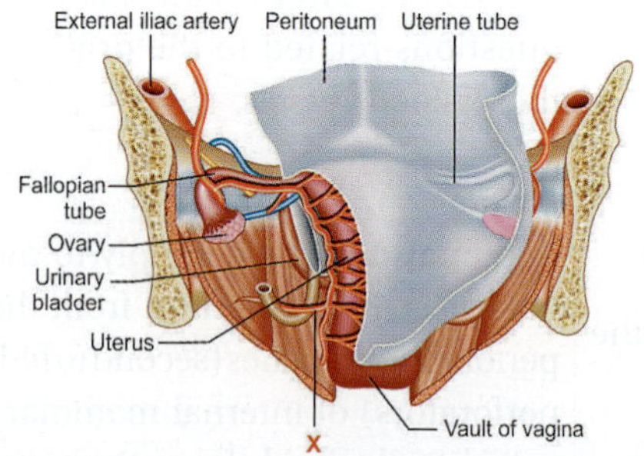

A. X is the ureter, which runs posterior to the uterine artery
B. X is the ureter, which runs anterior to the uterine artery
C. X is the uterine artery, which runs anterior to the ureter
D. X is the uterine artery, which runs posterior to the ureter
E. X is the uterine artery, which runs lateral to the ureter

</td>
<td>

Ans: C (X is the uterine artery, which runs anterior to the ureter)

In the anatomical course, the uterine artery passes above the ureter **(Fig. 4)**, a relationship often summarized by the mnemonic "water flows under the bridge" where "water" refers to the ureter and "bridge" to the uterine artery. This anatomical relationship is critical in gynecological surgeries to avoid ureteral injury.

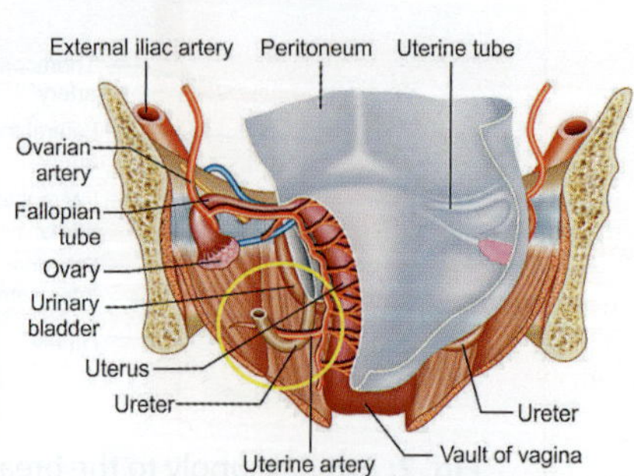

Fig. 4: Relationship of the uterine artery to ureters.

</td>
<td>

Explanation: The uterine artery, once it originates from internal iliac vessel, runs medially in the base of broad ligament to reach the uterus. While moving towards the internal os, the uterine artery passes above the ureter at right angles. Here, the uterine artery is closely related to the ureter. It is important for the gynecologist to know this relationship so that the ureter does not inadvertently get injured while clamping, cutting and ligating the uterine arteries.

Potential questions: The anatomical relationship between the uterine artery and ureter is of utmost importance and there can be questions pertaining to both at various landmark points throughout their course.

</td>
</tr>
</table>

<table>
<tr><th>Question</th><th>Answer</th><th>Comment</th></tr>
<tr>
<td>

Q5. In the image provided, identify, which color lymph nodes are responsible for draining the uterine body?

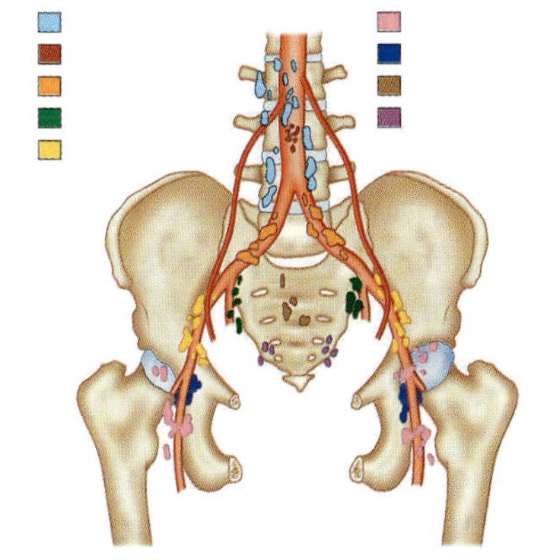

A. *Yellow:* External iliac lymph nodes
B. *Green:* Internal iliac lymph node
C. *Pink:* Superficial inguinal lymph nodes
D. *Orange:* Common iliac group
E. *Light blue:* Lumbar group

</td>
<td>

Ans: A (*Yellow:* External iliac lymph nodes)

As shown in **Figure 5**, the lymph node groups draining the female pelvis include the inguinal group, hypogastric group, external iliac group, internal iliac group, sacral group, common iliac group, pararectal group of lymph nodes, and lumbar group.

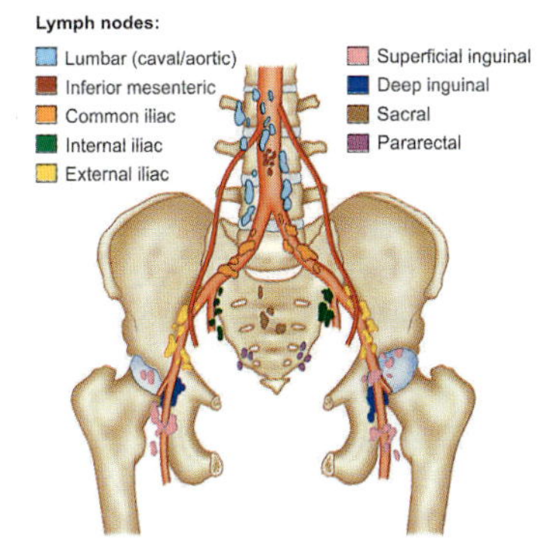

Fig. 5: Lymph drainage of pelvis: Frontal view.

</td>
<td>

Explanation: The cervix drains primarily into the external and internal iliac groups of lymph nodes, whereas the body of the uterus drains mainly into the external iliac and lumbar nodes. These drain into the common iliac group, which in turn drain into the paraaortic group of lymph nodes. Lymphatic drainage of ovaries is into the para-aortic group of lymph nodes.

Potential questions: There can be potential questions related to lymphatic drainage of various pelvic organs.

</td>
</tr>
<tr>
<td>

Q6. Identify the nerve marked with the letter X in the below image.

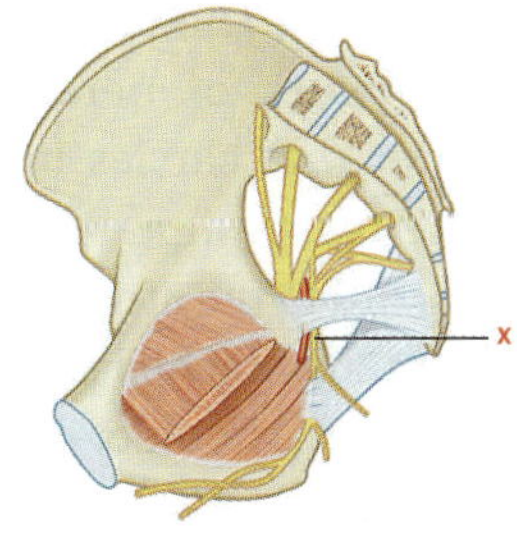

A. Levator ani nerve
B. Perineal nerve
C. Pudendal nerve
D. Inferior rectal nerve
E. Dorsal nerve of clitoris

</td>
<td>

Ans: C (Pudendal nerve)

Figure 6 presents a schematic illustration of the right half of pelvis showing the origin of pudendal nerve, its path along with its various branches.

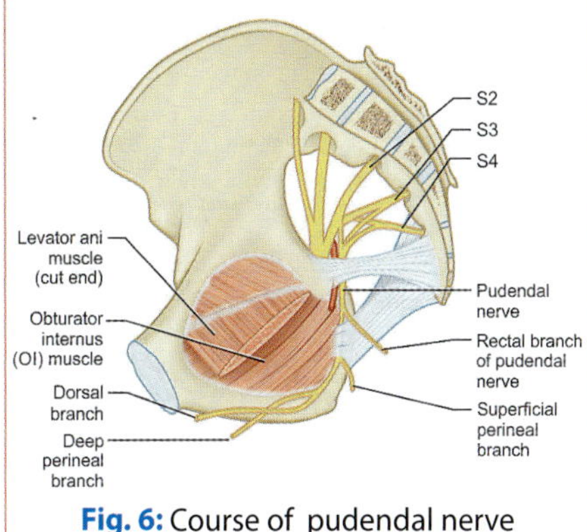

Fig. 6: Course of pudendal nerve and its branches.

</td>
<td>

Explanation: Most of the innervation of the perineum is by the pudendal nerve (ventral rami of S2, S3, and S4). It contains motor, sensory (pain and reflex), and postganglionic sympathetic fibers. The pudendal nerve (accompanied by internal pudendal vessels) traverses the greater sciatic foramen below the piriformis, crosses the back of the ischial spine, and enters the perineum through the lesser sciatic foramen. It traverses the pudendal canal in the lateral wall of the ischiorectal fossa, gives off the inferior rectal nerve, and divides into the perineal nerve and the dorsal nerve of the penis (or clitoris). The perineal nerve further divides into a deep and a superficial branch.

Potential questions: There can be questions pertaining to the branches of pudendal nerve.

</td>
</tr>
</table>

<table>
<tr><th>Question</th><th>Answer</th><th>Comment</th></tr>
<tr>
<td>

Q7. Identify the structure marked with the letter A in the below image

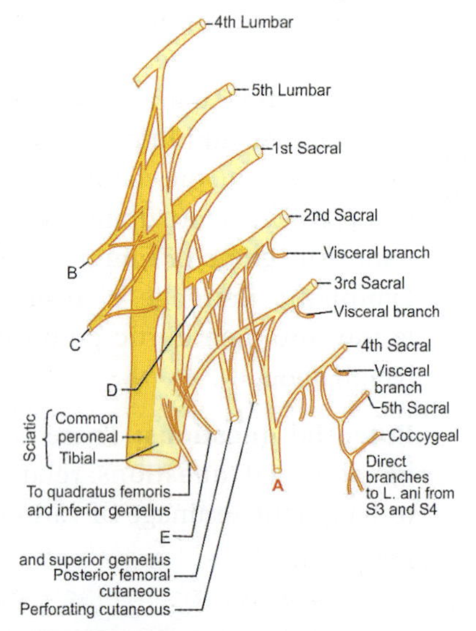

A. Superior gluteal nerve
B. Inferior gluteal nerve
C. Nerve to piriformis
D. Pudendal nerve
E. Nerve to obturator internus D

</td>
<td>

Ans: D (Pudendal nerve)

The sacral plexus **(Fig. 7)** supplies most of the pelvic structures, buttocks and lower limbs. It lies on the back of the pelvis between the piriformis muscle and the pelvic fascia.

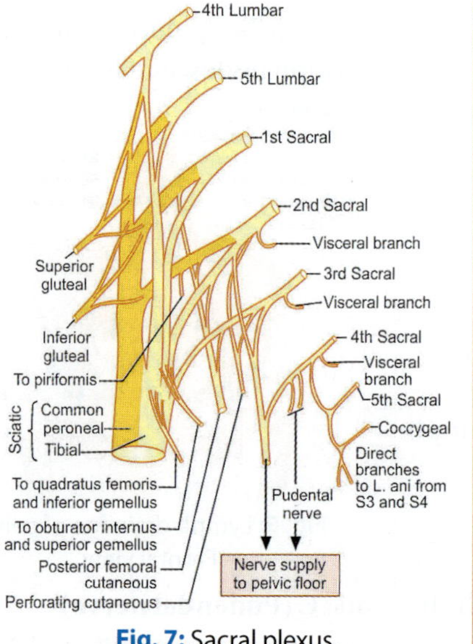

Fig. 7: Sacral plexus.

</td>
<td>

Explanation: Sacral plexus is formed by the lumbosacral trunk, comprising the whole of the anterior division of the V and a part of the IV lumbar nerve. It also includes, the ventral rami of S1 to S3, and the upper division of S4. Pudendal nerve, one of the major nerves supplying the pelvic floor, arises from the ventral rami (anterior divisions) of the spinal nerves S2, S3, and S4.

Potential questions: There can be questions related to identification of other major nerves arising from the sacral plexus.

</td>
</tr>
<tr>
<td>

Q8. What does the structure "D" represent in the given figure?

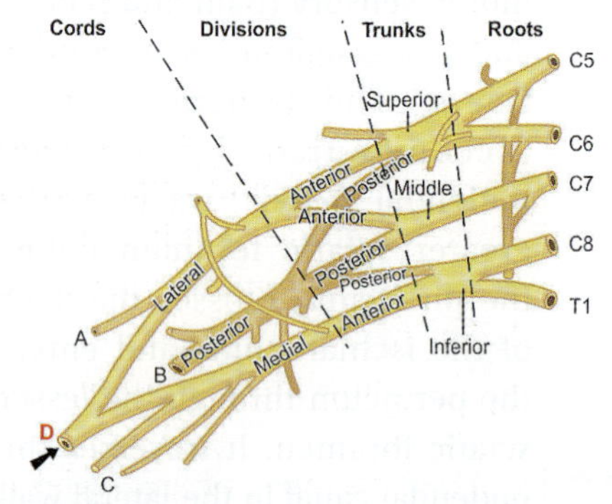

A. Axillary nerve
B. Median nerve
C. Musculocutaneous
D. Ulnar nerve
E. Radial nerve

</td>
<td>

Ans: B (Median nerve)

The figure in question represents the brachial plexus. Various nerves of brachial plexus are also shown in **Figure 8**.

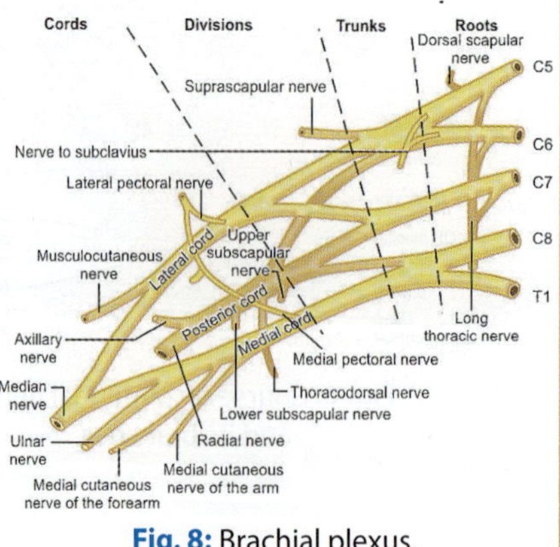

Fig. 8: Brachial plexus.

</td>
<td>

Explanation: The brachial plexus is a network of nerves in the shoulder that carries movement and sensory signals from the spinal cord to the arms and hands. Injury to the brachial plexus could occur during shoulder dystocia.

Potential questions: Besides the median nerve, it is also important to be familiar with the various other major nerves arising from the brachial plexus as well as the nerves arising from other plexuses such as the sacral and lumbar plexuses.

</td>
</tr>
</table>

Question	Answer	Comment
Q9. In the following anatomical figure of anal canal, identify J". 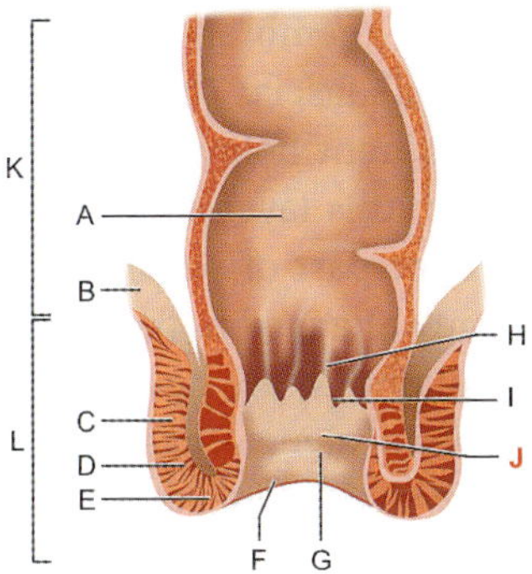 A. Rectal mucosa B. Columns of Morgagni C. Dentate line D. Squamous mucosa E. Skin	**Ans: D (Squamous mucosa)** **Figure 9** illustrates the anatomical structure of the anal canal. The anal canal is lined with stratified squamous nonkeratinized epithelium until the Hilton's line where the anal verge becomes continuous with the perianal skin containing keratinized squamous epithelium. 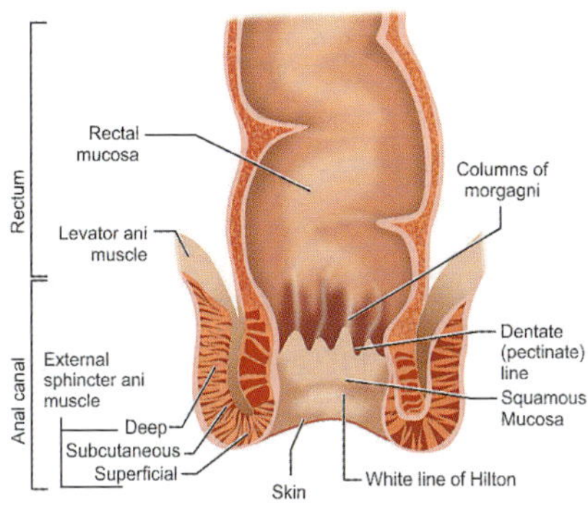 **Fig. 9:** Anatomical structure of anal canal.	**Explanation:** The transition from the columnar epithelium of the rectum to the squamous epithelium of the anal canal marks the pectinate line, a significant anatomical landmark, which has the following implications: ▪ Marks the mucocutaneous junction of the anal canal ▪ Corresponds with the position of anal valves ▪ Divides the anal canal into upper and lower areas, which are different in development, blood supply, lymph drainage, and nerve supply **Potential questions:** There can be questions related to other structures of the anal canal.
Q10. Identify X, Y, Z in the below image of epiploic foramen at the level of T12 vertebra. 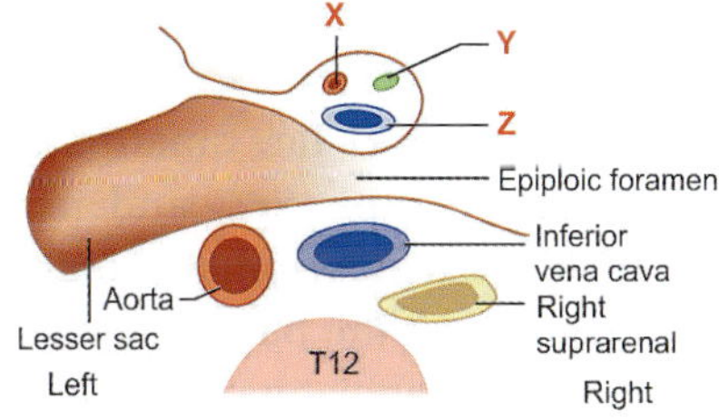 A. Common hepatic duct, proper hepatic artery, portal vein B. Common hepatic duct, proper hepatic artery, hepatic vein C. Proper hepatic artery, common hepatic duct, portal vein D. Proper hepatic artery, common hepatic duct, hepatic vein E. Hepatic vein, proper hepatic artery, common hepatic duct	**Ans: C (Proper hepatic artery, common hepatic duct, portal vein)** **Figure 10** demonstrates the epiploic foramen along with the contents of the right free margin of lesser omentum. 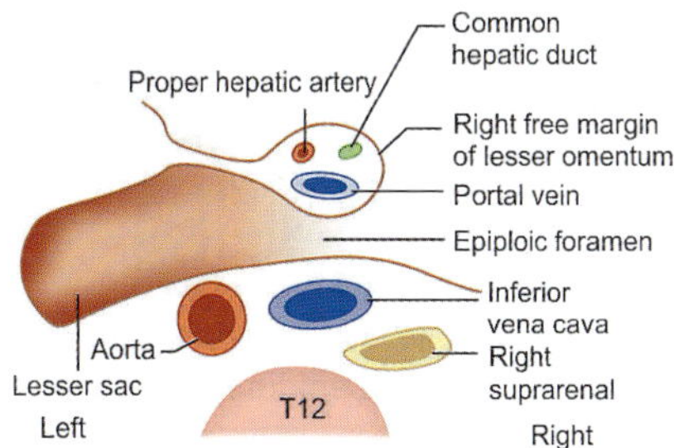 **Fig. 10:** Transverse section at the level of T12 vertebra showing the epiploic foramen.	**Explanation:** The epiploic foramen, also known as the foramen of Winslow, is an opening that connects the greater sac of the peritoneal cavity with the lesser sac. The anterior boundary of epiploic foramen is formed by the free edge of lesser omentum (hepatoduodenal ligament). Contents of the right free margin of the lesser omentum include the following: ▪ Common hepatic duct (at right) ▪ Hepatic artery proper (at left) ▪ Portal vein (posterior and between them) **Potential questions:** There can be potential questions related to the boundaries of the epiploic foramen.

Question	Answer	Comment
Q11. In the given picture of superficial fascia of abdominal wall, identify the parts labeled as A and B. 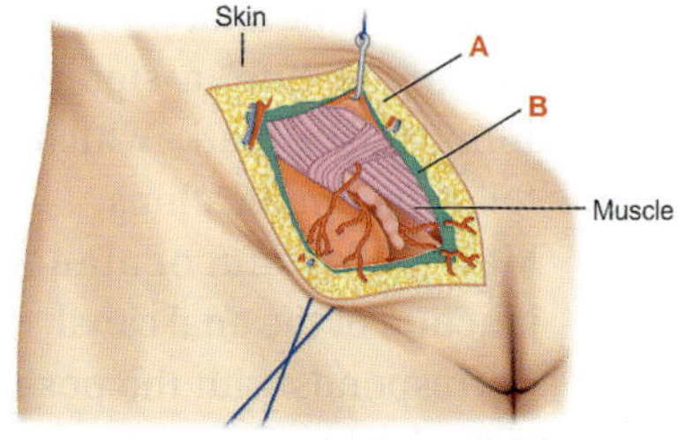 A: Aponeurosis; B: Colles' fascia A. A: Fat; B: Scarpa's fascia B. A: Scarpa's fascia; B: Camper's fascia C. A: Camper's fascia; B: Scarpa's fascia D. A: Scarpa's fascia; B: Colles' fascia E. A: Camper's fascia; B: Colles' fascia	**Ans: C (A: Camper's fascia; B: Scarpa's fascia)** **Figure 11** demonstrates the fascial layers of the anterolateral abdominal wall. The superficial fascia of abdominal wall is a layer of fatty connective tissue which forms two layers in the lower region of the anterior part of abdominal wall. 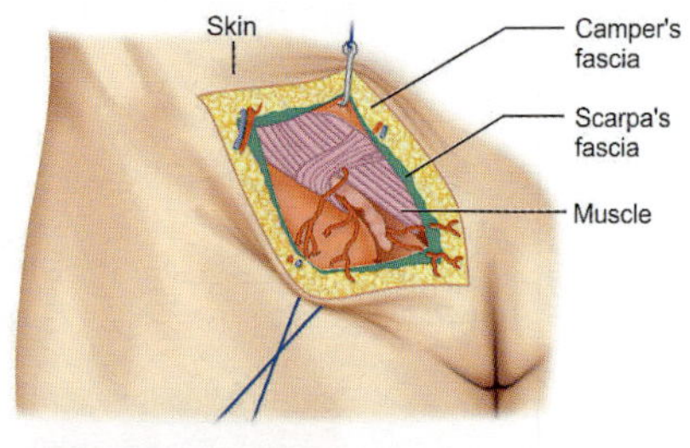 **Fig. 11:** Layers of the anterolateral abdominal wall.	**Explanation:** These two layers of superficial fascia are the outer fatty layer or Camper's fascia and the deeper membranous layer called Scarpa's fascia. This layer is more prominent below the umbilicus. When this layer continues in the deeper part of perineum, it gets firmly attached to the ischiopubic rami and to the posterior margin of perineal membrane. This is also known as Colles' fascia. **Potential questions:** There can be potential questions related to the fascial layer or the muscles of the anterior abdominal wall. There can also be questions related to the blood supply and nerve supply of the anterior abdominal wall.
Q12. In the below diagram of dura-arachnoid interface in relation to vertebral arch structures, identify the membranes A and B that are present alongside the epidural space. 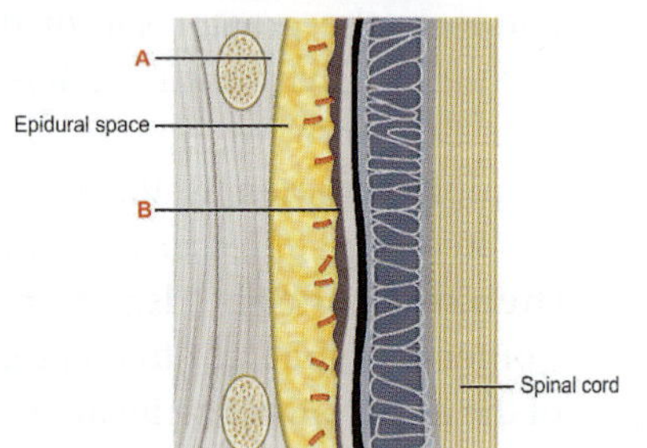 A. A: Dura mater; B: Ligamentum flavum B. A: Pia mater; B: Dura mater C. A: Arachnoid membrane; B: Pia mater D. A: Ligamentum flavum; B: Dura mater E. A: Dura mater; B: Subarachnoid space	**Ans: D (A: Ligamentum flavum; B: Dura mater)** The epidural space lies between the ligamentum flavum and the dura mater **(Fig. 12)**. 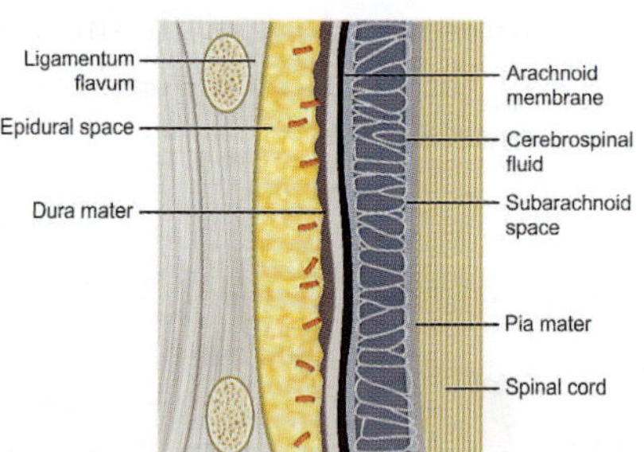 **Fig. 12:** Anatomical location of the epidural space.	**Explanation:** The epidural space is a clinically significant anatomical region located between the dura mater and the vertebral periosteum as well as ligamentum flavum (which connects the adjacent vertebrae). This space is filled with fat, small blood vessels, lymphatics, and nerve roots. It extends from the foramen magnum at the base of the skull to the sacral hiatus. The epidural space is important for performing procedures such as epidural anesthesia. **Potential questions:** There can be potential questions related to the meningeal layers surrounding the spinal cord as well as the spaces between them. There could be more questions related to the epidural block, its level, complications, etc.

Question	Answer	Comment
Q13. Given below is an image of superficial perineal pouch. Which of the following are correct options for muscles mentioned as A and B? 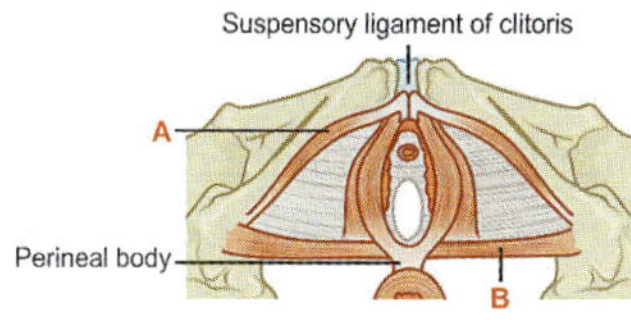 A. A: Ischiocavernosus muscle, B: Bulbospongiosus muscle B. A: Superficial transverse perineal muscle, B: Bulbospongiosus muscle C. A: Ischiocavernosus muscle, B: Superficial transverse perineal muscle D. A: Bulbospongiosus muscle, B: Ischiocavernosus muscle E. None of the above	**Ans: C (A: Ischiocavernosus muscle, B: Superficial transverse perineal muscle)** **Figure 13** shows various muscles present in the superficial perineal pouch. 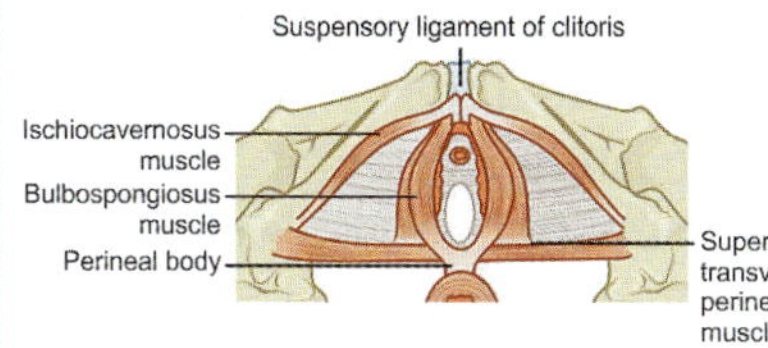 **Fig. 13:** Muscles in the superficial perineal pouch.	**Explanation:** Three muscles which make up the superficial perineal pouch include: Ischiocavernosus, bulbospongiosus, and superficial transverse perineal muscles. Other contents of the superficial perineal pouch include: ▪ Clitoris or corpus spongiosus of penis ▪ *Vessels:* Posterior scrotal arteries in males, labial arteries in females, artery to bulb/vestibule, urethral artery ▪ *Nerves:* Posterior scrotal nerves in males and posterior labial nerves in females ▪ *Other:* Crura of penis and bulb of penis in males, and crura of clitoris, bulb of vestibule, and Bartholin's glands in females **Potential questions:** There can be questions related to blood vessels, nerve, and other contents of superficial as well as deep perineal pouch.
Q14. The following diagram is of posterior view of the female reproductive tract. What does label "I" represent? 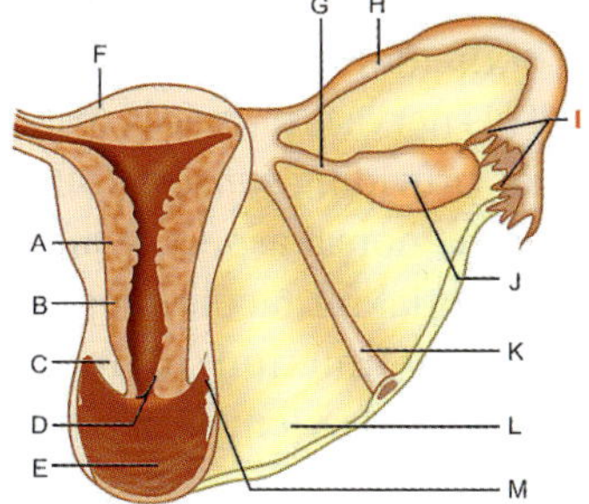 A. Ovaries B. Round ligament C. Ostium D. Fimbriae E. Cervix	**Ans: D (Fimbriae)** **Figure 14** shows the posterior view of the female reproductive tract. 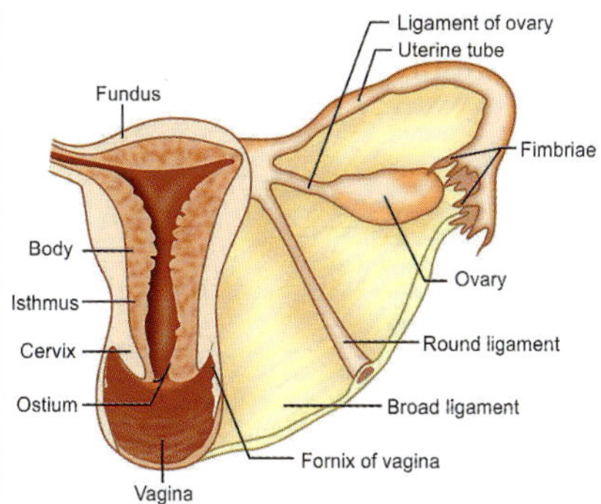 **Fig. 14:** Posterior view of the female reproductive tract.	**Explanation:** Fimbriae are finger-like projections traced at each end of the fallopian tube. It is a junction where the ovum enters and subsequently meets the sperm in the ampulla where fertilization commonly occurs. Transport between this region and implantation in the endometrium takes between 5 to 7 days. **Potential questions:** There can be potential questions related to other structures present in the posterior leaf of broad ligament.

<table>
<tr><th>Question</th><th>Answer</th><th>Comment</th></tr>
<tr><td>

Q15. Identify the structure marked by letter "A" in the image.

A. Posterior cerebral artery
B. Superior cerebellar artery
C. Anterior choroidal artery
D. Anterior cerebellar artery
E. Middle cerebral artery

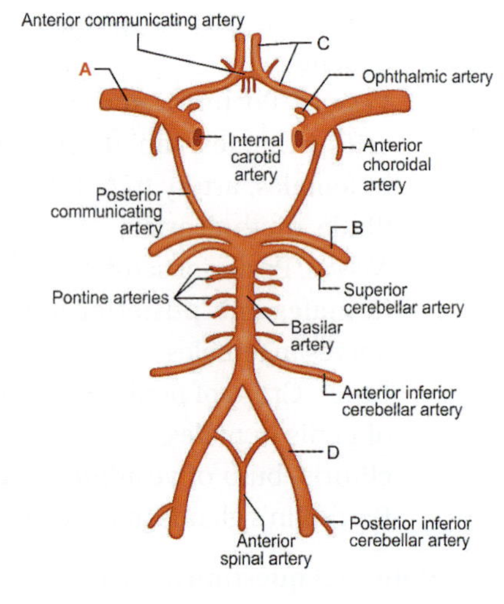

</td><td>

Ans: E (Middle cerebral artery)

Figure 15 shows the circle of Willis. Specifically, the circle is composed of the anterior cerebral arteries (branch of internal carotid artery), connected by the anterior communicating artery, middle cerebral artery (continuation of the internal carotid arteries), posterior cerebral arteries (branch of basilar artery, which arises from the vertebral artery), and posterior communicating arteries.

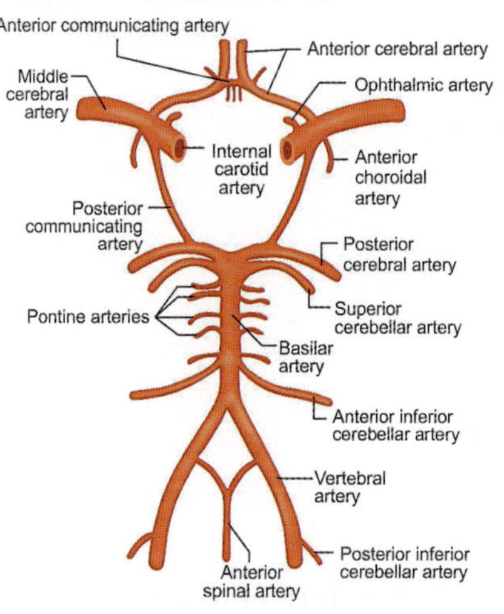

Fig. 15: Circle of Willis.

</td><td>

Explanation: The circle of Willis is a critical arterial structure located at the base of the brain, playing a key role in the brain's blood supply. This anastomotic ring allows for collateral circulation, implying that if there is a blockage or reduced blood flow in one part of the circle, other pathways can compensate, minimizing the risk of ischemic damage to the brain.

Potential questions: There can be questions on identification of any of the major blood vessels involved in the formation of circle of Willis.

</td></tr>
<tr><td>

Q16. Identify the nerve marked as A in the anatomical diagram. What is its primary function?

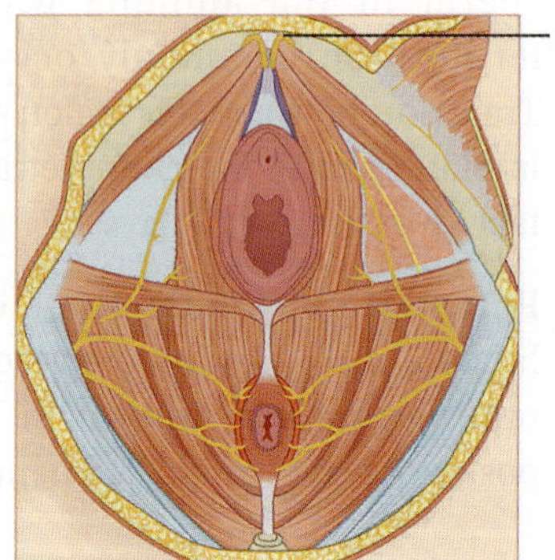

A. Dorsal perineal nerve
B. Perineal nerve
C. Pudendal nerve
D. Dorsal nerve of the clitoris
E. Genitofemoral nerve

</td><td>

Ans: D (Dorsal nerve of the clitoris)

Figure 16 illustrates various nerves supplying the perineum.

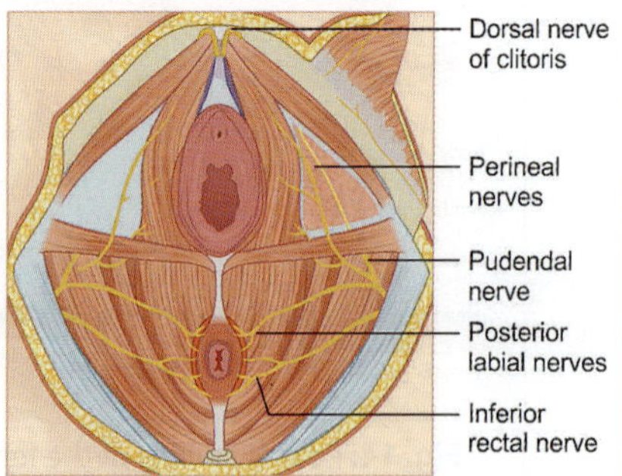

Fig. 16: Nerve supply to the perineum.

</td><td>

Explanation: The area represented by the letter A marks the location of the dorsal nerve of the clitoris. This nerve is primarily responsible for providing sensory innervation to the dorsal aspect of the clitoris, essential for tactile sensation and sexual function in individuals identified as female at birth.

Potential questions: There can be questions pertaining to other nerves innervating the perineum.

</td></tr>
</table>

ANATOMICAL/PHYSIOLOGICAL CHANGES DURING PREGNANCY

Question	Answer	Comment
Q17. A 28-year-old woman, unsure of her last menstrual period, comes to the clinic suspecting she might be pregnant. Home pregnancy test is positive. On examination, the obstetrician observes a bluish discoloration of the vaginal walls and cervix, as shown in this image. What is the name of the sign observed in the image? 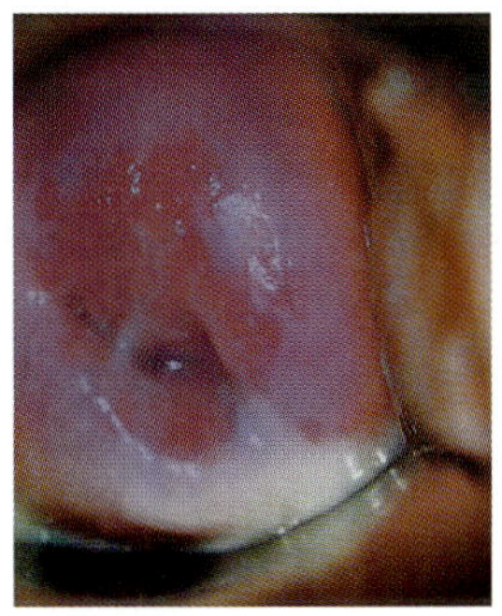 A. Goodell's sign B. McDonald's sign C. Hegar's sign D. Jacquemier's sign E. Piskacek's sign	**Ans: D (Jacquemier's sign)** This picture demonstrates Jacquemier's sign, also known as Chadwick's sign **(Fig. 17)**. 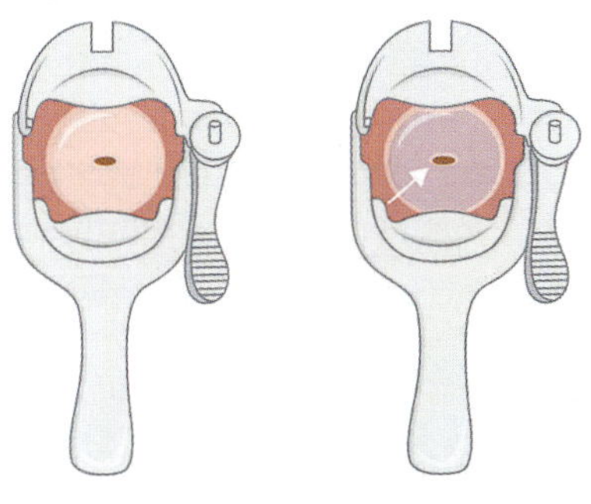 **Fig. 17:** Jacquemier's sign.	**Explanation:** This image shows dusky hue of the vestibule and anterior vaginal walls which is suggestive of Jacquemier's sign. It is associated with increased estrogen levels leading to increased vascularity and blood flow to the pelvic area. This sign can be observed by 8–10 weeks of gestation **Potential questions:** There can be questions related to various signs which appear at different stages of pregnancy, their pathogenesis, and clinical significance.
Q18. A 32-year-old woman, gravida 3, para 2, who believes she might be pregnant again, visits her obstetrician. She reports her last menstrual period was about 8 weeks ago. On examination, the obstetrician notes an unusual softening of the cervical tip, as shown in this image. 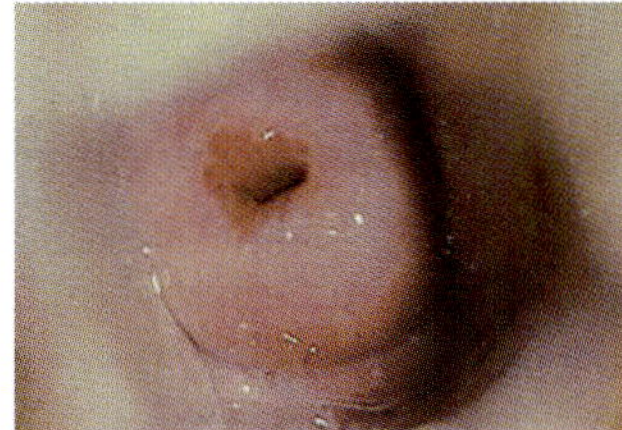 Around what time during pregnancy does this sign become noticeable? A. 7–8 weeks B. 5–6 weeks C. 10–12 weeks D. 16–18 weeks E. 20–24 weeks	**Ans: B (5–6 weeks)** Cervical sign, also known as Goodell's sign **(Fig. 18)**, usually is a sign which becomes apparent by 6th week of gestation in a primipara and even earlier in a multipara. 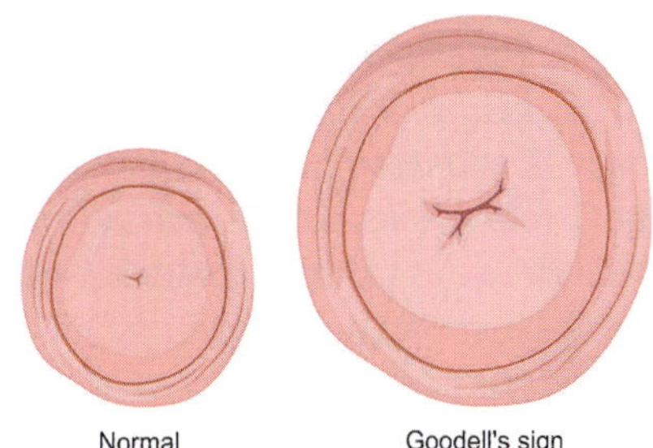 **Fig. 18:** Cervical sign (Goodell's sign).	**Explanation:** In this sign, softening of the cervix causes it to become like lips of the mouth. On the other hand, the nonpregnant cervix may feel like tip of the nose. During pregnancy, there occurs hypertrophy of the existing blood vessels as well as the growth of new blood vessels, which is responsible for these changes. **Potential questions:** There can be questions related to various signs which appear at different stages of pregnancy, their pathogenesis, and clinical significance.

Question	Answer	Comment
Q19. A 28-year-old woman with a positive home pregnancy test has a pelvic exam revealing a soft, compressible cervix at the junction with the uterine body as shown in the image. 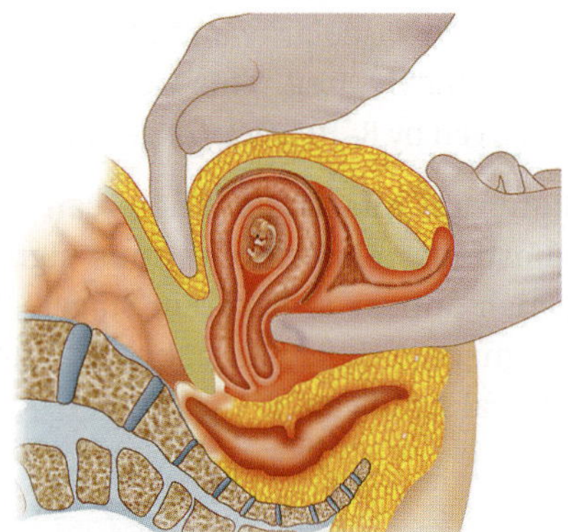 What is this sign known as? A. Positive Chadwick's sign B. Positive Hegar's sign C. Positive Goodell's sign D. Positive Braxton Hicks sign E. Positive Piskacek's sign	**Ans: B (Positive Hegar's sign)** **Figure 19** demonstrates Hegar's sign, which can be elicited in the first trimester of pregnancy. 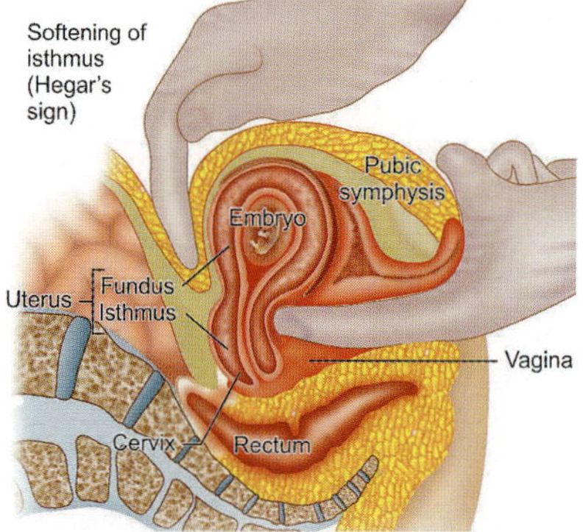 **Fig. 19:** Hegar's sign in the uterus.	**Explanation:** At 6–8 weeks of gestation, the cervix is firm in contrast to the soft isthmus and fundus. Due to the marked softness of uterine isthmus, the cervix and body of uterus may appear as separate organs. As a result, the isthmus of the uterus can be compressed between the fingers palpating vagina and abdomen, which is known as Hegar's sign. **Potential questions:** There can be questions related to various signs which appear at different stages of pregnancy, their pathogenesis, and clinical significance.
Q20. A 28-year-old primigravida came for antenatal checkup at 28 weeks of gestation. The fundal height was palpated at the level (highlighted by light brown shade) as shown in the image. What is the likely cause? 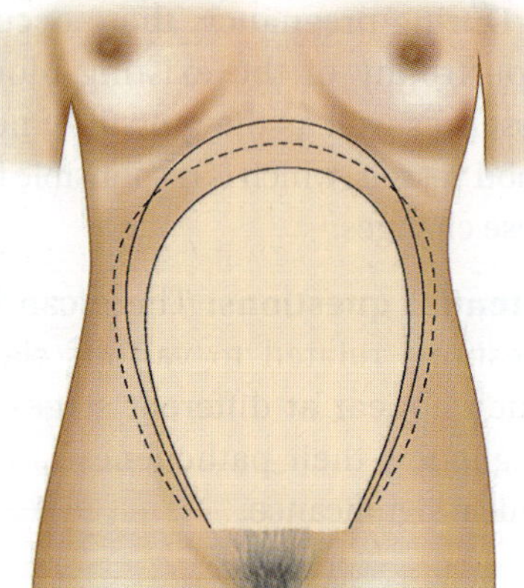 A. Oligohydramnios B. Intrauterine growth restriction C. Polyhydramnios D. Multiple pregnancy E. Incorrect calculation of POG	**Ans: E (Multiple pregnancy)** The rough estimation of fundal height with increasing period of gestation is shown in **Figure 20**. 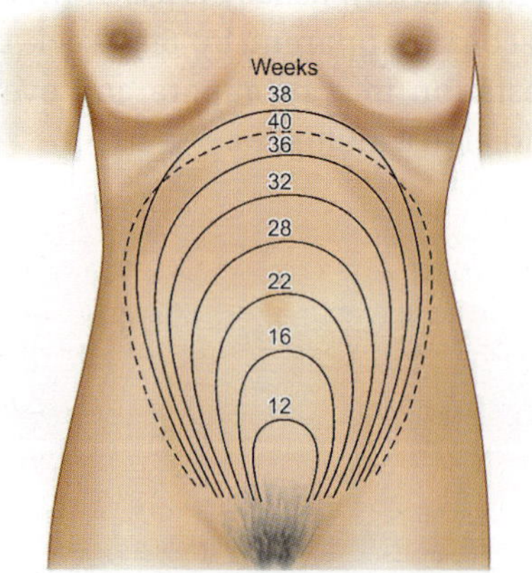 **Fig. 20:** Changes in fundal height with the period of gestation.	**Explanation:** In the given image, the area highlighted by light brown shade points towards the gestational age of 36 weeks, which is much greater than that expected to be at 28 weeks of gestation. The most likely cause for gestational height to be more than the period of gestation appears to be multiple gestation. Out of the choices given in the options, this appears to be the best option. Even though polyhydramnios can also result in fundal height to be more than the period of gestation, the discrepancy in fundal height with period of gestation would not be so much as in this case. **Potential questions:** There can be other potential questions related to fundal heights at different periods of gestation as shown in the image.

Question	Answer	Comment
Q21. Look at the image provided. It shows a clinician performing an external ballottement test on a pregnant woman. What is the primary clinical significance of a positive external ballottement during pregnancy? 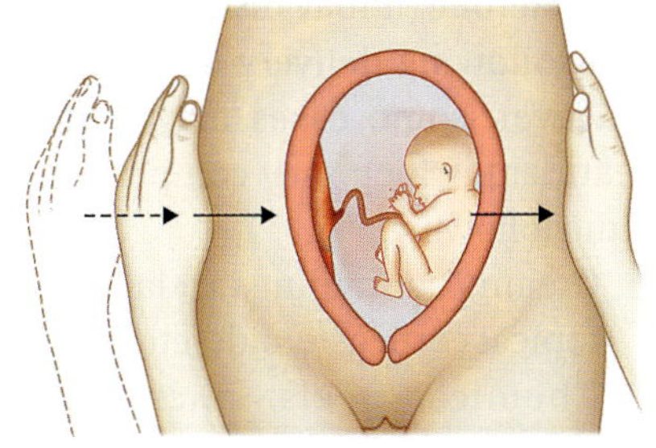 A. Confirms the presence of fetus B. Indicates the presence of a uterine tumor C. Confirms pregnancy and fetal viability D. Suggests the presence of poly-hydramnios E. Detects fetal malpresentation	**Ans: A (Confirms the presence of fetus)** In this test **(Fig. 21)**, a sharp tap is given with the forefingers of the clinician's right hand on the left side of the patient's abdominal wall. The presence of fetus can be felt by the return impact of the tossing fetus on the clinician's left hand placed on the patient's right abdominal wall. 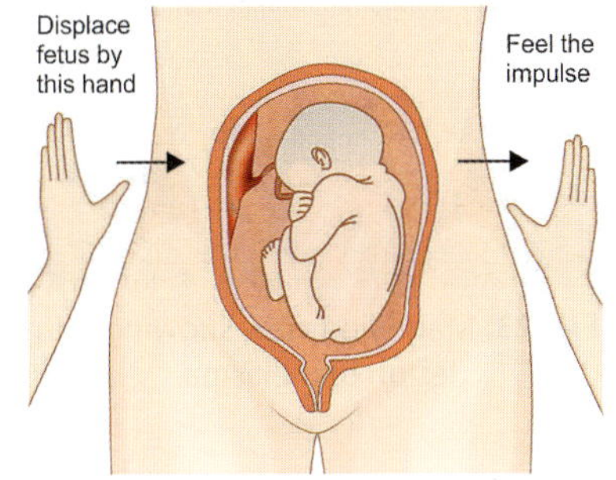 **Fig. 21:** External ballottement.	**Explanation:** Nowadays, external ballottement is rarely used for diagnosing pregnancy. External ballottement can be elicited as early as the 20th week of gestation because the size of the fetus is relatively smaller in comparison to the amount of amniotic fluid. It may be difficult to elicit this sign in woman who are obese or who have a reduced volume of amniotic fluid. **Potential questions:** There can be potential questions related to elicitation of other signs and tests specific to pregnancy.
Q22. The image shows the breast of a pregnant woman with small, raised bumps around the edge of the areola. What are these structures most likely to be? 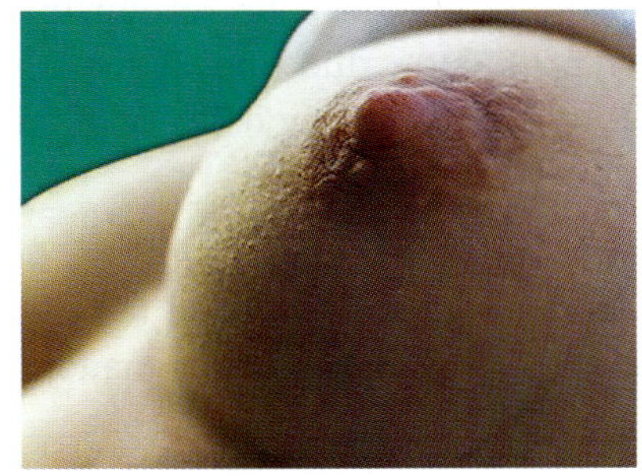 A. Sebaceous cysts B. Glands of Montgomery C. Acne vulgaris D. Malignant nodules A. Fungal infection	**Ans: B (Glands of Montgomery)** During pregnancy, there occur marked proliferation and hypertrophy of mammary ducts and alveoli **(Fig. 22)**. There also occur hypertrophy of the connective tissue stroma and formation of secondary areola during the second trimester. Increased vascularity of the tissues results in the appearance of bluish veins under the breast skin. The nipples become larger, erectile, and pigmented. There also occurs pigmentation of areola. Production of sticky, thick, yellowish secretions from the breasts occurs after about 12th week of pregnancy. 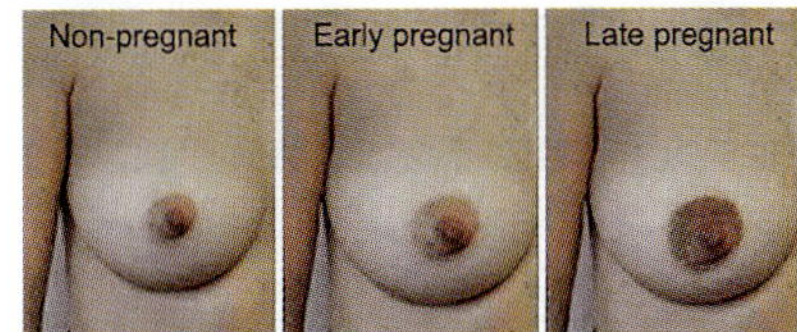 **Fig. 22:** Changes in the breasts, occurring during pregnancy.	**Explanation:** The figure in this question shows breast of a pregnant woman with full-term pregnancy. The small, raised bumps visible around the areola are known as Montgomery tubercles, which are related to the glands of Montgomery. These are modified sebaceous glands, which become more hypertrophied during pregnancy and lactation, serving to lubricate and protect the areola and nipple. They are a normal physiological change and are not indicative of any pathological condition such as cysts, acne, or malignancy. **Potential questions:** There can be questions related to physiological changes in internal genital organs such as uterus and cervix. Physiological changes occurring in various systemic organs could also be asked.

<table>
<tr><th>Question</th><th>Answer</th><th>Comment</th></tr>
<tr><td>Q23. A 29-year-old woman in her second trimester of pregnancy visits her dermatologist, concerned about dark, irregular patches that have developed on her forehead and cheeks, as shown in the image. She mentions that these changes began shortly after her pregnancy was confirmed. Which of the following is the most likely skin condition in this case?
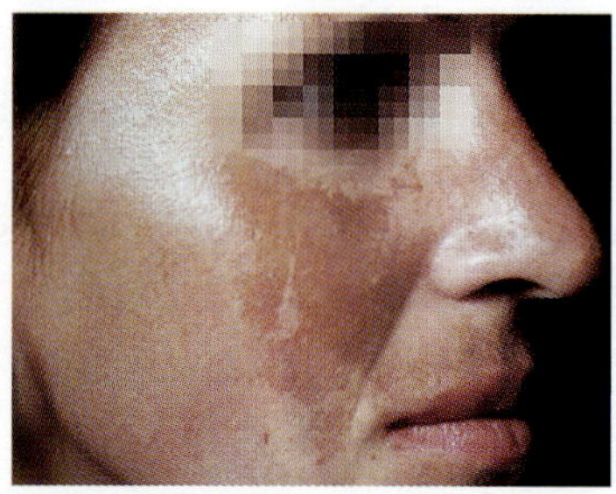
A. Melasma
B. Acne vulgaris
C. Solar lentigines
D. Atopic dermatitis
E. Polymorphic eruption of pregnancy</td><td>Ans: A (Melasma)
The figure in this question shows melasma (Fig. 23), also known as chloasma or mask of pregnancy which is a frequently encountered skin change during pregnancy.
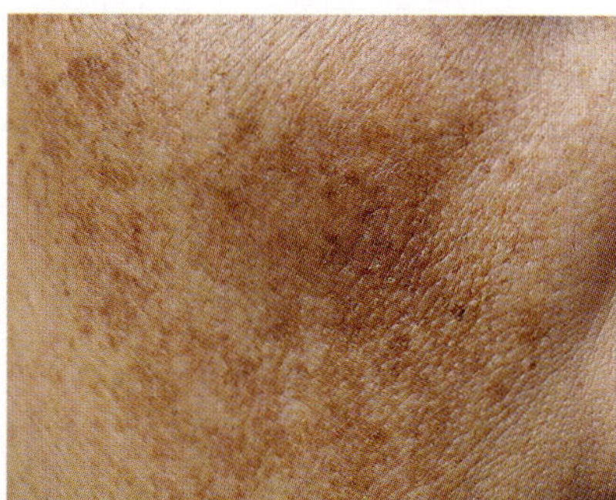
Fig. 23: Magnified view showing skin lesion of melasma.</td><td>Explanation: Melasma is characterized by the appearance of dark discolored patches on cheeks, forehead, bridge of nose, chin, etc., in pregnant women. This lesion is usually produced under the effect of hormones such as estrogen and progesterone. It may disappear on its own following delivery of the baby. However, some cases may require treatment, which may comprise one of the following:
▪ Creams containing, azelaic acid, topical corticosteroids, etc.
▪ Chemical peels, microdermabrasion
▪ Laser treatment (in extreme cases)
▪ Topical depigmentary agents
▪ Galvanic or ultrasonic facials
Potential questions: There can be potential questions related to various other skin changes in pregnancy.</td></tr>
<tr><td>Q24. A 28-year-old pregnant woman at 36 weeks of gestation notices a dark vertical line on her abdomen from her belly button to her pubic area. Based on the image and her description, what is the most likely explanation for this observation?
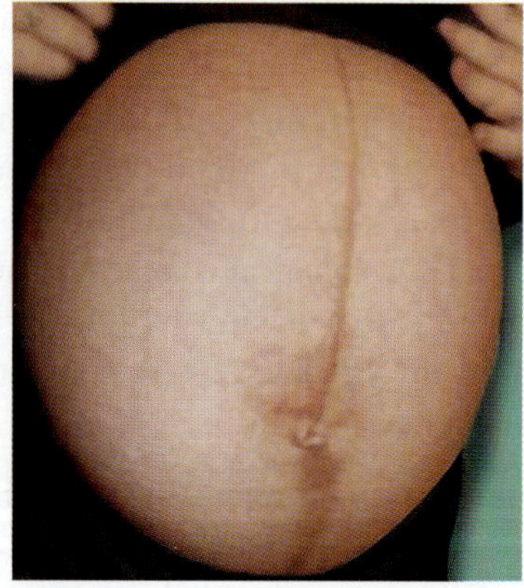
A. Striae gravidarum
B. Chloasma (Melasma)
C. Cushing's syndrome
D. Addison's disease
E. Linea nigra</td><td>Ans: E (Linea nigra)
Linea nigra is a blackish-brown line about 1 cm in width which runs in the midline from the xiphisternum to the pubic symphysis (Fig. 24) over the abdomen of a pregnant woman.
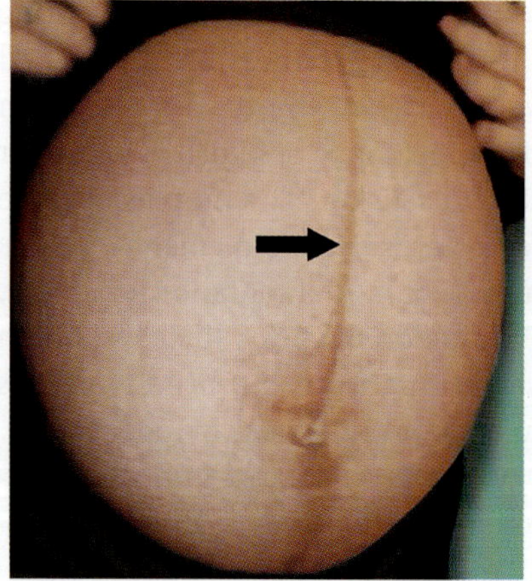
Fig. 24: Linea nigra (demonstrated by the arrow).</td><td>Explanation: This pigmentary change is probably related to the secretion of melanocyte-stimulating hormone from anterior pituitary. Production of estrogen and progesterone in the body may also be responsible for producing this line. It usually disappears following delivery of the baby.
Potential questions: There can be potential questions related to other physiological changes in pregnancy.</td></tr>
</table>

Question	Answer	Comment
Q25. A 32-year-old pregnant woman at 30 weeks' gestation has developed reddish streaks on her lower abdomen. Based on the image and her description, what is the most likely diagnosis? 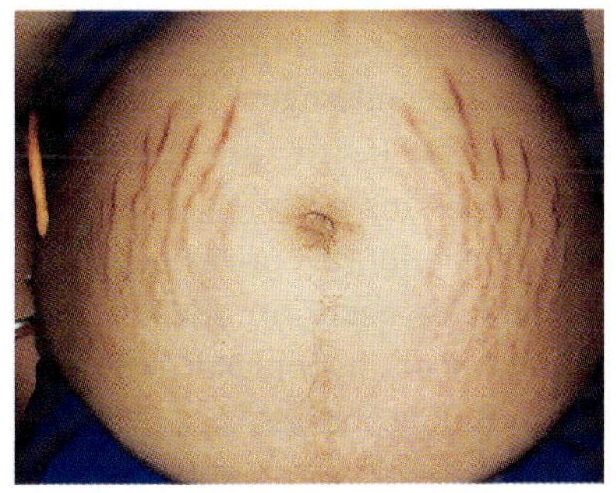 A. Linea nigra B. PUPPP (pruritic urticarial papules and plaques of pregnancy) C. Melasma D. Contact dermatitis E. Striae gravidarum	**Ans: E (Striae gravidarum)** Striae gravidarum are linear, slightly depressed marks varying in length and width, predominantly found over the lower anterior abdominal wall, usually below the umbilicus during pregnancy **(Fig. 25)**. 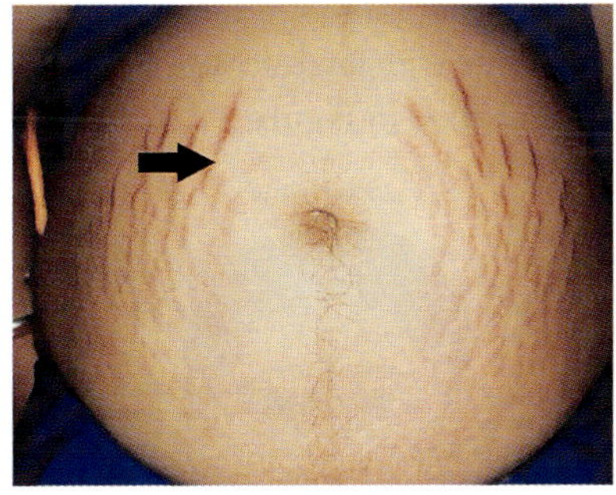 **Fig. 25:** Striae gravidarum.	**Explanation:** Occurrence of striae gravidarum is probably related to mechanical stretching of skin and production of aldosterone during pregnancy. Striae gravidarum develop when the elastic fibers in the skin stretch beyond their capacity. The rapid expansion of the skin due to hormonal changes, weight gain, and growing uterine contents contributes to this. Hormones like corticosteroids can weaken the skin's connective tissue, making it more prone to these marks. **Potential questions:** There can be potential questions related to other physiological changes in pregnancy.
Q26. Which lung volume is indicated by the arrows on the spirometry tracing in the given figure? How is this affected during pregnancy? 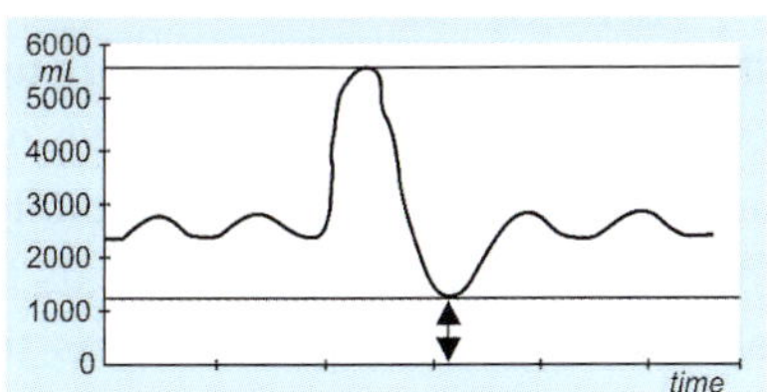 A. Residual volumes: Increases B. Tidal volume: Decreases C. Tidal volume: Increases D. Vital capacity: Decreases E. Residual volume: Decreases	**Ans: E (Residual volume: Decreases)** The arrow in the adjacent figure indicates residual volume, which refers to the air that cannot be expelled from the lungs, even with the hardest effort of expiration. Various lung volumes and capacities are illustrated in **Figure 26**. 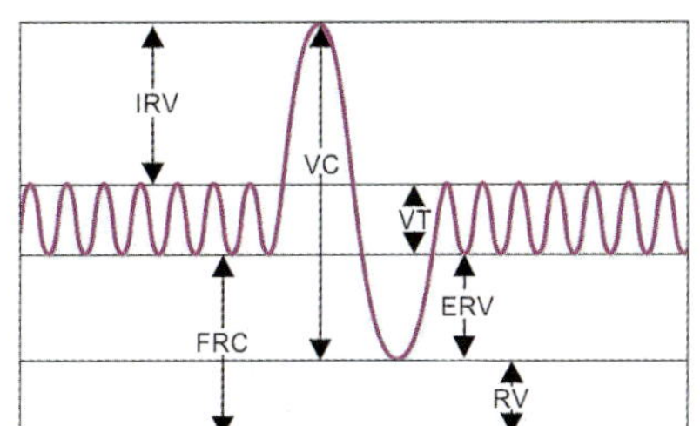 **Fig. 26:** Various lung volumes and capacities. (ERV: expiratory reserve volume; FRC: functional residual capacity; IRV: inspiratory reserve volume; RV: residual volume; VC: vital capacity; VT: tidal volume)	**Explanation:** Residual volume in lungs decreases during pregnancy due to elevated diaphragm and reduced functional residual capacity. Besides the residual volume, expiratory reserve volume also decreases during pregnancy. Pregnancy is a state of hyperventilation, resulting in an increase in tidal volume and respiratory minute volume by approximately 40%. **Potential questions:** There can be potential questions related to physiological changes occurring in various systemic organs in the body during pregnancy.

Question	Answer	Comment
Q27. The image shows a child with characteristic facial features including small eyes, epicanthal fold, a smooth philtrum, and a thin upper lip. What is the most likely diagnosis? 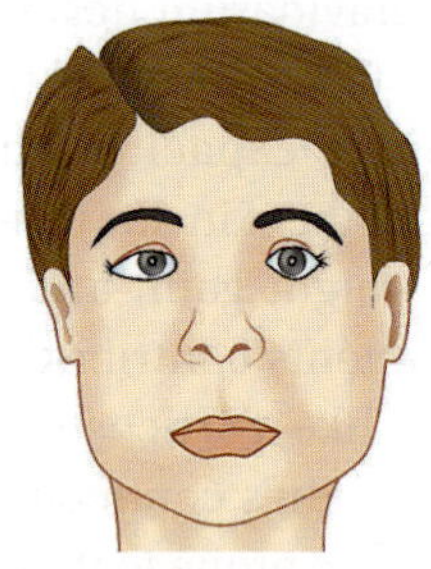 A. Down syndrome B. Turner syndrome C. Fragile X syndrome D. Noonan syndrome E. Fetal alcohol syndrome	**Ans: E (Fetal alcohol syndrome)** Prenatal alcohol exposure is associated with fetal complications such as the risk for fetal alcohol spectrum disorders, fetal alcohol syndrome (FAS), intraventricular hemorrhage, damage to white matter in preterm neonates, etc. The characteristic facial features in children with fetal alcohol syndrome are described in **Figure 27**. 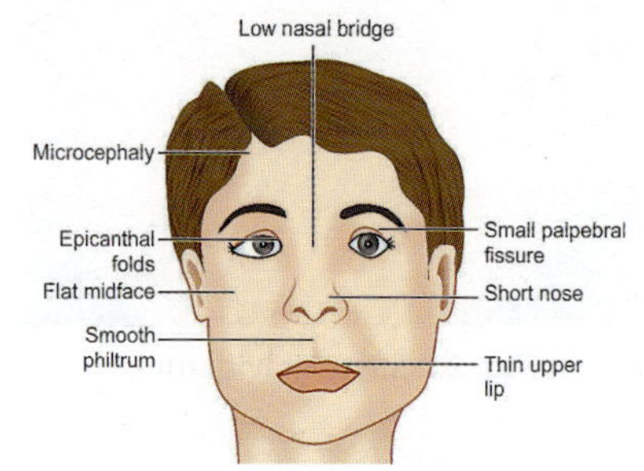 **Fig. 27:** Characteristic features of fetal alcohol syndrome.	**Explanation:** The child in **Figure 27** displays the characteristic facial features of FAS, which include small palpebral fissures (small eyes), a smooth philtrum, flat mid-face, epicanthal folds, thin upper lip, etc. Other facial anomalies (shown in **Figure. 27**) include short nose, flattened nasal bridge, micrognathia, maxillary hypoplasia (with prognathism), abnormalities of the premaxillary zone, flat midface, presence of epicanthal folds, ear anomalies, hemangiomas, ptosis, hypoplastic nails, cleft lip, protruding auricles, etc. **Potential questions:** There can be potential questions related to the characteristic phenotypic appearance in other syndromes, e.g. Down syndrome, Turner syndrome, etc.
Q28. A 32-year-old woman in her third trimester presents with leg pain, heaviness, and progressively worsening swollen veins after prolonged standing. The appearance of legs is shown in the image below. Which of the following statements is false regarding her diagnosis? 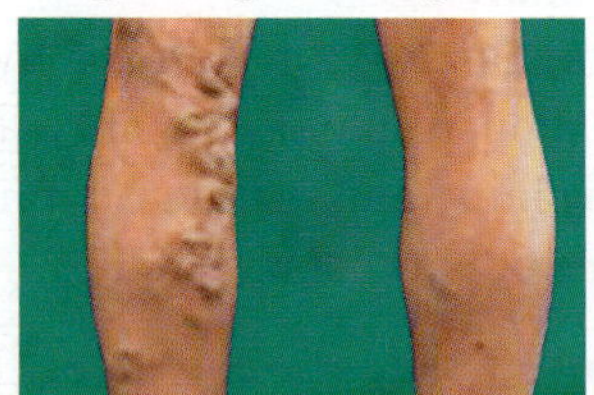 A. During pregnancy, it only occurs in the legs B. This condition usually resolves on its own after childbirth C. Exercises like walking or swimming can help reduce the risk during pregnancy D. This condition is caused by increased blood volume and pressure on the veins in the lower body during pregnancy E. Elevating the legs while resting can help reduce swelling and discomfort	**Ans: A (During pregnancy, it only occurs in the legs)** **Figure 28** shows the presence of dilated, tortuous veins over the left popliteal fossa and leg. This is likely to be related to the development of varicose veins, which can commonly develop during pregnancy due to pressure on the pelvic veins and inferior vena cava (IVC) by the gravid uterus. 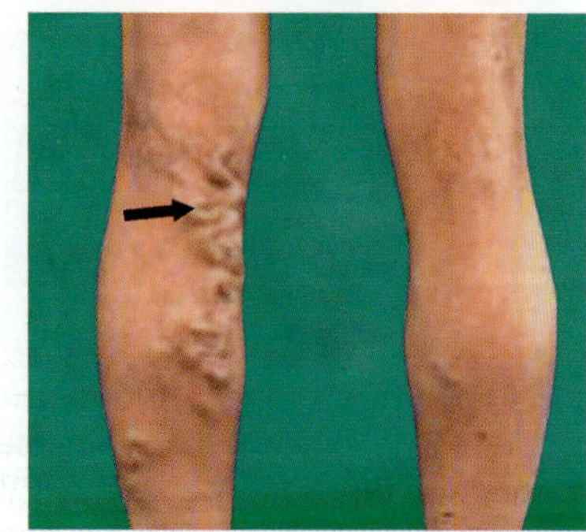 **Fig. 28:** Development of varicose veins during pregnancy (indicated by an arrow).	**Explanation:** While varicose veins are most common in the legs due to the pressure from the growing uterus, they can also occur in other areas, such as the vulva or rectum (hemorrhoids) during pregnancy. In most cases, varicose veins that develop during pregnancy are likely to improve or disappear after delivery, especially once the pressure from the uterus is relieved and blood flow returns to normal. To prevent the development of varicosities, the woman must be asked to do regular daily exercises during her pregnancy and elevate her legs and foot whenever possible. She should be advised not to sit or stand in the same position for a long time. Use of graded compression stockings also help. These strategies help in improving venous return and decreasing swelling and discomfort associated with varicose veins. **Potential questions:** There can be potential questions related to other physiological changes in pregnancy.

Question	Answer	Comment
Q29. A 32-year-old pregnant woman in her third trimester presents with complaints of rectal discomfort, itching, and bleeding during bowel movements. You perform a physical examination and observe the findings shown in the provided image. What is the most likely diagnosis? 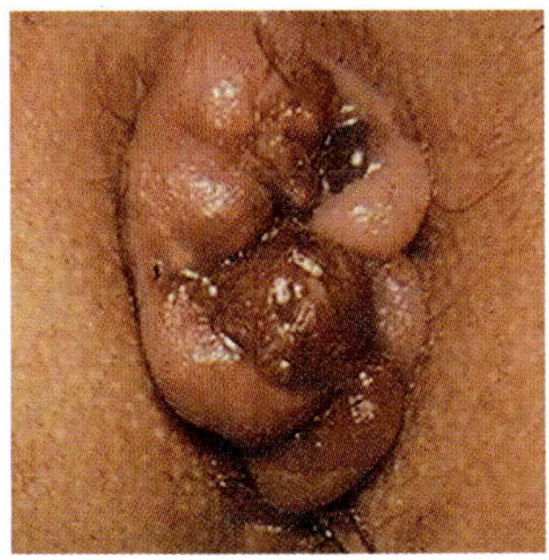 A. Anal fissure B. Rectal prolapse C. External hemorrhoids D. Perianal abscess E. Internal hemorrhoids	**Ans: C (External hemorrhoids)** Hemorrhoids are varicosities of the veins in the rectum, which develop due to pressure on the pelvic veins and IVC by the gravid uterus. These can commonly occur in pregnancy during the third trimester, during labor, and early postpartum period **(Fig. 29)**. 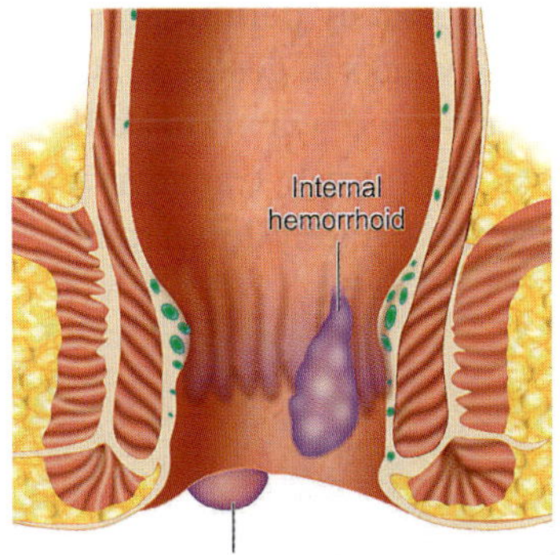 **Fig. 29 :** Development of hemorrhoids during pregnancy.	**Explanation: Figure 29** shows swollen, bluish, and tender masses that are consistent with external hemorrhoids. External hemorrhoids are dilated veins located under the skin around the anus. These hemorrhoids, which appear during pregnancy, generally disappear on their own following the baby's birth. The woman must be asked to avoid constipation by eating high fiber diet, drinking plenty of fluids, and doing regular Kegel exercises. Application of ice packs and use of warm sitz bath help. Cold and hot treatment must be regularly alternated. Application of witch hazel helps in providing relief from pain. The woman must be advised not to sit or stand for long periods of time. **Potential questions:** There can be potential questions related to other physiological changes in pregnancy.

DIAGNOSTIC PROCEDURES

Question	Answer	Comment
Q30. You are performing a procedure on a 38-year-old pregnant woman at 18 weeks' gestation with a family history of Down syndrome. The image below shows aspiration of fluid through a needle. What is the primary reason for performing this procedure in the patient? 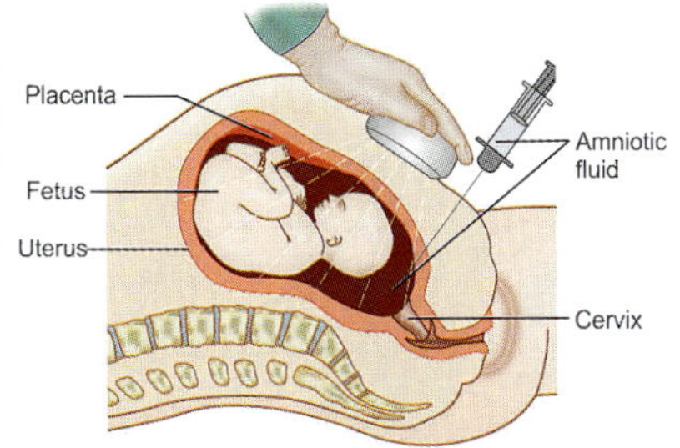 A. To assess fetal lung maturity B. To diagnose neural tube defects C. To determine the sex of the baby D. To detect chromosomal abnormalities E. To treat polyhydramnios	**Ans. D (To detect chromosomal abnormalities)** The procedure in the given scenario is amniocentesis, a prenatal diagnostic procedure, which involves the use of ultrasound-guided, needle-insertion technique for aspiration and sampling of amniotic fluid. It is usually performed between 16 and 18 weeks of gestation **(Fig. 30)**. 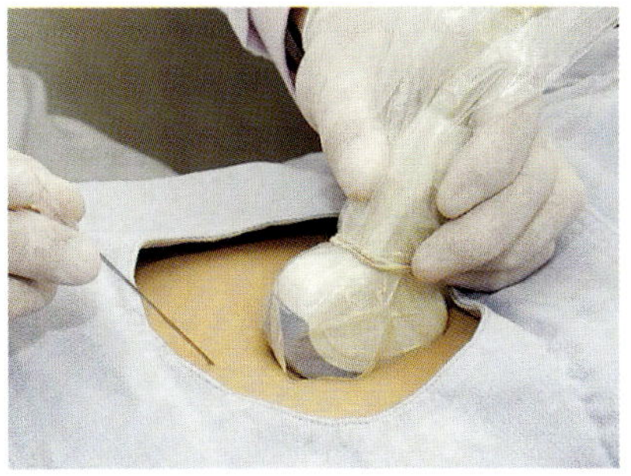 **Fig. 30:** Procedure of amniocentesis.	**Explanation:** Amniocentesis is a diagnostic procedure used primarily to detect chromosomal abnormalities, such as Down syndrome, especially in high-risk pregnancies. While it can also be used for other purposes, such as diagnosing neural tube defects and assessing fetal lung maturity, its primary indication in this scenario is to evaluate the risk of chromosomal abnormalities in the fetus, given the mother's age and associated risk factors. **Potential questions:** There can be potential questions pertaining to the indications and complications of various invasive and noninvasive diagnostic procedures which can be performed during pregnancy.

Question	Answer	Comment
Q31. A 32-year-old woman at 11 weeks' gestation undergoes a procedure involving the collection of a small sample of placental tissue for chromosomal testing. The procedure is shown in the image below. What is the most likely complication of this procedure? 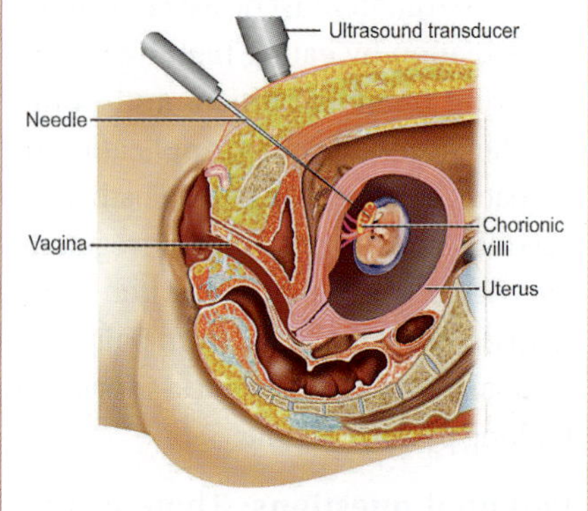 A. Amniotic fluid leakage B. Infection C. Limb defects D. Premature rupture of membranes E. Miscarriage	**Ans: E (Miscarriage)** The adjacent image shows the procedure of chorionic villus sampling (CVS), an invasive prenatal diagnostic technique, which involves collecting a sample of chorionic villi from chorion frondosum (future placenta) to test for chromosomal abnormalities **(Fig. 31)**. This test usually performed between 10 to 14 weeks of gestation. CVS can be performed via transabdominal (most common), transcervical, or transvaginal (rarely done) route. 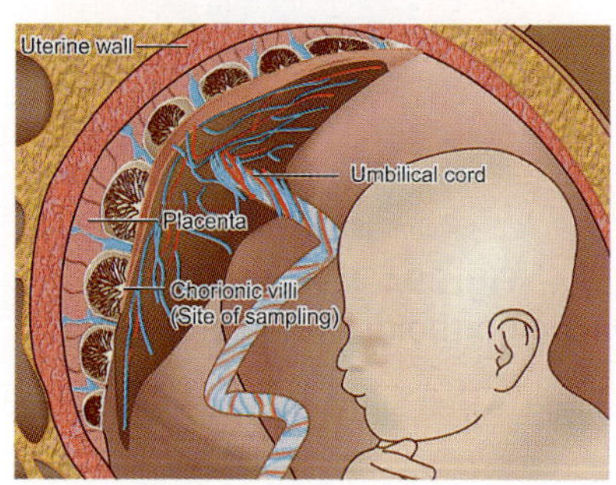 **Fig. 31:** Magnified view of the procedure of chorionic villus sampling.	**Explanation:** CVS carries a risk of miscarriage, with a rate slightly higher than that associated with amniocentesis. Miscarriage is the most common serious complication, typically occurring within 2 weeks of the procedure. Other risks include infection and limb defects, particularly when performed before 10 weeks' gestation. However, miscarriage remains the most significant concern in clinical practice. **Potential questions:** There can be potential questions pertaining to indications and complications of various invasive and noninvasive diagnostic procedures which can be performed during pregnancy.

Question	Answer	Comment
Q32. The image below shows a prenatal procedure being performed. What is the procedure and what is its primary use? 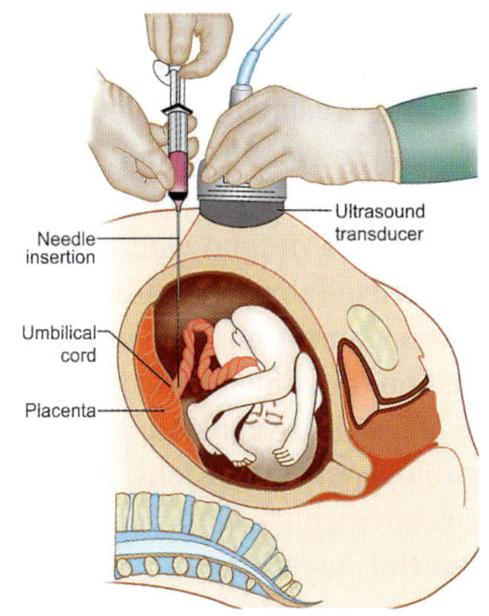 A. Cordocentesis—detect blood disorders B. Amniocentesis—detect genetic abnormalities C. Chorionic villus sampling (CVS)—diagnose chromosomal abnormalities D. Fetoscopy—inspect the fetus E. Ultrasound guided fluid aspiration—assess fetal abnormalities	**Ans: A (Cordocentesis—detect blood disorders)** Cordocentesis, also sometimes called percutaneous umbilical cord blood sampling (PUBS), is an invasive prenatal diagnostic test, which aims at detection of fetal blood disorders through direct examination of fetal blood obtained from the umbilical cord **(Fig. 32)**. 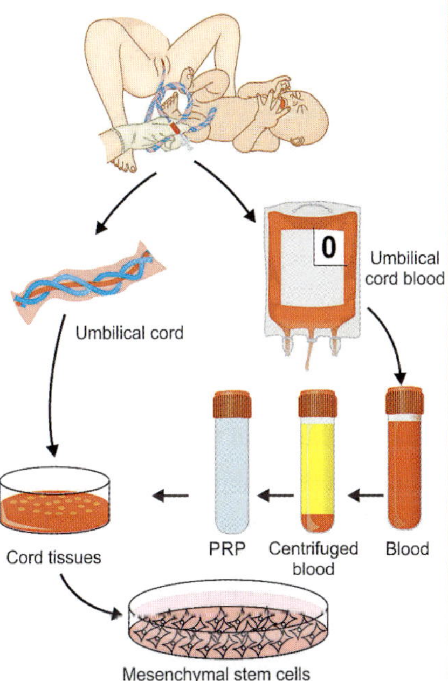 **Fig. 32:** Magnified view showing the procedure of cordocentesis. (PRP: platelet rich plasma)	**Explanation:** Cordocentesis is usually performed during 18–24 weeks of pregnancy. It is primarily used for detecting hematological disorders (e.g., thrombocytopenia), estimating the fetal hemoglobin and hematocrit levels, diagnosing fetal infections [rubella, cytomegalovirus (CMV), toxoplasmosis, etc.], for fetal blood gas analysis, and for therapeutic purposes such as intrauterine transfusion, drug therapy, and stem cell transplantation. Since this is an invasive procedure, associated with several risks, nowadays it is rarely used, only on occasions, when no alternative is available. **Potential questions:** There can be potential questions pertaining to various invasive and noninvasive diagnostic procedures which can be performed during pregnancy.

Question	Answer	Comment
Q33. The image below shows a monitor displaying fetal heart rate patterns during a prenatal test. What is this test and what does it primarily assess? 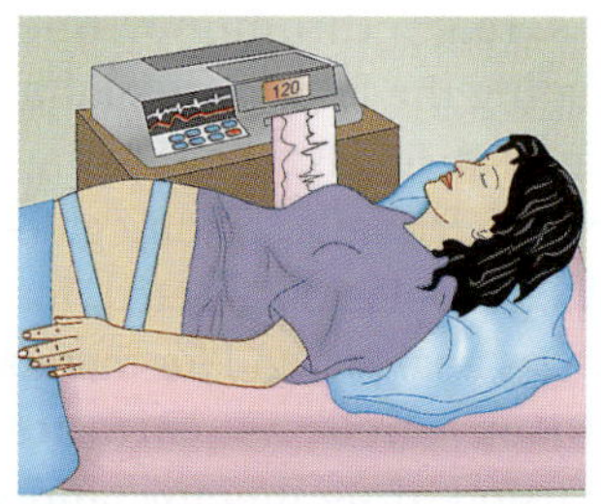 A. NST—assesses FHR with movement B. Biophysical profile—evaluates fetal well-being C. Contraction stress test—measures fetal heart rate with contractions D. Amniotic fluid index—assesses amniotic fluid volume E. Cardiotocography—monitors fetal heart rate and contractions	**Ans: A [Nonstress test (NST)—assesses fetal heart rate with movement]** The adjacent image shows NST, a common prenatal test to monitor the FHR in response to fetal movements. It is noninvasive and is typically used to assess fetal well-being, particularly in high-risk pregnancies. A normal result is characterized by an increase in the FHR with movement, indicating that the fetus is getting adequate oxygenation **(Fig. 33)**. 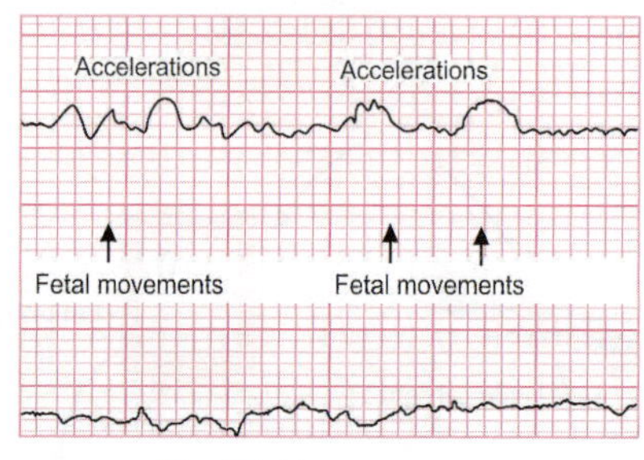 **Fig. 33:** Nonstress test.	**Explanation:** NST involves attaching one belt of an external tocodynamometer to the mother's abdomen to measure fetal heart rate and another belt to measure uterine contractions. Fetal movement, heart rate, and "reactivity" of fetal heart are measured for 20–30 minutes. The NST is classified as reactive (normal or indicative of fetal well-being) or nonreactive (abnormal or indicative of fetal compromise). The NST is based on the principle that the heart rate of a well-oxygenated, nonacidic, neurologically intact fetus normally accelerates with fetal movements. **Potential questions:** There can be potential questions pertaining to various invasive and noninvasive diagnostic procedures which can be performed during pregnancy.
Q34. The image below shows normal Doppler velocimetry waveform from the umbilical artery of a pregnant woman at 32 weeks' gestation. What does this waveform primarily assess? 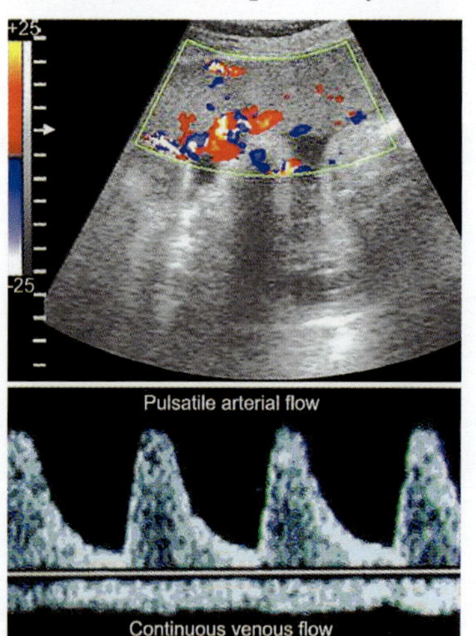 A. Fetal heart rate B. Uterine blood flow C. Placental function D. Amniotic fluid volume E. Fetal movements	**Ans: C (Placental function)** Doppler velocimetry is a noninvasive method for assessing fetal vascular impedance. Various types of Doppler waveforms are described in **Figures 34A to D**. Doppler indices, which help in evaluating the blood flow through uterine and umbilical blood vessels, include systolic/diastolic (S/D) ratio, pulsatility index, and resistance index. In normal pregnancy, due to an increase in the end-diastolic velocity as a result of reduced resistance in the umbilical artery with gestational age, S/D ratio and pulsatility index decrease. 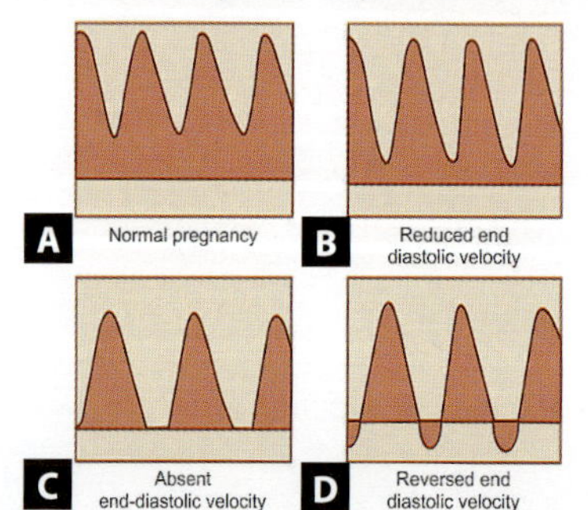 **Figs. 34A to D:** Types of Doppler waveforms.	**Explanation:** Doppler velocimetry of the umbilical artery assesses the resistance to blood flow in the placenta, which can indicate placental function. An increased resistance might suggest placental insufficiency, often linked to intrauterine growth restriction (IUGR) and preeclampsia. In cases of IUGR, there is a decrease in the end-diastolic velocity due to increased resistance to the blood flow with increasing gestational age. Umbilical artery indices are considered as abnormal if they become >95th percentile for gestational age or there may be early diastolic notching. The end diastolic flow may be either absent or reversed in extreme cases, prompting urgent delivery. **Potential questions:** There can be potential questions pertaining to various abnormalities in umbilical artery Doppler waveform, particularly in cases of IUGR.

FEMALE PELVIS

Question

Q35. The image below shows a ventral view of the pelvis. Which structure, labeled as X, forms the anterior boundary of the pelvic outlet?

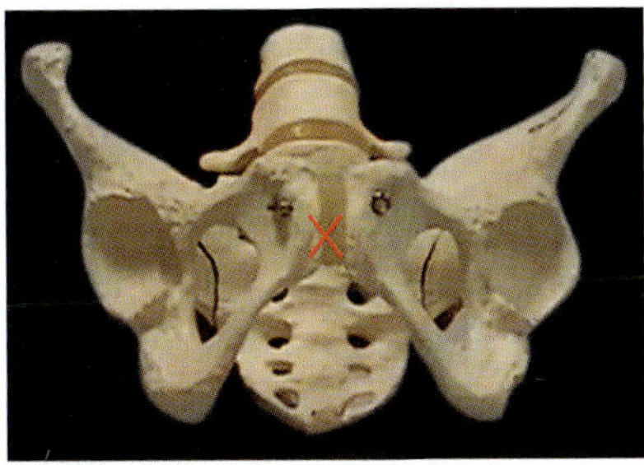

A. Ilium
B. Sacrum
C. Ischial spine
D. Pubic symphysis
E. Coccyx

Answer

Ans: D (Pubic symphysis)

Figure 35 illustrates the ventral view of female pelvis, which comprises four bones: Two innominate bones, one sacrum (which forms the rear of pelvis and articulates with the innominate bones on the two sides) and the other coccyx (which forms the base of the spine and pelvis).

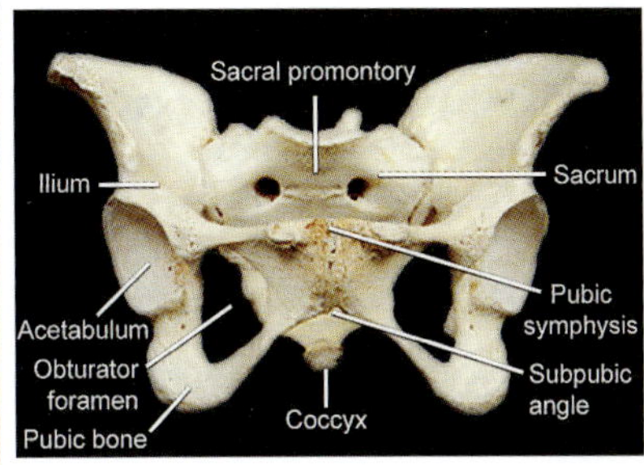

Fig. 35: Ventral/anterior view of pelvis.

Comment

Explanation: The four bones of the pelvis connect at four joints: Two sacroiliac joints, one pubic symphysis between the two innominate bone and one sacrococcygeal joint. Together, all these bones help in forming the true pelvis. This helps in forming the bony canal through which the fetus passes during the normal vaginal mechanism of childbirth. The true pelvis is composed of an inlet, cavity, and outlet.

Potential questions: There can be potential questions on any of the pelvic bones, joints, or anatomical landmarks

Question

Q36. In the image below, identify the parameter denoted by the letter C.

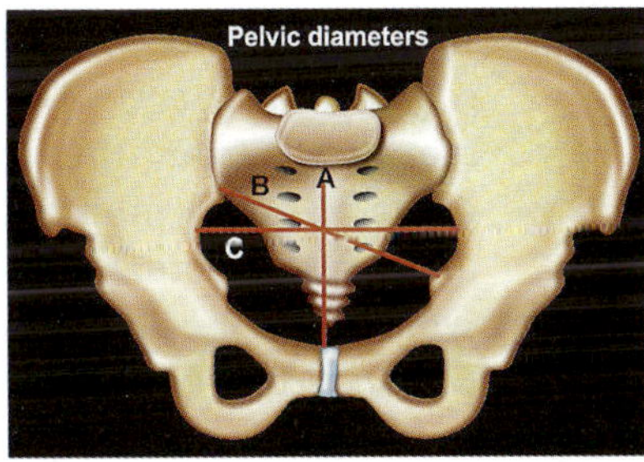

A. Obstetric conjugate
B. Anatomic conjugate
C. Diagonal conjugate
D. Transverse diameter of inlet
E. Transverse diameter of outlet

Answer

Ans: D (Transverse diameter of inlet)

The adjacent image shows superior view of the inlet or the pelvic brim, which helps in separating false pelvis above from the true pelvis below. Various diameters of pelvic brim, cavity, and outlet are summarized in **Figure 36**.

	Anteroposterior	Oblique	Transverse
Brim	11	12	13
Cavity	12	12	12
Outlet	13	12	11

Pelvic measurements given in centimeters

Fig. 36: Various pelvic diameters.

Comment

Explanation: The transverse diameter of the inlet is the distance between the farthest two points on the iliopectineal line and is the largest diameter of the pelvis. It measures about 13 cm (4 cm anterior to the promontory and 7 cm behind the symphysis).

Right and left oblique diameters of the inlet extend from right and left sacroiliac joints to the left and right iliopectineal eminences, respectively.

Potential questions: There can be questions pertaining to the various diameters of the pelvic inlet (anteroposterior, transverse, and oblique).

Question	Answer	Comment
Q37. The image below shows a ventral view of the pelvis. Which of the following best represents the measurement of the anatomical anteroposterior (AP) diameter of the pelvic outlet? 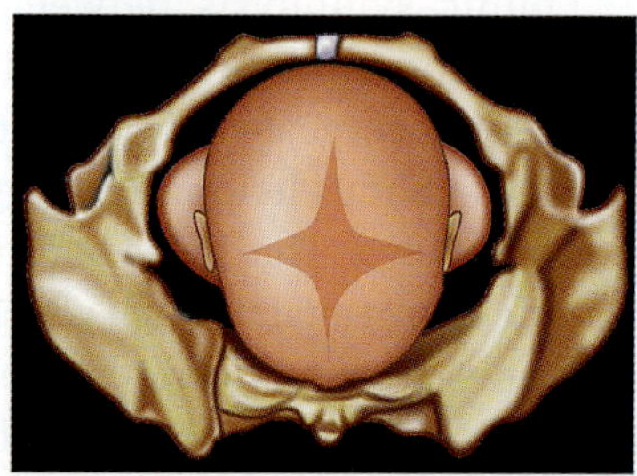 A. Anterior superior iliac spine to ischial tuberosity B. Sacral promontory to pubic symphysis C. Coccyx to pubic symphysis D. Posterior superior iliac spine to anterior superior iliac spine (ASIS) E. Left ischial spine to right ischial spine	**Ans: C (Coccyx to pubic symphysis)** The pelvic outlet as shown in **Figure 37** is lozenge-shaped and is bounded by the lower border of pubic symphysis, pubic arch, ischial tuberosities, sacrotuberous and sacrospinous ligaments, and tip of coccyx. 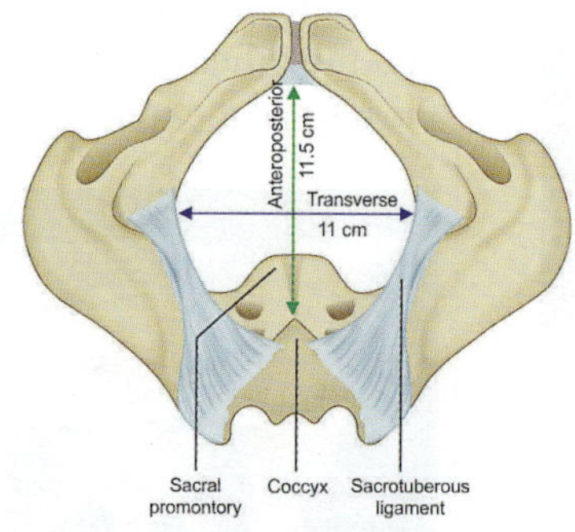 **Fig. 37:** View of pelvic outlet.	**Explanation:** Various diameters of pelvic outlet are as follows: ▪ *AP diameter:* Anatomical AP diameter (11 cm) extends from the tip of coccyx to the lower border of pubic symphysis. Obstetric AP diameter (13 cm) extends from the tip of sacrum to the lower border of symphysis pubis as the coccyx moves backward during the second stage of labor. ▪ *Transverse diameter:* This extends between the two ischial tuberosities and measures 11 cm. **Potential questions:** There can be potential questions related to various other diameters of the pelvic outlet as well.
Q38. In the image below, identify X and its dimensions. 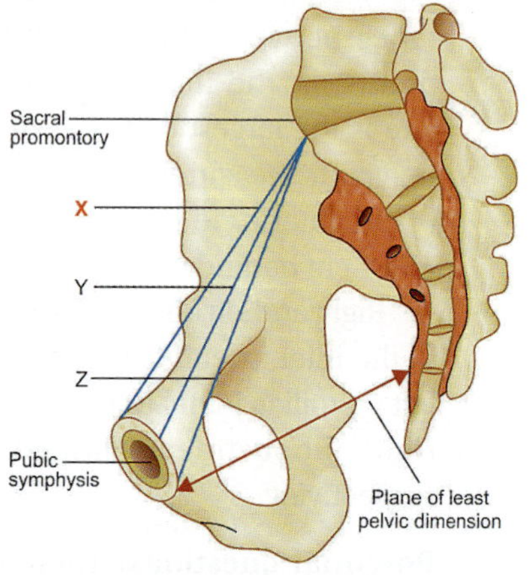 A. Anatomical conjugate, measures 11 cm B. Anatomical conjugate, measures 10 cm C. Obstetric conjugate, measures 10.5 cm D. Obstetric conjugate, measures 12.5 cm E. Diagonal conjugate, measures 12.5 cm	**Ans: A (Anatomical conjugate, measures 11 cm)** **Figure 38** shows the medial view of pelvis from left, illustrating various diameters of the pelvic inlet. 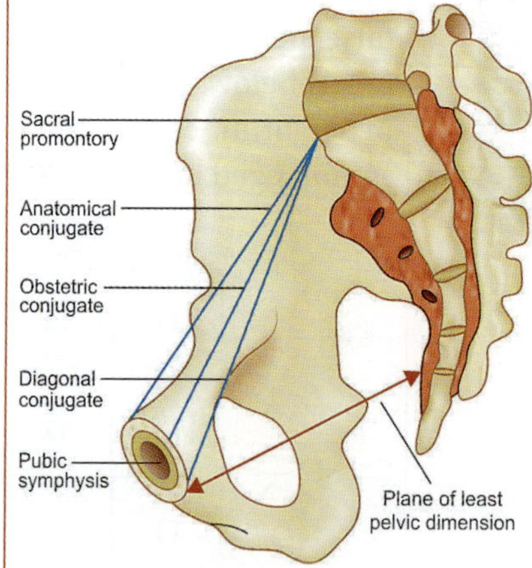 **Fig. 38:** Medial view of pelvis.	**Explanation:** Various anteroposteior (AP) diameters of pelvic inlet are as follows: ▪ *True conjugate or anatomical conjugate (11 cm):* This is measured from the midpoint of sacral promontory to the upper border of pubic symphysis. ▪ *Obstetric conjugate (10.5 cm):* This is measured from the midpoint of sacral promontory to the most bulging point on the back of symphysis pubic. ▪ *Diagonal conjugate (12.5 cm):* It is measured from the tip of sacral promontory to the lower border of pubic symphysis. **Potential questions:** There can be questions pertaining to the various other AP diameters of the pelvic inlet.

Question	Answer	Comment
Q39. In the image below, an obstetrician at the time of pelvic examination makes a measurement from the inferior border of the pubic symphysis to the sacral promontory. What anatomical measurement is being assessed? 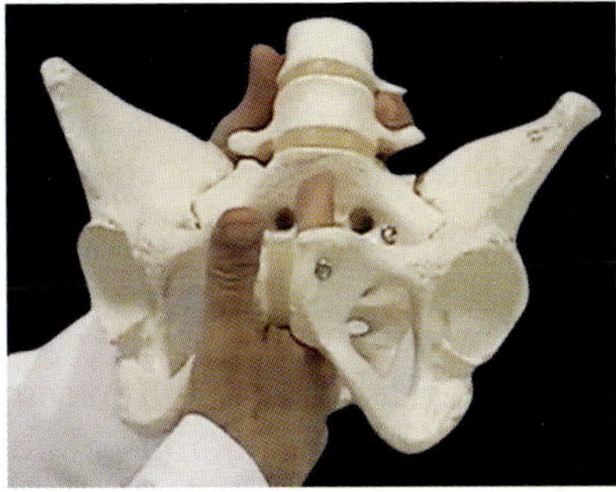 A. True conjugate B. Oblique diameter C. Diagonal conjugate D. Obstetric conjugate E. Anatomical conjugate	**Ans: C (Diagonal conjugate)** The method for measuring the diagonal conjugate is illustrated in **Figure 39**. The diagonal conjugate is the distance measured from the inferior border of the pubic symphysis to the sacral promontory. The diagonal conjugate is typically around 12.5 cm. 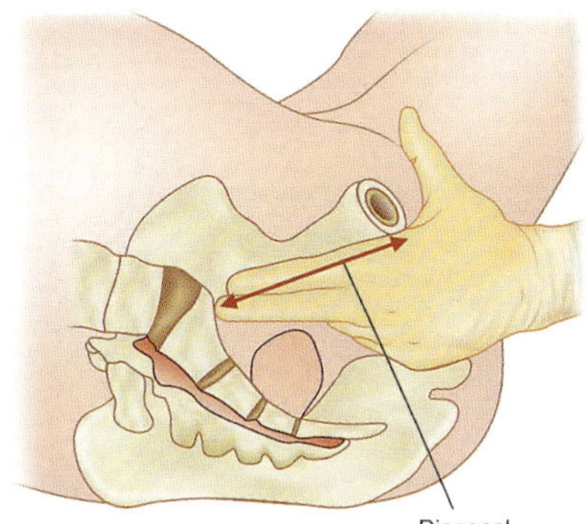 **Fig. 39:** Measurement of the diagonal conjugate.	**Explanation:** Measurement of diagonal conjugate is clinically important as it provides an estimate of the true conjugate, which cannot be measured directly during a pelvic examination. If the pelvis is adequate, the middle finger will not reach the sacral promontory. The clinician may be required to depress the elbow and wrist while mobilizing the fingers upward in order to reach the promontory. In normal cases, it will be difficult to feel the sacral promontory. **Potential questions:** There can be questions pertaining to other parameters which are assessed at the time of pelvic examination.
Q40. In the image below, the obstetrician measures the subpubic angle. What does this measurement help assess? 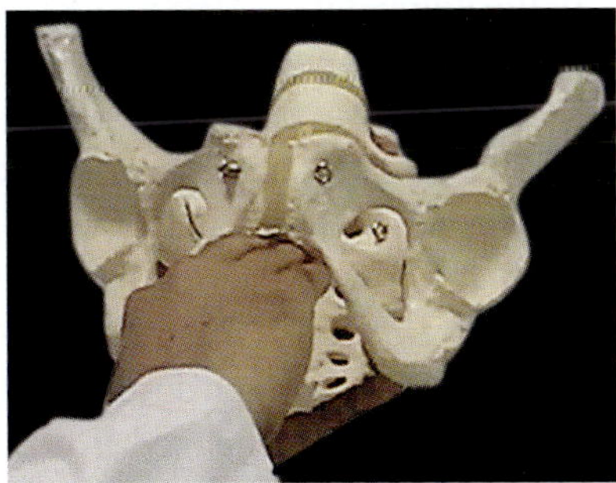 A. Fetal head engagement B. Pelvic inlet size C. Pelvic outlet size D. Ischial spine prominence E. Coccyx flexibility	**Ans: C (Pelvic outlet size)** **Figure 40** shows the assessment of subpubic angle. This is an important measure used for assessing the size of the pelvic outlet, which is important for evaluating the passage of the fetal head during childbirth. 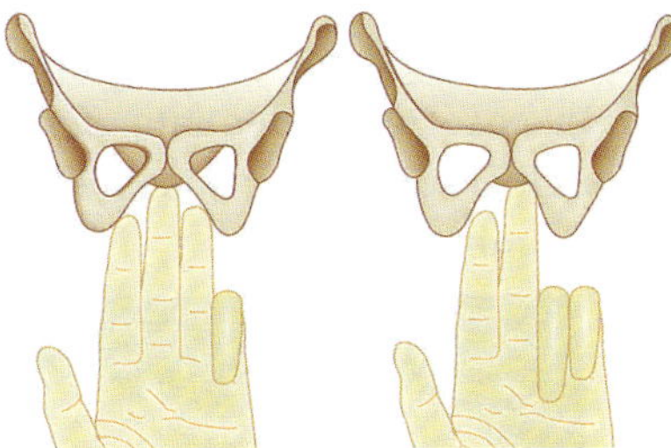 **Fig. 40:** Assessment of subpubic angle.	**Explanation:** Subpubic angle is the angle between two pubic rami. It varies from 85° ± 5°. Normal subpubic angle allows the placement of three to four fingers in the subpubic space. If at least three fingers can be placed under the pubis, the subpubic angle is approximately 90°, which can be considered as adequate. If the subpubic angle allows only two fingers, the subpubic angle is about 60°, which is indicative of an inadequate pelvic outlet. **Potential questions:** There can be questions pertaining to the various parameters which are assessed at the time of pelvic examination.

Question	Answer	Comment
Q41. An obstetrician is assessing the transverse diameter of the pelvic outlet in a pregnant woman as shown in the image below. Which of the following best describes the transverse diameter of the pelvic outlet? 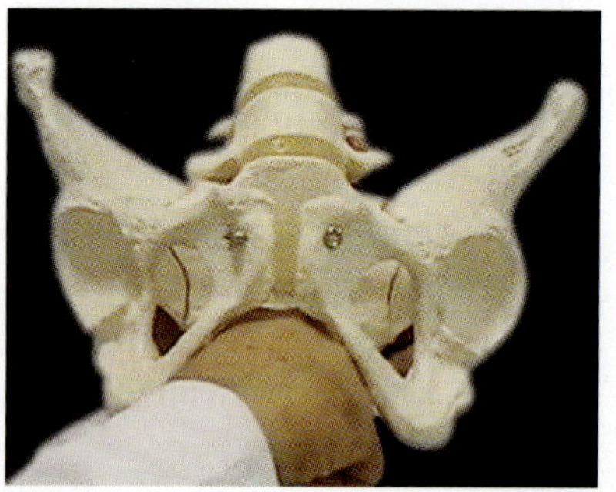 A. Distance between the ischial tuberosities B. Distance between the ischial spines C. Distance between the pubic symphysis and the sacral promontory D. Distance between the iliac crests E. Distance from the sacral promontory to the coccyx	**Ans: A (Distance between the ischial tuberosities)** The transverse diameter of the pelvic outlet is the distance between the inner borders of the ischial tuberosities **(Fig. 41)**. This measurement is important in obstetrics as it determines the transverse diameter of the pelvic outlet, which can affect the passage of the fetus during delivery. 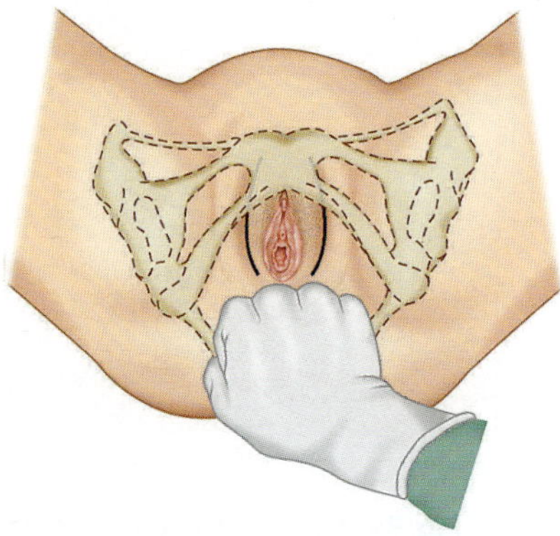 **Fig. 41:** Measurement of transverse diameter of the outlet.	**Explanation:** For assessment of the pelvic outlet, the subpubic angle, intertuberous diameter (transverse diameter of the outlet), and mobility of the coccyx are determined. After measuring the subpubic angle, as the obstetrician's hand is withdrawn from the vaginal introitus, the intertuberous diameter is measured with the knuckles of the closed fist of the hand placed between the ischial tuberosities. If the pelvis is adequate, the intertuberous diameter allows four knuckles. In case of an inadequate pelvis, the intertuberous diameter allows less than four knuckles. **Potential questions:** There can be questions pertaining to other parameters which are assessed at the time of pelvic examination.
Q42. In the below clinical image of the pelvis, what is the primary use of the ischial spines in obstetric assessments? 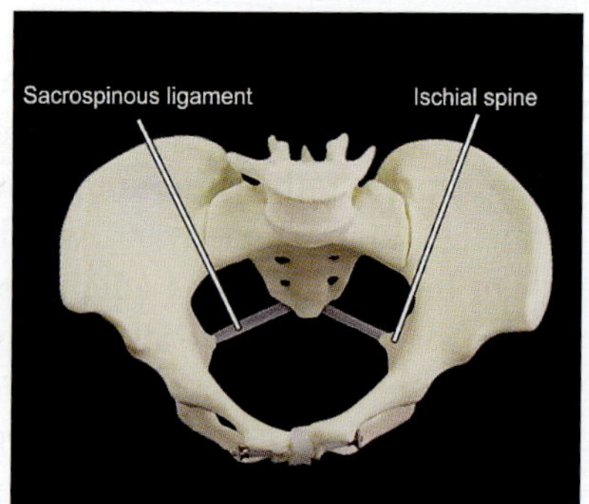 A. Assessing the midpelvis B. Determining the pelvic inlet diameter C. Measuring pelvic cavity depth D. Identifying the location of the sacroiliac joints E. Evaluating the position of the pubic symphysis	**Ans: A (Assessing the midpelvis)** **Figure 42** illustrates the palpation of ischial spines. Ischial spines are palpated for the assessment of midpelvis by evaluating the interischial diameter, also known as the plane of least pelvic dimensions or the plane of obstetric outlet. This should not be less than 9.5 cm. In case of inadequate pelvis, the ischial spines may appear sharp and prominent. 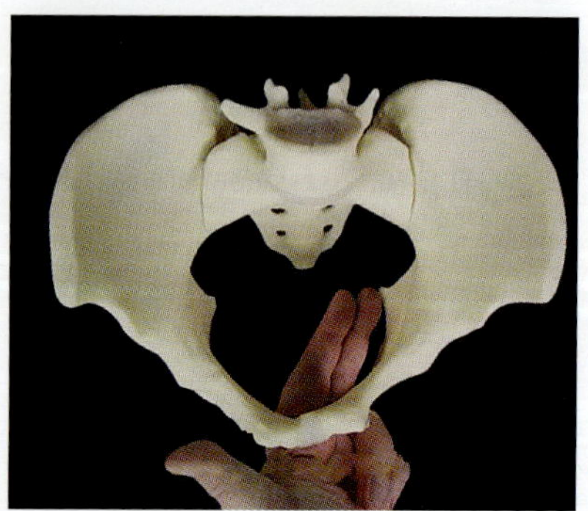 **Fig. 42:** Assessment of ischial spines.	**Explanation:** Ischial spine acts as an important landmark of pelvis because of the following: ▪ Ischial spines serve as key landmarks to assess the fetal head's descent during labor, marking the station in the pelvic canal and helping evaluate progress through the midpelvis. They indicate the fetal head's position during delivery. ▪ Fetal head is engaged if it is felt vaginally at or below this level. ▪ Internal rotation of fetal head occurs when occiput is at this level. ▪ Forceps are applied only when the head is at this level. ▪ Pudendal nerve block is carried out at this level. ▪ External os of cervix is at this level. **Potential questions:** There can be questions pertaining to the various parameters which are assessed at the time of pelvic examination.

Question	Answer	Comment
Q43. On a pelvic X-ray, which structure forms the posterior boundary of the pelvic brim (highlighted by green color)? 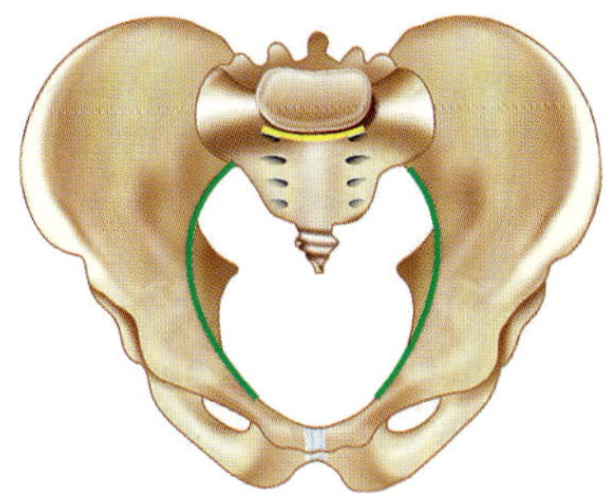 A. Sacrum B. Ischial tuberosity C. Pubic symphysis D. Iliac crest E. Greater sciatic notch	**Ans: A (Sacrum)** **Figure 43** shows margins of pelvic brim, which can be considered as the boundary line of pelvic inlet and divides the pelvis anatomically into false pelvis and true pelvis. 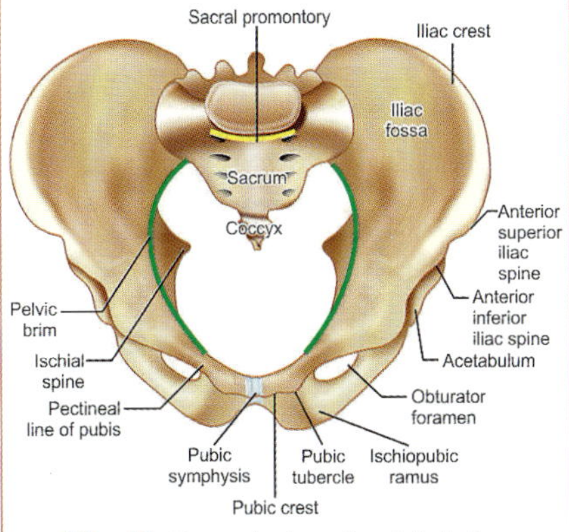 **Fig. 43:** Boundaries of pelvic brim.	**Explanation:** The boundaries of pelvic brim, also known as the pelvic inlet, are sacral promontory, alae of sacrum, sacroiliac joints, iliopectineal line, iliopectineal eminence, upper border of superior pubic rami, pubic tubercle, pubic crest, and upper border of symphysis pubis. The sacrum, including its promontory, contributes to the posterior edge of the pelvic brim, which is crucial for evaluating pelvic adequacy during labor and delivery. **Potential questions:** There can be questions pertaining to the various parameters which are assessed at the time of pelvic examination.
Q44. In the below image that shows the ventral view of pelvis, which diameter is most critical for assessing the engagement of the anteroposterior diameter of fetal head during labor? 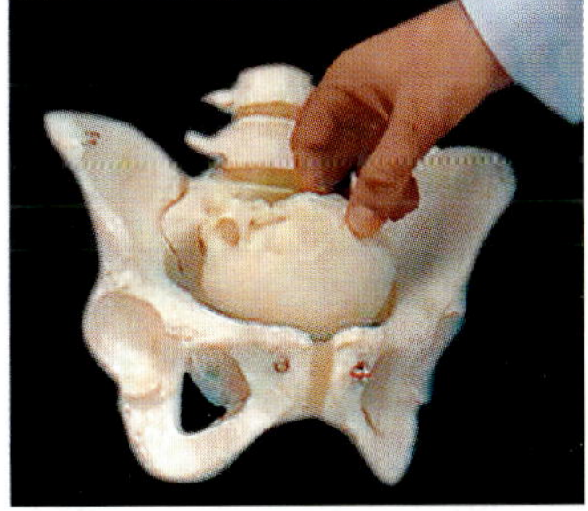 A. Anteroposterior diameter B. Transverse diameter C. Oblique diameter D. Pelvic outlet diameter E. Sacral diameter	**Ans: B (Transverse diameter)** **Figure 44** shows how the antero-posterior (AP) diameter of the fetal head engages into the transverse diameter of the pelvic inlet. 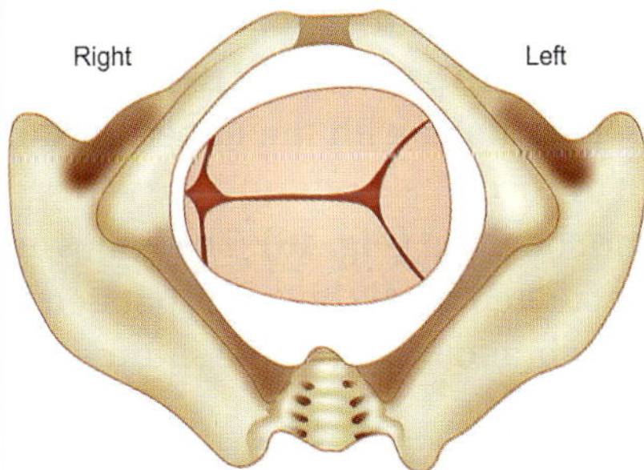 **Fig. 44:** Anteroposterior diameter of fetal head engages in the transverse diameter of the inlet resulting in the left occiput transverse (LOT) position.	**Explanation:** At the time of entry of fetal head into the maternal pelvis, the occipitofrontal diameter engages through the superior pelvic aperture in transverse diameter because it is the longest. As the fetal head descends downward and reaches the ischial spines, it undergoes rotation by 90° so that the longest diameter of fetal head engages in the AP diameter of the outlet, which is the largest diameter. **Potential questions:** There can be potential questions related to the movements of fetal presenting part as it negotiates through various pelvic diameters.

Question	Answer	Comment
Q45. In the below image showing different types of pelvis, which type of pelvis is denoted by letter B as per the Caldwell-Moloy classification? 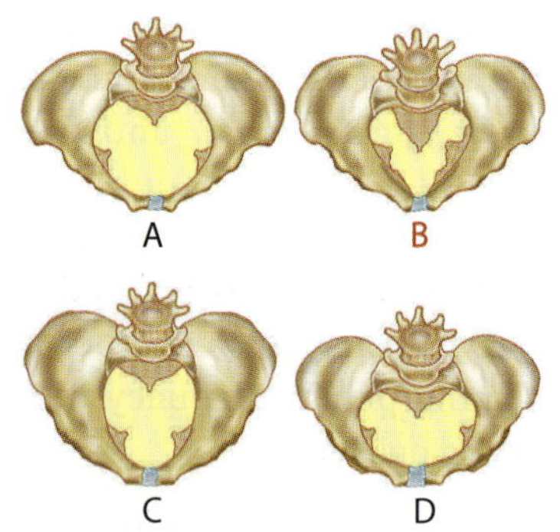 A. Gynecoid pelvis B. Android pelvis C. Anthropoid pelvis D. Platypelloid pelvis E. Mixed pelvis	**Ans: B (Android pelvis)** Using the "Caldwell-Moloy" system, the pelvic shape can be classified into four basic types **(Figs. 45A to D)**: Gynecoid (50%), android (20%), anthropoid (25%), and platypelloid (5%). 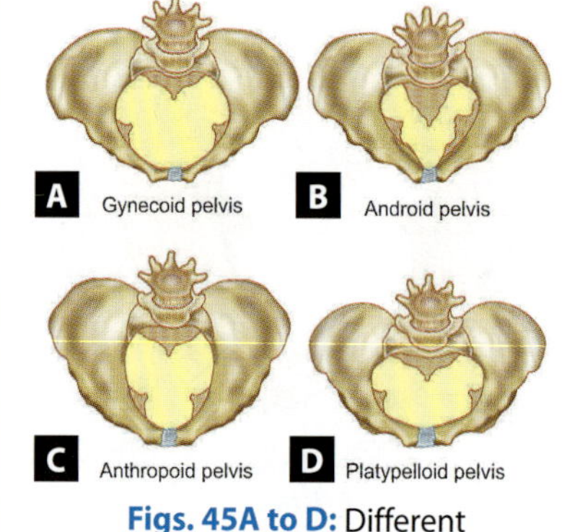 **Figs. 45A to D:** Different types of pelvis.	**Explanation:** Android pelvis is heart-shaped/triangular-shaped male type of pelvis with the base towards the sacrum. As a result, the posterior segment is short and anterior segment is narrow. The pelvic sidewalls are convergent with projecting ischial spines. Both the sacrosciatic notch and subpubic angles are narrow (<90°). These features of android pelvis make vaginal delivery more challenging. Android pelvis is more common in males but can also occur in females and often requires a cesarean section due to limited space for the fetus. **Potential question**: There can be questions pertaining to features of different types of pelves.

FETAL SKULL

Question	Answer	Comment
Q46. Identify the bone of the fetal skull in the figure below. 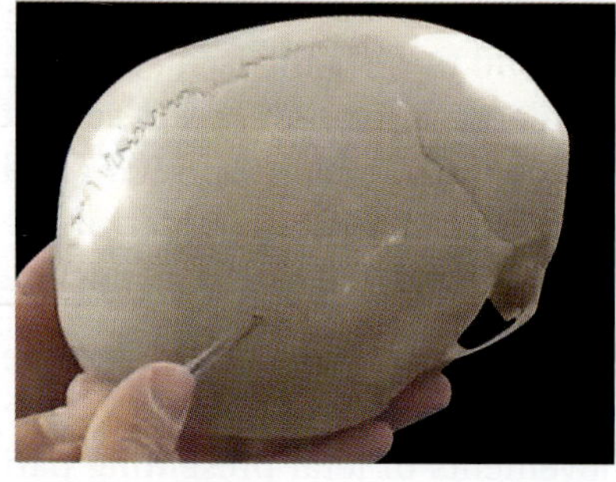 A. Frontal bone B. Parietal bone C. Occipital bone D. Temporal bone E. Sphenoid bone	**Ans: B (Parietal bone)** The fetal skull is made up of two frontal, two parietal, and two temporal bones, along with the upper portion of the occipital bone and the wings of the sphenoid **(Fig. 46)**. The bones are not united rigidly but are separated by membranous spaces, the sutures. 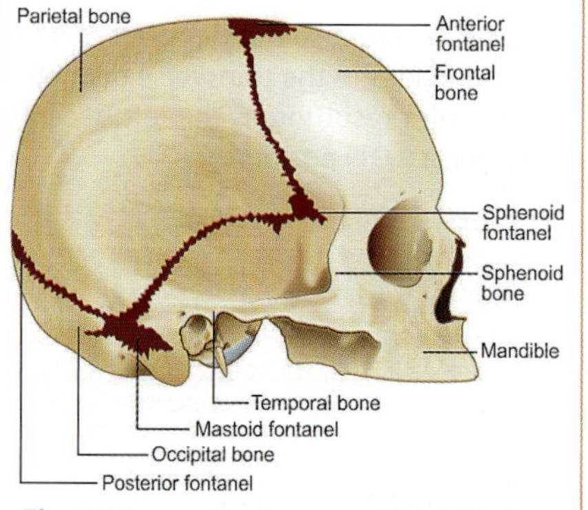 **Fig. 46:** Important bones of fetal skull as seen from the side.	**Explanation:** One parietal bone is located on each side of the skull just behind the frontal bone **(Fig. 46)**. Together, the parietal bones form the bulging sides and roof of the cranium. They are fused in the middle along the sagittal suture, and they meet the frontal bone along the coronal suture. **Potential questions:** Any of the skull bones, sutures, or landmarks can be asked as a question.

Question	Answer	Comment
Q47. Which bone of fetal skull is indicated by the arrow in the below image? 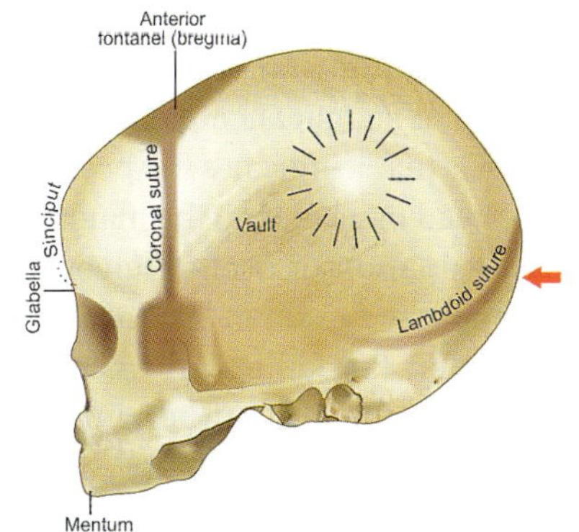 A. Frontal bone B. Parietal bone C. Temporal bone D. Occipital bone E. Sphenoid	**Ans: D (Occipital bone)** The arrow in the adjacent picture points towards the occipital bone. **Figure 47** shows important landmarks of the fetal skull. 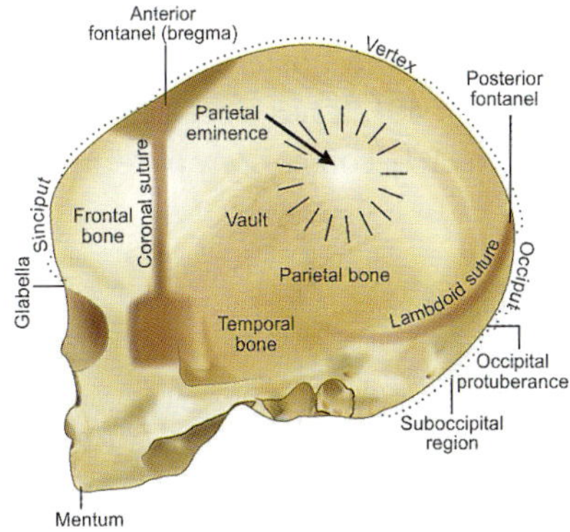 **Fig. 47:** Landmarks of fetal skull.	**Explanation:** The occipital bone is the primary bone forming the posterior part of fetal skull, known as the occiput. It is crucial for encasing and protecting the brain, especially during birth when the head passes through the birth canal. The occipital bone plays a critical role in obstetrics, particularly in determining the position of fetal head in relation to maternal pelvis during labor. **Potential questions:** Any of the skull bones, sutures, or landmarks can be asked as a question.
Q48. In the below image, the structure shown by the pointer corresponds to which of the following? 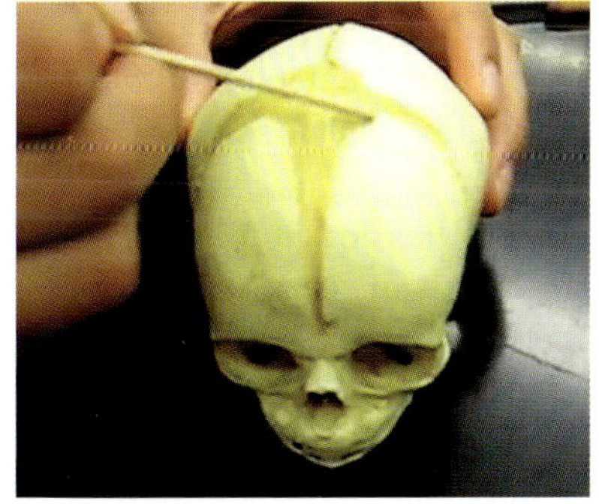 A. Junction of the frontal and parietal bones B. Junction of the parietal and occipital bones C. Junction of the temporal and parietal bones D. Junction of the frontal and temporal bones E. Junction of the parietal and sphenoid bones	**Ans: A (Junction of the frontal and parietal bones)** The pointer in the adjacent image is pointing towards a lozenge-shaped space which is a soft, membranous gap between the frontal and parietal bones and is known as the anterior fontanel **(Fig. 48)**. Fontanel can be identified as gaps which occur at the junctions where the cranial bones have not yet fully fused together. Anterior fontanel (measuring about 3 cm in each dimension) is formed by joining of four sutures: Frontal suture (anteriorly), sagittal suture (posteriorly), and coronal sutures on the two sides (laterally). 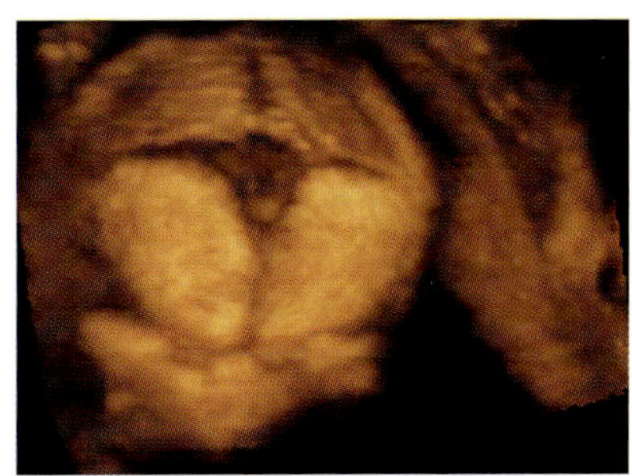 **Fig. 48:** Three-dimensional ultrasound view of the fetus showing anterior fontanel (bregma).	**Explanation:** The greater or anterior fontanel is situated at the junction of the sagittal and coronal sutures. The palpation of anterior fontanel on vaginal examination is of great obstetric significance. ▪ Palpation of anterior fontanel indicates degree of flexion of fetal head. ▪ Presence of this fontanel facilitates molding of fetal head. ▪ The membranous nature of anterior fontanel helps in accommodating the rapid growth of brain during the neonatal period. ▪ Floor of the anterior fontanel reflects the intracranial status. The floor may be depressed in case of dehydration and elevated in case of hydrocephalus. **Potential questions:** There can be potential questions related to the structural configuration and significance of both anterior and posterior fontanel.

Question	Answer	Comment
Q49. What is the clinical significance of the fontanel being pointed out in the below image? 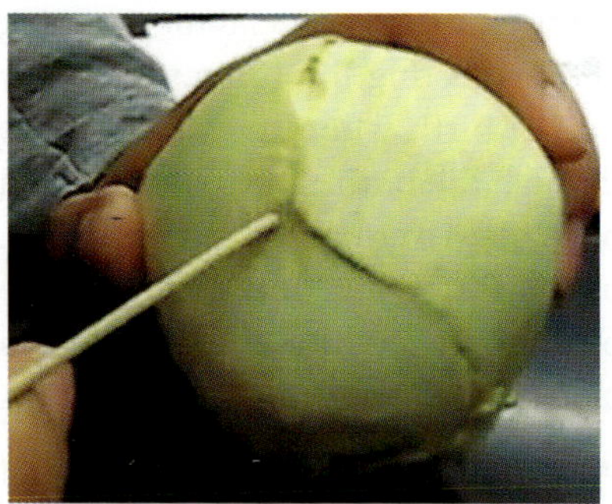 A. Indicates cerebral edema B. Indicates dehydration C. Indicates congenital malformation D. Indicates position of fetal head in relation to the maternal pelvis E. Indicates hydrocephalus	**Ans: D (Indicates position of fetal head in relation to the maternal pelvis)** The pointer in the adjacent figure shows the posterior fontanel which is triangular in shape (measuring about half inch in each dimension) and is present on the posterior aspect of skull **(Fig. 49)**. It has a membranous floor which becomes bony by term. 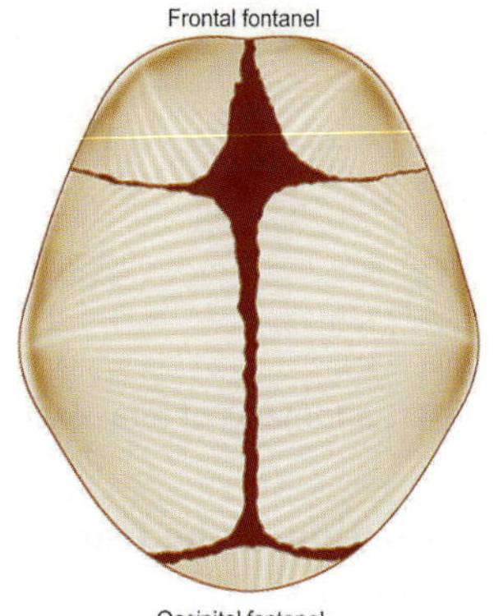 **Fig. 49:** Fontanels of fetal skull as seen from the top.	**Explanation:** Posterior fontanel is formed by the joining of three sutures: Sagittal suture (anteriorly) and lambdoid sutures on the two sides. The clinical significance of posterior fontanel is that it indicates the position of fetal head in relation to the maternal pelvis. Palpation of occiput gives an idea about the flexion of fetal head. In a completely flexed head, the occiput and posterior fontanel can be palpated. However, the anterior fontanel cannot be palpated. The more deflexed the fetal head, the more likely is the anterior fontanel to be palpated. **Potential questions:** There can be potential questions related to the structural configuration and significance of both anterior and posterior fontanel.
Q50. Identify the suture marked by the letter A in the below image. Which of the following statements regarding this suture is correct? 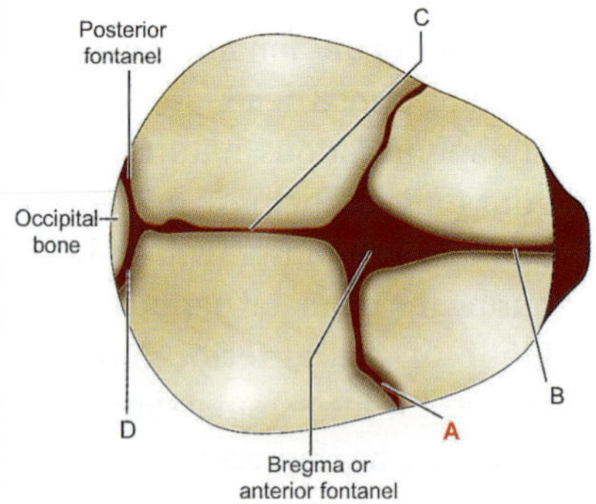 A. This suture separates the two parietal bones. B. This suture separates the frontal bone from the parietal bones. C. This suture separates the occipital bone from the parietal bones. D. This suture runs between the two frontal bones. E. This suture is located between the temporal and parietal bones.	**Ans: B (This suture separates the frontal bone from the parietal bones)** The letter A in the adjacent figure refers to the coronal suture. **Figure 50** shows all the important sutures of fetal skull. Sutures can be defined as narrow ridges of connective tissue joining the flat bones of the skull. 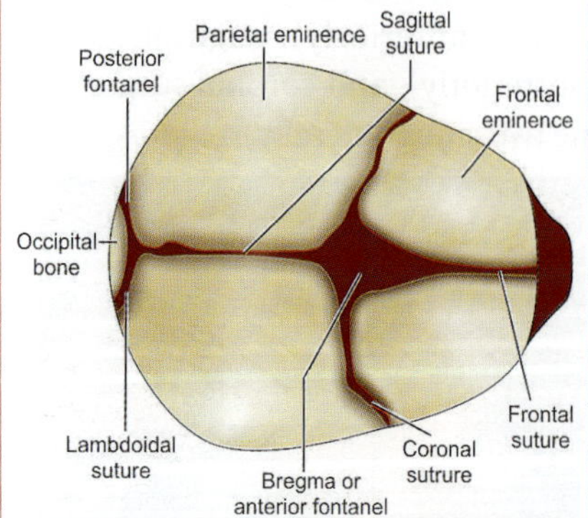 **Fig. 50:** Important sutures of fetal skull as seen from the top.	**Explanation:** The fetal skull has four main sutures as follows: 1. *Sagittal or longitudinal suture:* This suture lies longitudinally across the vault of the skull in midline between the two parietal bones 2. *Coronal sutures:* These sutures are present between the parietal and frontal bones and extend transversely on either side from the anterior fontanels. 3. *Lambdoid sutures:* These sutures separate the occipital bone from the two parietal bones and extend transversely on both sides from the posterior fontanel. 4. *Frontal suture:* This suture is present between the two halves of the frontal bone in the skull of babies and usually disappears by the age of 6 years. **Potential questions:** There can be a potential question related to any of the sutures on the fetal skull.

Question	Answer	Comment
Q51. Which anteroposterior (AP) diameter of fetal skull is represented by the letter X in the image below? 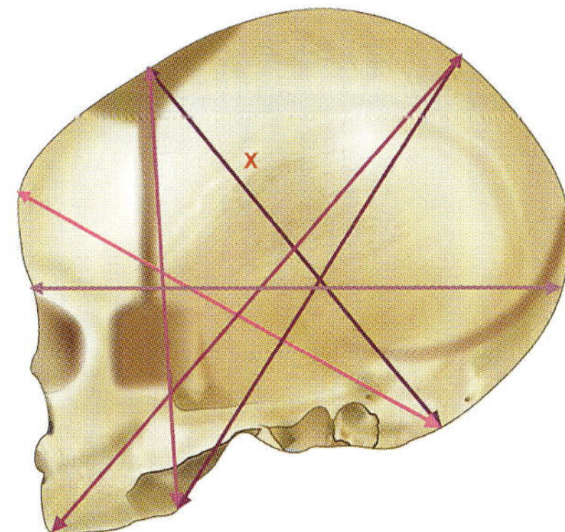 A. Suboccipitofrontal B. Suboccipitobregmatic C. Occipitofrontal D. Suboccipitofrontal E. Mentovertical	**Ans: B (Suboccipitobregmatic)** The important AP diameters of the fetal skull are shown in **Figure 51**. The letter X shows the suboccipitobregmatic diameter which represents a fully flexed fetal head. 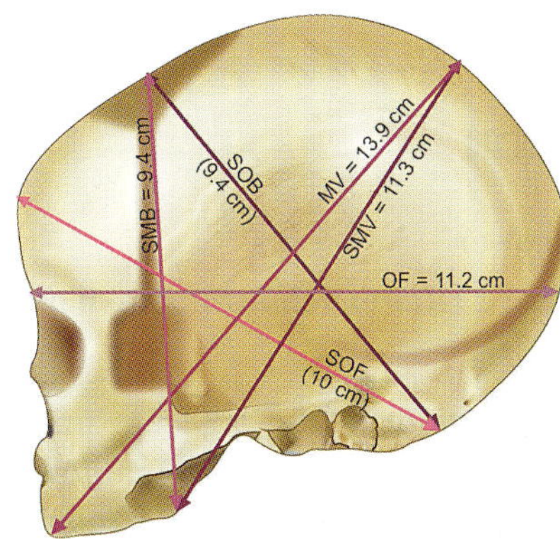 **Fig. 51:** Diameters of fetal skull. (MV: mentovertical; OF: occipitofrontal; SOF: suboccipitofrontal; SMB: Submentobregmatic; SMV: submentovertical; SOB: suboccipitobregmatic)	**Explanation:** Important AP diameters of the fetal skull are as follows: ▪ *Suboccipitobregmatic diameter:* Extends from the nape of the neck to the center of bregma ▪ *Suboccipitofrontal diameter:* Extends from the nape of the neck to the anterior end of anterior fontanel or center of sinciput ▪ *Occipitofrontal diameter:* Extends from the occipital eminence to the root of nose (glabella) ▪ *Mentovertical diameter:* Extends from the midpoint of the chin to the highest point on sagittal suture ▪ *Submentovertical diameter:* Extends from the junction of the floor of the mouth and neck to the highest point on sagittal suture ▪ *Submentobregmatic diameter:* Extends from the junction of the floor of the mouth and neck to the center of bregma **Potential questions:** There can be potential questions related to any of the AP or transverse diameters of the fetal skull.

CHAPTER 2

Labor and Delivery

GENERAL PHYSICAL EXAMINATION

Question	Answer	Comment
Q1. A 34-year-old primigravida patient presented to the antenatal clinic with complaints of extreme weakness at 16 weeks' gestation. On general physical examination, the appearance of conjunctiva is shown in the image below. From the following options, which nail change is most likely to be present in this case? 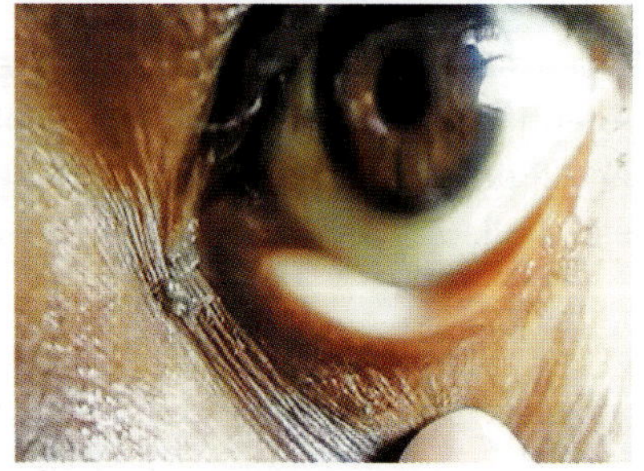 A. Clubbing B. Pitting: Small depressions C. Koilonychia: Spoon-shaped nails D. Leukonychia: White spots E. Horizontal ridges across the nails	**Ans: C (Koilonychia: Spoon-shaped nails)** The patient in the adjacent image has pallor in the lower palpebral conjunctiva due to anemia. The nail changes likely to be present in her case could be suggestive of koilonychia **(Fig. 1)**. This is a clinical finding where the nails lose their normal convexity and become depressed or flat or acquire a slight concavity. This results in appearance of spoon-shaped nails. 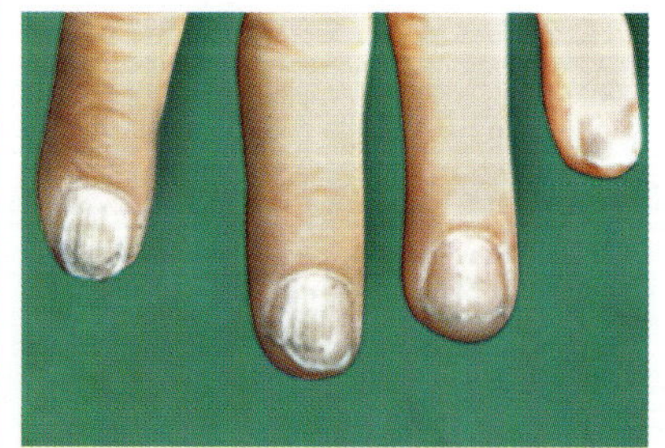 **Fig. 1:** Koilonychia.	**Explanation:** Presence of spoon-shaped nails or koilonychia is usually suggestive of hypochromic anemia, especially iron deficiency anemia. Reduced supply of oxyhemoglobin to the skin and mucous membranes is likely to result in their paleness, which can be detected on clinical examination. The areas in the body where pallor can be commonly observed include the lower palpebral conjunctiva, dorsal surface of tongue, palms of hand, and nail beds. **Potential questions:** There could be questions showing clinical findings suggestive of common medical disorders elicited during pregnancy on head-to-toe examination.

Question	Answer	Comment
Q2. A pregnant woman in her third trimester presents with swelling in both her feet and ankles, as shown in the image. Which of the following is the most likely cause of her condition? 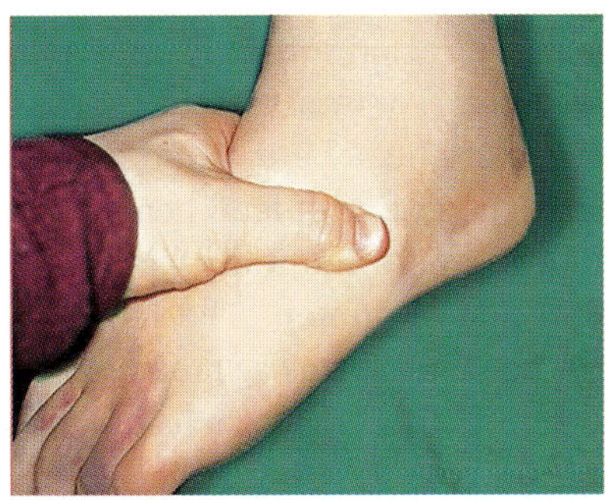 A. Pre-eclampsia B. Deep vein thrombosis (DVT) C. Heart failure D. Physiological edema of pregnancy E. Renal disease	**Ans: D (Physiological edema of pregnancy)** Physiological edema during pregnancy is a common finding, particularly in the dependent parts of the body such as feet/ankles or the sacral region. Pitting edema can be demonstrated as shown in **Figure 2**. 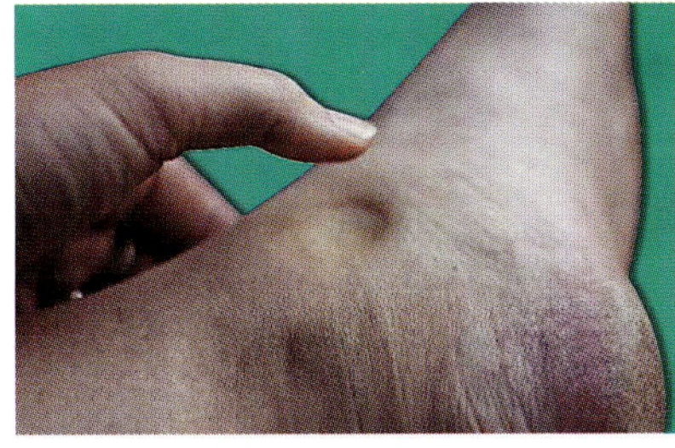 **Fig. 2:** Presence of pitting edema in the feet.	**Explanation:** Physiological changes in pregnancy such as increased blood volume, pressure from the growing uterus on the veins, and hormonal changes are likely to result in fluid retention, resulting in pedal edema. Physiological edema of pregnancy is generally benign and resolves postpartum, unlike the other conditions listed which may be associated with more severe symptoms and require immediate medical attention. **Potential questions:** There could be questions showing common clinical findings elicited during pregnancy on head-to-toe examination.

OBSTETRIC EXAMINATION

Q3. What maneuver is being performed by the obstetrician in the below image? 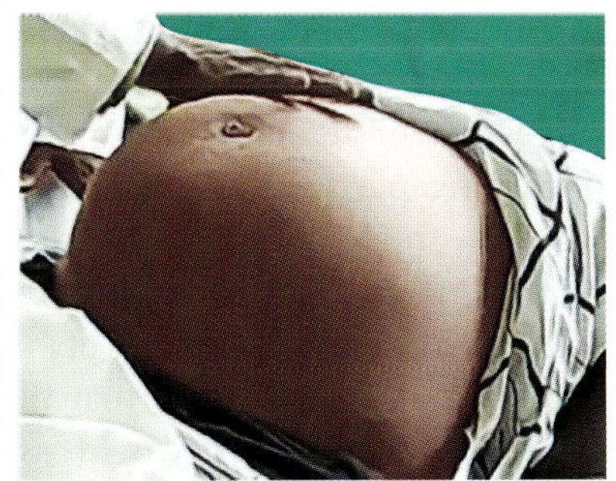 A. Leopold's first maneuver B. Leopold's second maneuver C. Leopold's third maneuver D. Leopold's fourth maneuver E. Pawlik's grip	**Ans: A (Leopold's first maneuver)** The adjacent image shows the obstetrician performing fundal grip (Leopold's first maneuver). The fundal area is palpated by placing both the hands over the fundal area **(Fig. 3)**. 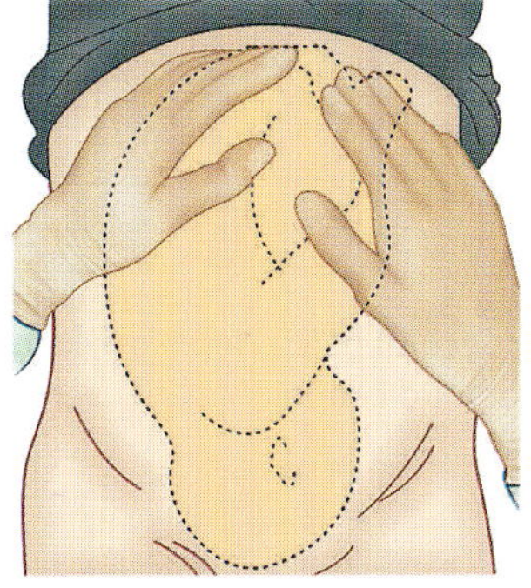 **Fig. 3:** Fundal grip (Leopold's first maneuver).	**Explanation:** Fundal grip helps the obstetrician to identify which of the fetal poles (head or breech) is present at the fundus. This maneuver can serve as an effective screening tool for detecting fetal malpresentation, particularly in settings where ultrasound may not be readily available. Palpation of broad, soft, irregular mass at the fundus is suggestive of fetal legs and/or buttocks, thereby pointing towards cephalic presentation. Palpation of a smooth, hard, globular, ballotable mass at the fundus is suggestive of fetal head and points towards breech presentation. **Potential questions:** There can be questions related to any of the four Leopold's maneuvers.

Question	Answer	Comment
Q4. What maneuver is being performed by the obstetrician in the below image? 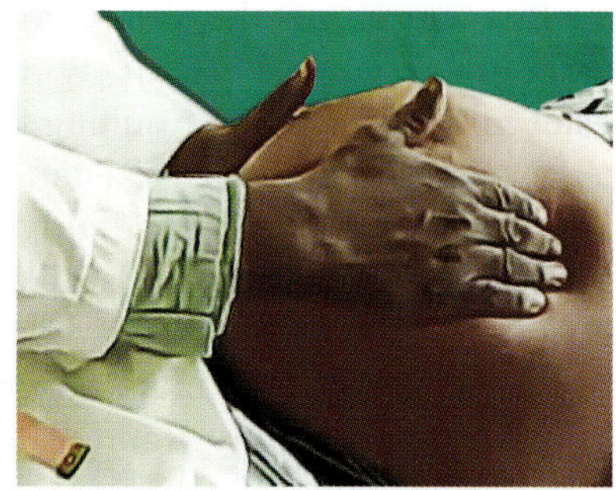 A. Leopold's first maneuver B. Leopold's second maneuver C. Leopold's third maneuver D. Leopold's fourth maneuver E. Pawlik's grip	**Ans: B (Leopold's second maneuver)** The adjacent image depicts Leopold's second maneuver or the lateral grip. In this grip, the obstetrician's hands are placed over the abdomen on either side of the umbilicus **(Fig. 4)**. 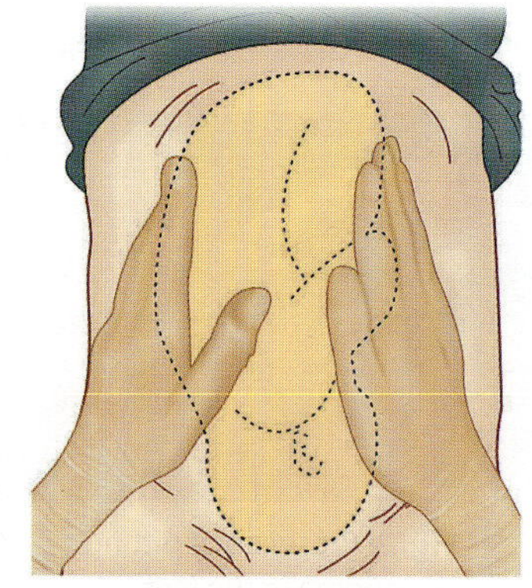 **Fig. 4:** Lateral grip (Leopold's second maneuver).	**Explanation:** Lateral grip helps the clinician in identifying the position of fetal back, limbs, and shoulder in case of vertex or breech presentation. The orientation of the fetus can be determined by noting whether the back is directed vertically (anteriorly, posteriorly) or transversely. In case of transverse lie, a hard round globular mass suggestive of fetal head can be identified horizontally across the maternal abdomen. The fetal back can be identified as a smooth curved structure with a resistant feel. **Potential questions:** There can be questions related to any of the four Leopold's maneuvers.
Q5. What maneuver is being performed by the obstetrician in the below image? 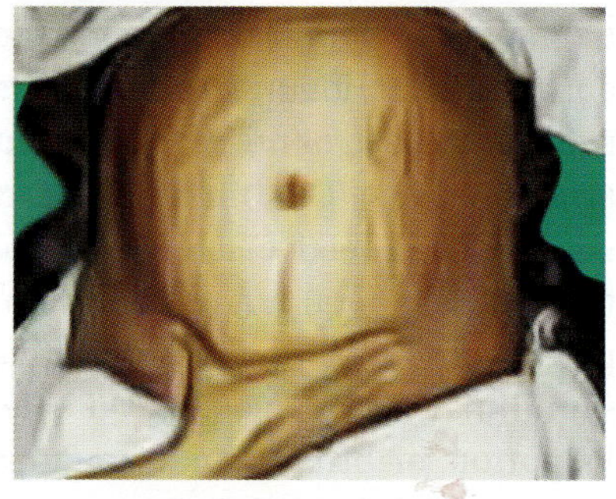 A. Leopold's first maneuver B. Leopold's second maneuver C. Leopold's third maneuver D. Leopold's fourth maneuver E. First pelvic grip	**Ans: C (Leopold's third maneuver)** The adjacent image depicts third Leopold's maneuver or second pelvic grip (Pawlik's grip). **Figure 5** depicts the method of performing this maneuver. 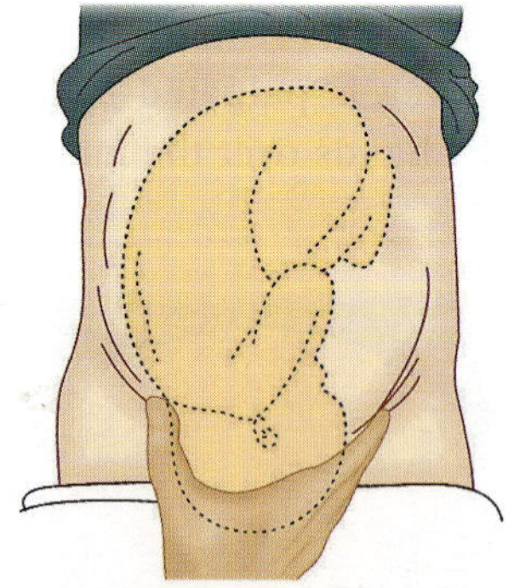 **Fig. 5:** Second pelvic grip (Pawlik's grip) or third Leopold's maneuver.	**Explanation:** In this grip, the obstetrician places the outstretched thumb and index finger of the right hand keeping the ulnar border of the palm on the upper border of the patient's pubic symphysis. If a hard globular mass is gripped during this maneuver, it implies vertex presentation. A soft broad part is suggestive of fetal breech. If the presenting part is not engaged, it would be freely ballotable between the two fingers. If the presenting part is deeply engaged, the findings of this maneuver simply indicate that the lower fetal pole is in the pelvis. In case of transverse presentation, the pelvic grip is empty. **Potential questions:** There can be questions related to any of the four Leopold's maneuvers.

Question	Answer	Comment
Q6. What maneuver is being performed by the obstetrician in the below image? 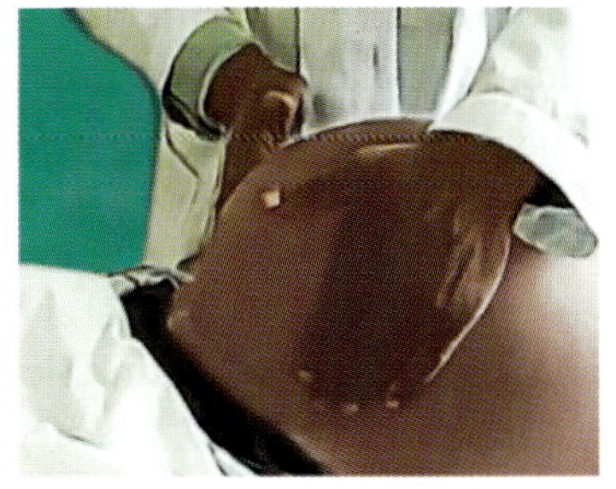 A. Leopold's first maneuver B. Leopold's second maneuver C. Leopold's third maneuver D. Leopold's fourth maneuver E. Pawlik's grip	**Ans: D (Leopold's fourth maneuver)** The adjacent image depicts Leopold's fourth maneuver or the first pelvic grip **(Fig. 6)**. 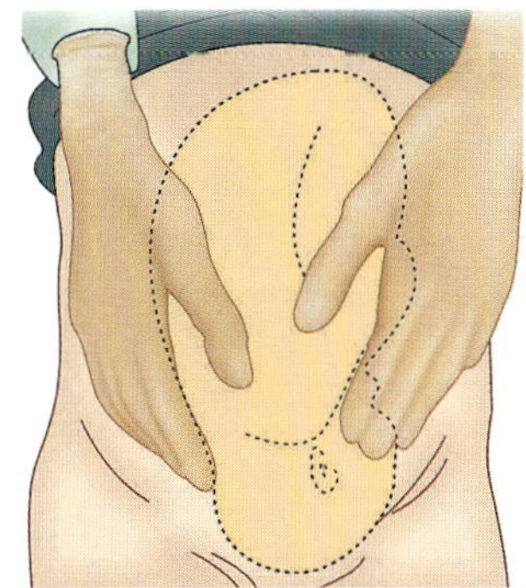 **Fig. 6:** First pelvic grip (fourth Leopold's maneuver).	**Explanation:** While performing this maneuver, tips of three fingers of each hand are placed on the either side of the midline in downward and backward direction in order to deeply palpate the fetal parts present in the lower pole of the uterus. In case of vertex presentation, a hard smooth globular mass suggestive of fetal head can be palpated on pelvic grip. In case of breech presentation, a broad soft, irregular mass is palpated. **Potential questions:** There can be questions related to any of the four Leopold's maneuvers.
Q7. A 32-year-old woman at term presents to the labor ward with uterine contractions. On abdominal examination using the fifth's formula as shown in the image, the obstetrician can palpate none of the fetal head per abdominally. She describes her finding as 0/5. What is the interpretation of the above finding in terms of the descent of the fetal head? 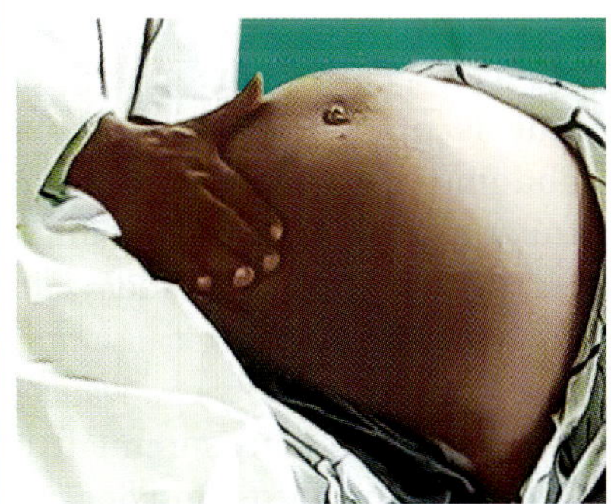 A. Fetal head is unengaged B. Fetal head is fixing C. Recently engaged fetal head D. Deeply engaged fetal head E. Free floating fetal head	**Ans: D (Deeply engaged fetal head)** As shown in **Figures 7A and B**, the assessment of fetal descent through the abdominal examination is done by using the Fifth's formula, which estimates the number of fifths of fetal head above the pelvic brim. 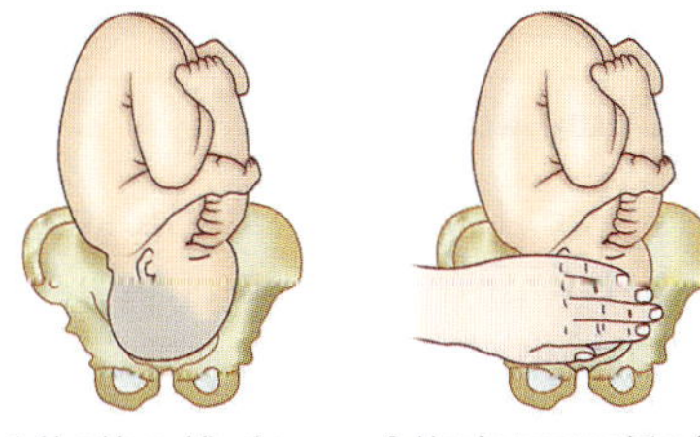 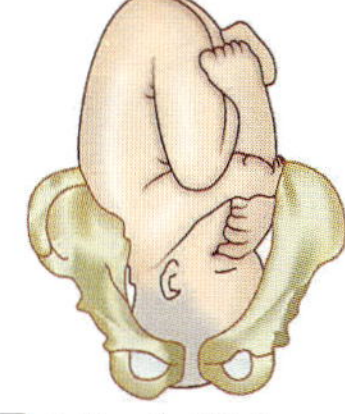 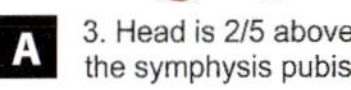 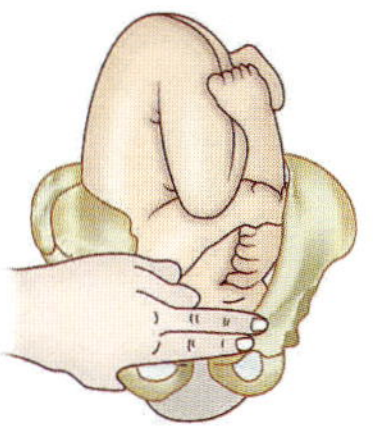 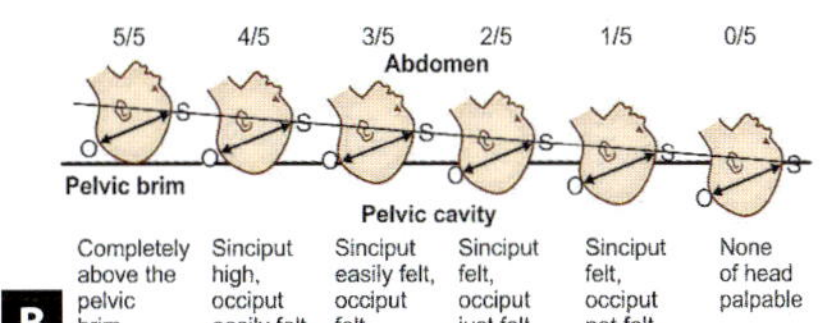 **Figs. 7A and B:** Abdominal examination for fetal descent using the Fifth's formula.	**Explanation:** In this method, the amount of fetal head that can be palpated per abdominally is estimated in terms of finger breadth which is assessed by placing the radial margin of the index finger above the symphysis pubis followed successively by other fingers. A free-floating head would be completely palpable per abdomen. This head accommodates full width of all the five fingers above the pubic symphysis and can be described as 5/5. A head which is fixing but not yet engaged may be three-fifths palpable per abdominally and is known as 3/5. A recently engaged fetal head may be two-fifths palpable per abdominally and is known as 2/5, while a deeply engaged fetal head may not be palpable at all per abdominally and may be described as 0/5. **Potential questions:** There can be questions related to interpretation of various abdominal and vaginal findings for assessment of progress of labor.

<table>
<tr><th>Question</th><th>Answer</th><th>Comment</th></tr>
<tr><td>

Q8. A 28-year-old second gravida presents in labor at 38 weeks of gestation. While examining the patient, the obstetrician auscultates the fetal heart sounds at the location marked by the red circle in the below image.

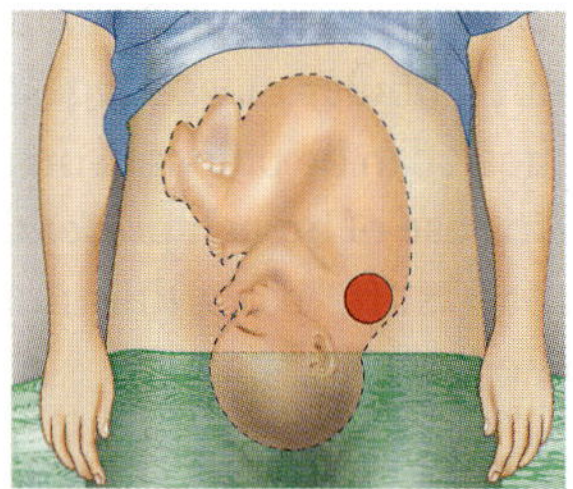

What is the likely fetal position in this case based on the location of fetal heartbeat?

A. Right occipitoanterior
B. Left occipitoanterior
C. Right occipitoposterior
D. Left occipitoposterior
E. Right mentoanterior

</td><td>

Ans: B (Left occipitoanterior position)

Figure 8 illustrates the location of fetal heart sounds based on the position of the fetal presenting part.

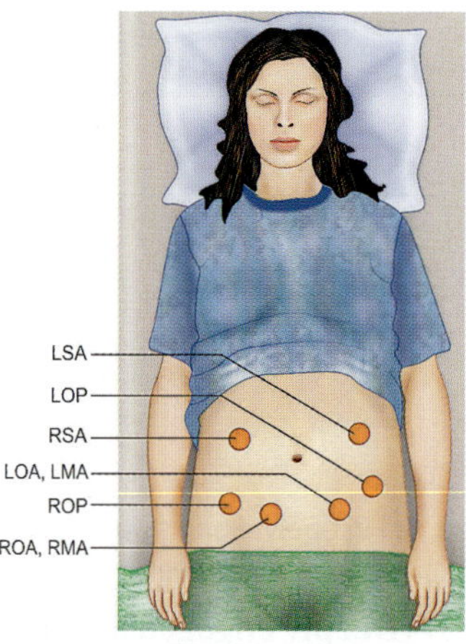

Fig. 8: Location of fetal heart rate based on the position of fetal head.
(LOA: left occipitoanterior; LOP: left occipito-posterior; LMA: left mentoanterior; LSA: left sacroanterior; ROP: right occipitoposterior; RMA: right mentoanterior; RSA: right sacroanterior)

</td><td>

Explanation: The region of maternal abdomen where the heart sounds are most clearly heard would vary with the presentation and extent of descent of the presenting part. In the LOA position, the fetal heart rate is typically best heard in the lower left quadrant of the maternal abdomen, just below the umbilicus. In the ROA position, it is heard in the same location on the right side. In both the occipitoanterior positions, the FHR is generally located closer to the midline of the maternal abdomen, reflecting the position of the fetal back, which is closest to the maternal abdominal wall in the OA positions.

Potential questions: There can be questions related to interpretation of various abdominal and vaginal findings for assessment of progress of labor.

</td></tr>
<tr><td>

Q9. Identify the instrument shown in the image below, commonly used in obstetrics.

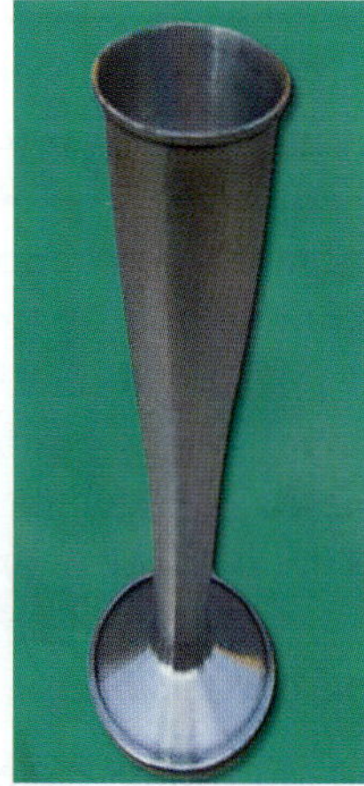

A. Doppler ultrasound device
B. Otoscope
C. Fetoscope
D. Sphygmomanometer
E. Stethoscope

</td><td>

Ans: C (fetoscope)

Fetoscope (Pinard's stethoscope) is an instrument previously used for auscultation of fetal heart rate **(Fig. 9)**.

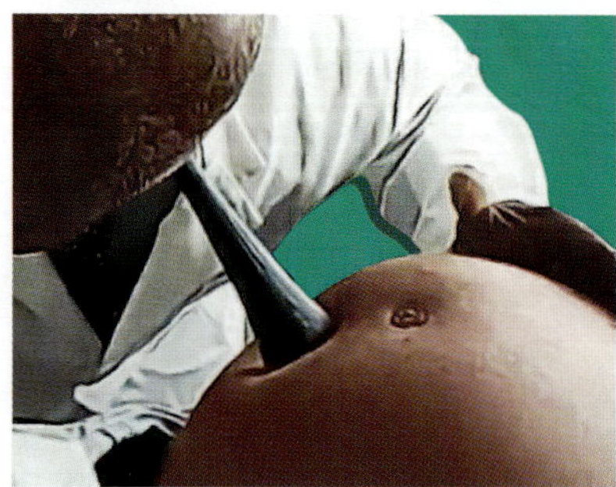

Fig. 9: Obstetrician using a fetoscope to measure the fetal heart rate in olden days

</td><td>

Explanation: It is a hollow tool made up of either wood or metal and is about 8 inches long. Tapering rim of the device is applied to the clinician's ear and the other wide side is pressed upon maternal abdomen. It functions like the trumpet by amplifying the sound.

This instrument is nowadays not commonly used in clinical settings due to the availability of advanced techniques for measurement of fetal heart rate. A stethoscope or a hand-held Doppler device can also be used instead of a fetoscope.

Potential questions: There can be other questions related to the common instruments used in obstetrics.

</td></tr>
</table>

Question	Answer	Comment
Q10. A 28-year-old pregnant woman in her 39th week of gestation is in active labor. On vaginal examination, the cervix appears to be as shown in the image B below. What is the likely interpretation of the findings? 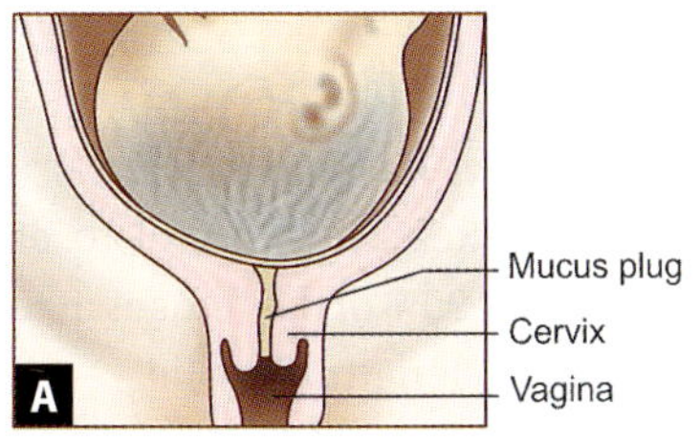 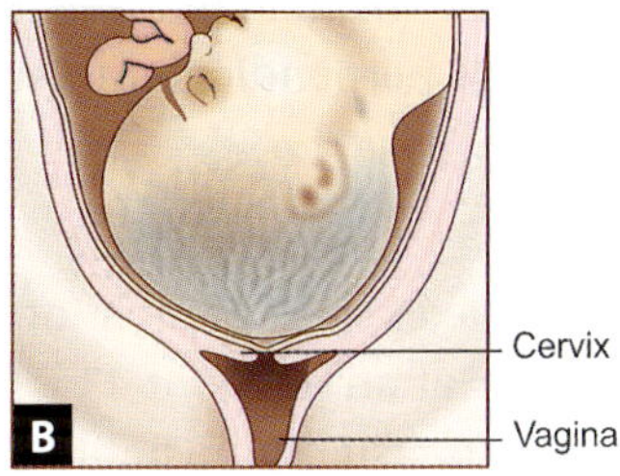 A. Uneffaced cervix B. 20% cervical effacement C. 50% cervical effacement D. 80% cervical effacement E. Fully effaced cervix	**Ans: E (Fully effaced cervix)** The image B in the adjacent picture shows that the cervix is fully effaced. Fully effaced cervix implies that it has thinned out to 100% of its original length, which is necessary for the baby to pass through the birth canal during delivery. As shown in **Figure 10**, cervical effacement can be defined as the gradual thinning, shortening, or drawing up of the cervix. It is usually measured in terms of percentage from 0% to 100%. 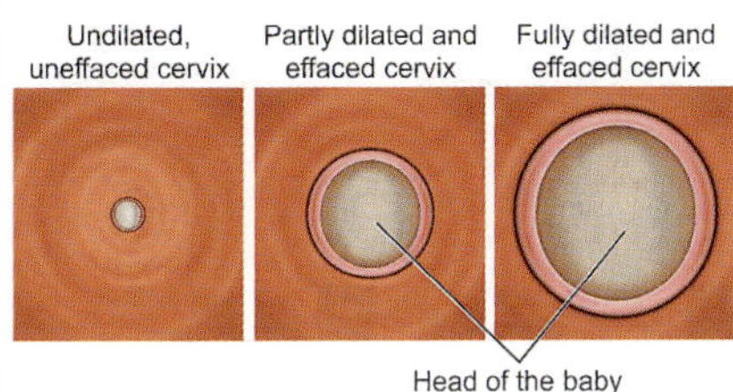 **Fig. 10:** Cervical effacement.	**Explanation:** Cervical effacement can be defined as obliteration or taking up of cervix resulting in conversion of cervical canal (about 2 cm in length) into a circular orifice with paper thin edges. This takes place from above downward. The cervical effacement primarily results due to taking up or pulling upward of the muscular fibers at the level of internal os into the lower uterine segment. **Potential questions:** There can be other questions related to the occurrence of various changes in the cervix and uterus at the time of labor and delivery to facilitate vaginal birth.
Q11. The clinical image below shows an anesthesiologist preparing to administer epidural analgesia to a patient in labor. 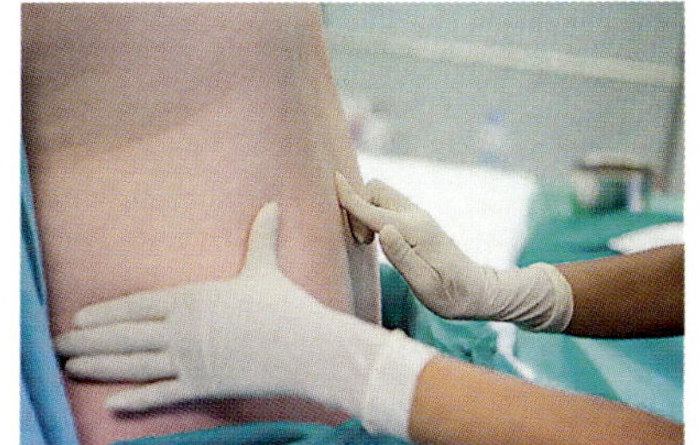 Which step is most critical for correct catheter placement? A. Proper positioning B. Aseptic technique C. Identifying epidural space (loss of resistance) D. Test dose administration E. Continuous vital monitoring	**Ans: C [Identifying epidural space (loss of resistance)]** Epidural analgesia has presently become a commonly employed technique for providing pain relief during labor. This technique involves injection of a local anesthetic agent into the epidural space (located between the dura mater and the vertebral periosteum as well as the ligamentum flavum, which connects the adjacent vertebrae.) at level of the space between the vertebrae L3 and L4 **(Fig. 11)**. 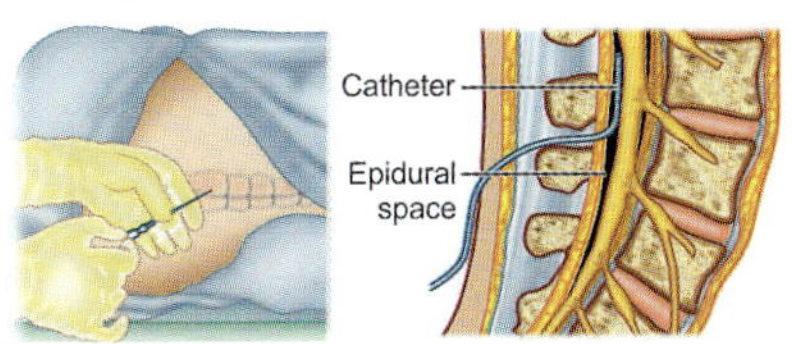 **Fig. 11:** Method for administration of epidural analgesia.	**Explanation:** Correct identification of the epidural space is the most important step in administering epidural analgesia. This is typically done using the "loss of resistance" technique, where the anesthesiologist carefully advances the needle and injects saline or air, feeling for a sudden loss of resistance that indicates entry into the epidural space. This step is essential to ensure that the anesthetic is delivered to the correct location for effective pain management during labor. **Potential questions:** There can be questions related to the technique of epidural analgesia as well as the associated complications and their management.

<table>
<tr><th>Question</th><th>Answer</th><th>Comment</th></tr>
<tr>
<td>

Q12. A 32-year-old woman in her 37th week of pregnancy undergoes an abdominal examination which reveals that the fetus is lying longitudinally, with the head positioned upwards as shown in the image below. What is the fetal lie in this case?

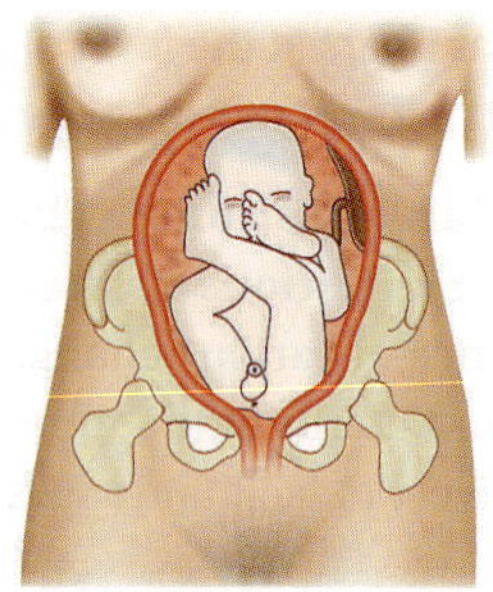

A. Transverse lie
B. Oblique lie
C. Longitudinal lie with breech presentation
D. Longitudinal lie with cephalic presentation
E. Transverse lie with shoulder presentation

</td>
<td>

Ans: C (Longitudinal lie with breech presentation)

As shown in the adjacent image, the long axis of the fetus lies parallel to maternal spine. This refers to a longitudinal lie. However, since the fetal buttocks are the presenting part on vaginal examination, this is a breech presentation.

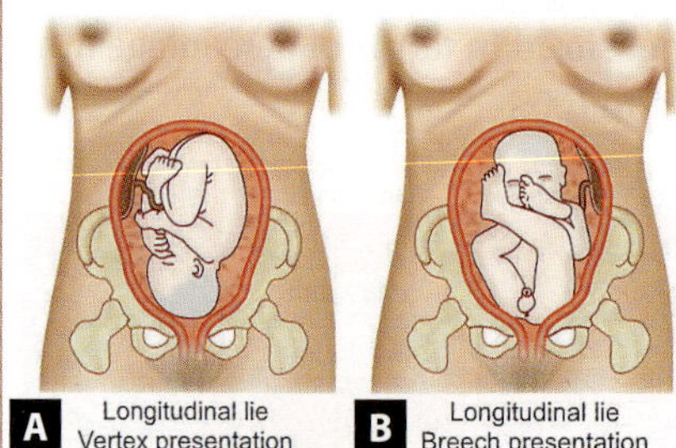

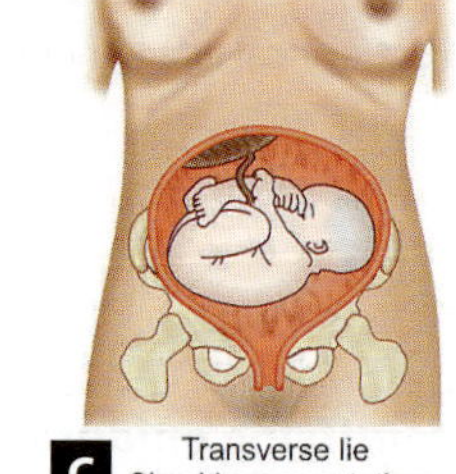

Figs. 12A to C: Types of fetal lie.

</td>
<td>

Explanation: Fetal lie refers to the relationship of cephalocaudal axis or long axis (spinal column) of fetus to the long axis of the centralized uterus or maternal spine.

Various types of fetal lie are as follows **(Figs. 12A to C)**:

Longitudinal lie: The maternal and fetal long axes are parallel to each other. About 99% of the fetuses at term present with longitudinal lie.

Transverse lie: The maternal and fetal long axes are perpendicular to each other.

Oblique lie: The maternal and fetal long axes cross each other obliquely or at an angle of 45°. The oblique lie is usually unstable and becomes longitudinal or transverse during the course of labor.

</td>
</tr>
</table>

Question	Answer	Comment
Q13. A 30-year-old woman at 38 weeks of gestation is in labor. An obstetrician performs a vaginal examination and finds the fetal head to be flexed with the occiput positioned anteriorly towards the mother's pelvis. What is the fetal presentation in this case? 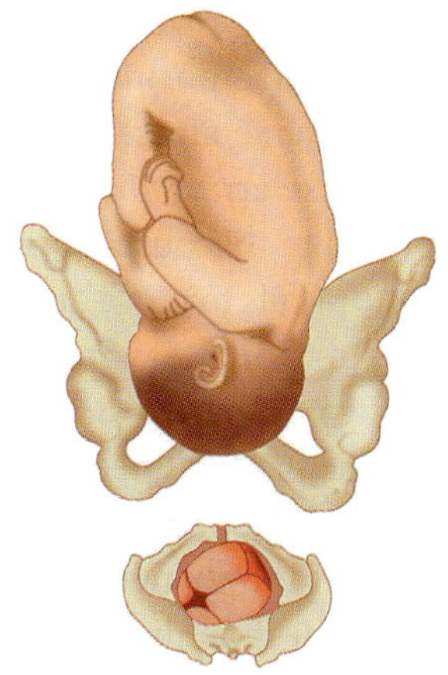 A. Occiput posterior (cephalic) B. Face presentation C. Brow presentation D. Occiput anterior (cephalic) presentation E. Transverse presentation	**Ans: D [Occiput anterior (cephalic)]** Fetal presentation can be described as the fetal body part, which occupies the lower pole of the uterus and thereby first enters the pelvic passage. Fetal presentation is determined by fetal lie and may be of three types: Cephalic, podalic (breech), or shoulder and is shown in **Figures 13A to E**. Cephalic or the head presentation is the most common and occurs in about 97% of fetuses. 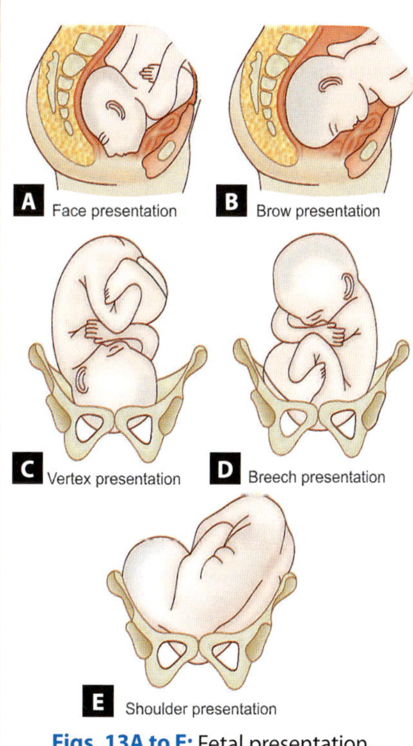 **Figs. 13A to E:** Fetal presentation.	**Explanation:** In the adjacent image, the baby is in cephalic presentation. The presenting part may be vertex, brow or face depending upon the degree of flexion of the fetal head. Since the fetal head is fully flexed in this image, the presenting part is the vertex, where occiput can be palpated by the fingers on vaginal examination. and the sagittal sutures lie in one of the oblique diameters (right or left) of the pelvic inlet. In left occiput anterior (LOA) position, the sagittal diameter lies in the right oblique diameter of the pelvic inlet. This position is most favorable for normal vaginal delivery. With the anterior rotation of the fetal head in occipitoanterior position, the sagittal diameter of the fetal head occupies the most spacious diameter of the outlet (AP diameter), thereby facilitating the movement of fetal head outside the pelvic outlet. **Potential questions:** There can be questions pertaining to various fetal presentations and different positions of the fetal presenting parts.

Question	Answer	Comment
Q14. A 25-year-old primigravida woman presents in advanced labor at 38 weeks' gestation. Vaginal examination shows the fetal head in a transverse position relative to the maternal pelvis, with both the fontanels palpable as shown in the image below. The occiput is directed towards the maternal left side. What is the correct description of this fetal position in this case? 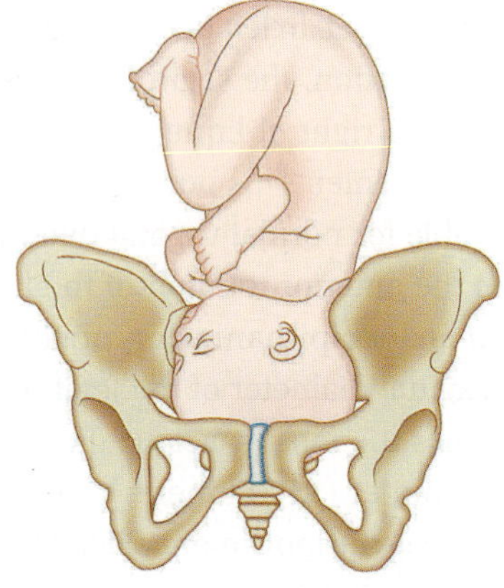 A. Left occiput anterior (LOA) B. Right occiput posterior (ROP) C. Left occiput posterior (LOP) D. Left occiput transverse (LOT) E. Right occiput transverse (ROT)	**Ans: D [Left occiput transverse (LOT)]** The baby's head in the adjacent image can be described to be in the occipitotransverse (OT) position, with the fetal head positioned transversely in the maternal pelvis. The sagittal sutures lie in the transverse diameter of the pelvis and both the fontanels are palpable **(Fig. 14)**. The occiput can either point towards the left or right side. When the occiput is directed towards the maternal left side, it is specifically termed "left occiput transverse (LOT)." 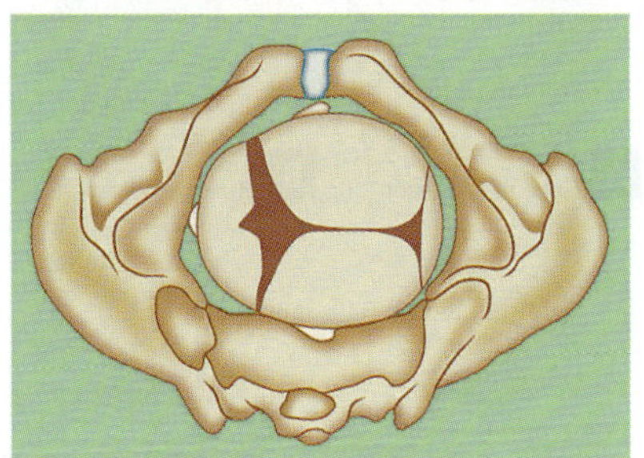 **Fig. 14:** Baby's head in occipitotransverse position.	**Explanation:** In most cases of occipitotransverse position, the sagittal sutures rotate anteriorly by 2/8th of a circle to occupy the anteroposterior (AP) diameter of the outlet. This is a position, which is the most favorable for normal vaginal delivery. Sometimes, the occipitotransverse position can lead to deep transverse arrest. In cases of deep transverse arrest, the fetal head gets captured in this position and the sagittal suture fails to move anteriorly, the position which favors normal vaginal delivery. Neither sinciput nor occiput leads the fetal head because of which further labor gets arrested and there is no advancement of fetal head. The head lies deep in the pelvic cavity at the level of ischial spines, and there is no progress in the descent of fetal head even after ½–1 hour following complete cervical dilatation. In these cases, the mother must not be encouraged to push down because it may not resolve the problem. Operative cesarean delivery appears to be the safest option for delivery in cases of deep transverse arrest. **Potential questions:** There can be questions pertaining to different positions of the fetal presenting parts and their outcomes in labor.

Question	Answer	Comment
Q15. A 36-year-old para 3 woman presents in advanced labor at 37 weeks' gestation. On abdominal examination, the fetal limbs can be palpated easily. The fetal back could not be located. Vaginal examination reveals the fetus to be in vertex presentation and the occiput positioned posteriorly towards the maternal sacrum. What is the most likely diagnosis? 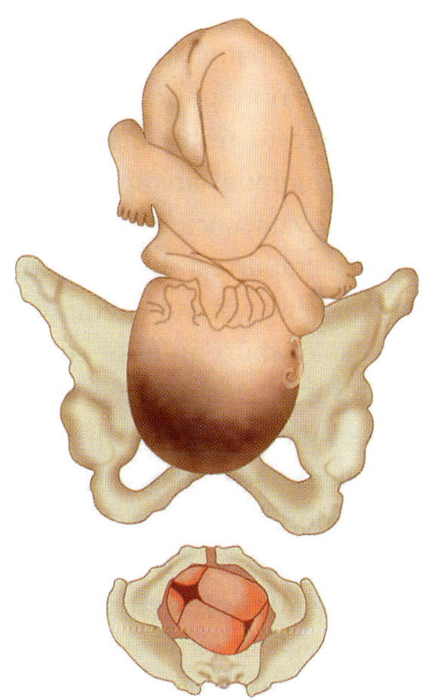 A. Occiput anterior position B. Occiput posterior position C. Occiput transverse position D. Face presentation E. Brow presentation	**Ans: B (Occiput posterior position)** On abdominal palpation, both the positions, occipitoanterior and occipitoposterior (OP), may present differently as shown in **Figures 15A and B**. In OP position, the fetal limbs are palpated more easily near the midline on either side. Also, fetal back and shoulders are far away from the midline. 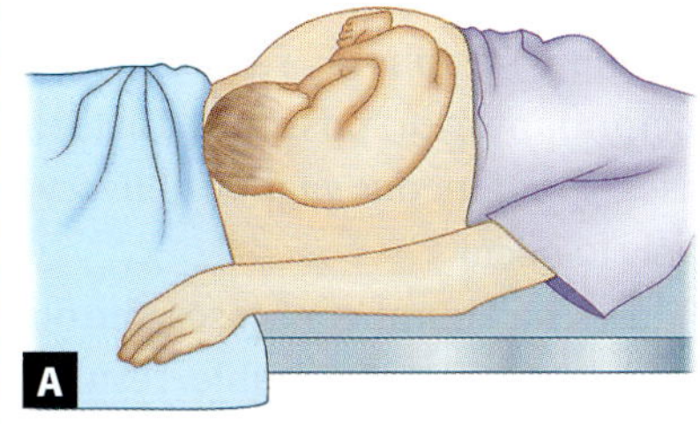 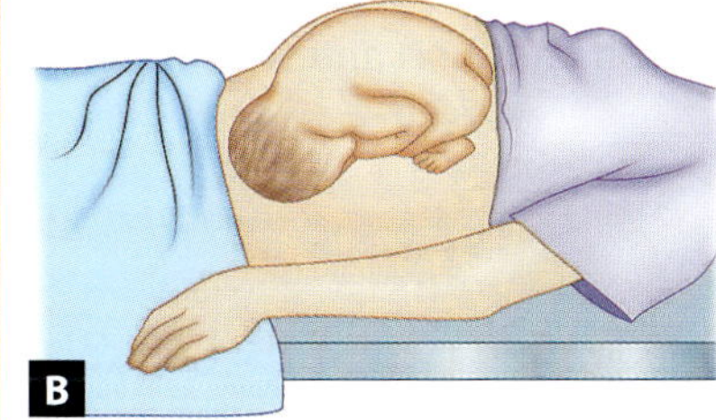 **Figs. 15A and B:** Comparison of abdominal examination. (A) Occipitoposterior position; (B) Occipitoanterior position.	**Explanation:** The adjacent image shows vertex in the OP position. This is a type of abnormal position of the vertex where the occiput may be placed over the left sacroiliac joint [left occipitoposterior (LOP)] or right sacroiliac joint [right occipitoposterior (ROP)] or directly over the sacrum (direct occipitoposterior position). In majority of cases, long anterior rotation of head occurs. Delivery, therefore, in majority of cases occurs spontaneously or with low forceps or ventouse. Cesarean section is the most used mode of delivery in cases where there is failure of instrumental delivery or there is failure of rotation of fetal head or there is presence of an obstetric indication for cesarean delivery. **Potential questions:** There can be potential questions related to the outcomes and consequences of OP position.

Question	Answer	Comment
Q16. In the same scenario as Q15, after 1 hour of active pushing in the second stage of labor, the vaginal examination shows the below image. The occiput can be palpated in the sacral bay. What is the fetal position now in this case? 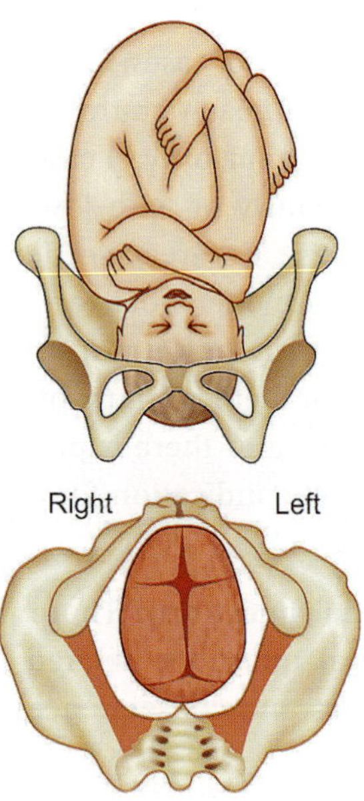 A. Persistent occipitoposterior position B. Deep transverse arrest C. Occipitoanterior position D. Oblique posterior arrest E. Occipitoposterior position	**Ans: A (Persistent occipitoposterior position)** The adjacent image shows persistent occipitoposterior position, one of the consequences of OP position. Other consequences related to OP position are depicted in **Figure 16**. In majority of cases of OP position, good uterine contractions result in the flexion of fetal head. Descent occurs and the occiput undergoes rotation by 3/8th of the circle to lie behind the pubic symphysis, resulting in an occipitoanterior position. In these cases, spontaneous vaginal delivery is likely to occur. In a small number of cases, the outcome may be less favorable, resulting in short posterior rotation, nonrotation and short anterior rotation. 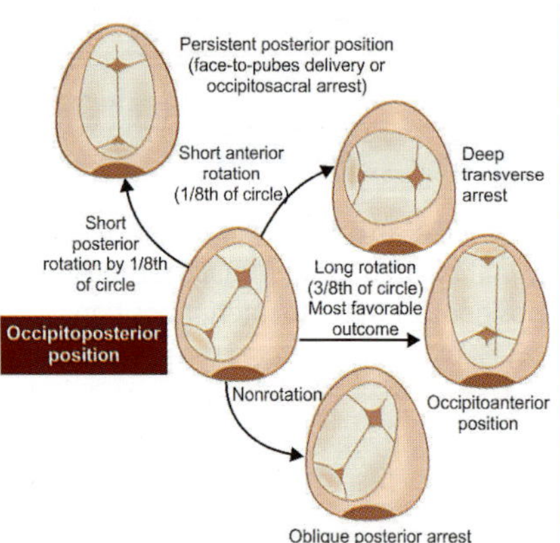 **Fig. 16:** Consequences related to occipitoposterior position.	**Explanation:** In case of short posterior rotation, posterior rotation of the sinciput may occur by 1/8th of the circle due to deflexed fetal head, putting the occiput in the sacral hollow. This position is known as persistent occipitoposterior position. Due to deflexed head, the occipitofrontal diameter (11.5 cm) enters the pelvis leading to delayed engagement. Under favorable conditions with an average sized baby, spacious pelvis, and good uterine contractions, spontaneous face to pubis delivery can occur. If conditions are not favorable, delivery may not occur, resulting in an occipitosacral arrest. In these cases, cesarean delivery may be required. In case of short anterior rotation, the occiput rotates through 1/8th of the circle anteriorly so that the sagittal sutures lie in the bispinous diameter. This position is known as the "deep transverse arrest". In case of nonrotation of the occiput, sagittal sutures lie in the oblique diameter. Further progress of labor is unlikely and this is known as oblique posterior arrest. **Potential questions:** There can be potential questions related to the outcomes, consequences of OP position, and their management.

Question	Answer	Comment
Q17. Upon vaginal examination of a 30-year-old second gravida in labor, the obstetrician feels the following structures: Alveolar margins of the mouth, nose, malar eminences, supraorbital ridges, and mentum. The clinical image of presentation is shown below. Which of the following is the most likely management option for this presentation? 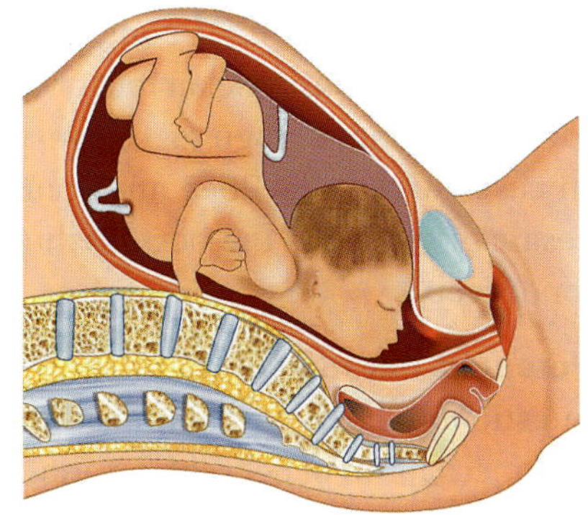 A. Immediate cesarean section in all cases B. Manual rotation to convert to vertex presentation C. Allowing labor to progress naturally with close monitoring D. Use of forceps for assisted delivery E. Performing an episiotomy to facilitate vaginal delivery	**Ans: C (Allowing the labor to progress with close monitoring)** The adjacent image and clinical findings point towards a face presentation. Face presentation is an abnormal fetal position characterized by an extreme extension of the fetal head so that the fetal face rather than the fetal head becomes the presenting part and the fetal occiput comes in direct contact with the back. Denominator in the cases of face presentation is mentum or chin. Four positions are possible depending on the position of the chin with left or right sacroiliac joints **(Figs. 17A to C)**: 1. Right mentoposterior position (deflexed LOA) 2. Left mentoposterior position [deflexed right occipitoanterior (ROA)] 3. Left mentoanterior position (deflexed ROP): Most common position 4. Right mentoanterior position (deflexed LOP) 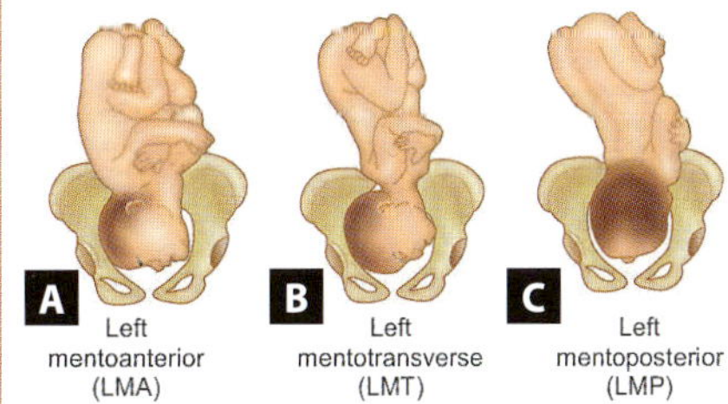 **Figs. 17A to C:** Different positions in case of face presentation.	**Explanation:** Delivery occurs spontaneously in most of cases of face presentation. In the presence of normal cervical dilatation and descent, there is no need for the obstetrician to intervene. Labor will be longer, but if the pelvis is adequate and the head rotates to a mentoanterior position, a vaginal delivery can be expected. The mechanism of delivery and corresponding body movements in case of anterior face presentations are like that of the corresponding occipitoanterior position. The only difference being that delivery of head occurs by flexion rather than extension. The engaging diameter is submentobregmatic in case of a fully extended head. Close monitoring is essential to ensure the safety of both the mother and the baby. If the head rotates backward to a mentoposterior position, a cesarean section may be required. In case of posterior face presentations, the mechanism of delivery is the same as that of occipitoposterior position except that the anterior rotation of the mentum occurs in only 20–30% of the cases. In the remaining 70–80% cases, there may be incomplete anterior rotation, no rotation, or short posterior rotation of mentum. There is no possibility of spontaneous vaginal delivery in case of persistent mentoposterior positions. Cesarean section may be required in these cases. **Potential questions:** There can be questions related to complications and mechanism of delivery in various abnormal positions of the fetal presenting part.

Question	Answer	Comment
Q18. A 24-year-old primigravida presents to the labor room at 37 weeks of gestation with strong uterine contractions. Her abdominal examination reveals a cephalic presentation. The cervix has been fully dilated and effaced for more than 2 hours. On vaginal examination, the anterior fontanel, brow, and orbits are palpable. The obstetrician also feels both the sinciput and the occiput at the same level. The clinical image in this case is shown below. What is the most appropriate management for this presentation? 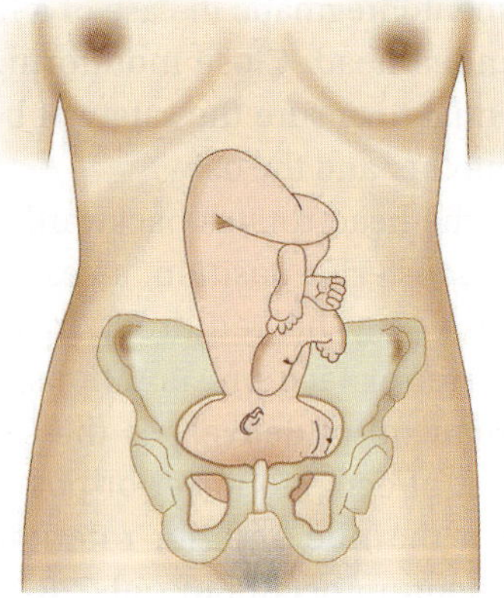 A. Proceed with a vacuum-assisted delivery B. Allow spontaneous delivery without intervention C. Attempt manual rotation to vertex presentation D. Perform a cesarean section E. Use of forceps for assisted delivery	**Ans: D (Perform a cesarean section)** The adjacent image and clinical findings point towards a brow presentation. Brow presentation is an abnormal fetal presentation where the fetal head is partially extended. The head is short of complete extension, which could have resulted in a face presentation. As a result, the presenting part becomes the brow. On vaginal examination, the occiput and sinciput are palpated at the same level. The following structures are palpable on vaginal examination: Brow, orbits, anterior fontanelle and, occasionally, the eyes and bridge of the nose **(Fig. 18)**. 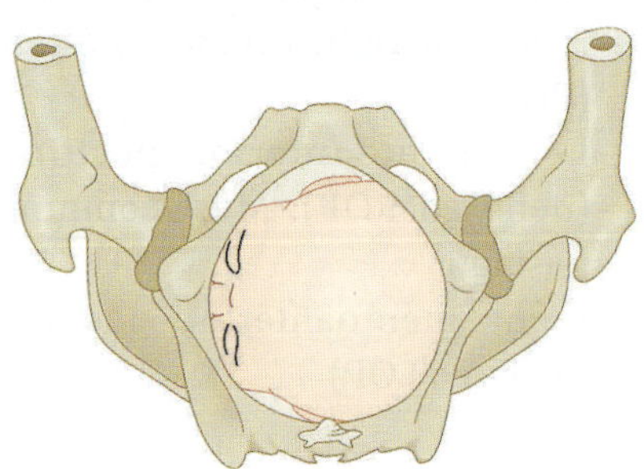 **Fig. 18:** Brow presentation.	**Explanation:** In brow presentation, the engaging diameter of the head is mentovertical (14 cm). As a result, there would be no mechanism of labor with an average-sized baby and a normal pelvis. Vaginal delivery may be the possible option only in cases where there is spontaneous conversion to face or vertex presentation. Therefore, after ruling out the cephalopelvic disproportion and fetal congenital anomalies, the obstetrician must wait for spontaneous vaginal delivery. In cases where this does not occur, cesarean section is the best method for delivery. **Potential questions:** There can be questions related to complications and mechanism of delivery in various abnormal positions of the fetal presenting part.

Question	Answer	Comment
Q19. The clinical image below is encountered at the time of delivery. What is the most appropriate management for this presentation? 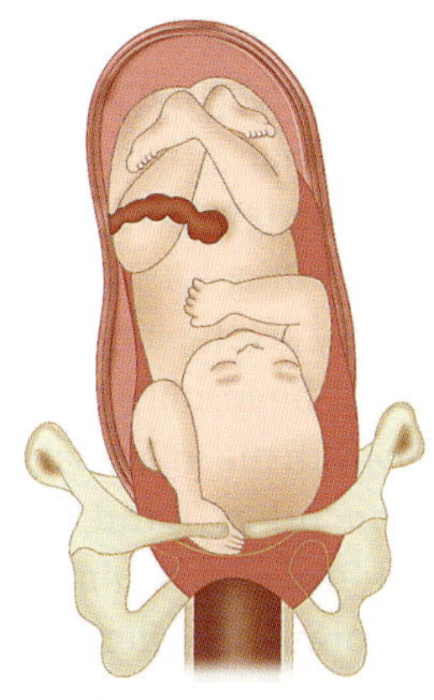 A. Proceed with vacuum-assisted delivery. B. Attempt to manually push the hand back. C. Perform a cesarean section. D. Allow spontaneous vaginal delivery with careful monitoring. E. Use forceps to assist delivery.	**Ans: D (Allow spontaneous vaginal delivery with careful monitoring)** The adjacent image shows the fetal hand presenting along with the head. The presentation in which one or two of the fetal extremities enter the pelvis simultaneously with the presenting part is known as the compound presentation **(Fig. 19)**. The most common combinations are head-hand, breech-hand, and head-arm-foot. 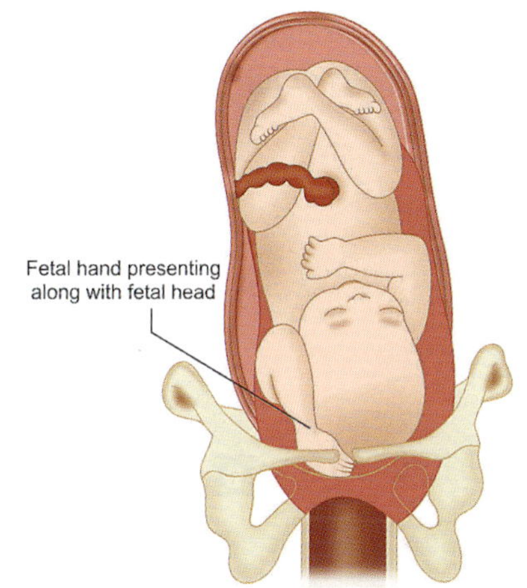 **Fig. 19:** Compound presentation.	**Explanation:** Close monitoring is important to ensure that there are no complications. In most cases, the prolapsed extremity does not cause any interference with the normal progress of labor and vaginal delivery. Moreover, the prolapsed limbs spontaneously rise up with the descent of the presenting part in most of the cases. In presence of cephalopelvic disproportion and/or cord prolapse, cesarean section is required. Manual repositioning of the hand or cesarean section may be necessary, if complications arise **Potential questions:** There can be questions related to complications and mechanism of delivery in various abnormal positions/presentations of the fetal presenting part.
Q20. A 35-year-old G3 presents to A&E with sudden rupture of membranes at home. On exam: partially dilated and effaced cervix, membranes absent, breech presentation, and a cord-like structure palpated alongside the fetal buttocks as shown in the image below. What is the most appropriate initial management? 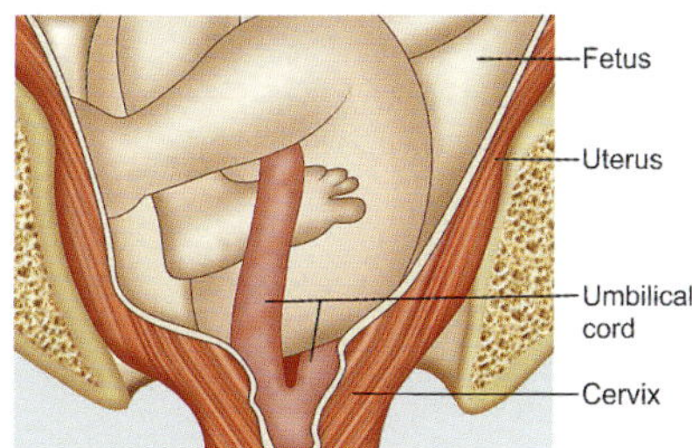 A. Immediate C-section B. Amnioinfusion C. Manual cord reduction D. Tocolytics + monitoring E. Trendelenburg + emergency C-section	**Ans: E (Trendelenburg position and an emergency cesarean section)** Cord presentation is the presence of the umbilical cord between the fetal presenting part and cervix with intact membranes. Cord prolapse is the descent of the umbilical cord through the cervix alongside the fetal presenting part (occult presentation) or past it (overt presentation) in the presence of ruptured membranes. In this case, color Doppler shows a dilated internal os with the cord inside, confirming cord prolapse **(Fig. 20)**. 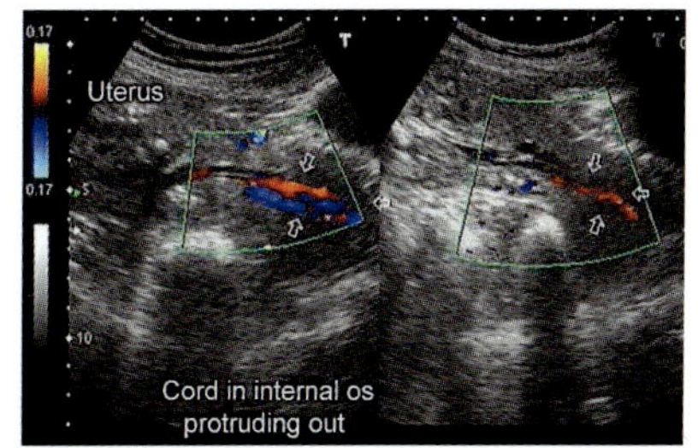 **Fig. 20:** Color Doppler ultrasound showing cord prolapse.	**Explanation:** Cord prolapse carries higher mortality than cord presentation due to fetal asphyxia. Definitive management is urgent delivery by the fastest route. In this case, since the patient is in early labor, an emergency cesarean section would be required. Meanwhile, Trendelenburg position and elevation of the presenting part either manually or via bladder filling would help relieve cord compression. **Potential questions:** There could be questions related to etiopathogenesis and management of cord prolapse in various clinical situations.

Question	Answer	Comment
Q21. A fetal ultrasound shows the head to be extended back, the spine is straight, and the limbs are partially extended away from the body as shown in the image below. What is the fetal attitude in this scenario? 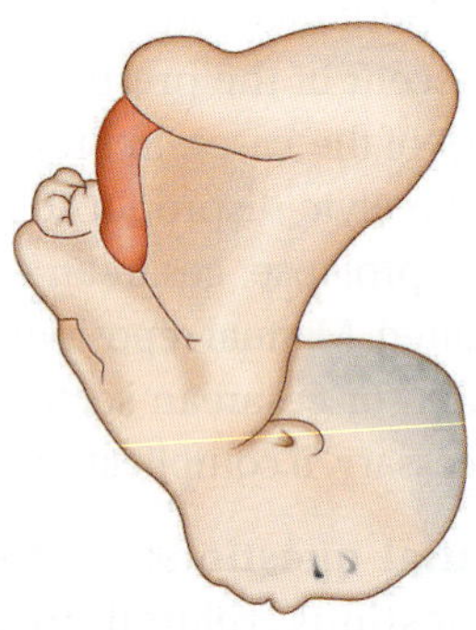 A. Flexed attitude A. Extended attitude B. Neutral attitude C. Hyperextended attitude D. Partially flexed attitude	**Ans: B (Extended attitude)** During the later months of pregnancy, the fetus adopts a characteristic posture called attitude. Usually, this posture is associated with flexion at all the fetal joints. Different types of attitudes which can be adopted by the fetus are depicted in **Figures 21A to D**. The adjacent image shows an extended attitude, which is characterized by the fetal head being tilted back, away from the chest, with a straighter spine and limbs that are partially or fully extended. 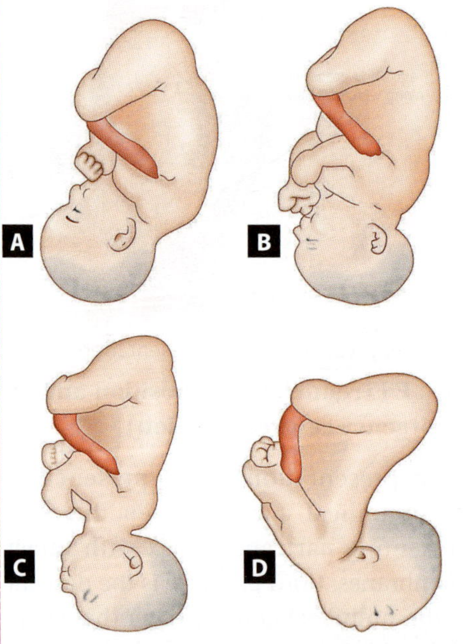 **Figs. 21A to D:** Different types of fetal attitudes: (A) Complete flexion; (B) Moderate flexion; (C) Poor flexion; (D) Hyperextension.	**Explanation:** The clinical significance of fetal attitude is that with the increasing degree of deflexion, the engaging diameter of fetal head progressively increases. In these cases, normal vaginal delivery may become difficult. Partially extended fetal attitude can create difficulties during labor and delivery, as the larger diameter of the fetal head may not align as favorably with the maternal pelvis. On the other hand, the engaging diameter is smallest in case of completely flexed head or completely extended head. In these cases, the fetal head can negotiate through the maternal pelvis and normal vaginal delivery is possible. **Potential questions:** There can be questions related to various other fetal attitudes and their clinical significance.

Question	Answer	Comment
Q22. An obstetrician detects face presentation on the vaginal examination. The engaging diameter of the fetal head is shown by the pink band in the below image. What are the most likely dimensions of this diameter? 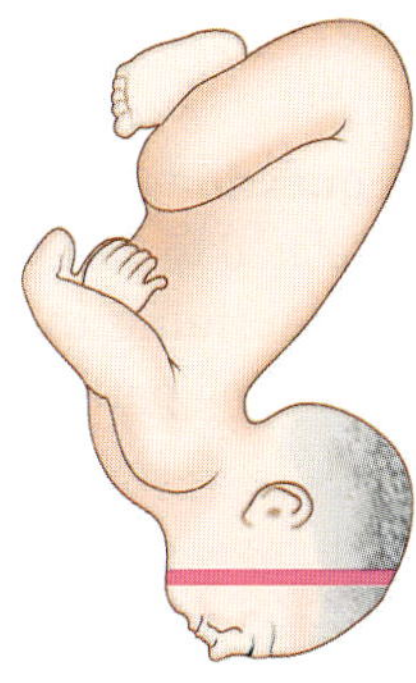 A. 9.4 cm B. 10.4 cm C. 11.4 cm D. 12.4 cm E. 13.4 cm	**Ans: A (9.4 cm)** **Figures 22A to D** show engaging diameters of fetal head depending upon the position of presenting part. The fetal head is engaged when the maximum transverse diameter of fetal head can pass through the pelvic brim. 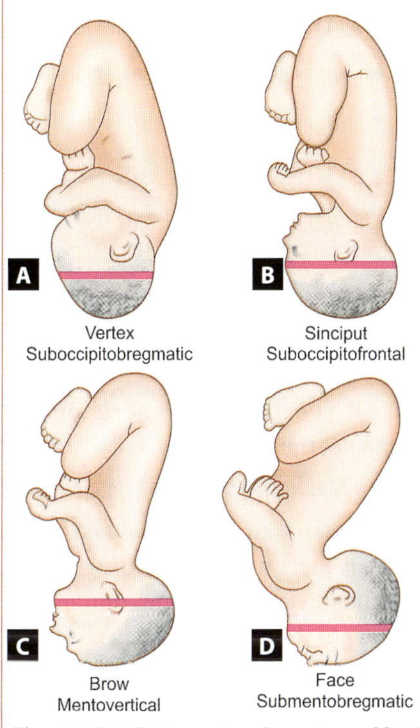 **Figs. 22A to D:** Engaging diameters of fetal head depending on the position of the presenting part.	**Explanation:** A normal pelvis would be easily able to permit the engagement of the fetal skull in vertex (fully flexed) and face (fully extended) presentations. This is so as in case of vertex and face presentations, the engaging AP diameters of fetal skull are respectively sub-occipitobregmatic (9.4 cm) and submentobregmatic (9.4 cm), both of which are equal in dimension. However, the passage of the fetal head in brow presentation would not be able to take place in a normal pelvis as the engaging AP diameter of fetal skull is mentovertical (13.9 cm) in this case. This can lead to the arrest of labor. **Potential questions:** There can be questions related to engagement and descent of various positions of the fetal presenting part in different clinical scenarios.

Question	Answer	Comment
Q23. On vaginal exam, the fetal head is at -2 station, as shown in the image. Which statement best describes the fetal head position in this scenario? 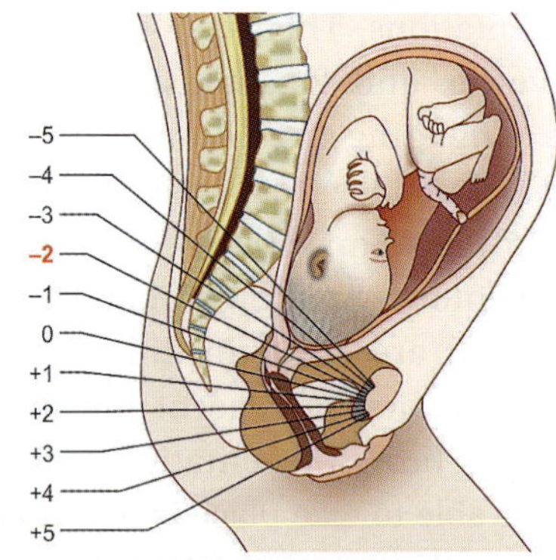 A. 2 cm below the ischial spine B. 2 cm above the ischial spines C. At the ischial spines D. 2.2 cm below the ischial spine E. 2.2 cm above the ischial spines	**Ans: B (2 cm above the ischial spines)** The station of the fetal head describes its position in relation to the ischial spines. When the fetal head is 2 cm above the ischial spines, it is assigned a station of-2. Negative stations indicate that the head is above the ischial spines, while positive stations indicate that the head is below them, moving towards delivery **(Fig. 23)**. 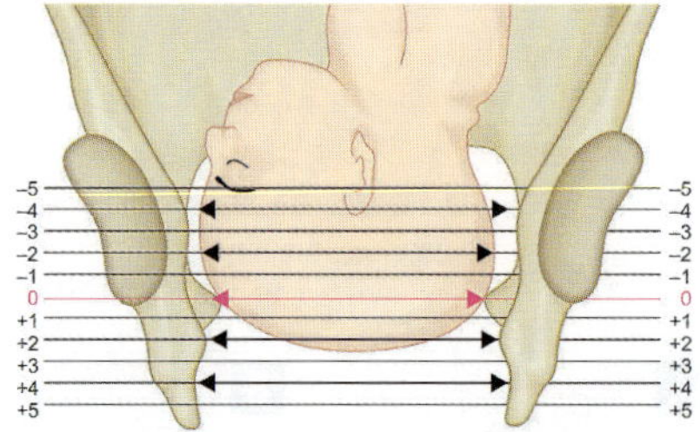 **Fig. 23:** Position of fetal head at various stations.	**Explanation:** ACOG classifies fetal head descent by dividing the pelvis into fifths above and below the ischial spines. Stations range from -5 at the inlet to 0 at the spines (engagement) and +5 at the introitus (head visible). Engagement means the biparietal diameter has passed the pelvic inlet. **Potential questions:** There can be questions related to various clinical scenarios describing the passage of fetal presenting part through the pelvis.
Q24. A 32-year-old third gravida in labor presents with severe abdominal pain and a visible ridge across her abdomen, just above the umbilicus. Fetal descent has stalled despite strong contractions. Upon examination, the ridge is identified as shown in the image below. What is the most appropriate next step in management? 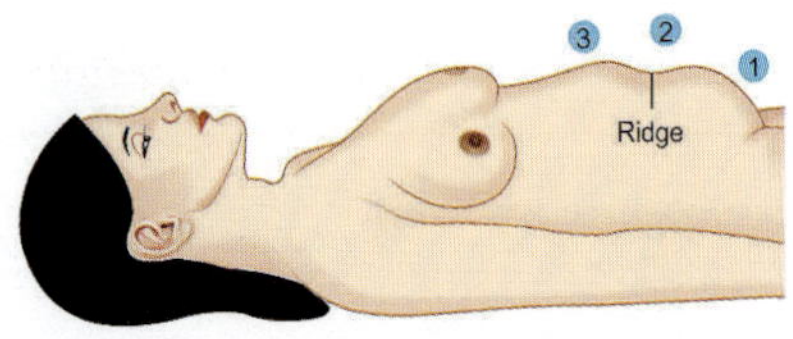 A. Administer uterotonic agents B. Perform an emergent cesarean section C. Apply forceps for vaginal delivery D. Wait and observe labor progression E. Initiate intravenous fluid therapy	**Ans: B (Perform an emergent cesarean section)** In primigravidas, obstructed labor causes maternal exhaustion and sepsis with an inert uterus. In multigravidas, obstruction triggers strong contractions, leading to thinning of the lower uterine segment and possible rupture. A pathological retraction ring (Bandl's ring) may form between the upper and lower segments. 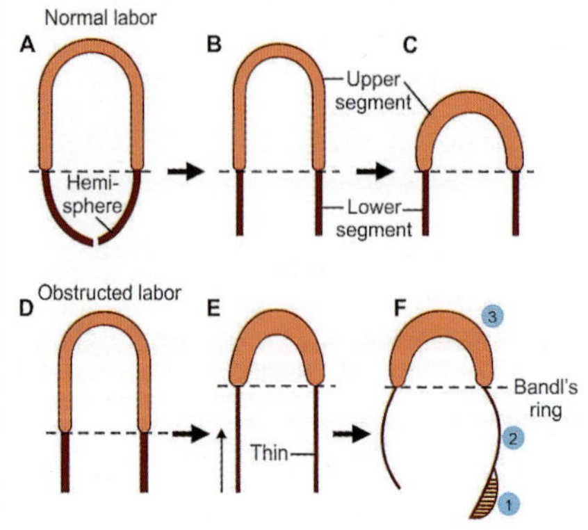 **Fig. 24:** Formation of Bandl's ring due to obstructed labor.	**Explanation:** The ridge shown in the adjacent image is Bandl's ring, also known as a pathological retraction ring. This is a late and serious sign of obstructed labor, indicating an impending uterine rupture. Obstructed labor can be defined as a condition in which the progressive descent of the fetal presenting part through the maternal genital tract is arrested despite strong uterine contractions. The presence of Bandl's ring suggests that the uterus is under extreme stress and unable to progress with labor naturally. An emergent cesarean section is necessary to prevent uterine rupture and ensure the safety of both mother and child.

Question	Answer	Comment
Q25. A 32-year-old second gravida in active labor with a transverse lie and a mass protruding through the cervix is in extreme pain. The finding on vaginal inspection is shown in the below image. If urgent cesarean is not performed, the most likely complication is: 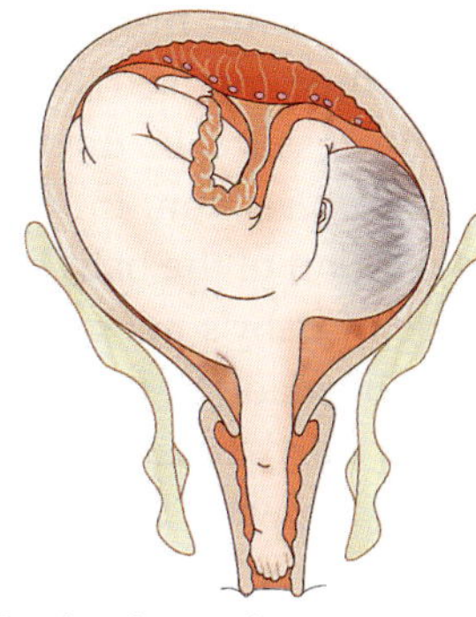 A. Uterine inversion B. Pathological retraction ring C. Uterine inertia D. Postpartum hemorrhage E. Colporrhexis	**Ans: B (Pathological retraction ring)** The adjacent image shows transverse lie with a prolapsed arm. If this is left neglected, a series of complications including obstructed labor can occur. Considering obstructed labor in this case, a pathological retraction ring or Bandl's ring develops **(Fig. 25)**. 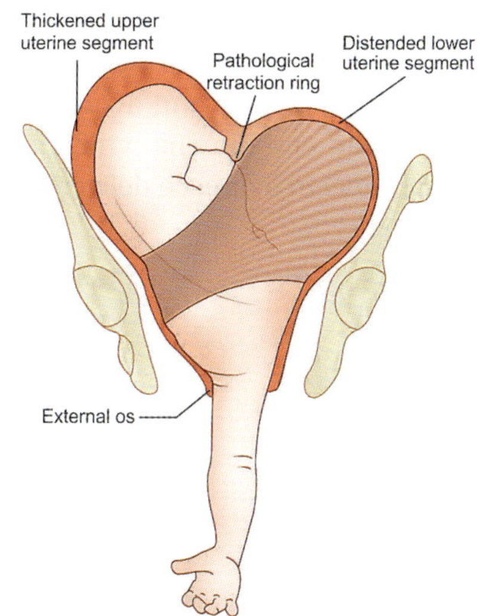 **Fig. 25:** Pathological retraction ring.	**Explanation:** In obstructed labor **(Fig. 25)**, a Bandl's ring forms at the upper-lower uterine segment junction and becomes prominent with increasing obstruction, eventually causing uterine rupture. Complications include dehydration, ketoacidosis, sepsis, hemorrhage, shock, peritonitis, and genital tract injury. In transverse lie with a prolapsed hand, cesarean section is the safest option for maternal and fetal safety. **Potential questions:** There can be questions related to complications associated with neglected transverse lie and their management.

BREECH VAGINAL DELIVERY

Question	Answer	Comment
Q26. In the below image, identify the type of breech presentation depicted. 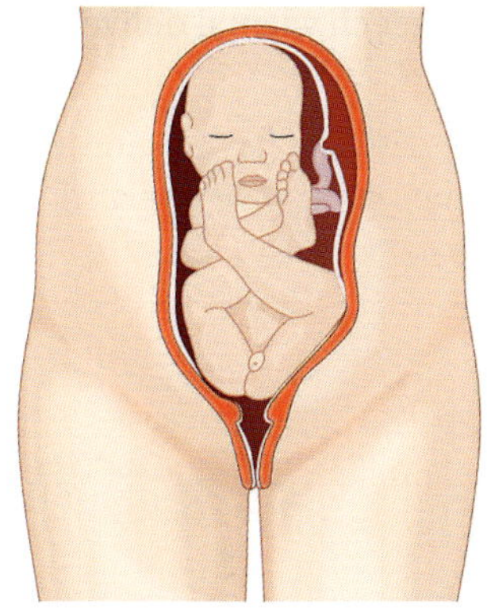 A. Frank breech B. Complete breech C. Footling breech D. Incomplete breech E. Transverse breech	**Ans: A (Frank breech)** **Figures 26A to C** show different breech types. The adjacent image depicts a frank breech (hips flexed, legs extended). Delivery choice—vaginal vs. cesarean—remains controversial; parents should be informed of maternal and neonatal risks and benefits. 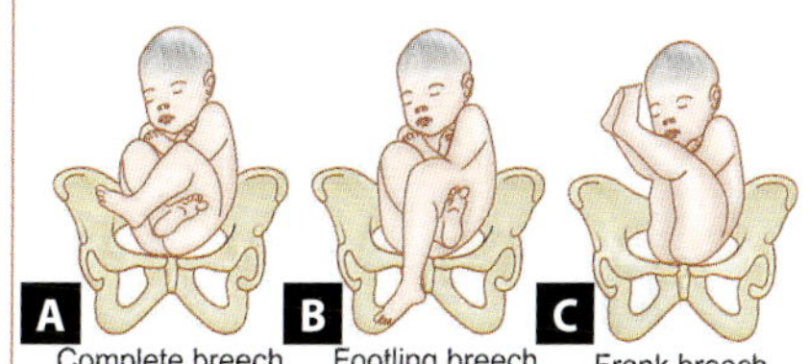 **Figs. 26A to C:** Different types of breech presentations.	In breech presentation, the fetus is longitudinal with the buttocks presenting. Types include: ▪ *Frank breech (most common):* Buttocks first, hips flexed, legs extended. ▪ *Complete breech:* Buttocks first, hips and knees flexed, feet not below buttocks. ▪ *Footling breech:* One or both feet first, hips and knees extended. **Potential questions:** There can be questions related to different types of breech presentation and their management strategies.

Question	Answer	Comment
Q27. A 32-year-old primigravida is in active labor with a breech presentation. The attending obstetrician decides to perform a vaginal breech delivery. During the delivery, after the fetal trunk is delivered, the obstetrician performs the maneuver shown in the image below to safely deliver the aftercoming fetal head. Which maneuver has been illustrated in the image below? 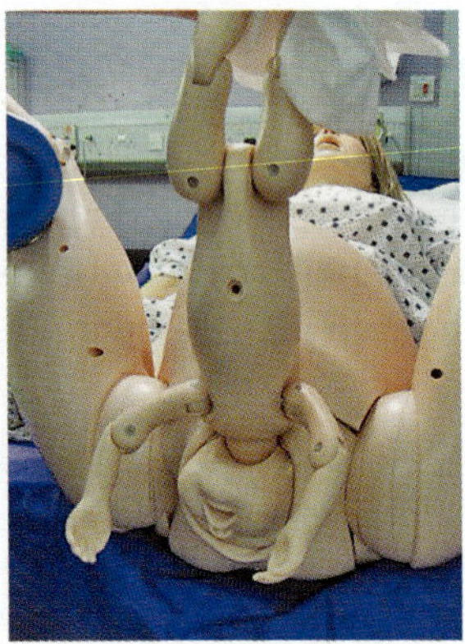 A. Mauriceau-Smellie-Veit maneuver B. Wood's corkscrew man euver C. Burns-Marshall maneuver D. Pinard maneuver E. Løvset maneuver	**Ans: C (Burns-Marshall technique)** The Burns-Marshall maneuver is specifically used during a breech delivery to deliver the aftercoming fetal head. In this technique, after the fetal trunk is delivered, the baby's feet are grasped and the fetal body is gently swung in a wide arc over the mother's abdomen **(Figs. 27A and B)**. This maneuver helps to deliver the fetal head smoothly and avoids the risk of head entrapment, which is a critical concern in breech deliveries. 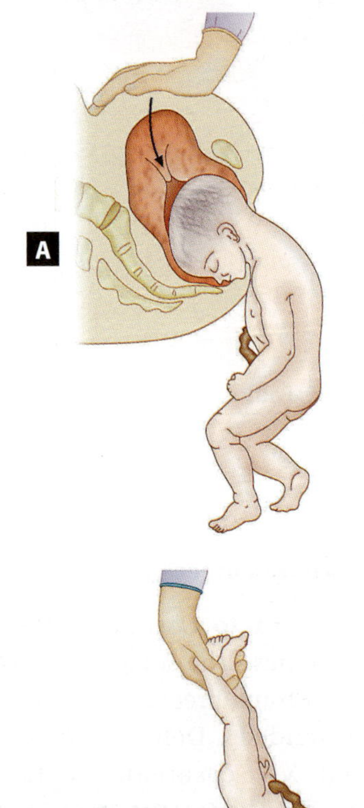 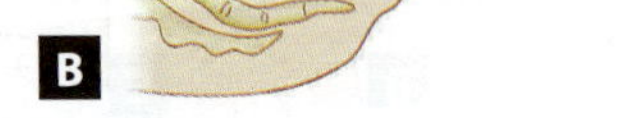 **Figs. 27A and B:** Burns-Marshall technique.	**Explanation:** The technique of performing Burns-Marshall technique is illustrated in **Figures 27A and B**. Following the delivery of shoulders and both the arms, the baby must be let to hang unsupported from the mother's vulva. This would help in encouraging flexion of fetal head. The nursing staff must be further advised to apply suprapubic pressure in downward and backward direction, in order to encourage flexion of the baby's head. As the nape of baby's neck appears, efforts must be made by the clinician to deliver the baby's head by grasping the fetal ankles with the finger of right hand between the two. Then the trunk is swung up forming a wide arc of the circle, while maintaining continuous traction when doing this. The obstetrician's left hand is used to provide pelvic support and to clear the perineum off successively from the baby's face and brow as the baby's head emerges out. **Potential questions:** There can be questions related to different maneuvers used for the delivery of fetal head, legs, or shoulders at the time of breech vaginal delivery.

Question	Answer	Comment
Q28. You are assisting in a vaginal breech delivery, and the fetal head remains in the pelvic cavity after the delivery of the body. The senior obstetrician instructs you to perform the Mauriceau-Smellie-Veit maneuver. You are shown the below image depicting the correct positioning of the hands during this procedure. Which of the following steps correctly describes the Mauriceau-Smellie-Veit maneuver for delivering the fetal head in a breech presentation? 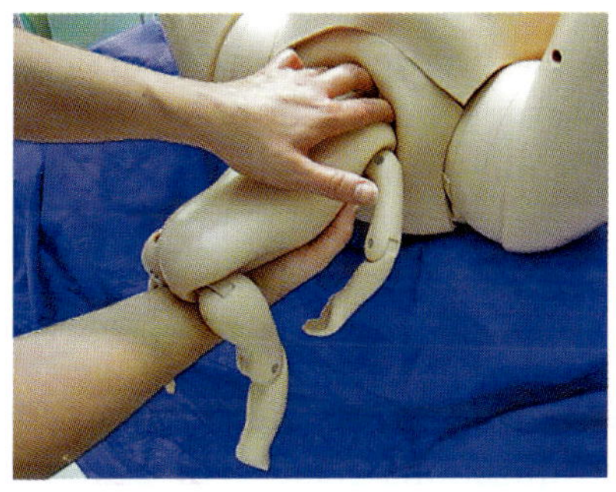 A. Downward traction on shoulders with neutral head B. Flexing head with one hand, upward traction with the other C. Fingers on maxilla and occiput, downward traction D. Suprapubic pressure, holding fetal feet E. Rotating fetal body 180	**Ans: C (Fingers on maxilla and occiput, downward traction)** Mauriceau-Smellie-Veit maneuver **(Fig. 28)** is another commonly used technique for the delivery of afte-rcoming fetal head of the breech and is named after the three clinicians who had described the method of using this grip. This maneuver comprises the following steps: ▪ The baby is placed face down with the length of its body over the supinated left forearm and hand of the clinician. ▪ As shown in the adjacent image, the clinician must then place the first (index) and second finger (middle finger) of this hand on the baby's cheekbones and the thumb over the baby's chin. This helps in facilitating flexion of the fetal head. The next steps to be followed are described in the adjacent column to the right. 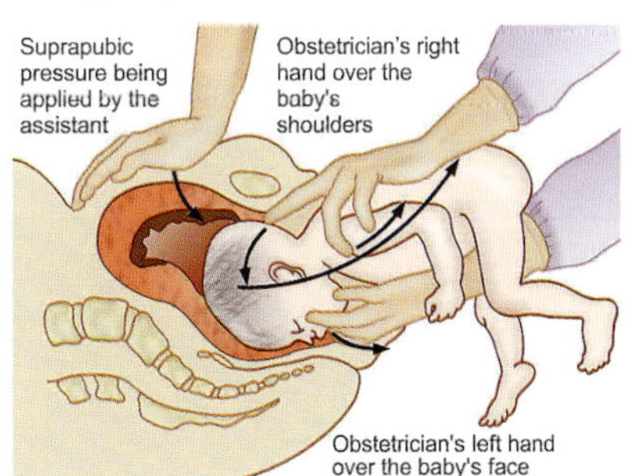 **Fig. 28:** Mauriceau–Smellie–Veit maneuver.	**Explanation:** The Mauriceau-Smellie-Veit maneuver involves placing the index and middle fingers on the maxilla and the other hand on the occiput to flex the fetal head while applying downward traction, facilitating the delivery of the after-coming head during a breech birth. An assistant may provide supra-pubic pressure to help the baby's head remain flexed. The right hand of the clinician is used for grasping the baby's shoulders. The little finger and the ring finger of the clinician's right hand are placed over the baby's right shoulder, the index finger over the baby's left shoulder, and the middle finger over the baby's suboccipital region. With the fingers of the right hand in this position, the baby's head is flexed towards the chest. At the same time, the left hand is used for applying downward pressure on the jaw to bring the baby's head down until the hairline is visible. Thereafter the baby's trunk is carried in upward and forward direction towards the maternal abdomen, till the baby's mouth, nose, and brow and lastly the vertex and occiput have been released. **Potential questions:** There can be questions related to different maneuvers used for the delivery of fetal head, legs, or shoulders at the time of breech vaginal delivery.

Question	Answer	Comment
Q29. Which of the following statements best describes the correct application of Piper's forceps during a breech delivery as shown in the image below? 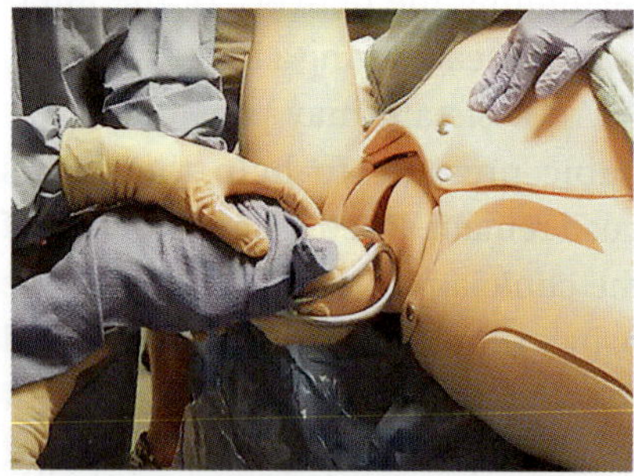 A. Piper's forceps are applied with the blades parallel to the fetal spine B. The forceps are applied while the fetus is rotated 90° C. Piper's forceps are applied after the fetal body is lifted to prevent head extension D. The forceps are applied with the mother in a supine position with knees flexed E. Piper's forceps are applied only after performing a midline episiotomy	**Ans: C (Piper's forceps are applied after the fetal body is lifted to prevent head extension)** Nowadays, Piper's forceps are commonly used to deliver the aftercoming head of the breech **(Fig. 29)**. Use of forceps helps in better maintenance of flexion of fetal head and in transmitting the force to the fetal head rather than the neck. This helps in reducing the risk of fetal injuries and prevents extension of the fetal head. 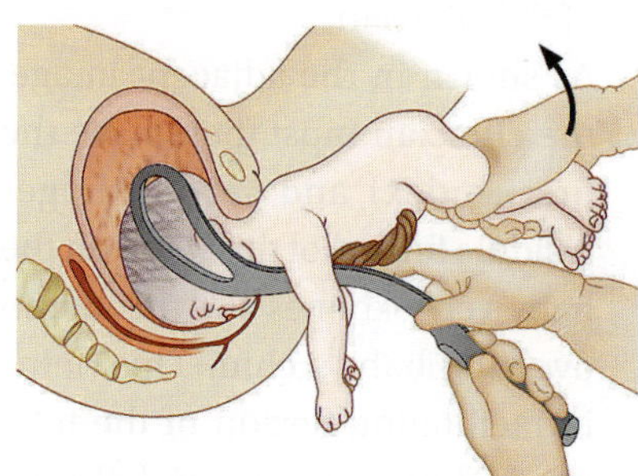 **Fig. 29:** Delivery of aftercoming head of breech using forceps.	**Explanation:** For delivery of fetal head using forceps, the following steps are required: ▪ Ordinary forceps or Piper's forceps (specially designed forceps with absent pelvic curve) can be used. ▪ While the clinician is applying forceps, the baby's body must be wrapped in a cloth or towel and held on one side by the assistant. The left blade of the forceps is applied first followed by the right blade and the handles are locked. ▪ The forceps are used for both flexing and delivering the baby's head. ▪ The head must be delivered slowly over 1 minute in order to avoid sudden compression or decompression of fetal head, which may be a cause for intracranial hemorrhage. **Potential questions:** There can be questions related to different maneuvers used for the delivery of fetal head, legs, or shoulders at the time of breech vaginal delivery.

Question	Answer	Comment
Q30. During a breech vaginal delivery, the obstetrician needs to deliver the fetal arms before the head and chooses to perform a maneuver by holding the baby by pelvifemoral grip as shown in the image. What is the purpose of rotating the fetal body 180° during this maneuver? 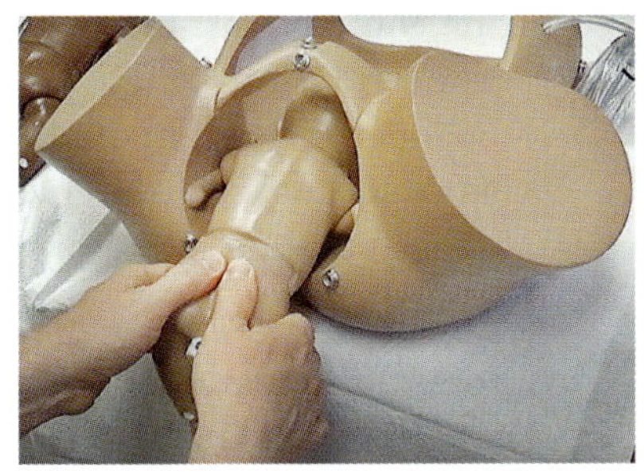 A. To align the fetal legs for easier delivery B. To reposition the fetal head for a smoother passage C. To bring one fetal arm into the anterior position for easier delivery D. To reduce the risk of umbilical cord prolapse E. To facilitate the delivery of both arms simultaneously	**Ans: C (To bring one fetal arm into the anterior position for easier delivery)** The maneuver demonstrated in the adjacent image is Løvset's maneuver. In case of breech presentation, if the baby's arms are stretched above the head or folded behind the neck (nuchal displacement), this maneuver is used for the delivery of fetal arms. Løvset's maneuver is based on the principle that due to the curved shape of the birth canal when the anterior shoulder is above the pubis symphysis, the posterior shoulder would be below the level of pubic symphysis. The maneuver should be initiated only when the fetal scapula becomes visible underneath the pubic arch and includes the steps shown in **Figures 30A to C**. 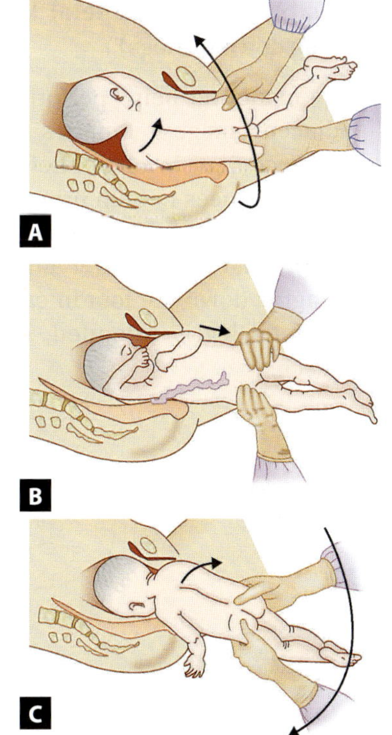 **Figs. 30A to C:** Løvset's maneuver.	**Explanation:** Løvset's maneuver is essential to safely deliver the fetal arms in a breech presentation, reducing the risk of complications associated with extended arms. This maneuver comprises the following steps: ▪ First, the baby is lifted slightly to cause lateral flexion of the trunk. ▪ Then the baby which is held by pelvifemoral grip is turned by 180°, keeping the back uppermost. Simultaneously, downward traction is applied so that the arm that was initially posterior and below the level of pubic symphysis now becomes anterior and can be delivered under the pubic arch. ▪ Delivery of the arm can be assisted by placing one or two fingers on the upper part of the arm. Then the arm is gradually drawn down over the chest as the elbow is flexed, with the hand sweeping over the face. ▪ In order to deliver the second arm, the baby is again turned by 180° in the reverse direction, keeping the back uppermost and applying downward traction and then delivering the second arm in the same way under the pubic arch as the first arm was delivered. **Potential questions:** There can be questions related to different maneuvers used for the delivery of fetal head, legs, or shoulders at the time of breech vaginal delivery.

Question	Answer	Comment
Q31. An obstetrician is performing a breech delivery and uses double groin traction as shown in the image below. What is the primary purpose of applying double groin traction during the delivery of the fetal buttocks in a breech presentation? 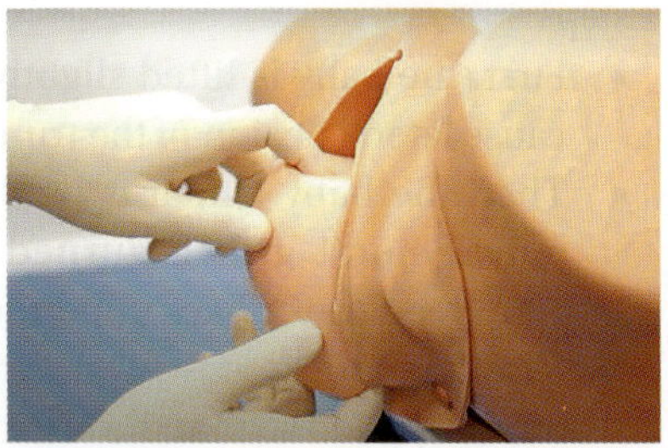 A. To rotate the fetus to an optimal position B. To ensure the fetal buttocks pass through the birth canal smoothly C. To prevent the umbilical cord from prolapsing D. To decrease the risk of shoulder dystocia E. To help in the delivery of the fetal head	**Ans: B (To ensure the fetal buttocks pass through the birth canal smoothly)** If the buttocks and hip do not deliver by themselves, the clinician can make use of simple maneuvers such as single or double groin traction **(Fig. 31)** to deliver the fetal legs. By applying controlled traction during this maneuver, the obstetrician ensures that the buttocks descend steadily and safely, reducing the risk of complications like entrapment. 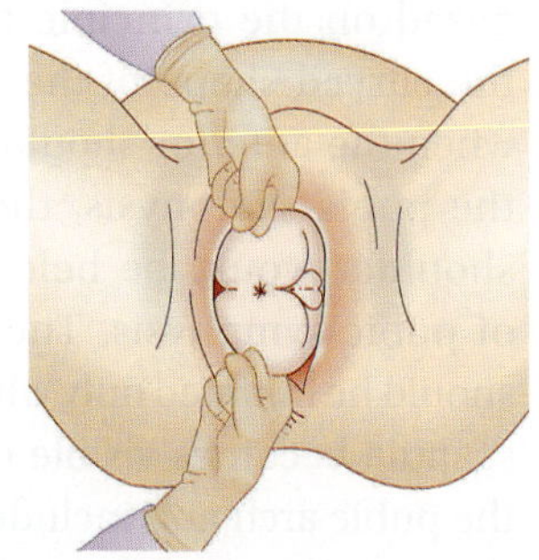 **Fig. 31:** Application of double groin traction.	**Explanation:** In single groin traction, the index finger of one hand is hooked in the groin fold and traction is exerted towards the fetal trunk rather than towards the fetal femur, in accordance with the uterine contractions. In double groin traction **(Fig. 31)**, the index fingers of both the hands are hooked in the groin folds and then traction is applied. **Potential questions:** There can be questions related to different maneuvers used for the delivery of fetal head, legs, or shoulders at the time of breech vaginal delivery.
Q32. An obstetrician is delivering a breech baby and uses a technique to aid in the delivery of the fetal legs as shown in the image below. What is the primary goal of using this technique during the delivery of fetal legs in a breech presentation? 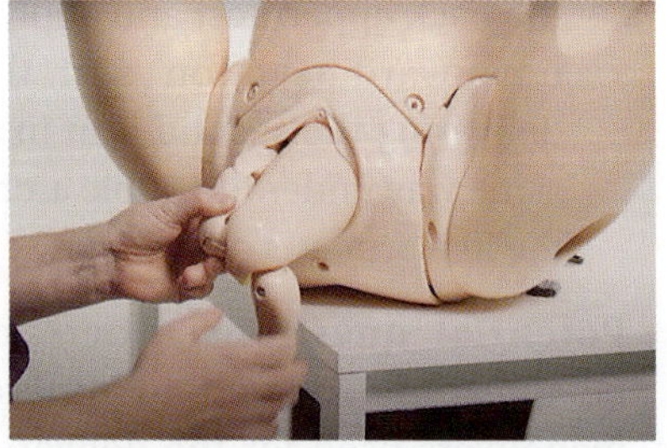 A. To flex the fetal knees and bring down the legs B. To rotate the fetus to a transverse lie C. To prevent umbilical cord compression D. To deliver the fetal head E. To assist in the delivery of the fetal arms	**Ans: A (To flex the fetal knees and bring down the legs)** The maneuver being performed in the adjacent image is Pinard's maneuver. This technique involves carefully flexing the fetal knees to help bring down the legs during a breech delivery **(Figs. 32A to C)**. Pinard's maneuver aims at safely bringing down the foot in cases where the fetal leg is extended, e.g., frank breech. 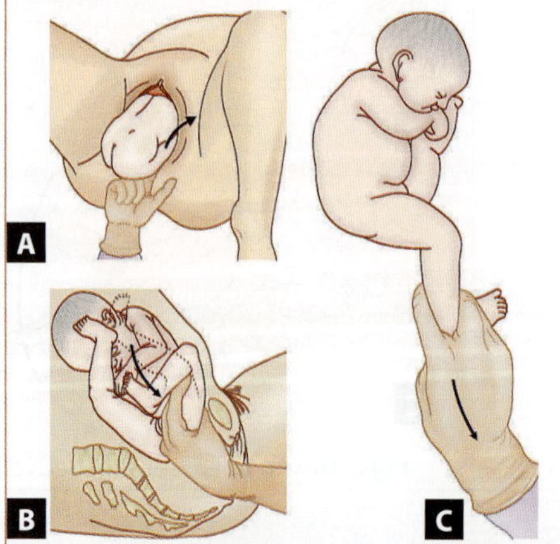 **Figs. 32A to C:** Steps for performing Pinard's maneuver.	**Explanation:** In this maneuver, pressure is exerted against the inner aspect of the knee (popliteal fossa), with help of the middle and index fingers of the clinician. As the pressure is applied, the knee gets flexed and abducted. This causes the lower leg to move downward, which is then swept medially and gently pulled out of the vagina. **Potential questions:** There can be questions related to different maneuvers used for the delivery of fetal head, legs, or shoulders at the time of breech vaginal delivery.

TRANSVERSE LIE

Question	Answer	Comment
Q33. A 28-year-old patient having strong uterine contractions presents at 38 weeks' gestation. The ultrasound image of the fetus is shown below. What is the next most appropriate step in managing this patient? 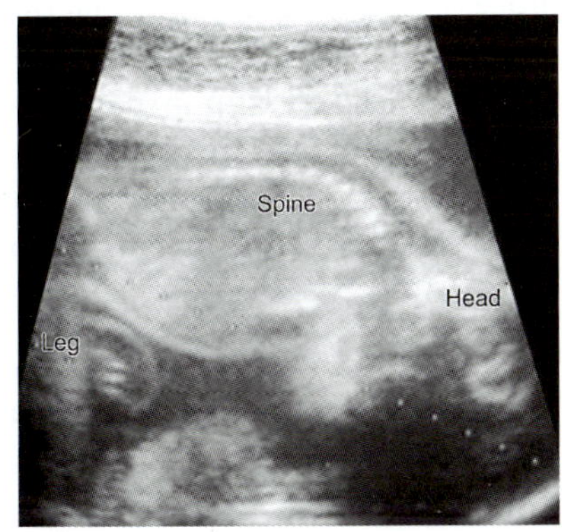 A. Attempt external cephalic version B. Proceed with an emergency cesarean section C. Perform internal podalic version D. Allow the patient to continue labor with close monitoring E. Use oxytocin to augment labor	**Ans: B (Proceed with an emergency cesarean section)** The adjacent image depicts an ultrasound image confirming the transverse lie with the fetal spine lying almost perpendicular to the maternal spine. Transverse lie is an abnormal fetal presentation in which the fetus lies transversely with the shoulders presenting in the lower pole of the uterus **(Fig. 33)**. In this presentation, the long axis of the fetus is perpendicular to the maternal spine. As a result, the presenting part becomes the fetal shoulder. 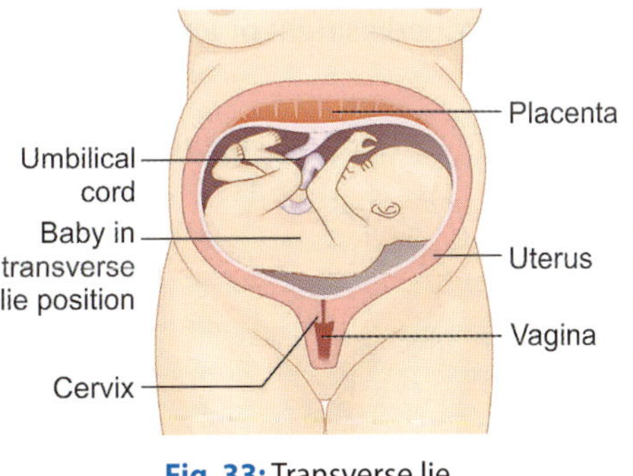 **Fig. 33:** Transverse lie.	**Explanation:** Shoulder presentation occurs when the fetus is in a transverse lie, making vaginal delivery impossible. Since the patient is in labor, the safest course of action is an emergency cesarean section to avoid various complications and ensure the safety of both the mother and the fetus. **Potential questions:** There can be questions related to the clinical finings, management, and complications related to transverse lie.

<table>
<tr><th>Question</th><th>Answer</th><th>Comment</th></tr>
<tr>
<td>Q34. A 32-year-old primigravida presents in labor at 38 weeks of gestation. On abdominal examination, the pelvic grip is empty and fetal head is palpated in the left iliac fossa. On vaginal examination, no definite fetal part can be identified. The vaginal touch picture in this case is shown below. What is the most common fetal position likely to be present in this case?
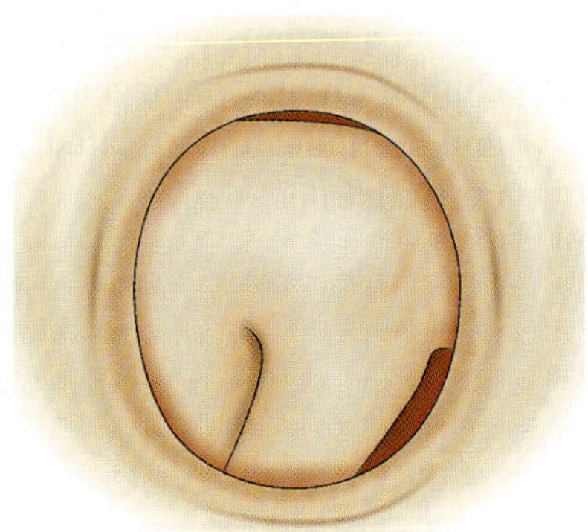
A. Right dorsosuperior
B. Left dorsoanterior
C. Dorsoanterior
D. Dorsoposterior
E. Dorsoinferior</td>
<td>Ans: C (Dorsoanterior)
In case of transverse lie, the denominator is the fetal back. Depending on the position of the fetal back, various positions are possible as follows (Figs. 34A and B):
▪ Dorsoanterior: The most common position where the fetal back is anterior
▪ Dorsoposterior: Fetal back is posterior
▪ Dorsosuperior: Fetal back is directed superiorly
▪ Dorsoinferior: Fetal back is directed inferiorly
Depending on the position of the fetal head, the fetal position can be described as right or left.
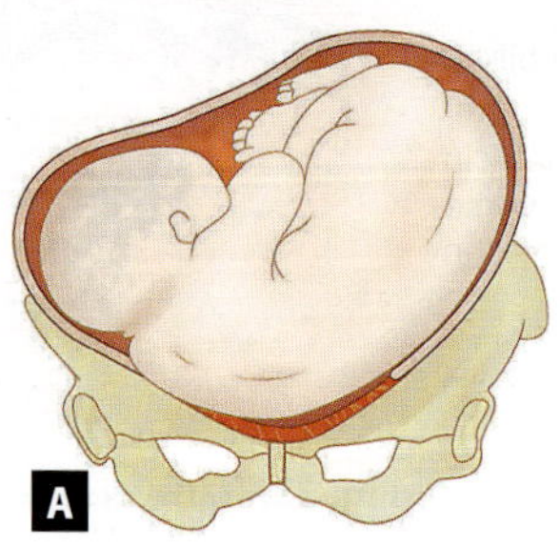

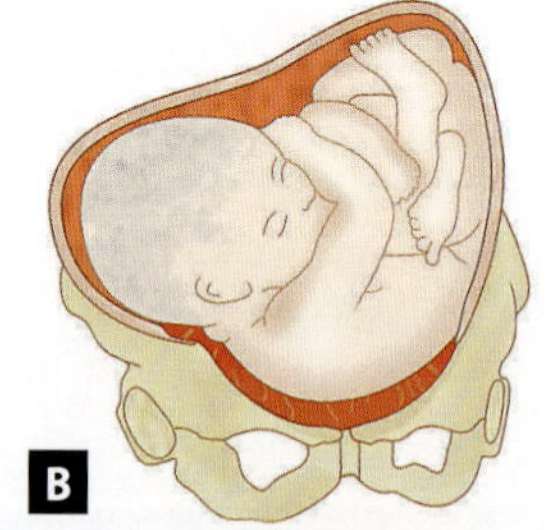

Figs. 34 A and B: (A) Dorsoanterior position; (B) Dorsoposterior position.</td>
<td>Explanation: In cases of transverse lie, at the time of labor, on vaginal examination, fetal shoulder including scapula, clavicle and humerus, and grid iron feel of fetal ribs can be palpated. If the membranes have ruptured, the fetal shoulder can be identified by feeling the acromion process, scapula, clavicle, axilla, ribs, and intercostal spaces. Ribs and intercostal spaces upon palpation give feeling of grid iron. If the arm prolapse has occurred, the fetal arm might be observed lying outside the vagina.
Potential questions: There can be questions related to the clinical finings, management, and complications related to transverse lie/shoulder presentation.</td>
</tr>
</table>

VERSION

Question	Answer	Comment
Q35. A 37-week-old pregnant patient presents with the fetus in a breech presentation during her antenatal visit. The obstetrician recommends an abdominal procedure to turn the fetus to a head-down position. Which of the following is most likely to increase the success rate of this procedure in a breech presentation? 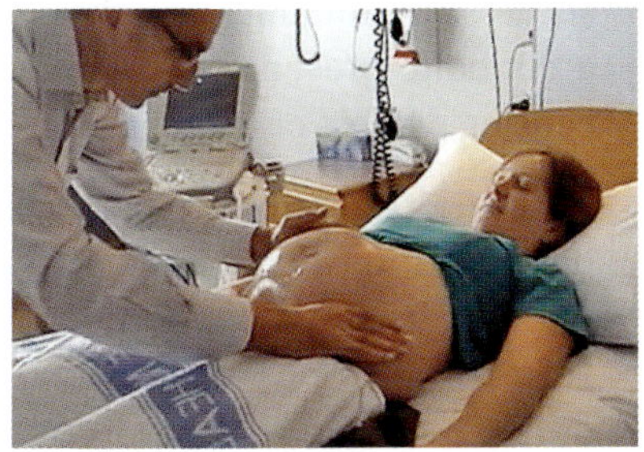 A. Adequate amniotic fluid volume B. Maternal body mass index BMI over 30 kg/m^2 C. Reduced amniotic fluid volume D. Fetal engagement in the pelvis E. Nulliparity	**Ans: A (Adequate amniotic fluid volume)** The procedure being performed in the adjacent image is external cephalic version (ECV). This is a procedure in which the clinician externally rotates the fetus from a breech presentation into cephalic presentation **(Figs. 35 A to D)**. 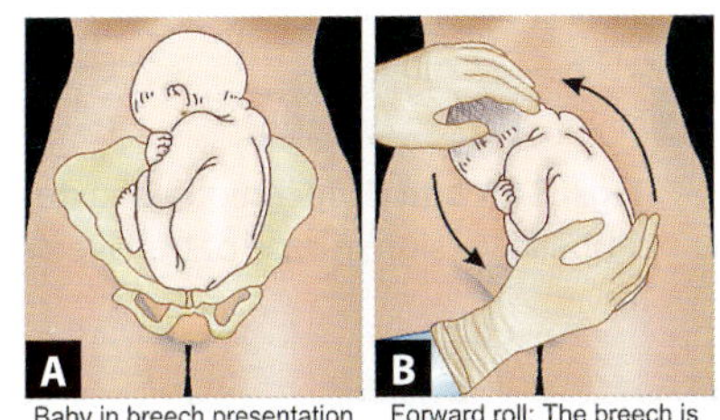 Baby in breech presentation Forward roll: The breech is disengaged and simultaneously pushed upward 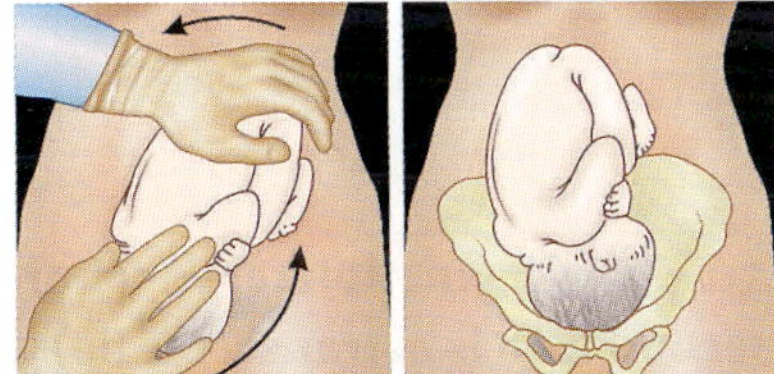 The vertex is gently pushed toward the pelvis Forward roll is completed **Figs. 35A to D:** External cephalic version through forward roll.	**Explanation:** While performing ECV, the clinician helps in gently manipulating the fetal head towards the pelvis, while the breech is brought up cephalad towards the fundus. The clinician must attempt a forward roll first and then a backward roll, if the initial attempt is unsuccessful. Adequate amniotic fluid volume is a key factor that increases the likelihood of successfully performing an ECV. The presence of sufficient fluid allows the fetus to move more freely within the uterus, making it easier for the obstetrician to manually turn the fetus from a breech to a cephalic position. Factors like low fluid levels, a high maternal BMI, or fetal engagement. Anterior placental placement, etc., can reduce the chances of a successful ECV. **Potential questions:** There can be questions pertaining to the indications and complications of various types of version procedures.

Question	Answer	Comment
Q36. A 37-week-old pregnant woman presents with a fetus in a transverse lie. The physician considers performing an external cephalic version (ECV) to reposition the fetus into a cephalic presentation. Which of the following is the most appropriate initial step before performing ECV? 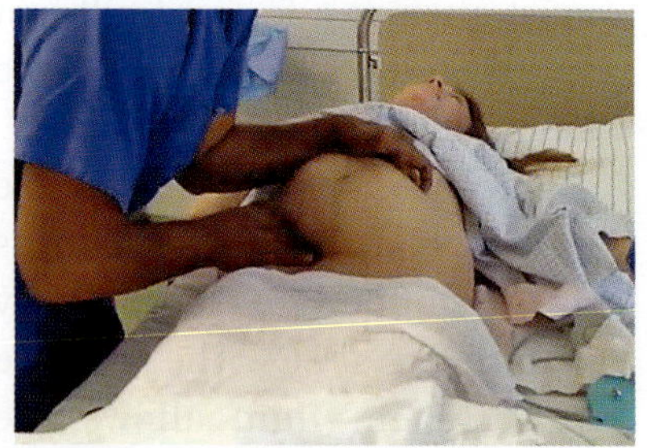 A. Administering a tocolytic agent B. Immediate induction of labor C. Performing an amniotomy D. Performing rupture of membranes E. Performing a digital vaginal examination	**Ans: A (Administering a tocolytic agent)** While performing the ECV, the clinician helps in gently manipulating the fetal head towards the pelvis while the podalic pole is brought up cephalad towards the fundus **(Figs. 36A and B)**. 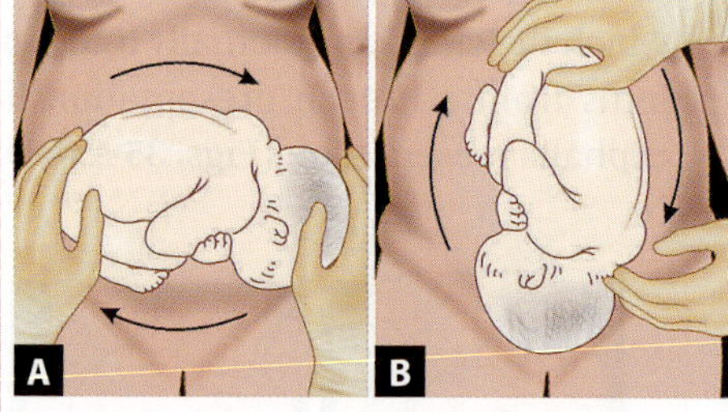 **Figs. 36A and B:** Technique of external cephalic version in case of transverse lie.	**Explanation:** External cephalic version is a procedure in which the clinician externally rotates the fetus from a transverse lie into a cephalic presentation. Before performing an ECV in a transverse lie, it is important to administer a tocolytic agent to relax the uterus and increase the likelihood of a successful version. This reduces uterine tone and enhances the chances of successfully rotating the fetus into a cephalic presentation without causing distress or complications. **Potential questions:** There can be questions pertaining to the indications and complications of various types of version procedures.
Q37. In the scenario being shown in the below image, what is the main indication for performing this maneuver? 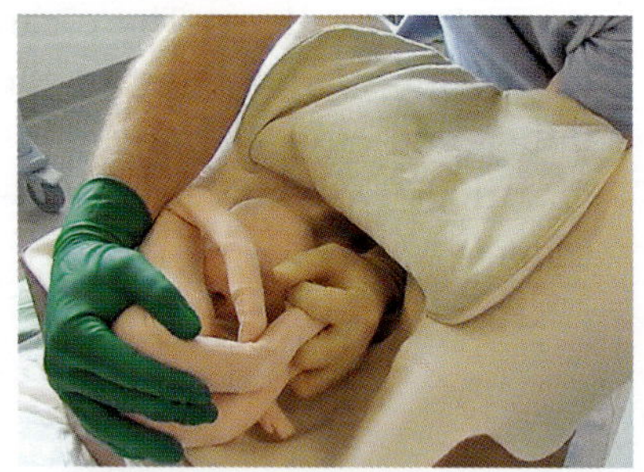 A. Breech presentation in the second trimester B. Transverse lie with a prolapsed umbilical cord C. Twin delivery, where the second twin is in transverse lie D. Fetal distress in cephalic presentation E. Placenta previa with a transverse lie	**Ans: C (Twin delivery, where the second twin is in transverse lie)** The technique of internal podalic version is shown in the adjacent figure. As demonstrated in **Figure 37**, This maneuver involves the obstetrician reaching into the uterus to grasp and bring down one or both feet, converting the fetus into a breech presentation for delivery. It is a highly specialized and rarely performed procedure, typically reserved for emergent situations where rapid delivery is needed. 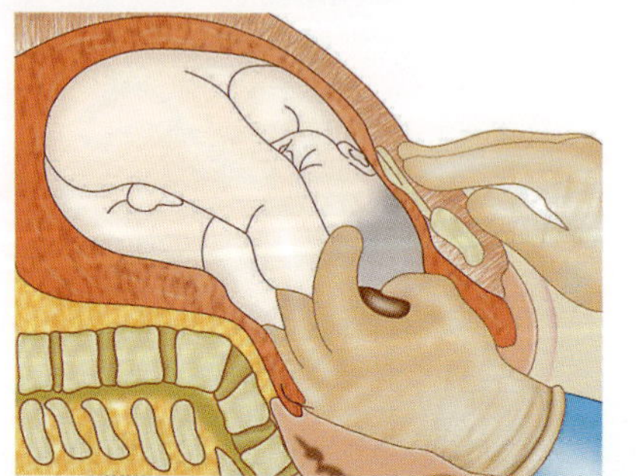 **Fig. 37:** Technique of internal podalic version.	**Explanation:** The only indication for using internal podalic version in modern obstetrics is during the delivery of twins, particularly when the second twin is in a transverse lie following the delivery of the first twin. Besides this indication, the procedure of internal version has no place in modern obstetrics. In case of vaginal delivery for twin gestation, following the delivery of the first twin in vertex presentation, the lie of second fetus is checked through abdominal examination. If the lie of second twin is transverse, external version must be attempted to correct the fetal lie. If the external version fails, internal version under general anesthesia can be attempted. **Potential questions:** There can be questions related to indications, technique, and complications of any of the version procedures.

SHOULDER DYSTOCIA

Question	Answer	Comment
Q38. A 28-year-old G2P1 woman at 39 weeks' gestation was in active labor. After delivering the fetal head, the shoulders became impacted behind the maternal pubic symphysis. The depicted maneuver was performed to resolve the dystocia. Which of the following is the primary purpose of this maneuver during delivery? 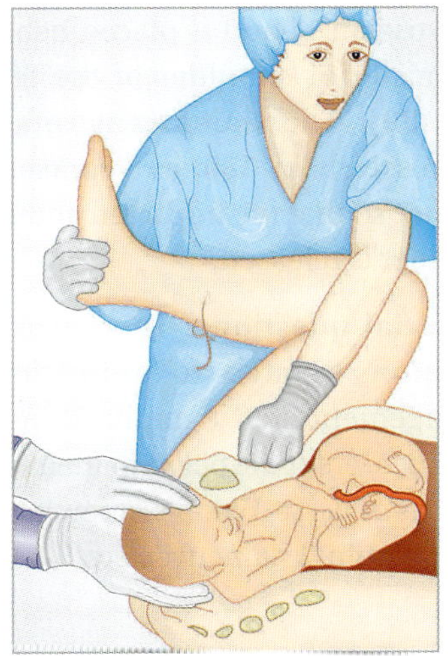 A. To rotate the fetal head during breech delivery B. To reduce maternal discomfort during labor C. To widen the pelvic outlet and relieve shoulder dystocia D. To facilitate the descent of the umbilical cord E. To expedite the second stage of labor	**Ans: C (To widen the pelvic outlet and relieve shoulder dystocia)** The scenario in the given question is suggestive of shoulder dystocia and the maneuver being performed in the adjacent image is McRobert's maneuver. Shoulder dystocia can be defined as the inability to deliver the fetal shoulders after the delivery of delivery fetal head without the aid of specific maneuvers (other than the gentle downward traction on the head). McRobert's maneuver along with the application of suprapubic pressure is the first-line maneuver which must be employed in cases of shoulder dystocia. This maneuver is likely to be successful in nearly 90% women. 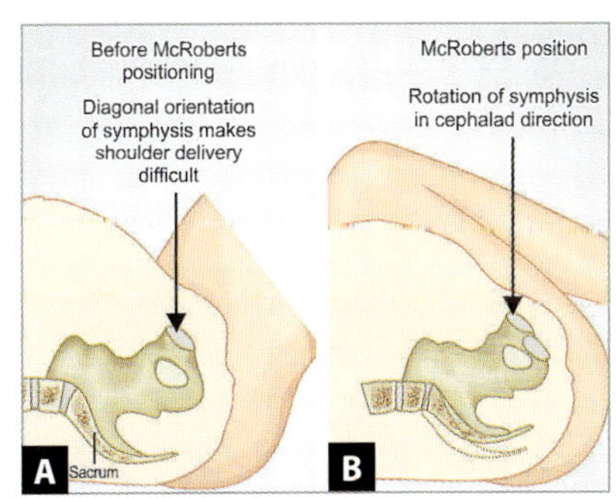 **Figs. 38A and B:** Mechanism by which McRobert's maneuver works.	**Explanation:** McRobert's maneuver involves sharp flexion and abduction of the maternal hips and positioning the maternal thighs on the woman's abdomen. This maneuver helps in cephalad rotation of the symphysis pubis and the straightening of lumbosacral angle **(Figs. 38A and B)**. This maneuver, by straightening the sacrum, tends to widen the pelvic outlet, thereby helping to free the impacted anterior shoulder. The American College of Obstetricians and Gynecologists (ACOG) has recommended that an estimated fetal weight of over 4.5 kg should be considered as an indication for delivery by cesarean section in order to reduce the potential morbidity and mortality in pregnancies complicated with maternal diabetes mellitus since macrosomia is an important risk factor for the development of shoulder dystocia. **Potential questions:** There can be various questions related to risk factors, clinical diagnosis, and management of shoulder dystocia under different clinical circumstances. There can also be questions related to various maneuvers used for resolving this problem.

Question	Answer	Comment
Q39. During a vaginal delivery, a 31-year-old, gravida 2, para 1, encounters difficulties delivering the fetal shoulder. First-line maneuvers like McRobert's maneuver and suprapubic pressure do not resolve the issue. The obstetrician then uses a manual method involving a corkscrew-like rotation to rotate the baby's shoulders as shown in the image below. What is the main goal of this technique in cases of shoulder dystocia? 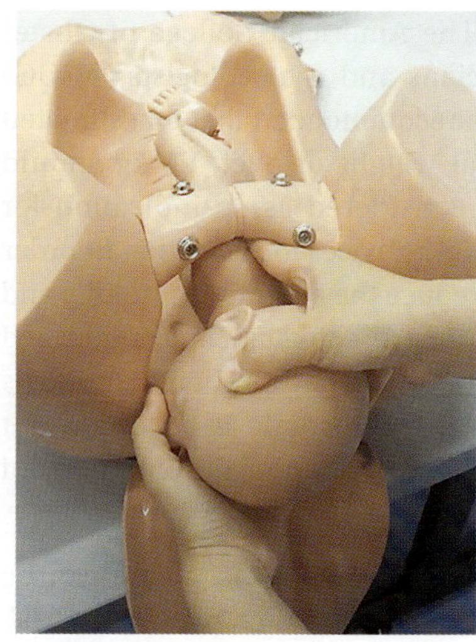 A. To rotate the anterior shoulder by 180° B. To increase the space in the birth canal by abducting the fetal arm C. To deliver the posterior arm first D. To apply suprapubic pressure E. To rotate the posterior shoulder by 180°	**Ans: A (To rotate the anterior shoulder by180°)** The adjacent image demonstrates the Wood's screw maneuver. In case of the failure of first-line maneuvers, such as McRobert's maneuver and the application of suprapubic pressure, the second-line maneuvers for resolution of shoulder dystocia must be employed. These include "enter the pelvis maneuvers" (internal rotation), such as Rubin II maneuver, Wood's screw maneuver **(Fig. 39)**, and reverse Wood's screw maneuver. 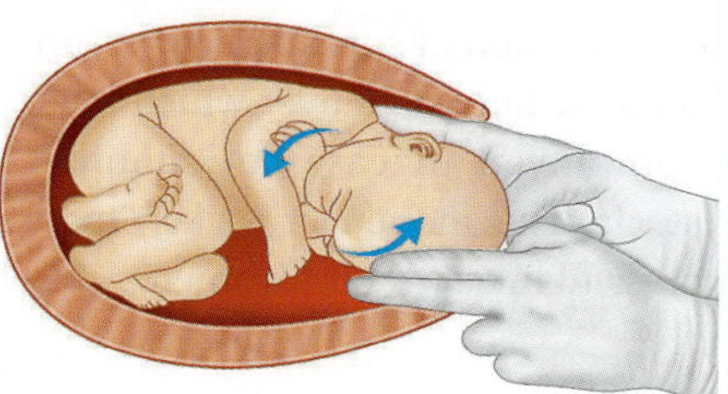 **Fig. 39:** Wood's screw maneuver.	**Explanation:** Wood's screw maneuver is used during shoulder dystocia to relieve the obstruction of the anterior shoulder by rotating it 180°. This rotation helps to free the shoulder from behind the pubic symphysis, allowing for easier delivery of the fetus. It is an important technique in managing shoulder dystocia, aiming to prevent complications such as brachial plexus injury. *Procedure:* In this maneuver, the obstetrician's hand is placed behind the posterior shoulder of the fetus **(Fig. 39)**. The shoulder is rotated progressively by 180° in a corkscrew manner so that the impacted anterior shoulder is released. **Potential questions:** There can be questions related to indications, management, and complications of the other "enter the pelvis maneuvers" such as reverse Wood's screw maneuver, Rubin II maneuver, etc.

Question	Answer	Comment
Q40. A 28-year-old primigravida presents to the labor ward in second stage of labor. After successfully delivering the fetal head, the obstetrician observes the turtle sign and fetal shoulders remain undelivered. First-line maneuvers like McRobert's maneuver and application of suprapubic pressure are unsuccessful. The obstetrician tries doing a maneuver as depicted in the image below. What is this maneuver? 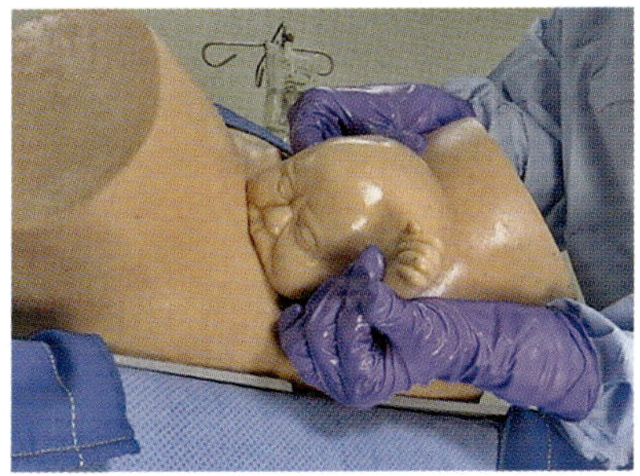 A. Suprapubic pressure B. Zavanelli maneuver C. Delivery of the posterior arm D. Rubin's maneuver E. Wood's screw maneuver	**Ans: C (Delivery of the posterior arm)** The maneuver being demonstrated in the adjacent image is "delivery of posterior arm" which is another effective maneuver for resolving shoulder dystocia. The steps for performance of this maneuver are described in **Figures 40A to C**. 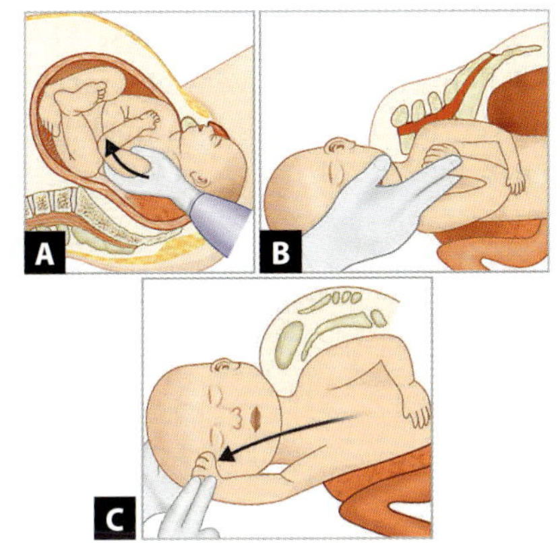 **Figs. 40A to C:** Delivery of posterior arm: (A) The clinician's hand is introduced into the vagina along the posterior shoulder. Keeping the arm flexed at the elbow, it is swept across the fetal chest. (B) The fetal hand is grasped and the arm is extended out along the side of the face. (C) The posterior arm and shoulder are delivered from the vagina.	**Explanation:** In cases of shoulder dystocia, first-line maneuvers such as application of suprapubic pressure and McRobert's maneuvers are likely to work in most of the cases. However, if these maneuvers are unsuccessful, the obstetrician can try the second-line maneuvers, where there are two options: Delivery of the posterior arm or enter the pelvis maneuvers (Rubin II, Wood's screw maneuver, and reverse Wood's screw maneuver). *Procedure:* In this maneuver, the obstetrician places his or her hand behind the posterior shoulder of the fetus and locates the arm. This arm is then swept across the fetal chest and delivered. With the posterior arm and shoulder now delivered, it is relatively easy to rotate the baby, dislodge the anterior shoulder, and allow delivery of the remainder of the baby. **Potential questions:** There can be questions related to the indications, techniques, and complications of the various second-line or third-line maneuvers.

<table>
<tr><th>Question</th><th>Answer</th><th>Comment</th></tr>
<tr>
<td>Q41. During normal vaginal delivery, a 31-year-old woman, gravida 2, para 1, faces complications while delivering the baby's shoulder. As shown in the below image, the obstetrician decides to employ a specific maneuver involving repositioning the baby's head back into the birth canal for a cesarean delivery. What is the name of this maneuver?
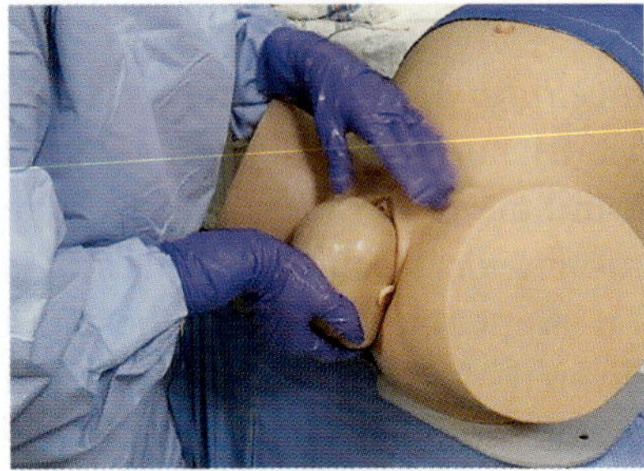
A. McRobert's Maneuver
B. Wood's corkscrew maneuver
C. Rubin maneuver
D. Zavanelli maneuver
E. Reverse Wood's corkscrew maneuver</td>
<td>Ans: D (Zavanelli maneuver)
The maneuver being demonstrated in the adjacent image is Zavanelli maneuver. Several third-line methods have been described for cases of shoulder dystocia, which are resistant to all simple measures (including the first- and the second-line maneuvers). Some of the third-line maneuvers include cleidotomy, symphysiotomy, and Zavanelli maneuver (Figs. 41A and B). These maneuvers are rarely employed in today's modern obstetric practice.
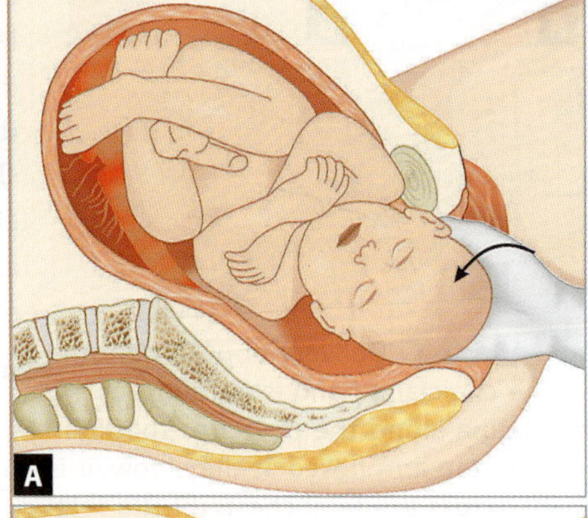
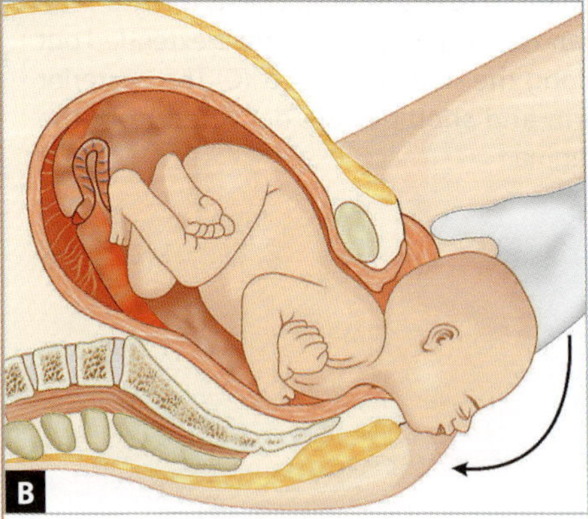
Figs. 41A and B: Zavanelli maneuver.</td>
<td>Explanation: Zavanelli maneuver involves cephalic replacement of the head followed by cesarean section. In this maneuver, firstly the fetal head is rotated back into its prerestitution position, i.e., occiput anterior. Following this, the head is flexed and pushed back up into the vagina. Once the fetal head gets back into the pelvis, an emergency cesarean section is performed to deliver a live baby.
It is typically used as a last resort when other maneuvers for resolving shoulder dystocia have failed. The maneuver requires careful execution and is associated with significant maternal and fetal risks and is rarely used.
Potential questions: There can be questions related to the indications, techniques, and complications of the various second-line or third-line maneuvers.</td>
</tr>
</table>

INSTRUMENTAL DELIVERY

Question	Answer	Comment
Q42. The image shows a pair of short, lightweight obstetric forceps used for outlet deliveries in the second stage of labor. Identify the forceps. 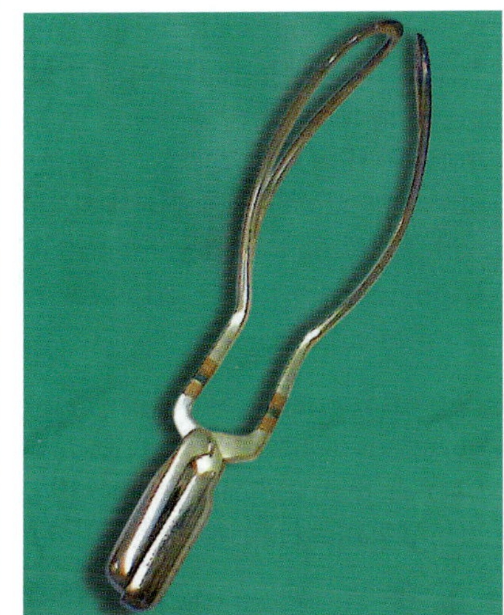 A. Kielland's forceps B. Simpson's forceps C. Neville Barnes forceps D. Wrigley's forceps E. Tucker-McLane forceps	**Ans: D (Wrigley's forceps)** The adjacent image shows Wrigley's forceps. **Figure 42** illustrates different types of forceps employed in the clinical practice. 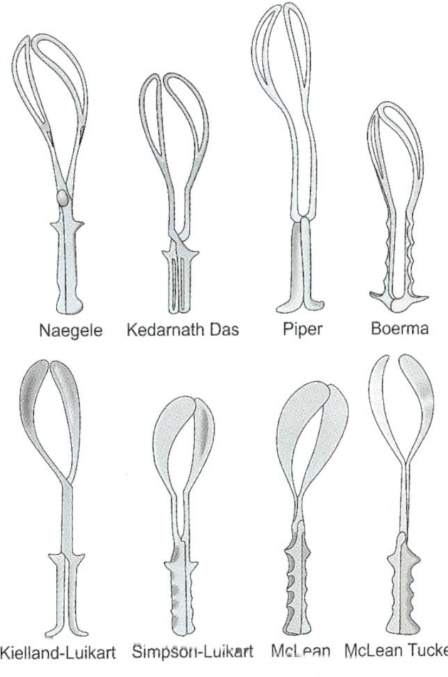 **Fig. 42:** Different types of forceps.	**Explanation:** Wrigley's forceps is one of the most commonly used forceps in the routine practice. It is a short, light instrument having pelvic and cephalic curves and an English lock. These forceps are designed specifically for outlet deliveries, often during the second stage of labor. Their short length and lightweight construction make them ideal for such situations, where more extensive forceps would be unnecessary or inappropriate. They are not suitable for high-cavity or rotational deliveries. **Potential questions:** There can be questions related to different types of forceps, their indications, technique of application, and complications.

Question	Answer	Comment
Q43. In which situation would forceps with a minimal pelvic curve as shown in the image below be most appropriate? 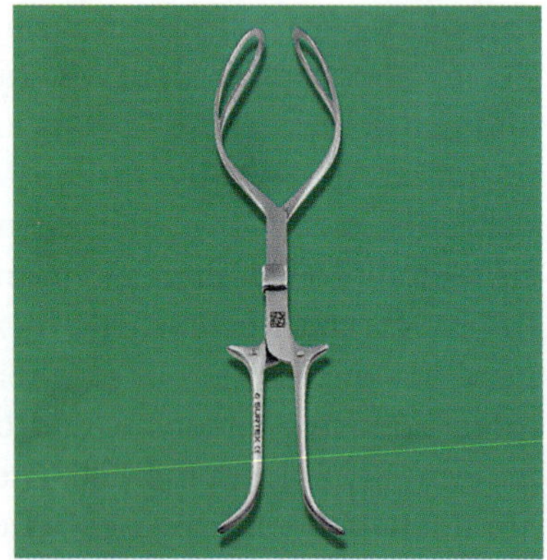 A. Breech presentation in the second stage of labor B. Cephalic presentation with occiput transverse in the second stage C. Fully dilated cervix in the first stage of labor D. Cephalic presentation with posterior asynclitism E. Compound presentation in the second stage of labor	**Ans: B (Cephalic presentation with occiput transverse in the second stage)** The forceps shown in the adjacent image is the Kielland forceps, introduced by Dr Christian Kielland in 1915. This forceps was originally designed to facilitate rotation and extraction of the fetal head, arrested in the deep transverse or occipitoposterior position. **Figure 43** demonstrates different parts of the Kielland forceps. 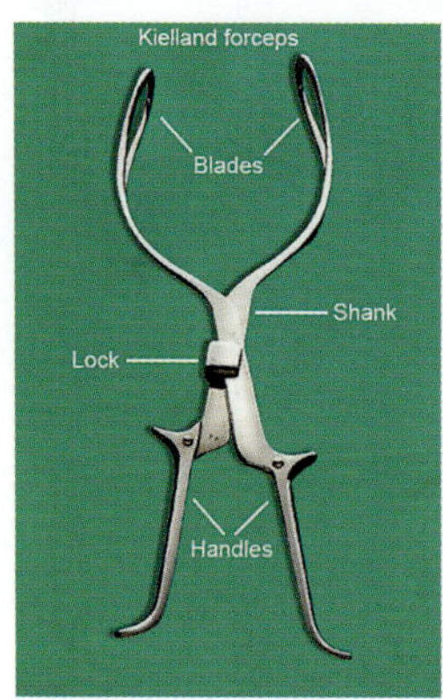 **Fig. 43:** Parts of Kielland forceps.	**Explanation:** Kielland forceps are designed for malpositioned fetal heads, especially when the occiput is transverse or posterior, requiring rotation for an anterior position. They have a minimal pelvic curve, which enables the operator to safely rotate the blades during delivery. The anterior blade is applied first in the second stage of labor. Unlike nonrotational forceps, Kielland forceps feature overlapping shanks with a sliding lock and identifiable knobs on the finger grips for the anterior surface. **Potential questions:** There can be questions related to different types of forceps, their indications, technique of application, and complications.

Question	Answer	Comment
Q44. The image below shows a hand-held vacuum device with a soft silastic cup used during delivery. Which of the following describes the best option for the placement of vacuum cup? 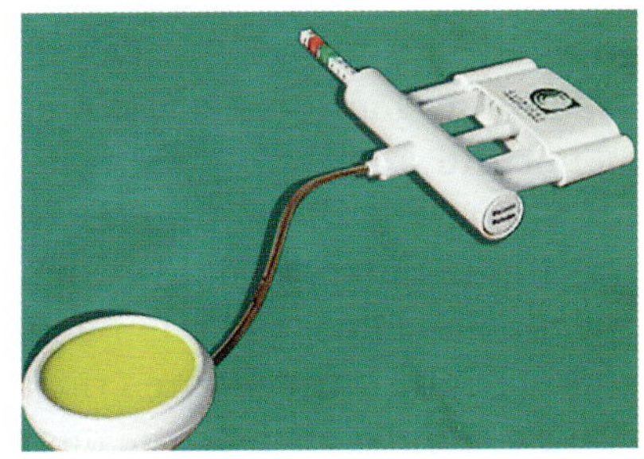 A. Edge of the cup is approximately located over the posterior fontanel B. Edge of the cup is located 2 cm in front of the posterior fontanel C. Edge of the cup is located 2 cm behind the posterior fontanel D. Edge of the cup is located approximately over the anterior fontanel E. Edge of the cup is located approximately 2 cm in front of the anterior fontanel	**Ans: A (Edge of the cup is located approximately over the posterior fontanel)** Ventouse is an instrument, which assists in delivery of the fetus by creating a vacuum force between it and the fetal scalp. The pulling force in case of vacuum extraction helps in dragging the cranium. The correct placement of vacuum cup over the fetal head is described in **Figure 44**. 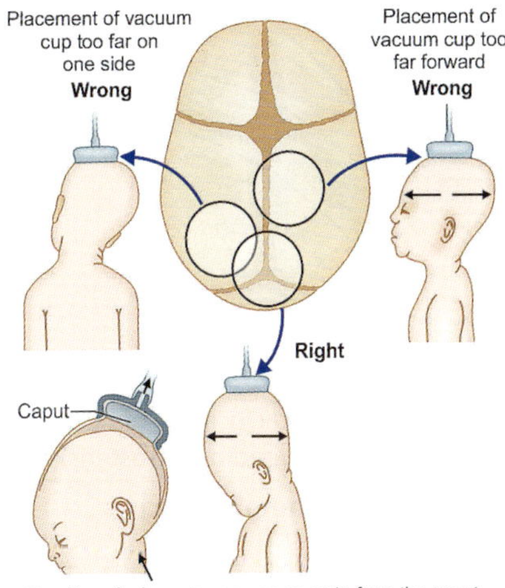 **Fig. 44:** Correct placement of vacuum cup over the fetal head.	**Explanation:** The vacuum cup should be so positioned so as to prevent the deflexion and asynclitism of fetal head. In case of an occipitoanterior position, the cup should be placed in such a way that the center of the cup lies directly over the flexion point or the pivot point which can be defined as a point over the sagittal suture, about 6 cm behind the anterior fontanel or 3 cm in front of the posterior fontanel. Generally, the cup must be placed as far posteriorly as possible. This implies that the edge of the cup having a diameter of 5–7 cm would be approximately 3 cm from the anterior fontanel and would lie over the posterior fontanel. If the cup is placed anteriorly on the fetal cranium near the anterior fontanel rather than over the occiput, this may result in undue extension of the cervical spine. Similarly, if the cup is asymmetrically placed in relation to the sagittal suture, it is likely to worsen asynclitism. **Potential questions:** There can be questions related to indications, technique of application, and complications of vacuum application.

Question	Answer	Comment
Q45. The image below illustrates a significant swelling in a newborn head that crosses the suture lines on the scalp. 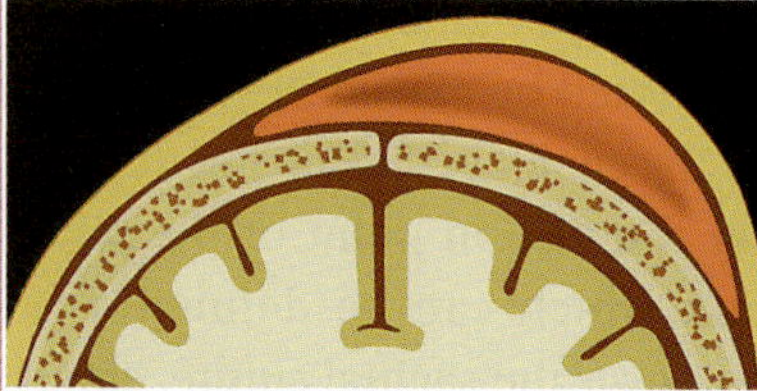 Based on this clinical presentation, which of the following is the most likely diagnosis? A. Caput succedaneum B. Cephalohematoma C. Subgaleal hematoma D. Epidural hematoma E. Scalp edema	**Ans: C (Subgaleal hematoma)** Subgaleal or subaponeurotic hematomas occur as a result of bleeding in the potential space between the skull periosteum and epicranial aponeurosis **(Fig. 45)**. Since the collection occurs above the periosteum, it can cross the sutures lines. Subgaleal hematoma must be suspected in case of boggy scalp swelling, swelling crossing the suture lines, and an expanding head circumference. 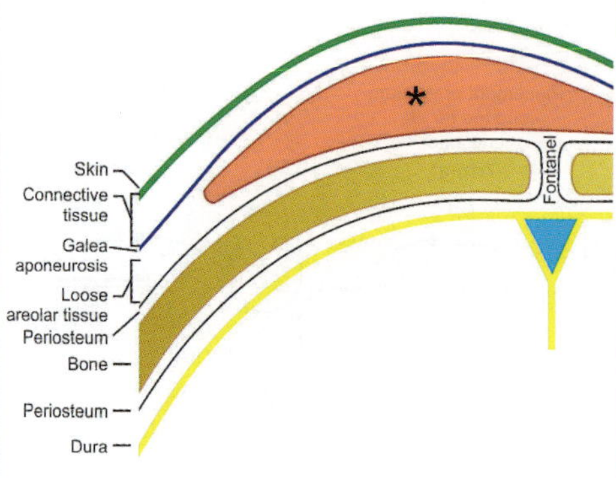 **Fig. 45:** Anatomical location of subgaleal hematoma [indicated by the asterisk (*)].	**Explanation:** Diagnosis of subgaleal hematoma is established based on history and physical examination. The diffuse, progressive, fluctuant, head swelling related to subgaleal hematoma shifts with repositioning, indents on palpation and is not limited by suture lines. Optimal clinical diagnosis is made through CT or MRI scan. Subgaleal hematomas can be life-threatening due to significant blood loss, and prompt diagnosis and treatment are critical. This condition often occurs due to traction during vacuum-assisted deliveries. **Potential questions:** There can be questions related to anatomical location and characteristic features of common vacuum-related injuries such as subgaleal hematoma and cephalohematoma.
Q46. The image below illustrates a soft, well-defined swelling over the parietal bone in a newborn that does not cross the suture lines on scalp. Which of the following is the most likely diagnosis? 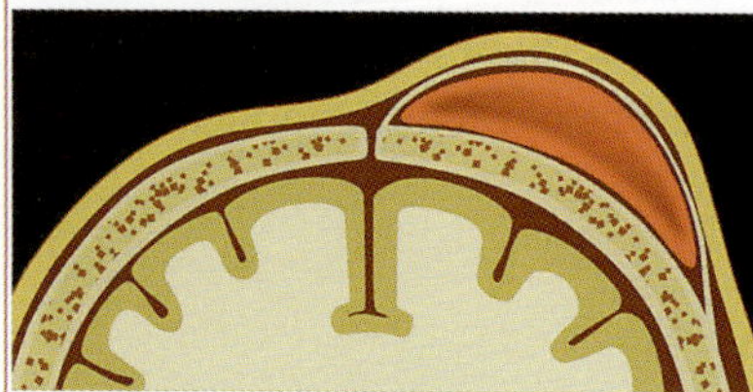 A. Caput succedaneum B. Cephalohematoma C. Subgaleal hematoma D. Epidural hematoma E. Scalp edema	**Ans: B (Cephalohematoma)** Cephalohematoma is a scalp swelling, which may occur during a difficult vaginal delivery, including the use of vacuum extractors. In case of cephalohematoma, bleeding occurs beneath the periosteum, between the skull and the periosteum **(Fig. 46)**. As a result, the boggy swelling associated with cephalohematoma is limited by the suture lines in contrast to the subgaleal hematomas, which are not limited by the suture lines. 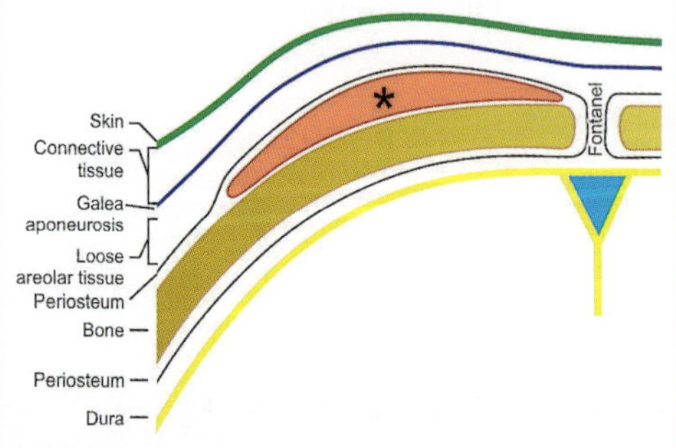 **Fig. 46:** Anatomical location of cephalohematoma [indicated by the asterisk (*)].	**Explanation:** Cephalohematoma also needs to be differentiated from caput succedaneum, which is a swelling of the scalp occurring due to pressure from the uterus or vaginal wall at the time of delivery in case of vertex presentation. This is present above the periosteum in contrast to cephalohematoma, which is present below the periosteum. Cephalohematoma usually disappears on its own, and conservative management is usually sufficient. **Potential questions:** There can be questions related to anatomical location and characteristic features of common vacuum-related injuries such as subgaleal hematoma and cephalohematoma.

CESAREAN SECTION

Question	Answer	Comment
Q47. The image shown below demonstrates two different uterine incisions. Which of the following statements is false? 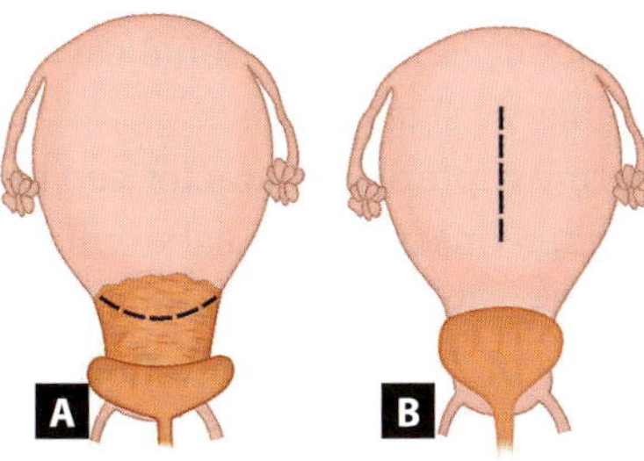 A. Incision in Figure A is associated with a lower likelihood of adhesion formation involving bowel or omentum B. Incision in Figure A is more commonly used than that in Figure B C. Incision in Figure B allows for easy entry into the uterus when there is fibroid in the lower segment D. Figure B is associated with a higher risk of uterine rupture during subsequent pregnancy E. Figure A is indicated in the presence of carcinoma of the cervix	**Ans: E (Figure A is indicated in the presence of carcinoma of the cervix)** Figure A in the adjacent image shows a transverse incision in the lower uterine segment (Pfannenstiel incision), whereas figure B shows a vertical incision in the upper uterine segment (classical incision). Pfannenstiel incision is most commonly used in the clinical practice. Various types of uterine incisions and their variations are illustrated in **Figure 47**. Classical cesarean delivery is rarely performed nowadays due to a high risk of scar rupture in future pregnancy (2% risk) in comparison to the Pfannenstiel incision (0.5% risk). Classical incision may be rarely administered in cases where the lower uterine segment may not be accessible. This could be in cases of invasive carcinoma cervix, densely adherent bladder in the lower uterine segment, presence of a myoma in the lower uterine segment, transverse lie of the fetus with the shoulder impacted in the birth canal, cases of placenta previa where the placenta penetrates through the lower uterine segment (placenta percreta), cases where the lower uterine segment has not formed (e.g., small fetus having a breech presentation), postmortem cesarean delivery, etc. 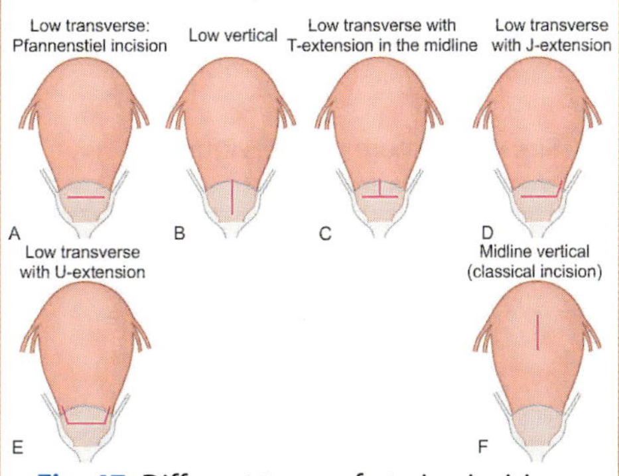 **Fig. 47:** Different types of uterine incisions.	**Explanation:** A classical cesarean delivery is associated with a weaker scar in comparison to a transverse incision. Therefore, rather than performing a classical cesarean section, the clinicians nowadays prefer to use some kind of variations in the lower segment uterine incision. Mostly, the surgeon is able to decide the exact incision only at the time of surgery. Variations of the lower segment incision are commonly used, in cases where there is requirement for an extended surgical field, to avoid scar extension, e.g., transverse lie with hand prolapse and large baby, etc. Some of the variations of Pfannenstiel incision include the following: ▪ *An inverted T-shaped incision:* This incision involves cutting upward from the middle of the transverse incision. ▪ *J-shaped or hockey-stick incision:* This incision involves extension of one end of the transverse incision upward. ▪ *U-shaped or trap-door incision:* This incision involves extension of both ends of the transverse scar upward. Of all these various choices, T-shaped scar is the worst choice due to its difficult repair, poor healing, and chances of scar rupture during subsequent pregnancies. Also, the classical scar is likely to be associated with a higher risk of development of adhesions with the bowel or the omentum. **Potential questions:** There can be questions related to the indications, technique, and complications associated with cesarean delivery.

Question	Answer	Comment
Q48. A 28-year-old woman with a history of previous cesarean section presents at 26 weeks' gestation with sharp abdominal pain. The ultrasound image demonstrates some abnormal findings which are shown below. 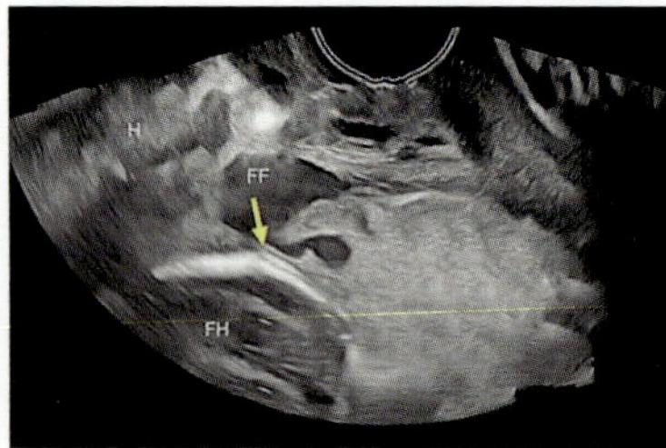 What is the most likely diagnosis? A. Uterine rupture B. Placenta previa C. Placenta accreta D. Preterm labor E. Vasa previa	**Ans: A (Uterine rupture)** The adjacent image shows the features of scar rupture. The yellow arrow in adjacent image points towards a defect in the uterine wall, indicative of the scar giving way. There is presence of hematoma (H) and free fluid (FF) in the peritoneal cavity. Fetal head (FH) can be seen lying within the uterus. All these features are indicative of scar rupture. Other features of uterine scar rupture on ultrasound include protruding portion of the amniotic sac through the uterine wall, endometrial or myometrial defect, intraperitoneal fetal parts (lying outside the uterine cavity), etc. As previously discussed, a classical scar is associated with the highest risk of rupture in case of TOLAC (trial of labor after cesarean). **Figure 48** depicts the appearance of rupture uterus in case of a previous classical uterine scar. 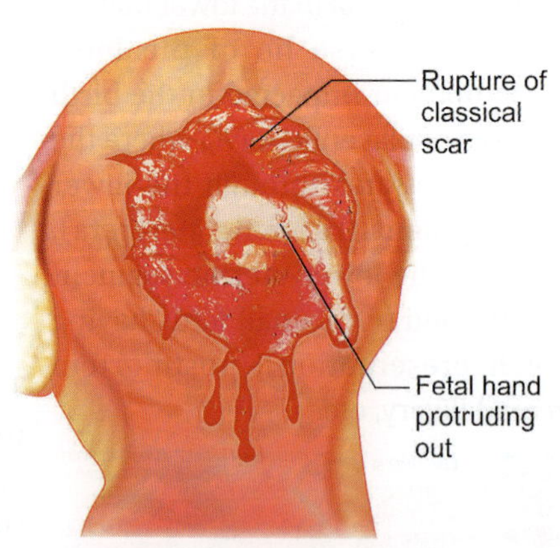 **Fig. 48:** Rupture of a previous classical uterine scar.	**Explanation:** Uterine rupture is a rare but life-threatening complication of TOLAC. Clinical signs include sudden onset of severe abdominal pain, abnormal fetal heart rate patterns, loss of uterine contractions, and free fluid (blood) in the abdominal cavity. There may be signs of shock. Uterine rupture is characterized by the sudden onset of sharp abdominal pain, cessation of contractions, and evidence of fetal distress. Prompt recognition and surgical intervention are critical for preventing severe maternal and fetal complications associated with uterine rupture. **Potential questions:** There can be questions related to the indications, technique, and complications associated with cesarean delivery.

INTRAUTERINE FETAL DEATH

Question	Answer	Comment
Q49. During a routine ultrasound of a 32-year-old woman, gravida 2, para 1, at 30 weeks of gestation, the sonographer observes overlapping skull bones in the fetus. The ultrasonographic image is shown below. What does this finding most likely indicate? 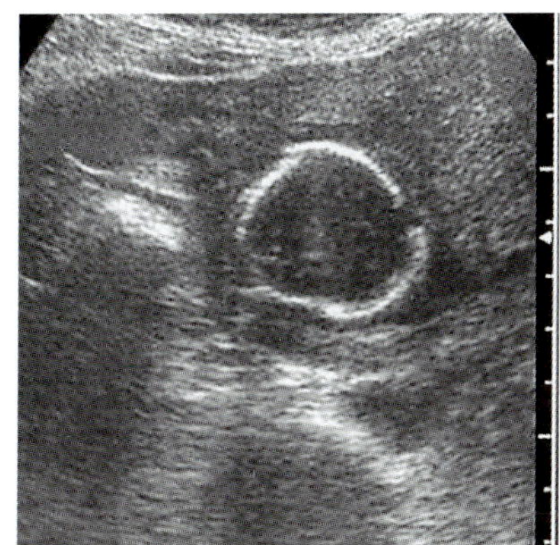 A. Normal fetal development B. Hydranencephaly C. Fetal demise D. Contusion of fetal skull E. Skull fracture	**Ans: C (Fetal demise)** The adjacent ultrasound image demonstrates overlapping of the fetal skull bones, also known as the Spalding sign. Intrauterine fetal death can be defined as the diagnosis of the stillborn infant (with the period of gestation being >24 weeks and fetal weight > 500 g). 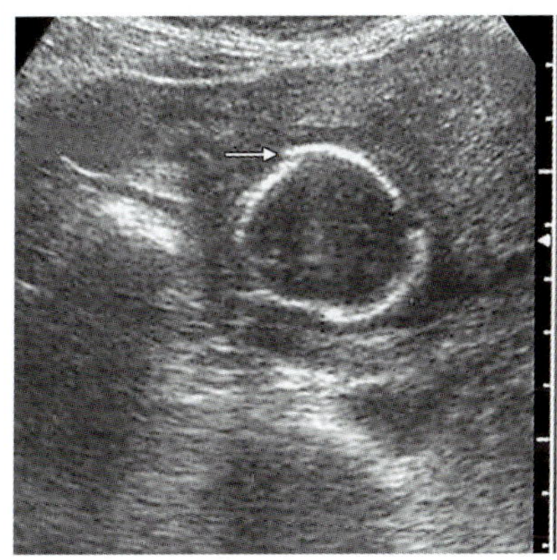 **Fig. 49:** Spalding sign, showing overlapping of the fetal skull bones (indicated by arrow).	**Explanation:** The Spalding sign, characterized by overlapping fetal skull bones (indicated by an arrow in **Figure 49**), is a radiological indicator of fetal demise. This sign occurs due to the collapse of the fetal brain and is typically observed a week or more after the fetal death. Definitive diagnosis is made by observing the lack of fetal cardiac motion during a 10-minute period of careful examination with real-time ultrasound. Other signs of fetal death may include hyperflexion of the spine, crowding of ribs, and appearance of gas shadows in the heart and great vessels (Robert's sign). **Potential questions:** There can be questions related to causes, diagnosis and management of intrauterine fetal demise.

MONITORING DURING LABOR

<table>
<tr><th>Question</th><th>Answer</th><th>Comment</th></tr>
<tr><td>

Q50. What does the line A on the WHO partograph in the below image primarily indicate?

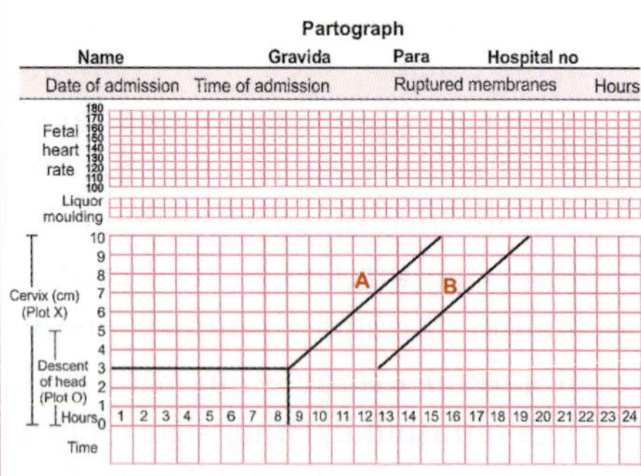

A. The need for immediate delivery
B. The transition from the latent to the active phase of labor
C. The normal rate of cervical dilation
D. The onset of fetal distress
E. The need for augmentation of labor

</td><td>

Ans: C (The normal rate of cervical dilation)

Normal labor should be plotted graphically on a partogram as shown in **Figure 50**. Partogram is the graphical record of the progress of labor. Dilatation of cervix and descent of fetal presenting part are plotted, which gives an estimate about the progress of the first stage of labor. The partograph clearly identifies women showing abnormal progress of labor who are likely to benefit from early intervention (medical or surgical induction of labor). The partograph is divided into a latent phase and an active phase. Line A on the partogram refers to the alert line and line B refers to the action line.

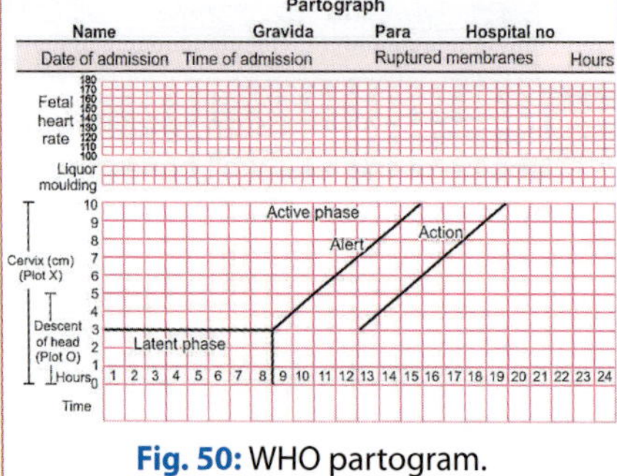

Fig. 50: WHO partogram.

</td><td>

Explanation: The latent phase ends while the active phase begins when the cervix is 3 cm dilated. Cervical dilation and descent of the presenting part are plotted in relation to an alert line and an action line. Alert line starts at the end of latent phase and ends with the full dilation of the cervix (10 cm) within 7 hours (at the rate of 1 cm/h). The action line is drawn 4 hours to the right of the alert line. Labor is considered to be abnormal when the cervicograph crosses the alert line and intervention is required when it crosses the action line.

The alert line on a partograph is a guide to monitor the progress of labor. It represents the expected normal rate of cervical dilation, usually about 1 cm/h in active labor. If the labor curve crosses to the right of the alert line, it may indicate slow progress, requiring closer monitoring or intervention.

Potential questions: There can be questions regarding the various components of the partogram as well as the labor care guide.

</td></tr>
</table>

<table>
<tr><th>Question</th><th>Answer</th><th>Comment</th></tr>
<tr>
<td>

Q51. A 28-year-old primigravida woman at 40 weeks of gestation presents to the labor ward with regular contractions. On examination, her cervix is 4 cm dilated, and the fetal heart rate is normal. Which of the following assessments should be performed next according to the WHO Labour Care Guide (LCG), cropped part of which is shown in the image below?

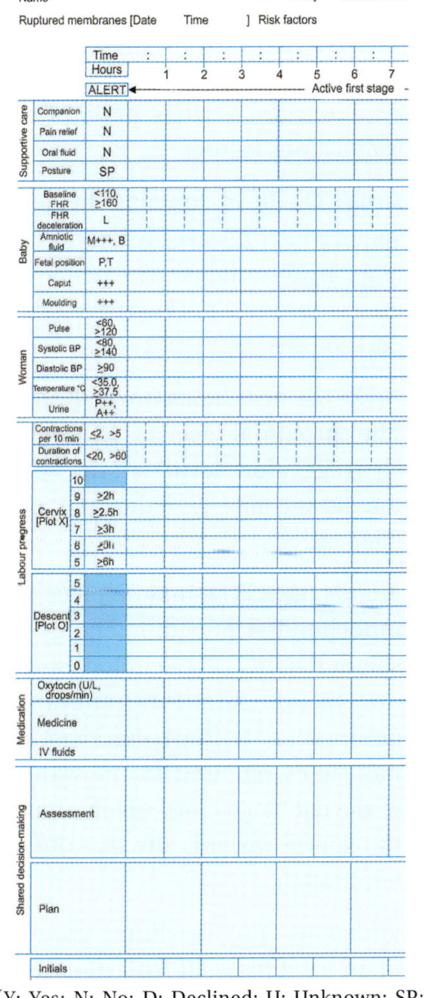

(Y: Yes; N: No; D: Declined; U: Unknown; SP: Supine; MO: Mobile; E: Early; L: Late; V: Variable; I: Intact; C: Clear; M: Meconium; B: Blood; A: Anterior; P: Posterior; T: Transverse; P+: Protein; A+: Acetone)

A. Continuous electronic fetal monitoring
B. Vaginal examination every 2 hours
C. Immediate amniotomy
D. Administering oxytocin infusion
E. Encouraging upright positions and mobility

</td>
<td>

Ans: E (Encouraging upright positions and mobility)

Normal labor was previously plotted graphically on a modified WHO partograph (as shown in Q50). The WHO has now devised a new monitoring tool called the WHO Labour Care Guide as shown in the adjacent image. Both the tools are graphical representations of progress of labor in terms of the woman's cervical dilatation and descent of the fetal presenting part against time. Both the tools involve formal regular monitoring of important clinical parameters describing the well-being of the mother as well as the baby. This new Labor Care Guide comprises seven sections, some of which were adapted from the previous partograph design. These are demonstrated in **Figure 51**.

For all observations, there is a horizontal time axis where the clinician can document the corresponding time of observation. There is a vertical reference value axis for determination of any deviation from normal observations.

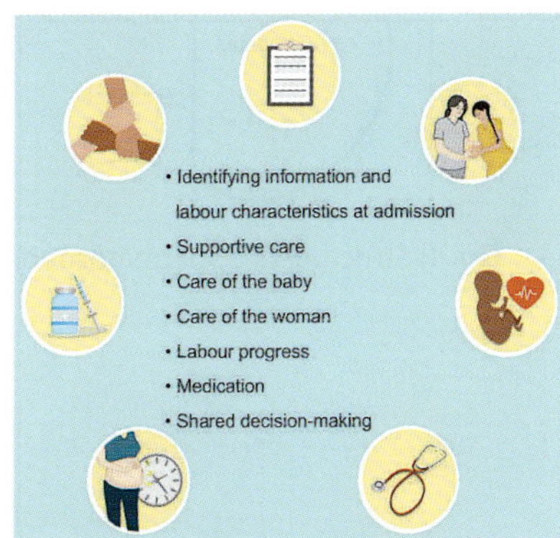

Fig. 51: Structure of the Labor Care Guide (LCG).

</td>
<td>

Explanation: While in the modified WHO partograph, alert and action lines are fixed at 1 cm/h, in LCG there are evidence-based time limits at each centimeter cervical dilatation. There are no action or alert lines. Observations during labor are compared with reference values in the "Alert" column.

The WHO LCG emphasizes women-centered supportive care, involving her in shared-decision-making and employing evidence-based practices.

In this scenario, encouraging upright positions and mobility is recommended. Upright positions (such as walking, standing, or sitting) during labor can improve maternal comfort, facilitate progress, and reduce the risk of interventions.

LCG discourages unnecessary interventions. For example, continuous electronic fetal monitoring is not routinely recommended for low-risk pregnancies

Vaginal examinations every 2 hours may increase the risk of infection and unnecessary interventions and therefore must be avoided. Immediate amniotomy is not indicated unless there are specific medical indications. Administering oxytocin infusion should be reserved for cases of inadequate uterine contractions.

Potential questions: There can be questions regarding the various components of the partogram as well as the labor care guide.

</td>
</tr>
</table>

CHAPTER 3

Embryology

GAMETOGENESIS

Question	Answer	Comment
Q1. You are observing the structure of a spermatozoon under the microscope. The image below shows a diagrammatic image of a sperm. Which part of the spermatozoon contains the mitochondria, responsible for providing energy for motility? 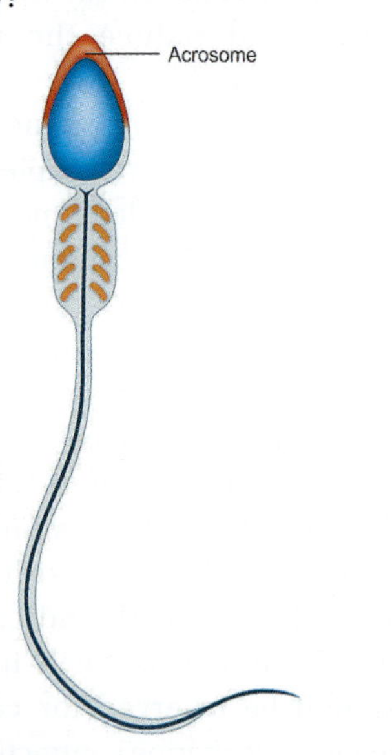 A. Acrosome B. Nucleus C. Midpiece D. Tail (Flagellum) E. Plasma membrane	**Ans: C (Midpiece)** **Figure 1** demonstrates the structure of a human spermatozoon, which comprises four main parts: Head, neck, middle piece, and tail. 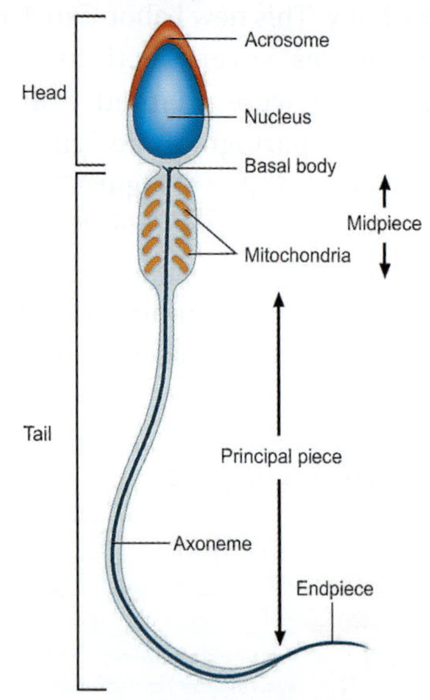 **Fig. 1:** Structure of a spermatozoon.	**Explanation:** Various parts of the sperm are as follows: *Head:* The head contains the acrosome, which releases lytic enzymes (e.g., hyaluronidase) to penetrate the ovum, and a nucleus with tightly packed DNA. *Neck:* The neck holds two centrioles: The proximal assists in zygote cleavage after fertilization, while the distal connects to the tail's axial filament. *Middle piece:* The middle piece has mitochondria providing energy for sperm motility. These mitochondria are responsible for generating adenosine triphosphate (ATP) molecules required for movement of the tail (flagellum), which propels the sperm towards the egg during fertilization. *Tail:* The tail (flagellum) consists of an axial filament with nine pairs of longitudinal fibers, enabling movement. **Potential questions:** There can be different questions related to different parts of sperm and their functions.

Question	Answer	Comment
Q2. Identify the structure labeled "C" in the below diagrammatic image of the testis. 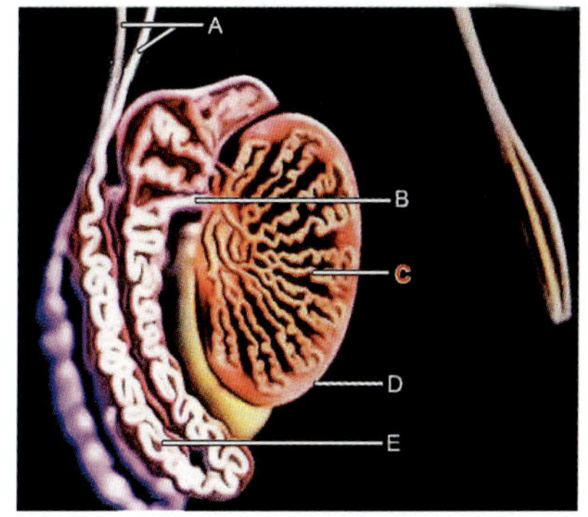 A. Seminiferous tubules B. Rete testis C. Epididymis D. Tunica albuginea E. Leydig cell	**Ans: A (Seminiferous tubules)** The testes are male gonads, responsible for producing sperms and male hormone, mainly testosterone. The internal structure of testis is shown in **Figure 2**. In males two testis are present, one in each scrotal sac. 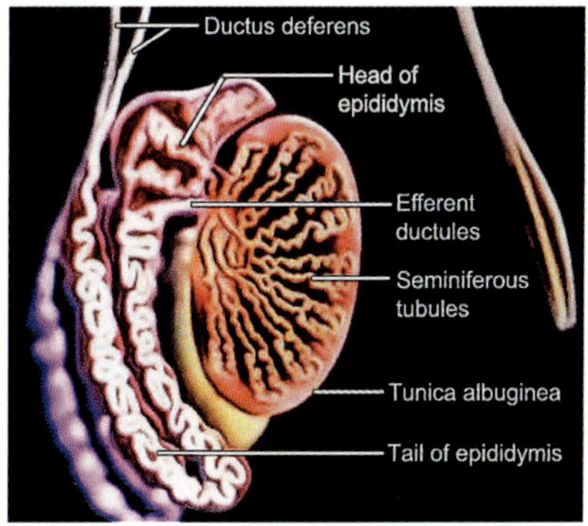 **Fig. 2:** Internal structure of testis.	**Explanation:** Each testis is surrounded by a fibrous capsule or tunica albuginea and comprises numerous lobules. Each lobule contains one or more convoluted tubules known as the seminiferous tubule, where spermatogenesis occurs. These tubules are lined with Sertoli cells that support and nourish the developing sperm cells. Various seminiferous tubules join to form approximately 20 small ducts, which pierce the fibrous capsule to enter the head of epididymis. These ducts eventually join up and become continuous with ductus deferens, which begins at the lower end of epididymis or its tail. **Potential questions:** There can be questions pertaining to various internal structures of testis.
Q3. Identify the stage of spermatogenesis labeled "A" in the below image of male gametogenesis. 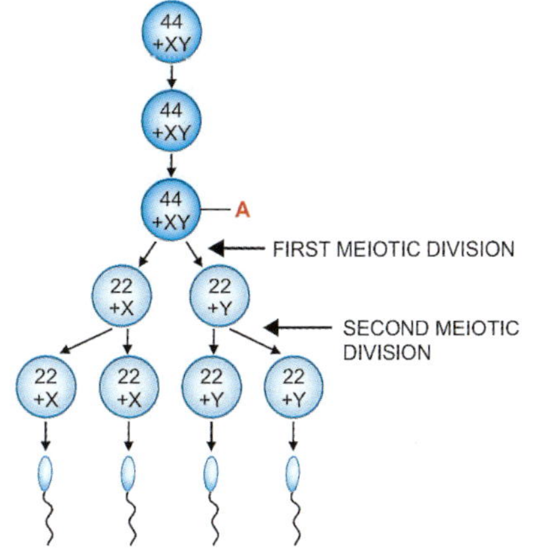 A. Spermatogonia B. Primary spermatocytes C. Secondary spermatocytes D. Spermatids E. Spermatozoa	**Ans: B (Primary spermatocytes)** The process in which spermatogonia gets transformed into spermatozoon is known as spermatogenesis and is primarily under the control of follicle stimulating hormone (FSH) and testosterone. It involves the production of sperms. Stages of spermatogenesis are described in **Figure 3**. 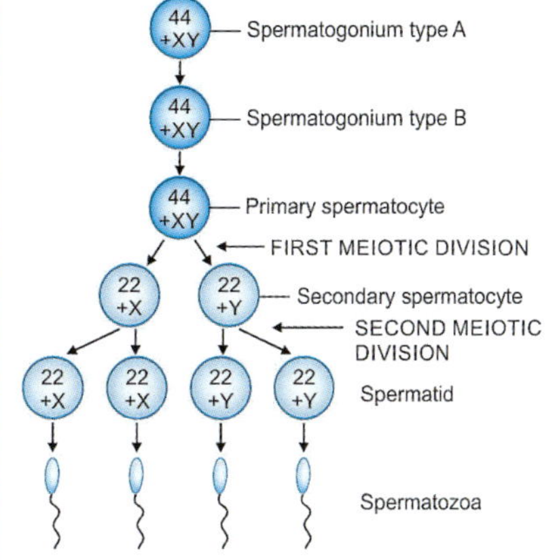 **Fig. 3:** Stages of spermatogenesis.	**Explanation:** Primary spermatocytes are diploid cells that arise from spermatogonia through mitotic division. The spermatozoa then develop through a process of meiosis so that eventually diploid spermatocytes get converted into four haploid spermatids. The spermatids eventually transform into spermatozoa by a process known as spermiogenesis. Testosterone, which plays an important role in the facilitation of spermatogenesis, is synthesized in the interstitial Leydig cells from where it diffuses into the seminiferous tubules. **Potential questions:** There can be questions pertaining to different stages of spermatogenesis.

Question	Answer	Comment
Q4. Identify the structure labeled A in the below image that surrounds the ovum and plays a key role in sperm binding during fertilization. 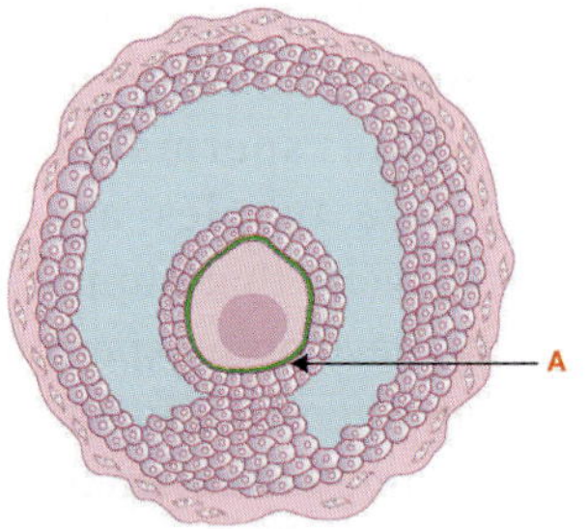 A. Zona pellucida B. Corona radiata C. Ooplasm D. Granulosa cells E. Cumulus oophorus	**Ans: A (Zona pellucida)** The ovum is a haploid cell with a nucleus (germinal vesicle) and cytoplasm (ooplasm). It is surrounded by a thick envelope, the zona pellucida, and covered by a layer of follicle-derived cells called the corona radiata, which remains attached even after the ovum is released **(Fig. 4)**. 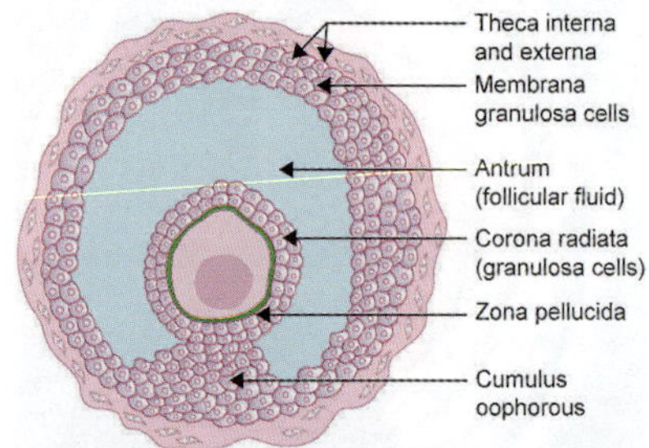 **Fig. 4:** Tertiary (Graafian follicle) showing structure of the female gamete (ovum).	**Explanation:** The zona pellucida is a glycoprotein-rich layer surrounding the ovum, which is crucial for sperm binding during fertilization. It acts as a barrier that ensures species-specific sperm attachment and triggers the acrosome reaction in sperm, allowing penetration. Once a sperm penetrates, the zona undergoes changes to prevent further sperm from binding, ensuring monospermy. On the other hand, cumulus oophorus is a cluster of cells surrounding the oocyte in the ovarian follicle, supporting and nourishing it as it matures and facilitating its release during ovulation. It connects the oocyte to the granulosa cells lining the follicle. **Potential questions:** There can be questions related to other structures related to the female gamete such as corona radiata, cumulus oophorus, etc.
Q5. The diagrammatic image of an ovary shown below is displaying follicles at various stages of maturation. Identify the stage at which the follicle marked as A is present in. An antrum is present in this follicle as seen in the image. 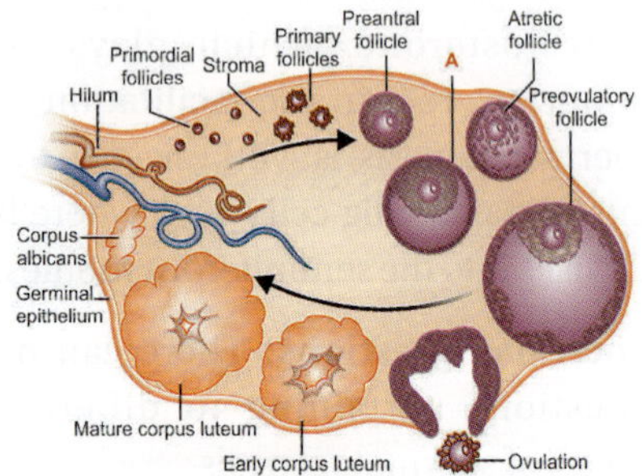 A. Primordial follicle B. Primary follicle C. Secondary follicle D. Graafian follicle E. Atretic follicle	**Ans: C (Secondary follicle)** Inside the ovary, various follicles are present in different stages of development (as shown in **Figure 5**). This may include primordial follicle, primary follicle, secondary/antral follicle, preantral follicle, preovulatory/Graafian follicle, etc. 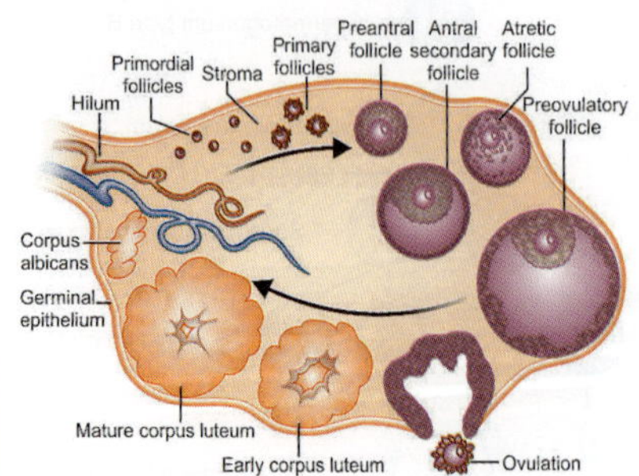 **Fig. 5:** Internal structure of an ovary.	**Explanation:** The secondary/antral follicle is characterized by the presence of a fluid-filled cavity known as the antrum. As the follicle matures from the primary stage, granulosa cells multiply, and the follicular fluid accumulates to form the antrum. The Graafian follicle also has an antrum, but it is larger and closer to ovulation. In contrast, primordial and primary follicles lack an antrum, and the atretic follicle represents a degenerated follicle. Out of the various developing follicles, only one single (preovulatory/Graafian) follicle is destined to develop into a dominant follicle, which eventually undergoes ovulation. **Potential questions:** There can be questions related to various stages of ovarian follicles as well as ovulation.

Question	Answer	Comment
Q6. A 22-year-old female presents with concerns about her fertility. During a discussion about oogenesis, the doctor explains the stages of oocyte development as described in the image below. Which of the following statements accurately describes a key event in the process of oogenesis? 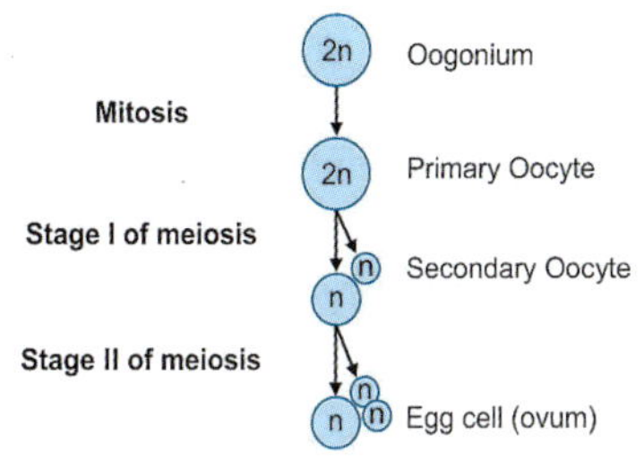 A. Primary oocytes are arrested in metaphase I until ovulation B. Oogonia undergo mitosis after birth to replenish the pool of oocytes C. Secondary oocytes complete meiosis II after fertilization D. Primary oocytes are arrested in prophase II until ovulation E. Meiosis I is completed before birth and meiosis II is completed before ovulation	**Ans: C (Secondary oocytes complete meiosis II after fertilization.)** Various stages of oogenesis are shown in **Figure 6**. The primordial germ cells, after arriving in the female gonad, differentiate into oogonia by around the 9th week of gestation. These enter the first meiotic division and are converted into primary oocytes. 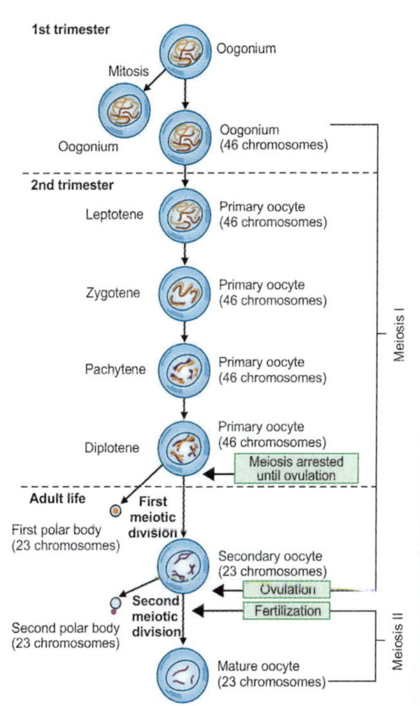 **Fig. 6:** Female gametogenesis (oogenesis).	**Explanation:** Oogenesis begins during fetal development, where oogonia differentiate into primary oocytes. These primary oocytes start meiosis I. However, in the last week before birth, all the primary oocytes get arrested in the diplotene stage of prophase. The primary oocytes remain arrested at this stage and do not undergo the completion of the first meiotic division till the age of puberty, when the completion of the first meiotic division occurs at the time of ovulation. The second meiotic division starts, but gets arrested in the metaphase, which is completed only at the time of fertilization, resulting in the formation of the ovum and the second polar body. **Potential questions:** There can be questions related to different steps of oogenesis.

DEVELOPMENT OF HUMAN EMBRYO

Question	Answer	Comment
Q7. What is the structure pointed by the arrow in the given figure? 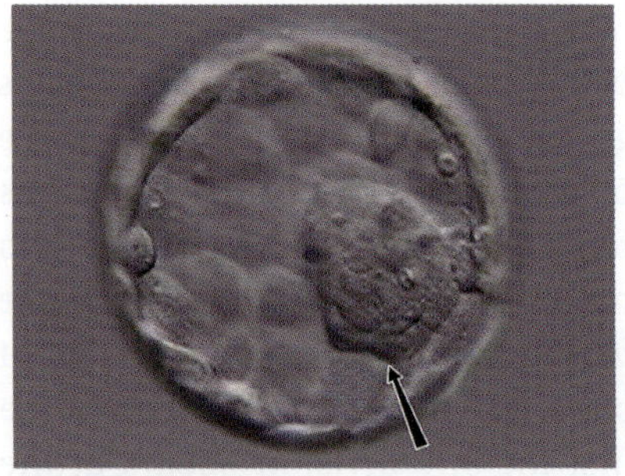 A. Trophoblast B. Amniocytes C. Polar body from zygote D. Inner cell mass E. Blastocyst cells	**Ans: D (Inner cell mass)** The arrow in the adjacent figure points toward the mass of cells known as the inner mass. The inner cell mass would eventually give rise to the definitive structures of the fetus. 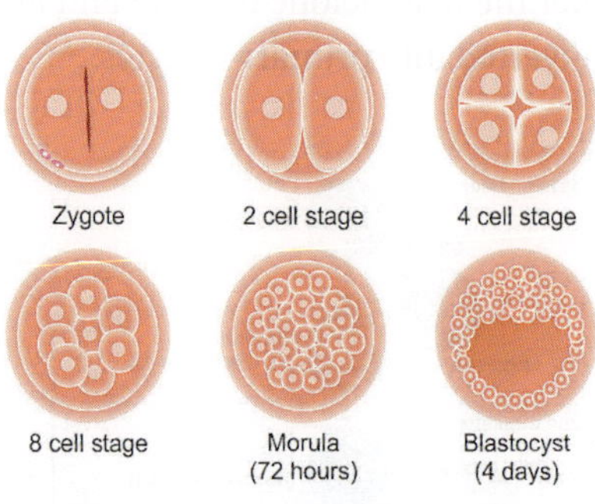 **Fig. 7:** Formation of blastocyst.	**Explanation:** Following the fertilization of the male and the female gametes, the zygote is formed. In the zygote, the cells continue to divide to form a morula. Fluid gradually accumulates between the morula's cells, transforming the morula into a blastocyst. Blastocyst gets transformed into two types of cells: Trophoblast cells and an inner cell mass at about 4th to 5th day of fertilization **(Fig. 7)**. While the trophoblast forms the future placenta, the inner cell mass is responsible for the formation of embryo proper. **Potential questions:** There could be potential questions pertaining to the structure of morula, blastocyst, and zygote.
Q8. The below diagram shows a 12-day-old blastocyst. Which of the following regions is represented by the arrow in the figure below? 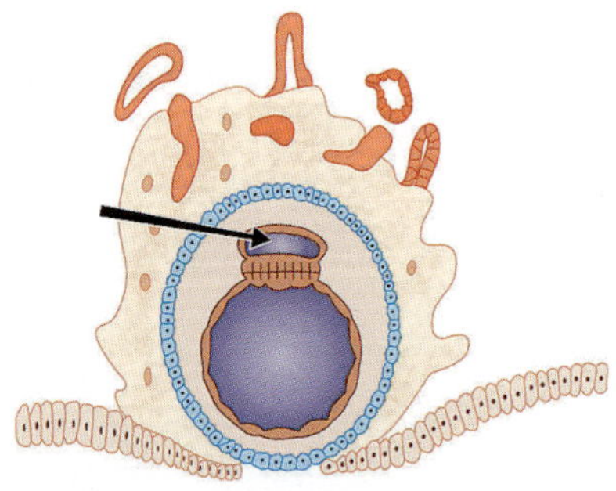 A. Allantois B. Yolk sac C. Amniotic cavity D. Chorionic cavity E. Extraembryonic coelom	**Ans: C (Amniotic cavity)** On the 12th day after fertilization, the blastocyst undergoes implantation. The changes occurring in the blastocyst during this stage **(Fig. 8)** set up the foundation for placental development and early embryonic growth. 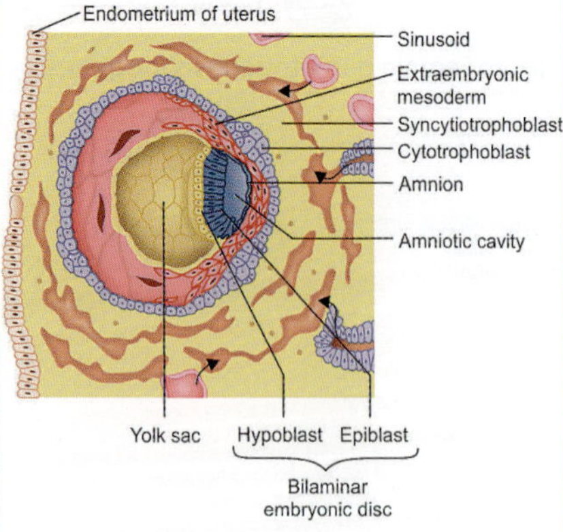 **Fig. 8:** Blastocyst at 12th day after fertilization.	**Explanation:** During this stage, the following changes occur in the blastocyst: Trophoblast differentiates into the cytotrophoblast and syncytiotrophoblast, with the latter invading the uterine wall. Lacunae form in the syncytiotrophoblast, which later develop into spaces for nutrient exchange. The inner cell mass forms the epiblast and hypoblast, with the amniotic cavity developing in the epiblast. The extraembryonic mesoderm forms between the cytotrophoblast and embryonic structures. The primary yolk sac, or primary umbilical vesicle, forms from proliferating hypoblast cells after implantation. **Potential questions:** There can be questions related to various structures present in the blastocyst at 12th day after fertilization.

Question	Answer	Comment
Q9. The below image is obtained from the intracytoplasmic sperm injection (ICSI) procedure. What is the structure represented by the arrows? 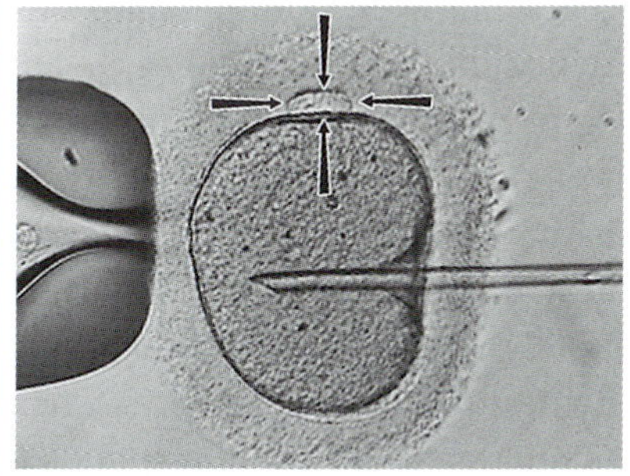 A. Oocyte B. First polar body C. Second polar body D. Cumulus oophorus E. Zona pellucida	**Ans: B (First polar body)** Changes occurring in the ovum following fertilization by a sperm are depicted in **Figure 9**. 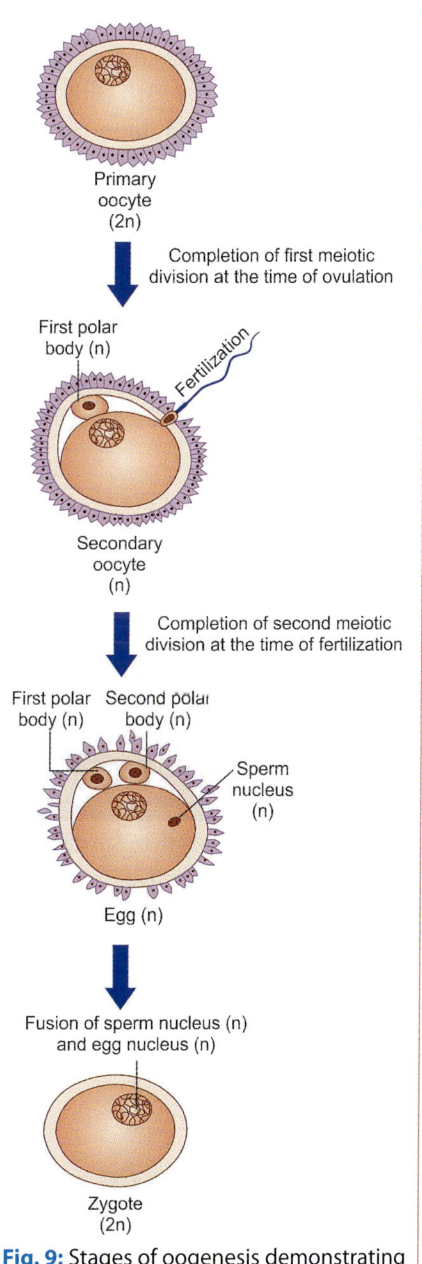 **Fig. 9:** Stages of oogenesis demonstrating the formation of polar bodies.	**Explanation:** The structure represented by the arrow in the given figure is the first polar body. In the last week before birth, all the primary oocytes get arrested in the diplotene stage of prophase. The primary oocytes remain arrested at this stage and do not undergo the completion of the first meiotic division till the age of puberty, when the completion of the first meiotic division occurs at the time of ovulation. The second meiotic division starts, but gets arrested in the metaphase, which is completed only at the time of fertilization. Since the figure in the above question is demonstrating the procedure of ICSI, where the sperm is injected into the ovum, the fertilization has yet not occurred. Therefore, the formation of the second polar body has not yet occurred. However, the first meiotic division has occurred, resulting in the formation of the first polar body. **Potential questions:** There can be questions related to changes occurring during various stages of oogenesis.

Question	Answer	Comment
Q10. A blastocyst has successfully travelled through the fallopian tube and has attached to the endometrium. It has now started penetrating into the endometrium as shown in the image below. Which of the following events occurs first during the process of implantation? 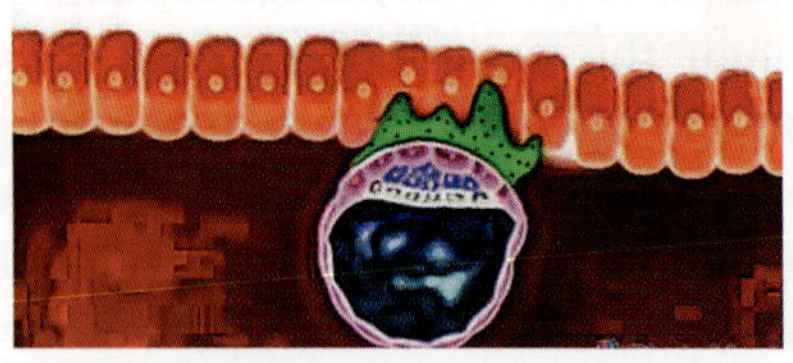 A. The trophoblast differentiates into cytotrophoblast and syncytiotrophoblast B. The blastocyst completely embeds into the endometrium by day 14 C. Decidual reaction begins in response to the invasion of syncytiotrophoblast D. The zona pellucida remains intact during implantation E. The inner cell mass differentiates into the epiblast and hypoblast before implantation	**Ans: A (The trophoblast differentiates into cytotrophoblast and syncytiotrophoblast)** Prior to implantation, the blastocyst starts getting attached to the surface endometrium. Attachment of the blastocyst to the surface endometrium occurs by 5th–6th day postfertilization. Implantation begins with the burrowing and penetration of the blastocyst into the endometrium, which occurs by about 6–7 days after fertilization. The most common site of implantation is upper posterior wall of the uterine cavity. Changes in the blastocyst by 4th to 5th day of implantation are depicted in **Figure 10**. 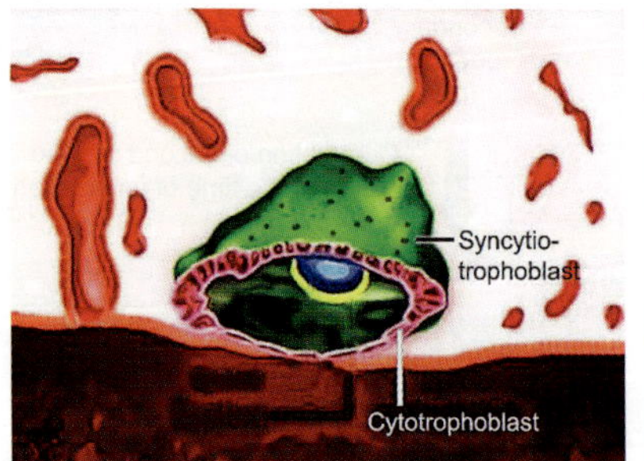 **Fig. 10:** Blastocyst at 4th to 5th day of implantation.	**Explanation:** During implantation, the trophoblast differentiates into two layers: Cytotrophoblast (inner) and syncytiotrophoblast (outer). During the process of implantation, this is the first key event which occurs. The syncytiotrophoblast then extends into the maternal tissue and begins the process of embedding the blastocyst. The zona pellucida disintegrates prior to implantation, allowing the blastocyst to attach directly to the endometrial lining. The decidual reaction follows, where the endometrial stroma responds to support the embryo. The inner cell mass eventually gets differentiated into a top layer: Ectoderm (epiblast) and an underlying layer of endoderm (hypoblast). **Potential questions:** There can be questions related to various structures developing in the blastocyst at the time of implantation and few days after implantation has occurred.

<table>
<tr><th>Question</th><th>Answer</th><th>Comment</th></tr>
<tr>
<td>

Q11. The image shown below demonstrates early stages of development around the 9th day post fertilization. Which structure forms the primary yolk sac?

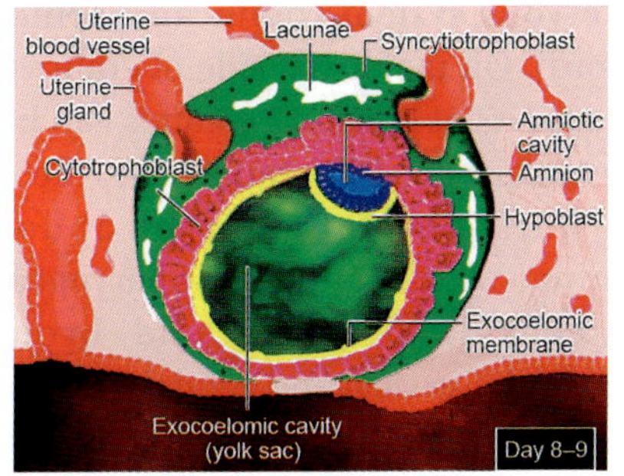

A. Hypoblast cells lining the blastocoel
B. Trophoblast layer
C. Amniotic cavity
D. Extraembryonic mesoderm
E. Syncytiotrophoblast

</td>
<td>

Ans: A (Hypoblast cells lining the blastocoel)

By the 9th day of implantation, the endodermal germ layer (hypoblast) produces additional cells which form a new cavity, known as the primary umbilical vesicle or definitive yolk sac. By the 10th day of implantation **(Fig. 11)**, small embryonic mesenchymal cells also start appearing as isolated cells within the cavity of blastocyst.

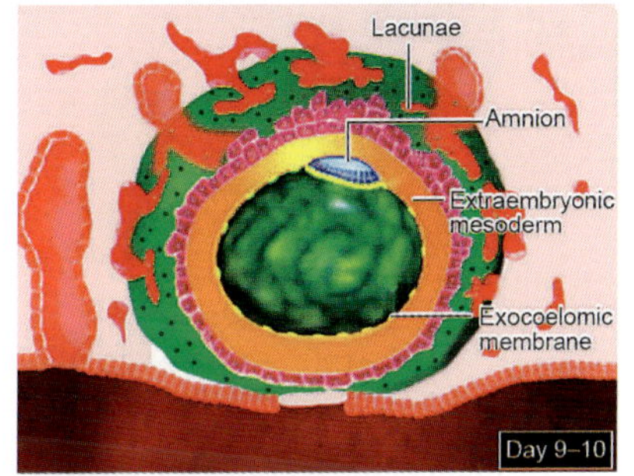

Fig. 11: Tenth day of implantation.

</td>
<td>

Explanation: The primary yolk sac forms when hypoblast cells migrate and line the inner surface of the blastocoel, creating a primitive structure known as the exocoelomic membrane. This will later contribute to the formation of the primary yolk sac. By the 9th day of implantation, the syncytiotrophoblast continues to expand into the surrounding endometrium. Lacunar spaces start appearing within the syncytiotrophoblast and these start filling with maternal blood. Also, during this period, primary villi start extending from the trophoblast into the surrounding endometrium.

Potential questions: There can be questions related to various structures developing in the blastocyst at the time of implantation and few days after implantation has occurred.

</td>
</tr>
<tr>
<td>

Q12. The image below shows the formation of extraembryonic mesoderm on the 11th day post implantation. Which of the following is formed after the extraembryonic mesoderm splits into two layers?

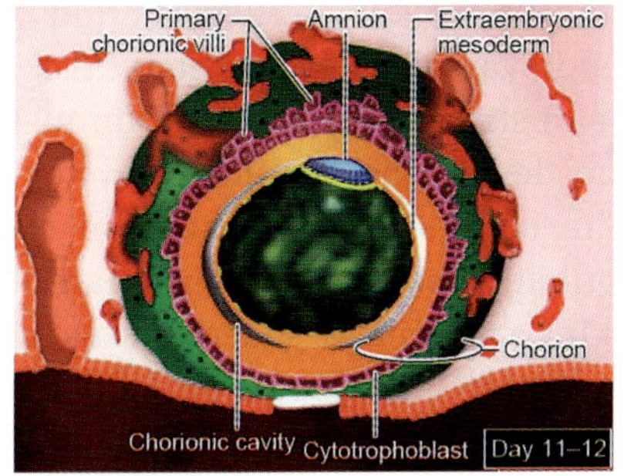

A. Amniotic cavity
B. Primary yolk sac
C. Secondary yolk sac
D. Chorionic cavity
E. Exocoelomic cavity

</td>
<td>

Ans: D (Chorionic cavity)

By the 10th day of implantation, small embryonic mesenchymal cells appear as isolated cells within the cavity of blastocyst. They soon line the cavity of blastocyst. When the blastocyst is completely lined with mesoderm, it is termed chorionic vesicle. By the 12th day of implantation, numerous small cavities appear within the extraembryonic mesoderm **(Fig. 12)**. These cavities soon become confluent and form the extraembryonic coelom or the chorionic cavity.

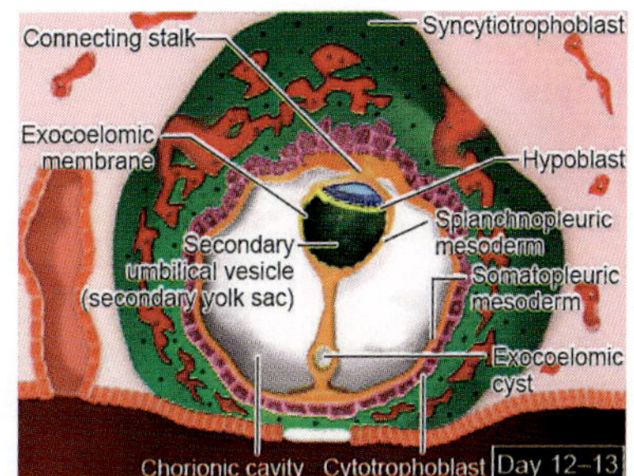

Fig. 12: Twelfth to thirteenth day of implantation.

</td>
<td>

Explanation: The extraembryonic coelom or the chorionic cavity splits extraembryonic mesoderm into two layers: (1) Extraembryonic somatopleuric mesoderm, lining the trophoblast and amnion, and (2) extraembryonic splanchnopleuric mesoderm, covering the yolk sac. The chorionic cavity surrounds the amniotic cavity and yolk sac and plays a vital role in establishing the connection between the embryo and the trophoblast. With the development of extraembryonic coelom, the yolk sac becomes much smaller and is known as the secondary yolk sac.

Potential questions: There can be questions related to various structures developing in the blastocyst at the time of implantation and few days after implantation has occurred.

</td>
</tr>
</table>

Question	Answer	Comment
Q13. The image below shows an embryo during the 3rd to 4th week of development. Which of the following is the most prominent feature seen during this stage? 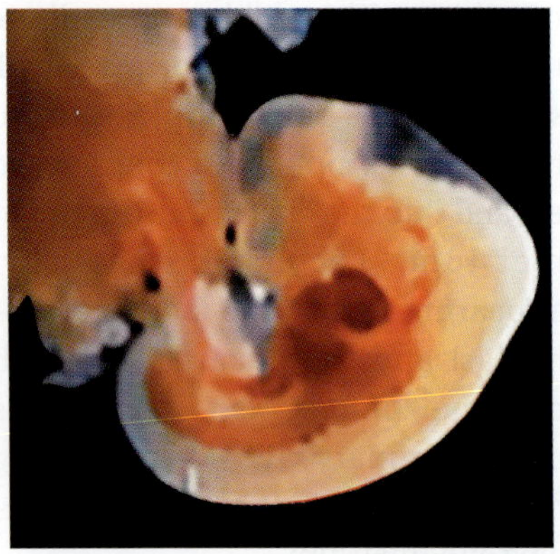 A. Formation of the limb buds B. Development of the neural tube C. Appearance of the heart chambers D. Closure of the oropharyngeal membrane E. Formation of the somites	**Ans: B (Development of the neural tube)** As the embryo grows, there is enlargement of the amniotic cavity, resulting in progressive reduction in the size of extraembryonic coelom. Structures present in the embryo at 4 weeks of development are depicted in **Figure 13**. 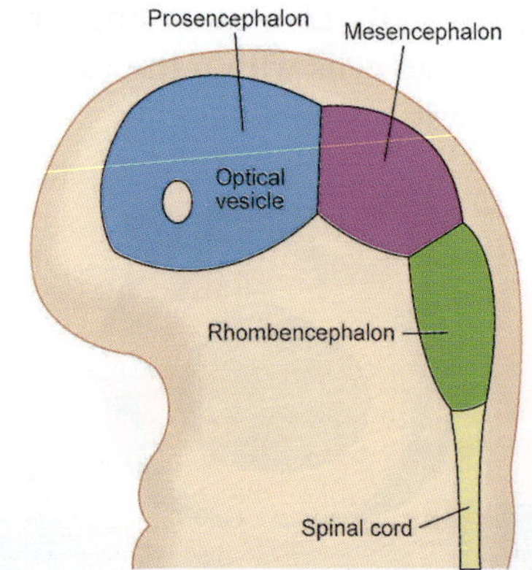 **Fig. 13:** Brain of the embryo at 4 weeks of development.	**Explanation:** During the 3rd to 4th week of embryo development, the most significant process is the formation and closure of the neural tube, which will give rise to the central nervous system (brain and spinal cord). On the dorsal side of embryo, contours of first 4–12 somites can be recognized. At the same time, there occurs development of abdominal wall and first two pharyngeal arches (mandibular and hyoid arches). Cervical and caudal flexures appear in the embryo, which give it a characteristic C-shape. The heart and limb buds develop later in the 5th–6th weeks. Closure of oro-pharyngeal membrane occurs after neural tube formation. **Potential questions:** There can be questions related to the development of important milestones at different stages of fetal development.
Q14. The image below shows an embryo at 5–6 weeks' gestation. Which key feature of development would be visible during this stage? 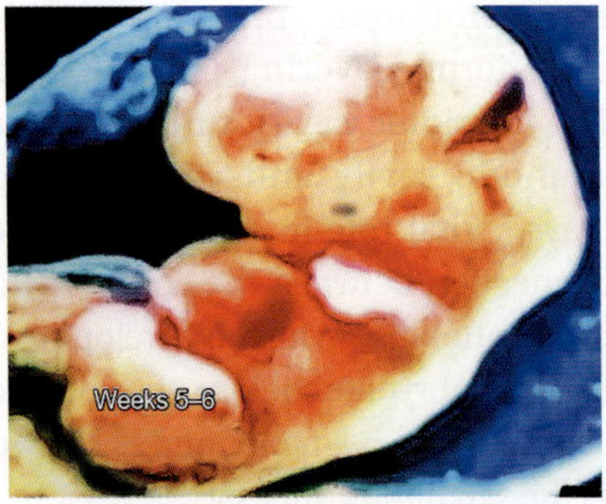 A. Formation of limb buds B. Closure of the neural tube C. Appearance of the primitive heartbeat D. Formation of the optic vesicle E. Development of pharyngeal arches	**Ans: C (Appearance of the primitive heartbeat)** In the early stages, the embryo acquires the form of three-layered disc or germ layers; from outside to inward, they are: Ectoderm, mesoderm, and endoderm. Structures present in the embryo at 6 weeks of development are depicted in **Figure 14**. 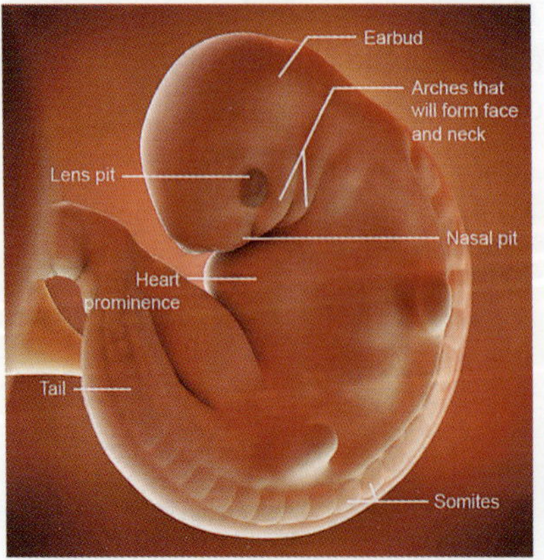 **Fig. 14:** Appearance of embryo at about 6 weeks of gestation.	**Explanation:** At 5–6 weeks of gestation, the embryo's heart begins to beat, which is one of the earliest detectable signs of life in the embryo. This is a crucial period of cardiovascular development, as the heart starts pumping blood through the developing circulatory system. The ectoderm also results in the formation of nails, tooth, enamel, skin, and hair. Mesoderm forms the heart, circulatory system, cartilage, bone, etc. Limb buds and other features like the optic vesicle begin to form around this time. **Potential questions:** There can be questions related to the development of important milestones at different stages of fetal development.

Question	Answer	Comment
Q15. The image below shows an embryo at the 7th week of development. What is the most significant structural change occurring during this period? 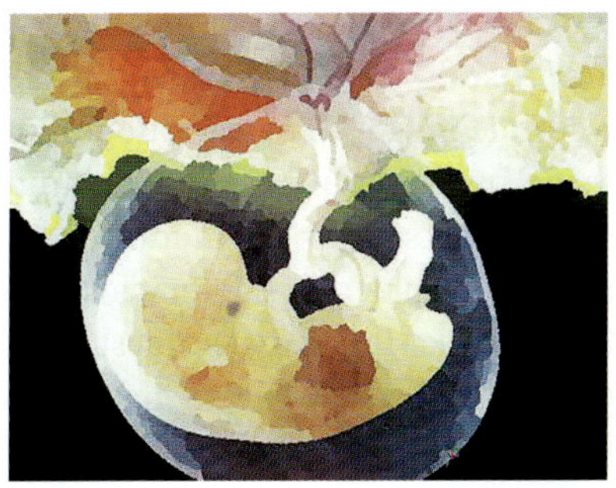 A. Formation of the external genitalia B. Fusion of the palatal shelves C. Formation of digital rays in the limbs D. Development of the lungs E. Rotation of the intestines into the umbilical cord	**Ans: C (Formation of digital rays in the limbs)** By the 7th week of development, the limb buds start growing, the mouth opening appears, and the inner ear is formed. During this period of development, the digestive tract starts developing and the organs such as lungs, liver, pancreas, and thyroid glands are formed. Structures present in the embryo at 7 weeks of development are depicted in **Figure 15**. 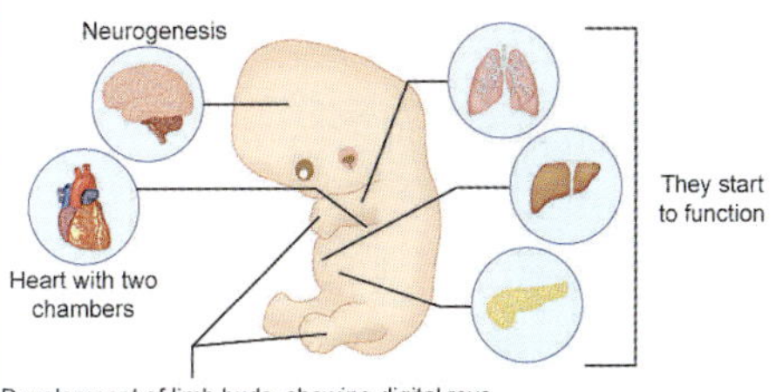 **Fig. 15:** Appearance of embryo at about 7 weeks of gestation.	**Explanation:** By the 7th week, the embryo's limbs begin to show digital rays, which are the early outlines of fingers and toes. This is a critical event during this week. The external genitalia and palatal fusion occur later, while lung development starts earlier but continues throughout gestation. The intestinal rotation begins but is more prominent by the 8th to 10th weeks. By the end of 9th week, formation of fingers and toes is almost complete. **Potential questions:** There can be questions related to the development of important milestones at different stages of fetal development.
Q16. The below image shows a 12-week-old embryo. Which of the following changes is expected by this stage? 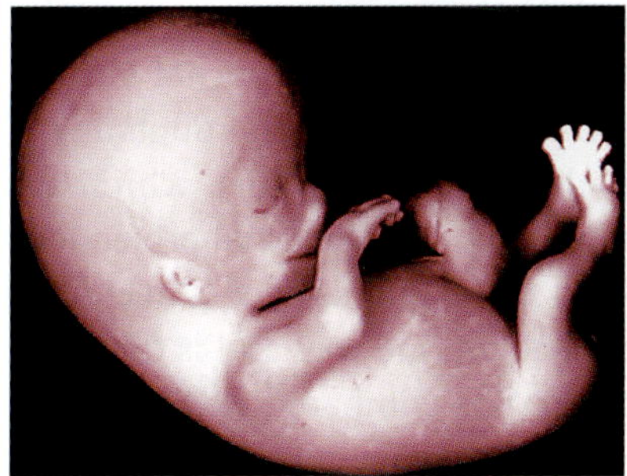 A. External genitalia are distinguishable B. Neural tube is formed C. Lung alveoli are functional D. First heart chambers are developing E. Limbs are forming as buds	**Ans: A (External genitalia are distinguishable)** During the 12th week of gestation, the fetus becomes about 6 cm in size and starts moving spontaneously. By 12 weeks of gestation, fetal sex can also be distinguished. The fetus now starts resembling the baby's face. The fetal heart can be heard using a Doppler ultrasound. Structures present in the embryo at 12 weeks of development are depicted in **Figure 16**. 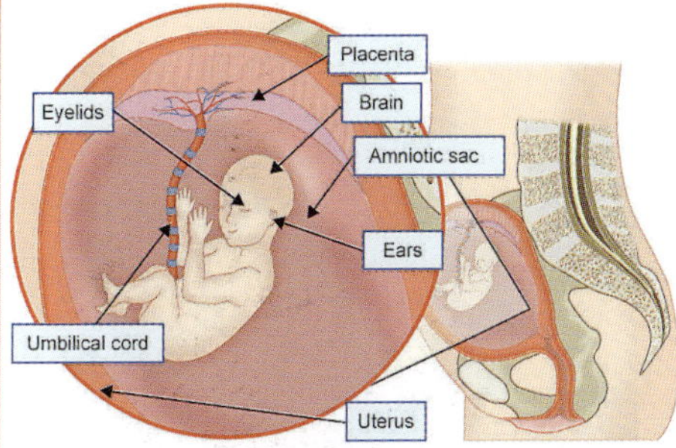 **Fig. 16:** Appearance of embryo at about 12 weeks of gestation.	**Explanation:** By the 12th week of development, the external genitalia can be differentiated, though they are not fully developed. The neural tube forms much earlier, and lung alveoli develop much later in pregnancy. Heart chambers start forming in earlier weeks, and limb buds appear around the 4th week. By 12 weeks, the number of fetal fingers and toes can be counted. The baby's fingers and toenails also appear during this time. The pancreas starts functioning and producing insulin. Since the baby's brain has started developing during this time, it can feel pain. **Potential questions:** There can be questions related to the development of important milestones at different stages of fetal development.

Question	Answer	Comment
Q17. The image below shows a fetus at 20 weeks' gestation. Which of the following developmental features is most likely to be observed? 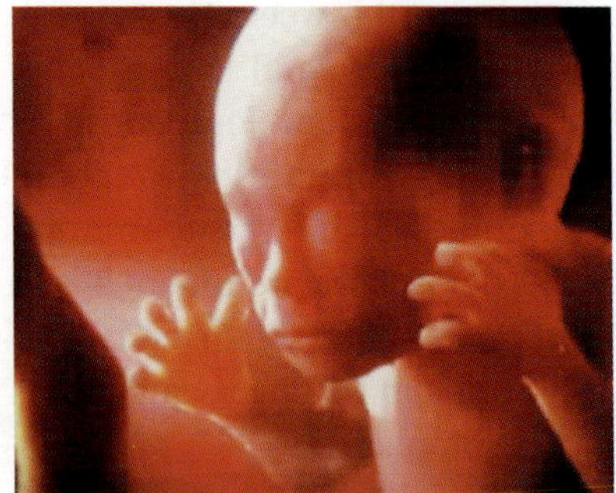 A. Fetal heartbeat is detectable using a Doppler ultrasound B. Eyelids are open C. Kidneys have begun producing urine D. The lungs have started producing surfactant E. The fetus exhibits spontaneous movements	**Ans: E (The fetus exhibits spontaneous movements)** By 20 weeks of pregnancy, the mother is likely to start perceiving the fetal movements. The growth of hair begins on the rest of the body. The skin starts getting thicker and development of various sense organs starts occurring. 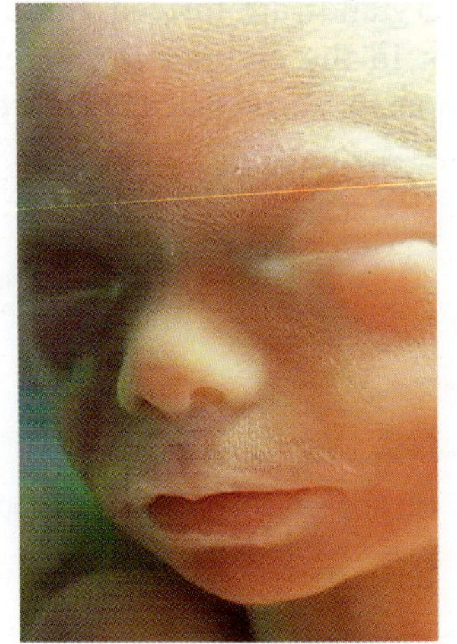 **Fig. 17:** Face of the fetus as seen at 20 weeks of gestation.	**Explanation:** At 20 weeks, the fetus is active, with spontaneous movements noticeable on ultrasound. Fetal heartbeat can be detected much earlier (around 8–12 weeks) through Doppler ultrasound. Eyelids are fused shut until around 26 weeks **(Fig. 17)**. The production of urine by the kidneys starts around 9–12 weeks, and surfactant production begins much later, closer to 24–28 weeks. By 20 weeks of gestation, the baby is also able to hear and recognize the mother's voice. Until 20 weeks of gestation, the baby's crown-rump length is measured, following which the baby's crown-heel length is measured. **Potential questions:** There can be questions related to the development of important milestones at different stages of fetal development.

DEVELOPMENT OF PLACENTA

Question	Answer	Comment
Q18. An image shows the maternal surface of the placenta post delivery. Which of the following is a common feature found on this surface? 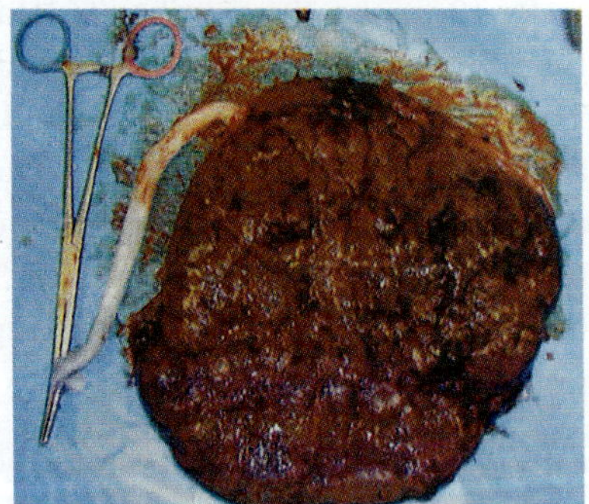 A. Amniotic membrane on surface B. Radiating umbilical cord vessels C. Cotyledons separated by septa D. Presence of Wharton's jelly E. Shiny, smooth appearance	**Ans: C (Cotyledons separated by septa)** **Figure 18** shows the maternal surface of placenta. The placental cotyledons are visible on the maternal side of the placenta. 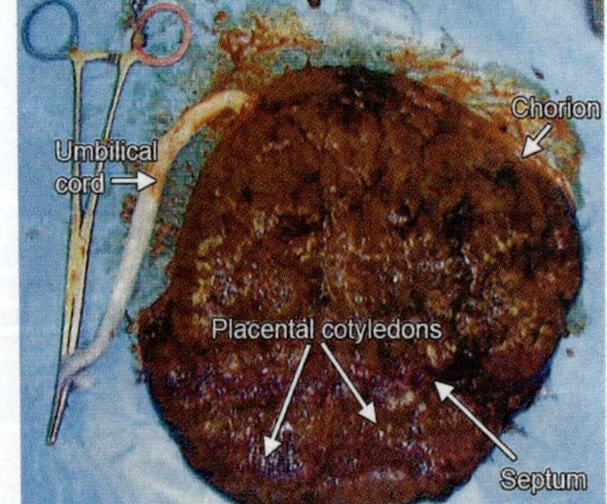 **Fig. 18:** Maternal surface of placenta.	**Explanation:** The maternal surface of the placenta appears rough and is divided into cotyledons, which are separated by endometrial projections called septa. This surface is in contact with the uterine wall and is darker in appearance compared to the smooth fetal surface covered by the amniotic membrane. The central umbilical cord attachment is typically seen on the fetal side of the placenta. **Potential questions:** There can be questions related to different structures present on both the maternal and fetal surface of placenta.

Question	Answer	Comment
Q19. An image of the fetal surface of the placenta is presented. Which of the following best describes the membrane covering this surface? 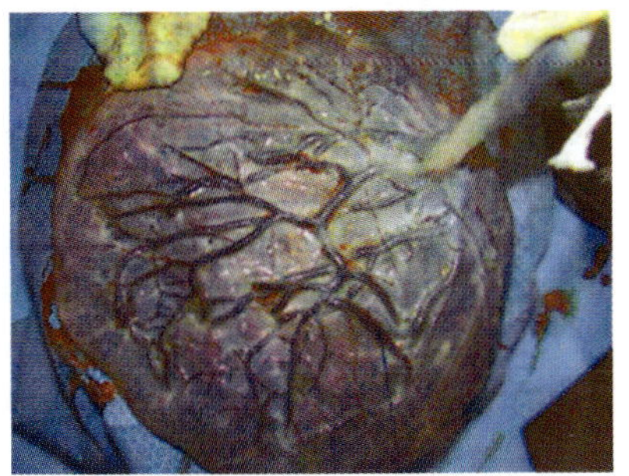 A. Decidua basalis B. Amnion C. Chorion D. Yolk sac E. Decidua capsularis	**Ans: B (Amnion)** **Figure 19** shows the fetal surface of placenta. On the fetal side, the placenta shows a flat surface due to the presence of a smooth and transparent membrane, the amnion. 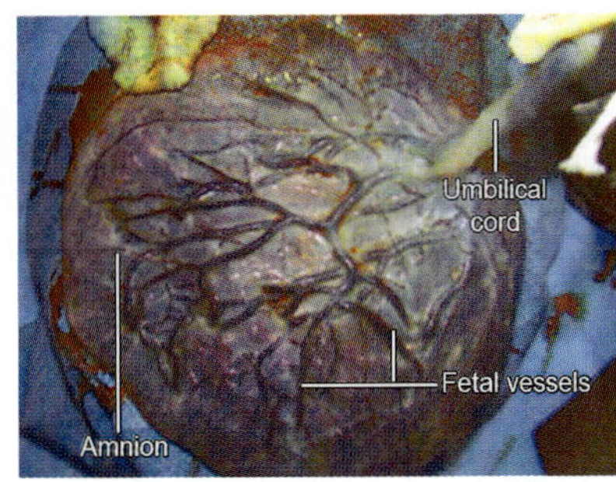 **Fig. 19:** Fetal surface of placenta.	**Explanation:** The amnion provides a protective barrier and is responsible for containing the amniotic fluid surrounding the fetus. Another membrane, called chorion, is located on the fetal surface of the placenta, directly beneath the amnion, which forms the outermost layer covering the placenta on the fetal side. The umbilical cord is attached at the center of the fetal surface of placenta. **Potential questions:** There can be questions related to different structures present on both the maternal and fetal surface of placenta.
Q20. The image below displays cross-section of the uterine wall during early pregnancy. Which type of decidua labeled as "C" is directly involved in the maternal-fetal exchange and forms part of the placenta? 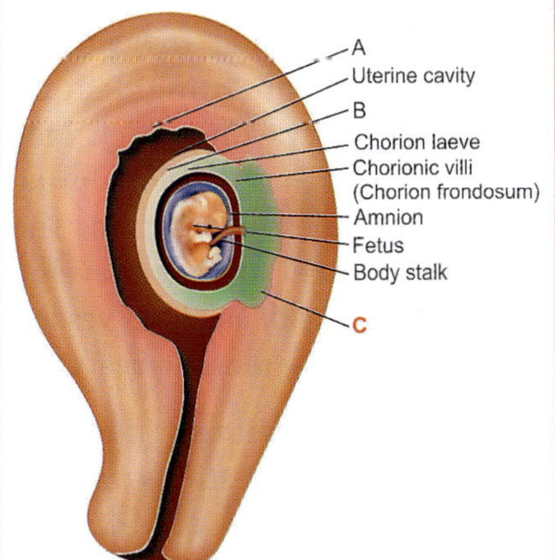 A. Decidua basalis B. Decidua parietalis C. Decidua capsularis D. Decidua marginalis E. Decidua vera	**Ans: (A) Decidua basalis** Following implantation, the syncytiotrophoblast starts secreting the hormone human chorionic gonadotropin (hCG). Under the influence of this hormone, the cells of endometrial lining are converted into specialized cells, known as the decidua. This reaction is known as decidual reaction and the endometrium is known as decidua. Different portions of decidua are shown in **Figure 20**. By the 10th day of implantation, the blastocyst completely penetrates below the surface of decidua. 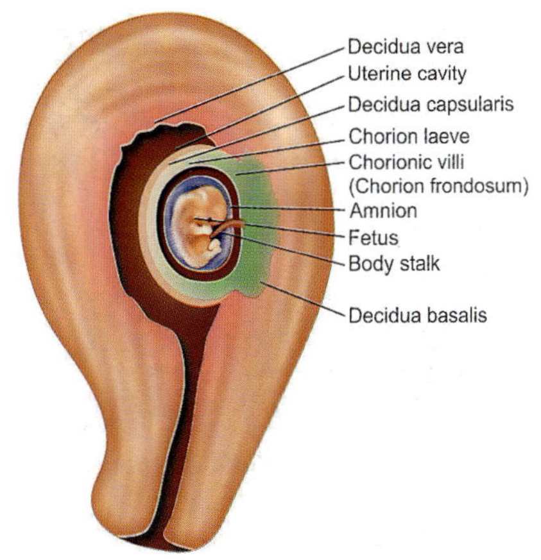 **Fig. 20:** Process of decidua formation.	**Explanation:** The decidua at this stage can be classified into three portions. The decidua basalis is the portion of the decidua that is in direct contact with the chorionic villi and plays an important role in forming the maternal part of the placenta, supporting the exchange of nutrients and gases between mother and fetus. The decidua lying over the surface of the implanted blastocyst is the decidua capsularis, and the remainder of the decidua lining the inside of the uterus is the decidua vera. **Potential questions:** There can be questions pertaining to any of the different portions of decidua.

Question	Answer	Comment
Q21. Blood circulation in the umbilical cord is shown in the image below. Which of the following statements correctly describes the circulation in the umbilical cord? 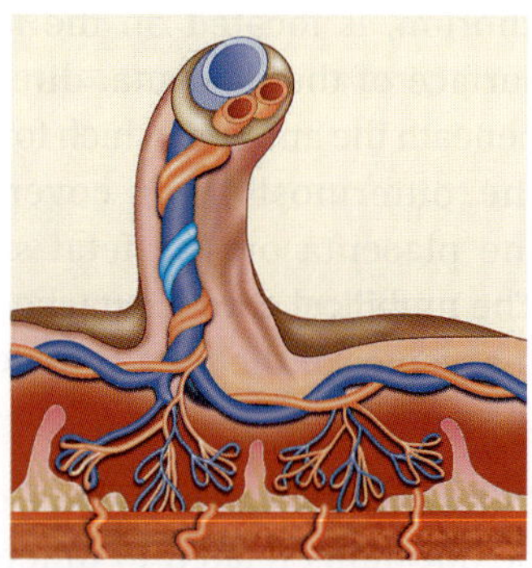 A. One artery, two veins B. Two arteries, one vein C. Two veins, two arteries D. One artery, one vein E. Three arteries, no veins	**Ans: B (Two arteries, one vein)** The anatomical structure of the umbilical cord is shown in **Figure 21**. The umbilical cord contains two umbilical arteries and one umbilical vein. 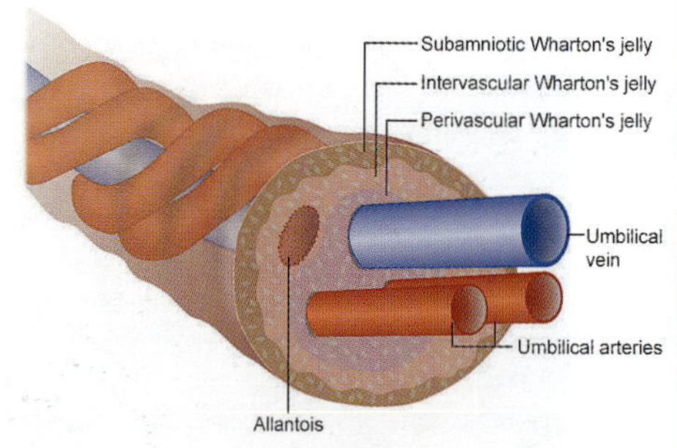 **Fig. 21:** Anatomical structure of the umbilical cord.	**Explanation:** In the umbilical cord, the umbilical arteries carry deoxygenated blood from the fetus to the placenta, while the vein carries oxygenated blood from the placenta to the fetus. This unique arrangement ensures that the fetus receives oxygen and nutrients necessary for development. Umbilical arteries are the only arteries in the body which carry deoxygenated blood and umbilical veins are the only veins in the body carrying oxygenated blood. **Potential questions:** There can be questions related to functions and various structures present in the umbilical cord.
Q22. Identify the stage of placental villi development shown in the image below. 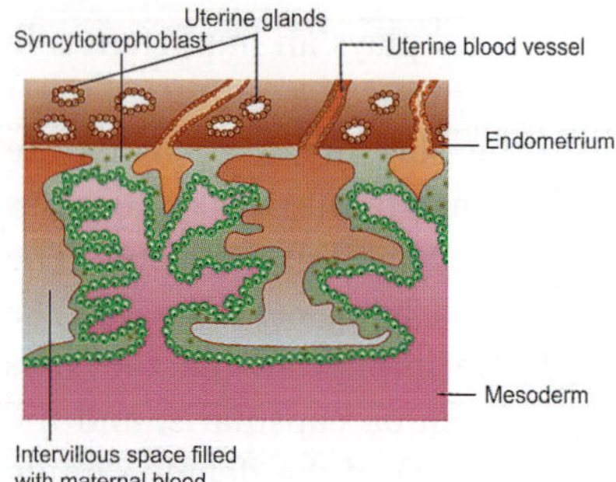 A. Primary villi B. Tertiary villi C. Mature villi D. Secondary villi E. Anchoring villi	**Ans: D (Secondary villi)** The development of chorionic villi passes through three stages: Primary, secondary, and finally tertiary. Primaryvilliprogressto secondary villi, which then progress to tertiary villi. **Figure 22** illustrates development of placental villi in these three stages. Primary villi comprises solid villi composed of cytotrophoblast core, which is surrounded by syncytium. In tertiary villi, there is occurrence of angiogenesis in the mesenchymal core of secondary villi. 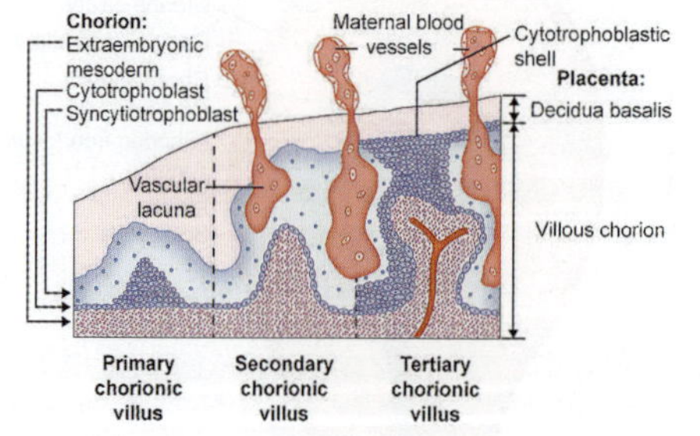 **Fig. 22:** Development of three stages of placental villi.	**Explanation:** Secondary placental villi are characterized by the invasion of extraembryonic mesoderm into the core of the primary villi, forming a loose connective tissue core. This mesodermal invasion is a key differentiating feature from primary villi, which lack mesoderm. They develop during the third week of gestation. The secondary villi will later develop into tertiary villi as blood vessels form within the mesodermal core. **Potential questions:** There can be different questions related to the structure of different types of placental villi: Primary, secondary, and tertiary.

Question	Answer	Comment
Q23. Identify the type of placentation shown in the image below. 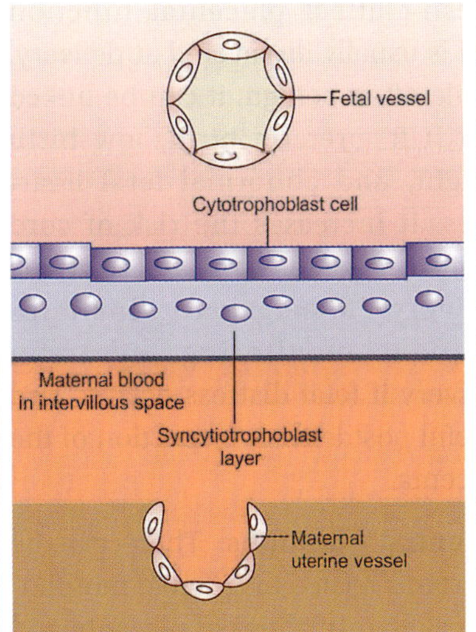 A. Epitheliochorial B. Endotheliochorial C. Hemochorial D. Syndesmochorial E. Hemotrophic	**Ans: C (Hemochorial)** In hemochorial placenta, the word "hemo" stands for maternal blood, which directly bathes the lacunae present in syncytiotrophoblast. On the other hand, the word "chorio" stands for chorion placenta, which in turn is separated from fetal blood by the endothelial lining of fetal capillaries that traverse the villous core. 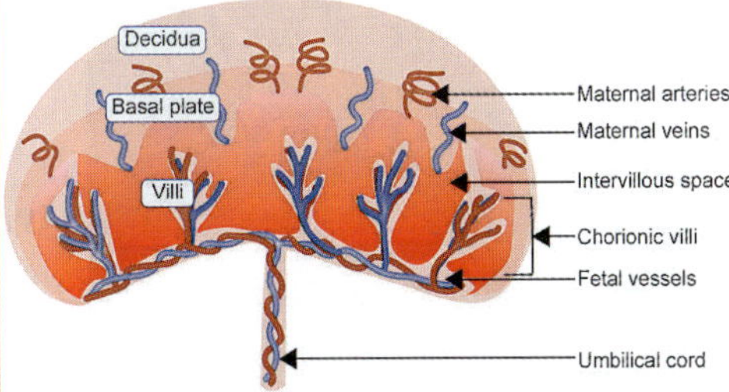 **Fig. 23:** Maternal circulation in the human placenta.	**Explanation:** The hemochorial placenta is characterized by direct contact between maternal blood and the chorionic villi of the fetus **(Fig. 23)**. This type of placentation is seen in humans, monkeys, and some other primates. In the hemochorial placenta, the trophoblast cells invade the maternal endometrium and erode the maternal blood vessels, allowing maternal blood to bathe the chorionic villi directly. This facilitates efficient exchange of nutrients, gases, and waste products between the mother and the fetus. **Potential questions:** There can be different questions related to the placental physiology and different types of placental villi: Primary, secondary, and tertiary.
Q24. Identify the abnormality in the placenta shown in the image below. 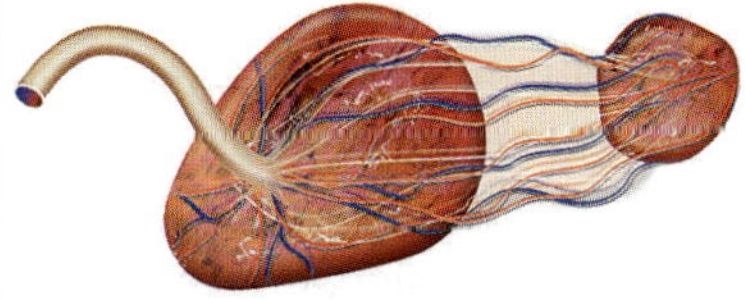 A. Circumvallate placenta B. Placenta previa C. Succenturiate lobe D. Placenta accreta E. Bilobed placenta	**Ans: C (Succenturiate lobe)** Succenturiate lobe can be identified on ultrasound as two separate placental masses without bridging placental tissue between them. As shown in **Figure 24**, there is rolling and shouldering of the placental margins on ultrasound examination. Also, the chorionic plate (fetal surface) is smaller than the basal plate (surface interacting with the uterus). 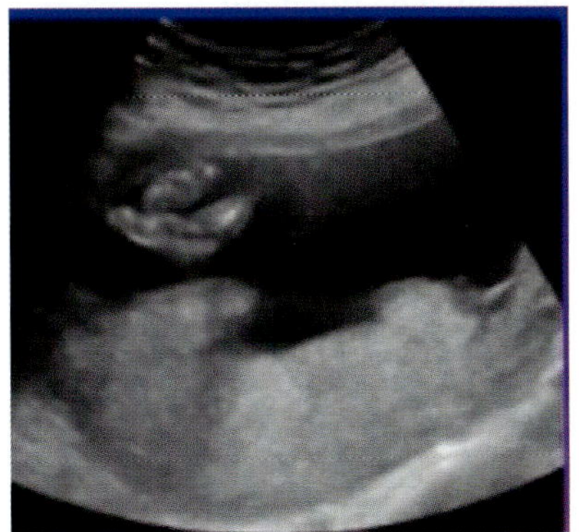 **Fig. 24:** Ultrasound image in case of the succenturiate lobe of placenta.	**Explanation:** As shown in the adjacent diagram, the main part of placenta is connected to one or more accessory lobes (which are smaller than the main lobe) through blood vessels. This morphological anomaly of placenta is known as the succenturiate lobe. Presence of the succenturiate lobe of placenta is not associated with an increased risk of fetal anomalies. It can, however, increase the risk of complications such as vasa previa, retained placenta, and postpartum hemorrhage. Rupture of the connecting vessels at the time of labor may result in fetal death. Proper antenatal diagnosis and management are important for ensuring maternal and fetal safety during delivery. **Potential questions:** There can be questions related to different abnormalities of placenta and umbilical cord

Question	Answer	Comment
Q25. Identify the abnormality in the placenta shown in the image below. 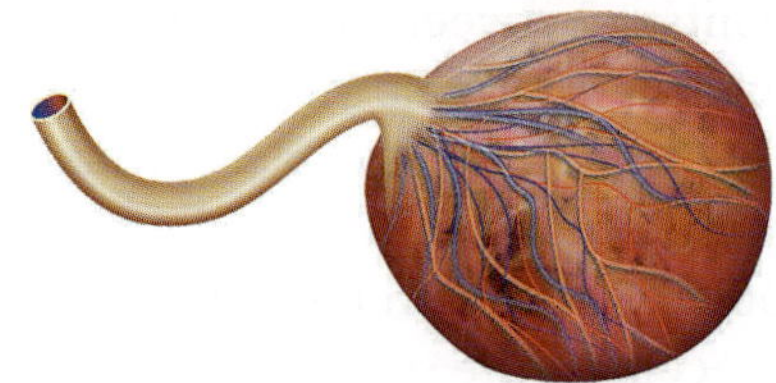 A. Velamentous cord insertion B. Circumvallate placenta C. Battledore placenta D. Placenta accreta E. Bilobed placenta	**Ans: C (Battledore placenta)** The adjacent image shows a morphological anomaly of placenta where the umbilical cord is attached to the placental edge. This type of placenta is known as the battledore placenta and can be identified on ultrasound as cord attachment within 2 cm of the placental margin **(Fig. 25)**. 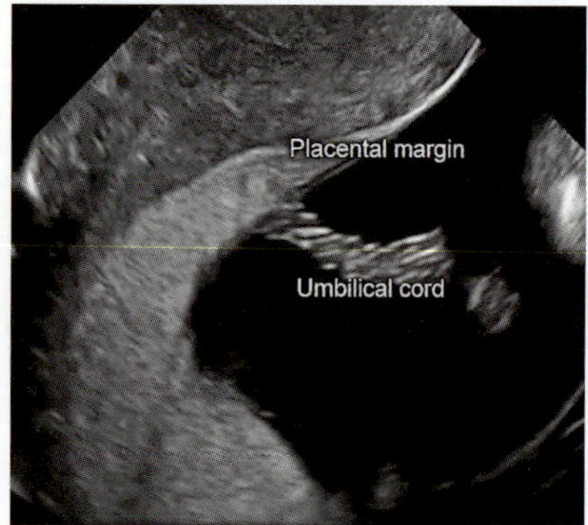 **Fig. 25:** Battledore placenta.	**Explanation:** Battledore placenta is a rare placental abnormality that doesn't affect placental function and is usually discovered at delivery. While often benign, it can be linked to IUGR, preterm birth, low birth weight, and abnormal fetal heart rates. It increases the risk of cord rupture and massive PPH during delivery. Management includes frequent monitoring, cesarean delivery if fetal distress occurs, and careful postdelivery inspection of the placenta. **Potential questions:** There can be questions related to different morphological abnormalities of placenta and umbilical cord.
Q26. Identify the abnormality in the umbilical cord shown in the image below. 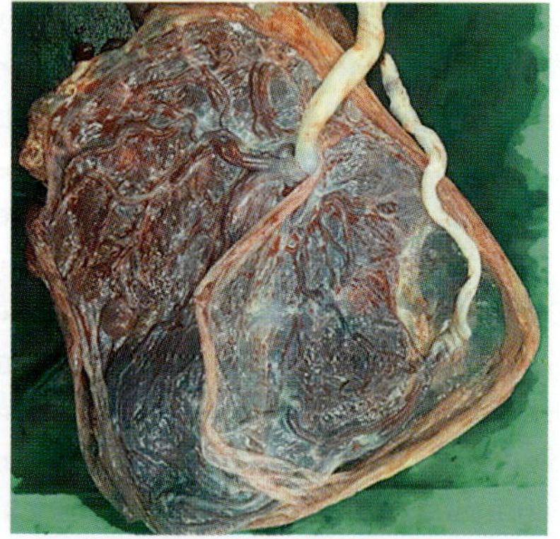 A. Marginal cord insertion B. Velamentous cord insertion C. Circumvallate placenta D. Battledore placenta E. Placenta previa	**Ans: B (Velamentous cord insertion)** The adjacent image shows the velamentous cord insertion. This condition can be identified on ultrasound by the presence of membranous vessels at the placental insertion site on ultrasound **(Fig. 26)**. Ultrasound is able to accurately diagnose these cases in the second trimester, with a specificity of 100%. In these cases, presence of vasa previa must be ruled out. 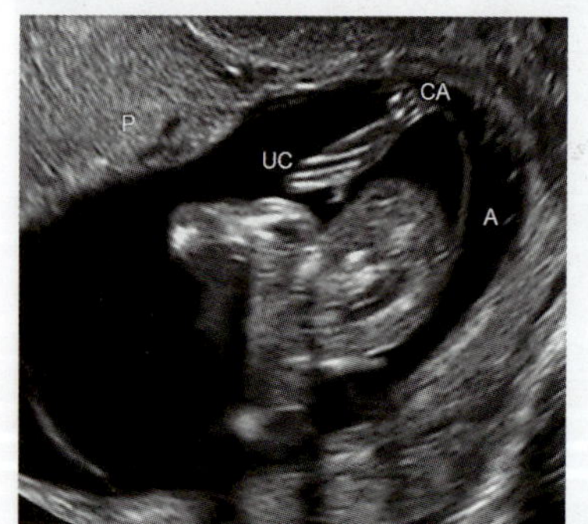 **Fig. 26:** Transvaginal scan showing the umbilical cord attached to the amnion. (A: amnion; UC: umbilical cord; CA: cord insertion into the amnion; P: placenta)	**Explanation:** Velamentous cord insertion occurs when the umbilical cord inserts into the fetal membranes and travels within them to the placenta. The exposed vessels are at risk of rupture, particularly if near the cervical os (vasa previa). This condition is linked to risks such as fetal growth restriction, preterm birth, and increased perinatal morbidity and mortality. Close fetal monitoring is required in the third trimester, and elective cesarean delivery is recommended if vasa previa is present to prevent fetal death. **Potential questions:** There can be questions related to different morphological abnormalities of placenta and umbilical cord.

ORGANOGENESIS

Question	Answer	Comment
Q27. In a clinical image showing the development of female internal genitalia from the paramesonephric ducts, which of the following structures is derived from these ducts? 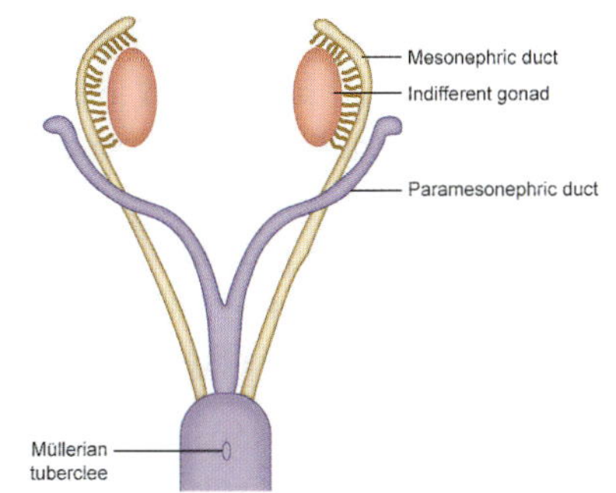 A. Ureter B. Fallopian tubes C. Prostate gland D. Epididymis E. Seminiferous tubules	**Ans: B (Fallopian tubes)** Differentiation of Müllerian ducts occurs in a cephalocaudal direction to form the female internal genital organs. In females, due to the absence of Müllerian inhibiting substance (MIS), produced by the Sertoli cells of testis, Müllerian ducts develop passively to form the female internal genitalia which includes fallopian tubes, uterus, and upper vagina **(Fig. 27)**. 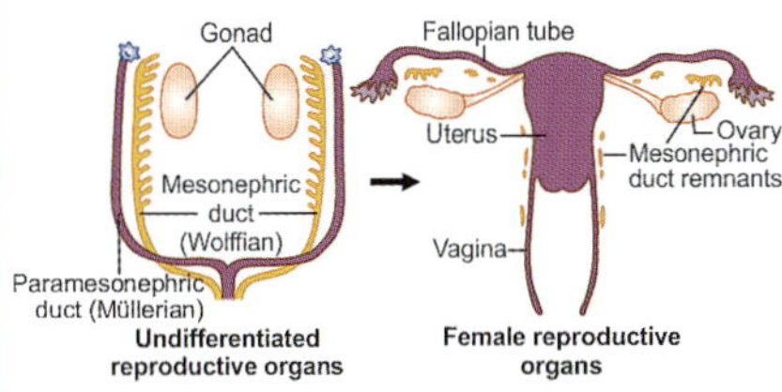 **Fig. 27:** Development of female internal genitalia from paramesonephric ducts.	**Explanation:** The paramesonephric (Müllerian) ducts give rise to key female internal genitalia, including the fallopian tubes, uterus, and the upper portion of the vagina. These ducts are essential for the development of female internal genitalia. On the other hand, the male internal genitalia (epididymis, seminal vesicles, and vas deferens) arises from the mesonephric (Wolffian) ducts under the influence of testosterone produced by the Leydig cells of testis. **Potential questions:** There can be questions related to the embryological origin of the various structures comprising the female internal as well as external genitalia.
Q28. Identify the structures derived from the genital tubercle, urethral folds, and genital swellings in the image below. 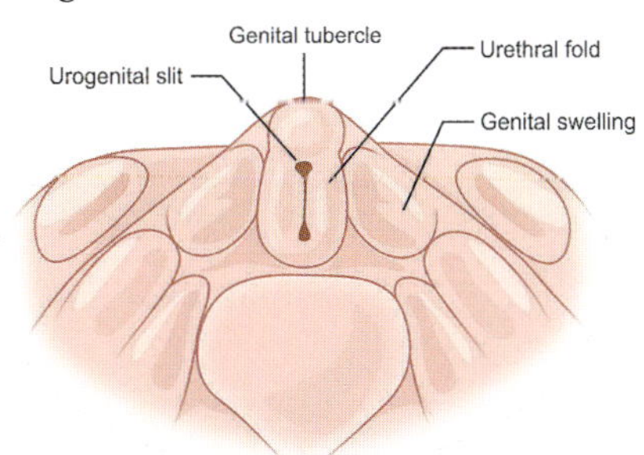 A. Clitoris, labia minora, and labia majora B. Urethra, labia minora, and labia majora C. Clitoris, urethra, and labia majora D. Clitoris, labia minora, and vestibule E. Urethra, clitoris, and labia minora	**Ans: A (Clitoris, labia minora, and labia majora)** In females in the absence of masculinizing effect of dihydrotestosterone, the undifferentiated external genitalia develop along the female lines, resulting in the formation of female external genitalia as shown in **Figure 28.** 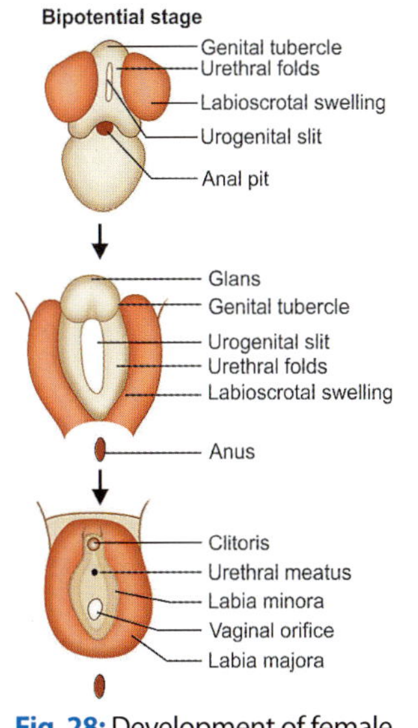 **Fig. 28:** Development of female external genitalia.	**Explanation:** External genitalia persist in a bipotential state until 9 weeks of gestation at which time it consists of a genital tubercle, urogenital sinus (UGS), and lateral labioscrotal folds or swellings. Dihydrotestosterone, produced by the testes, determines the development of male external genitalia. In its absence in females, the genital tubercle elongates slightly to form the clitoris. The urethral folds do not fuse and instead form the labia minora. The genital swellings or the labioscrotal folds also do not fuse and develop into the labia majora. **Potential questions:** There can be questions related to the embryological origin of the various structures comprising the female internal as well as external genitalia.

Question	Answer	Comment
Q29. A clinical image shows the embryonic development stages of the female genital tract. Based on the image, what is the correct embryological origin of the vagina? 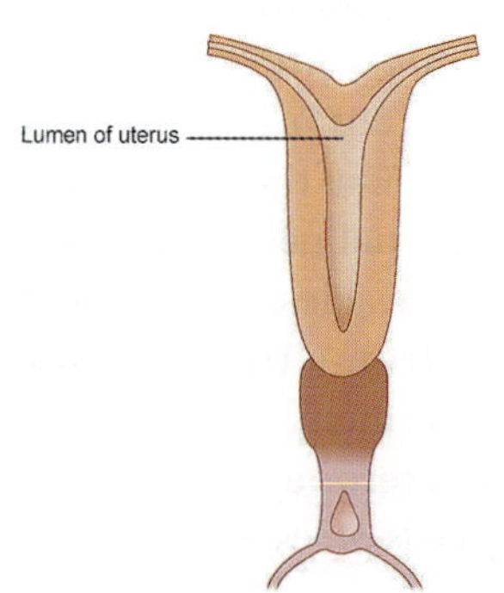 A. Entirely from the urogenital sinus B. Entirely from the paramesonephric ducts C. Upper part from the paramesonephric ducts and lower part from the urogenital sinus D. Upper part from the mesonephric ducts and lower part from the urogenital sinus E. Upper part from the urogenital sinus and lower part from the paramesonephric ducts	**Ans: C (Upper part from the paramesonephric ducts and lower part from the urogenital sinus)** **Figures 29A to D** show the development of vagina. The vagina has a dual embryological origin: *Upper one-third:* Derived from the paramesonephric ducts (Müllerian ducts), which also form the uterus and fallopian tubes *Lower two-thirds:* Arises from the urogenital sinus (UGS), which is of endodermal origin and is derived from the cloaca 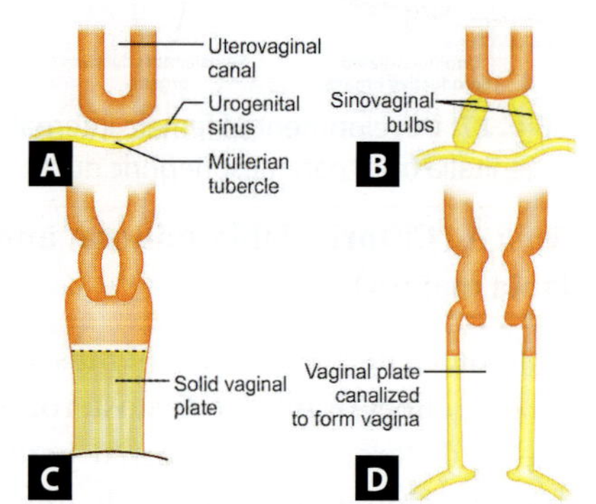 **Figs. 29A to D:** Development of vagina (part derived from mesoderm is brown; part derived from endoderm is yellow).	**Explanation: Figure 29A** demonstrates the mesoderm of uterovaginal canal pressing on the posterior wall of the endodermal UGS forming Müllerian tubercle. Proliferation of the endoderm of UGS results in the formation of sinovaginal bulbs **(Fig. 29B)**. Solid vaginal plate is formed due to fusion of mesoderm of uterovaginal canal and endoderm of sinovaginal bulbs **(Fig. 29C)**. Vagina is eventually formed by canalization of this vaginal plate **(Fig. 29D)**. **Potential questions:** There can be questions related to the embryological origin of the various structures comprising the female internal as well as external genitalia.

Question	Answer	Comment
Q30. The embryology of the developing genitourinary system is shown in the below figure. In this figure, what does "A" represent? 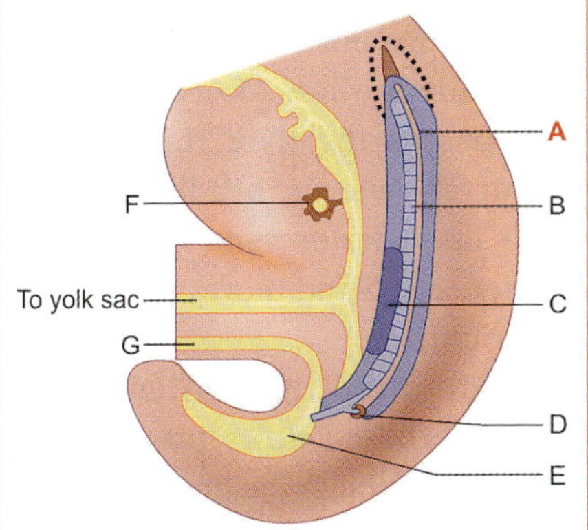 A. Mesonephric tubules B. Mesonephric duct C. Allantois D. Primordial gonad E. Ureteric bud	**Ans: B (Mesonephric duct)** Permanent kidney develops from two sources: Ureteric bud or the metanephros diverticulum and metanephrogenic blastema. **Figure 30** shows primordium of metanephros which is the permanent kidney. 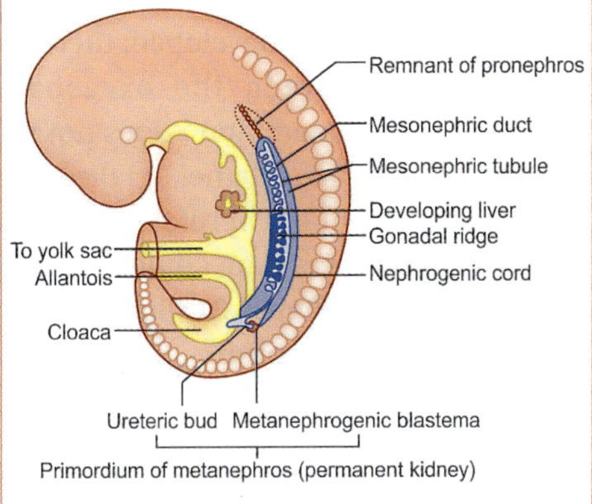 **Fig. 30:** Primordium of metanephros which is the permanent kidney.	**Explanation:** Ureteric bud or the metanephros diverticulum is the diverticulum or an outgrowth from the mesonephric duct near its entrance into the cloaca during the development of urinary and reproductive organs. The derivatives of ureteric bud include the following: Collecting tubules and ducts, minor and major calyces, and ureters. Metanephrogenic blastema (metanephric part of mesenchyme) comprises a mass of intermediate mesodermal cells around the distal end of the ureteric bud, giving rise to the nephrons. **Potential questions:** There could be other questions pertaining to embryonic development of kidneys.

Question	Answer	Comment
Q31. Below is the image depicting the fetal circulatory system. Identify the structure labeled "A" in the image that allows blood to bypass the fetal liver. 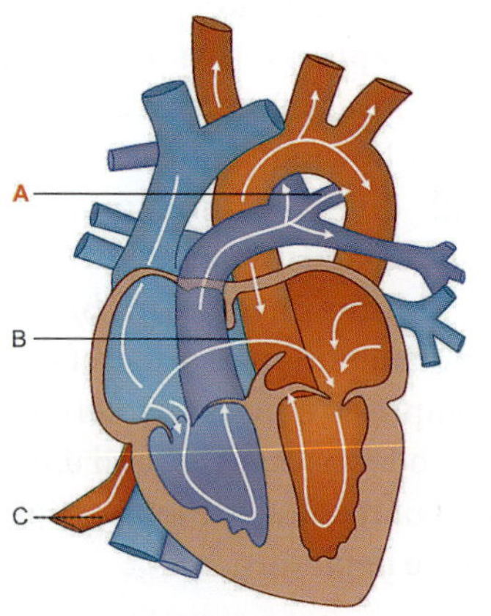 A. Foramen ovale B. Ductus arteriosus C. Ductus venosus D. Umbilical vein E. Umbilical artery	**Ans: C (Ductus venosus)** Fetal circulation is characterized by presence of three shunts: Ductus venosus, foramen ovale, and ductus arteriosus. These shunts permit the blood to bypass the liver and lungs and shunt the most oxygenated blood from the right to the left side of the heart. These shunts disappear following the birth of the baby. Also, in the fetus the lungs are not fully developed; therefore, exchange between the oxygenated and deoxygenated blood does not take place in the lungs. Rather, it takes place in the placenta. Therefore, the fetal circulation differs from adult circulation in many ways. **Figure 31** illustrates fetal circulation before birth. 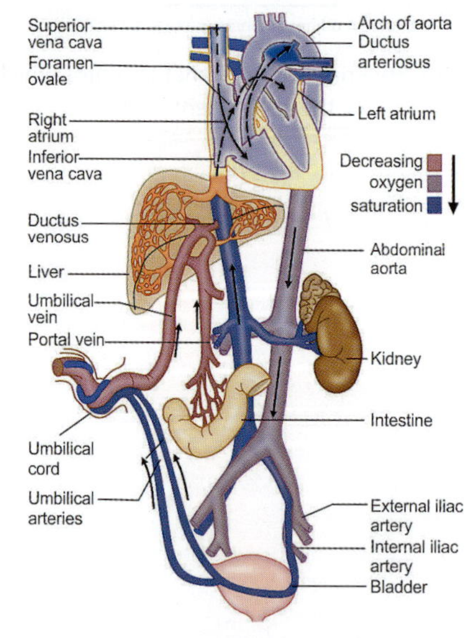 **Fig. 31:** Fetal circulation just before birth.	**Explanation:** Fetal circulation is a unique system that supports the developing baby in utero. Oxygenated blood from the placenta enters through the umbilical vein, bringing oxygen and nutrients. This blood travels towards the liver. Most of the blood bypasses the liver through the ductus venosus, heading directly to the inferior vena cava. From there the blood moves to the right atrium. From the right atrium, most of the blood flows into the left atrium through the foramen ovale, skipping the lungs because the pulmonary system in not well developed in the fetus and there is high resistance in the pulmonary vessels before birth. From the left atrium, blood moves to the left ventricle to supply the oxygenated blood to brain, heart and other parts of the body. Small amount of blood which moves from the right atrium to right ventricles, moves through the pulmonary arteries to the lungs. However, most of this blood is shunted through the ductus arteriosus into the descending aorta thereby bypassing the pulmonary circulation. **Potential questions:** There can be questions related to any of the shunts present in the fetal circulatory system.

CHAPTER 4

Pregnancy Complications

ECTOPIC PREGNANCY

Question	Answer	Comment
Q1. A 28-year-old woman at 7 weeks of gestation presents with severe pelvic pain and vaginal bleeding. Ultrasound shows no intrauterine pregnancy but reveals an adnexal mass. The doctor draws a diagram to explain the condition to the patient. Based on the image shown below, what is the pathophysiology of this condition? 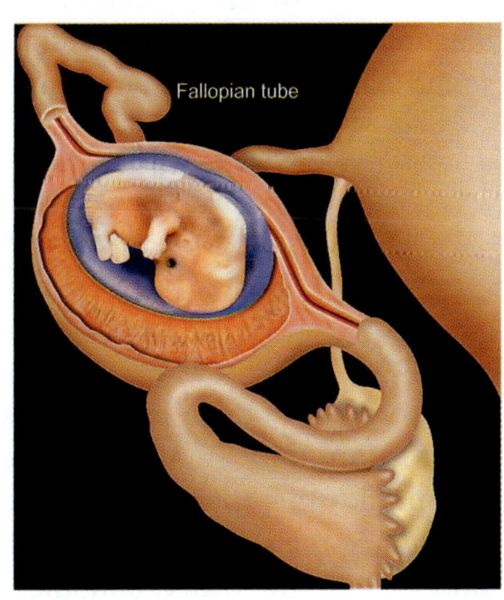 A. Implantation in the uterine cavity B. Tubal damage leading to flawed egg migration C. Myometrial implantation D. Implantation at the cervical os E. Abnormal placental attachment with normal uterine implantation	**Ans: B (Tubal damage leading to flawed egg migration)** The adjacent image demonstrates the presence of a gestational sac in the fallopian tube. When a fertilized egg implants outside the uterine cavity, the pregnancy is termed ectopic **(Fig. 1)**. The fallopian tube is the most common site for an ectopic pregnancy. 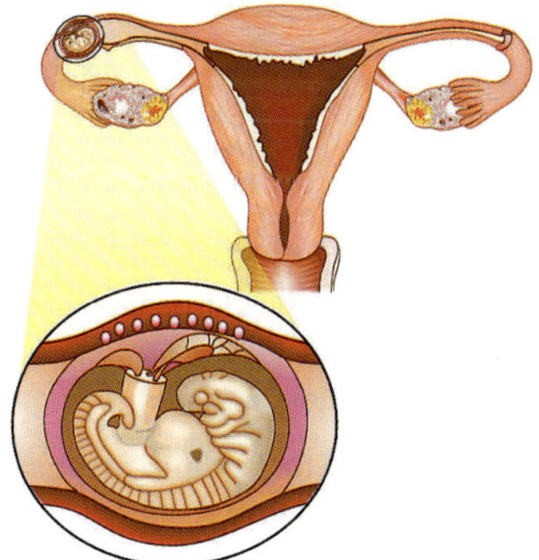 **Fig. 1:** Section through the fallopian tube showing an ectopic pregnancy.	**Explanation:** The primary pathophysiological mechanism for the development of an ectopic pregnancy involves flawed migration of the fertilized egg, often due to damage or scarring of the fallopian tube. This damage may result from infections (pelvic inflammatory disease), previous surgeries, or congenital abnormalities, etc. Following implantation, as the trophoblastic cells start invading the walls of the fallopian tube, there is a high risk of choriodecidual hemorrhage and rupture or erosion of the tubal wall. Therefore, early diagnosis and management of these cases is of utmost importance. **Potential questions:** There could be questions related to various locations, clinical presentation, diagnosis, management, and identification of the ultrasound features of ectopic pregnancy.

Question	Answer	Comment
Q2. A 30-year-old woman presents with severe lower abdominal pain and vaginal bleeding. She has missed her last menstrual period by 6 weeks. The ultrasound shows a gestational sac located in the left adnexa with no intrauterine pregnancy. What is the most likely location of this pathology? 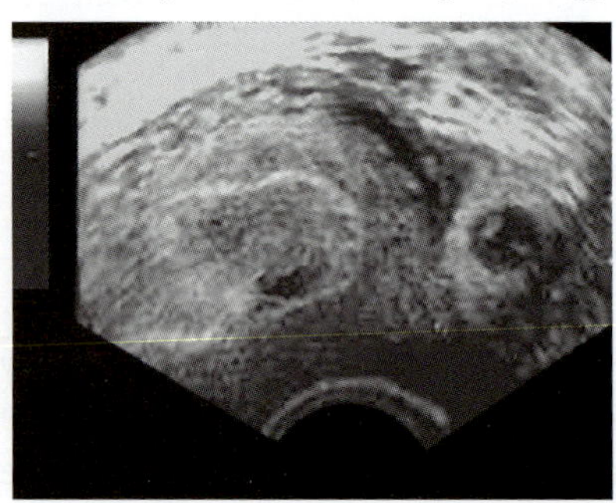 A. Ovarian B. Cervical C. Tubal D. Abdominal E. Cornual	**Ans: C (Tubal)** The presentation of a gestational sac in the adnexa with the absence of an intrauterine pregnancy on ultrasound strongly suggests a tubal ectopic pregnancy. The average incidence for occurrence of ectopic pregnancy at various locations is as follows **(Fig. 2)**: ▪ *Fallopian tube:* 95–96% • Ampulla: 70% • Isthmus: 12% • Fimbria/infundibulum: 11% • Cornua: 2% • Cornual/ interstitial: 2% ▪ Ovarian < 3% ▪ Cervical < 1% ▪ Abdominal 0.9–1.4% ▪ Cesarean scar < 1% ▪ Intramural < 1% ▪ Heterotopic 1–3% 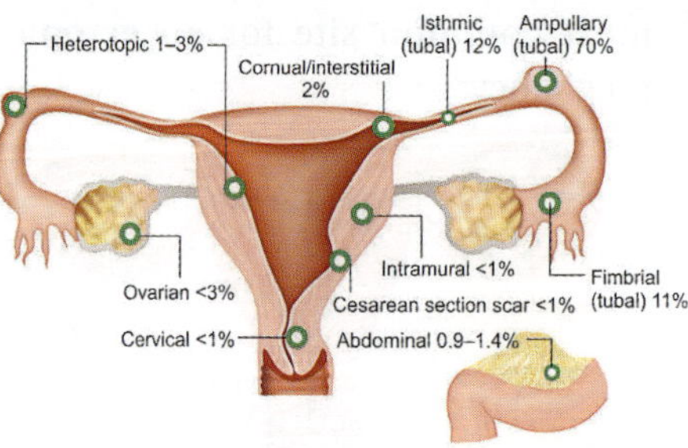 **Fig. 2:** Common sites for occurrence of ectopic pregnancy.	**Explanation:** The most common location for an ectopic pregnancy is the fallopian tube, specifically the ampullary segment, which accounts for approximately 96% of ectopic pregnancies. Most commonly, i.e., in nearly 95% of cases, the fertilized ovum gets implanted inside the fallopian tube. The ovum buries into the tube and induces a decidual reaction in the cells of endosalpinx. However, this reaction is feeble. Also, there occurs invasion of the trophoblastic cells into the wall of the fallopian tube. As a result, there is a high risk of choriodecidual hemorrhage and of erosion or rupture of the tubal wall. **Potential questions:** There could be questions related to various locations, clinical presentation, diagnosis, management, and ultrasound features of ectopic pregnancy.
Q3. Identify site A of ectopic pregnancy. 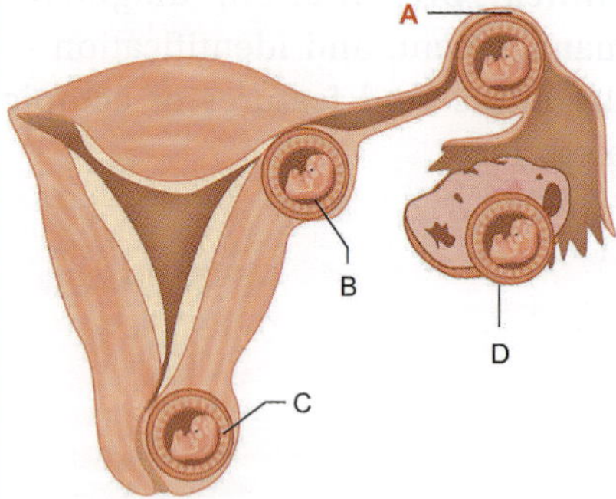 A. Cornual ectopic B. Ampullary ectopic C. Cervical ectopic D. Ovarian ectopic E. None of the above	**Ans: B (Ampullary ectopic)** Common sites for ectopic pregnancy are depicted in **Figure 3**. 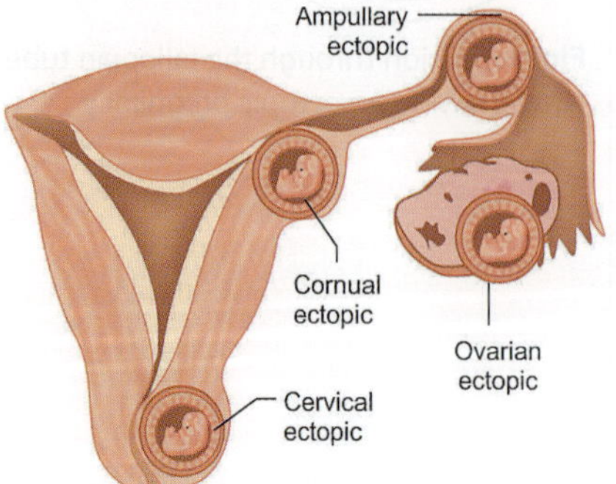 **Fig. 3:** Common sites of occurrence of ectopic pregnancy.	**Explanation:** Ectopic pregnancies most commonly implant in the fallopian tube, particularly the ampullary region. Other possible sites include the ovary, abdomen, cervix, etc. These locations cannot support a growing pregnancy, leading to potential rupture, severe bleeding, and life-threatening risks. **Potential questions:** There could be questions related to various locations, clinical presentation, diagnosis, and management of ectopic pregnancy.

Question	Answer	Comment
Q4. An ultrasound image shows a gestational sac located in the upper lateral aspect of bicornuate uterus with a thin surrounding myometrium. Which of the following is the most likely diagnosis? 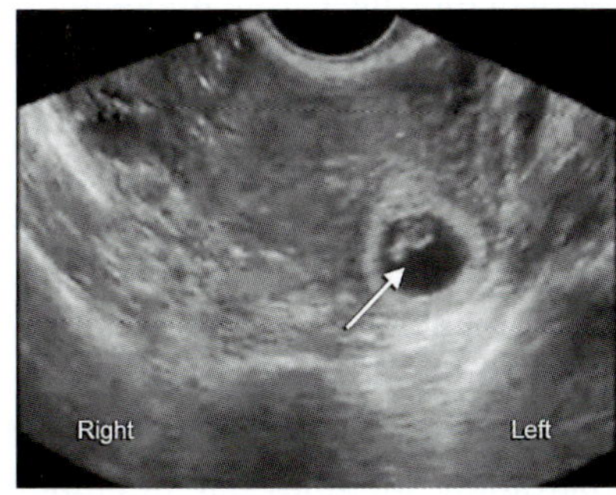 A. Interstitial ectopic pregnancy B. Cornual ectopic pregnancy C. Cervical ectopic pregnancy D. Tubal ectopic pregnancy E. Abdominal ectopic pregnancy	**Ans: B (Cornual ectopic pregnancy)** The adjacent image shows the presence of a gestational sac in the left horn of the bicornuate uterus. A gestational sac with a sonolucent center can be identified. It is surrounded by a thick, concentric, echogenic ring and contains a fetal pole. Cornual pregnancy occurs in the cornual part or the upper lateral part of the uterus **(Fig. 4)**. Since this portion of the tube is surrounded by uterine myometrium, it can expand significantly when it hosts a pregnancy. The cornu of the uterus usually ruptures between 12 to 16 weeks of pregnancy. 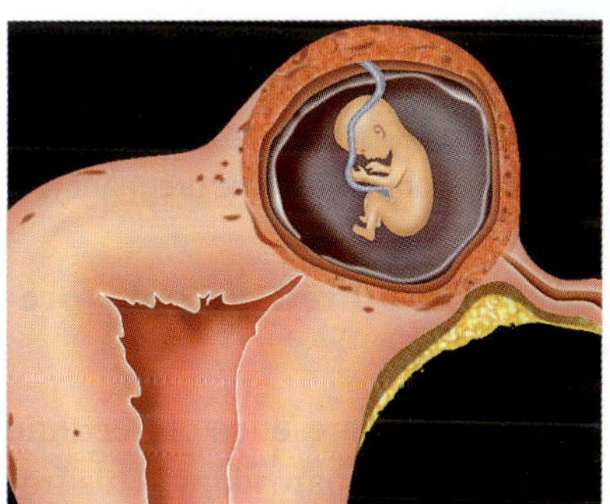 **Fig. 4:** Cornual ectopic pregnancy.	**Explanation:** The diagnostic features of a cornual pregnancy on ultrasound include the following: Dearth of myometrium around the gestational sac (<5 mm), an empty uterine cavity, gestational sac separate from the uterine cavity, and presence of an echogenic line, extending from the endometrial cavity to the corner next to the gestational mass (interstitial line sign). This type of ectopic pregnancy is rare and can be confused with an interstitial pregnancy. In a cornual ectopic, the gestational sac is located more laterally within the upper lateral part of the uterus. On the other hand, interstitial pregnancy occurs when the fertilized egg implants in the interstitial part of the fallopian tube (tubal segment that passes through the muscular wall of the uterus). The treatment is primarily surgical and involves removal of the products of conception (POC) and surgical repair of the uterus. **Potential questions:** There could be questions related to various locations, clinical presentation, diagnosis, and management of ectopic pregnancy.

Question	Answer	Comment
Q5. An ultrasound shows gestational sac located outside the uterus, adjacent to the bowel loops, with no surrounding myometrium. The schematic image of the ultrasound findings is shown below. Which of the following is the most likely diagnosis? 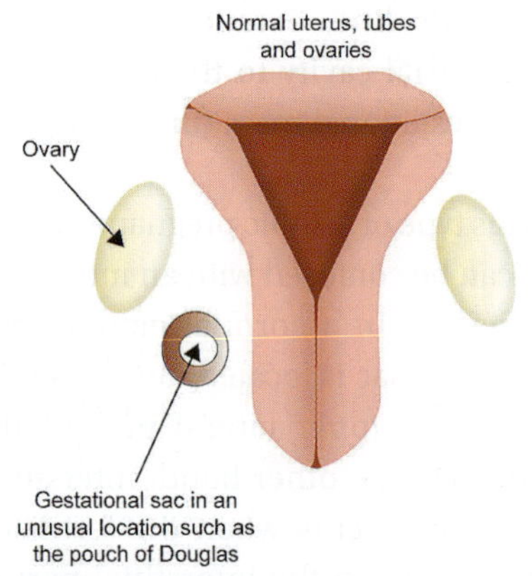 A. Interstitial ectopic pregnancy B. Cornual ectopic pregnancy C. Cervical ectopic pregnancy D. Tubal ectopic pregnancy E. Abdominal ectopic pregnancy	**Ans: E (Abdominal ectopic pregnancy)** In abdominal pregnancy, the pregnancy gets implanted in the peritoneal cavity, outside the fallopian tubes and ovary **(Fig. 5)**. These pregnancies can rarely result in the delivery of a viable infant, though the outcome can be equally fatal as compared to ectopic pregnancy at other locations. 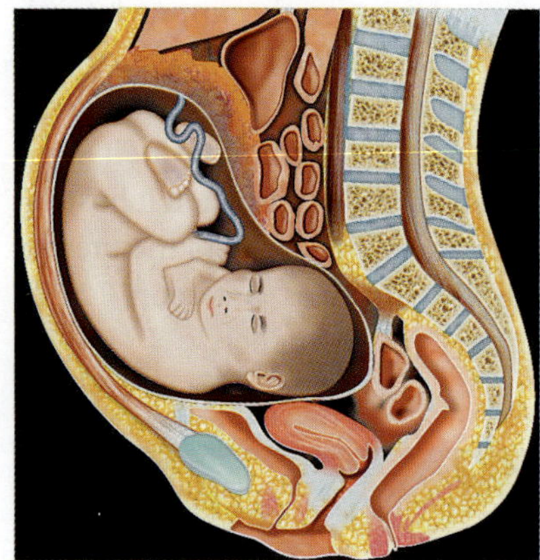 **Fig. 5:** Abdominal ectopic pregnancy.	**Explanation:** Abdominal ectopic pregnancy occurs when a fertilized egg implants in the abdominal cavity, outside of the uterus, often near the bowel or other abdominal organs. This type of ectopic pregnancy is rare but can be life-threatening due to the risk of hemorrhage from implantation in highly vascularized areas. The key ultrasound finding is the absence of myometrium surrounding the gestational sac and its location away from the uterus, often near bowel loops or other abdominal structures. Treatment is primarily surgical involving the removal of fetus through laparotomy. Methotrexate or embolization can also be used for termination of pregnancy. **Potential questions:** There could be questions related to various locations, clinical presentation, diagnosis, and management of ectopic pregnancy.
Q6. In a patient with a suspected ectopic pregnancy, an ultrasound reveals the presence of free fluid in the pouch of Douglas (POD). What does this finding most likely indicate? 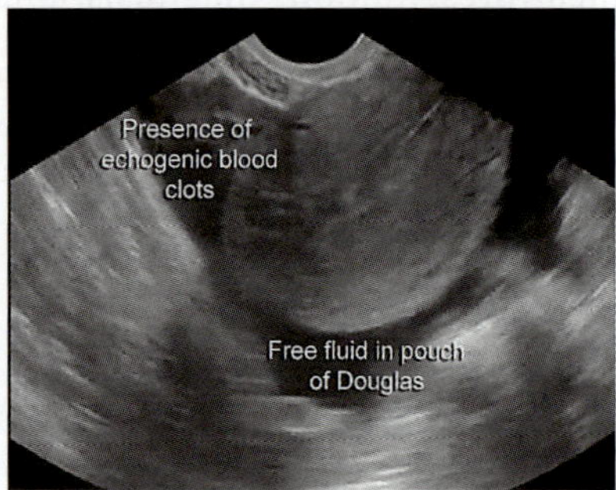 A. Normal early pregnancy B. Miscarriage in progress C. Ruptured ovarian cyst D. Ruptured ectopic pregnancy E. Physiological fluid collection	**Ans: D (Ruptured ectopic pregnancy)** **Figure 6** shows presence of free fluid in the POD on laparoscopy. This free fluid comprises blood and blood clots, probably resulting from the rupture of ectopic pregnancy, which accumulate in the most dependent part of pelvis, i.e., rectouterine pouch or POD or the intraperitoneal gutters (Morrison pouch). 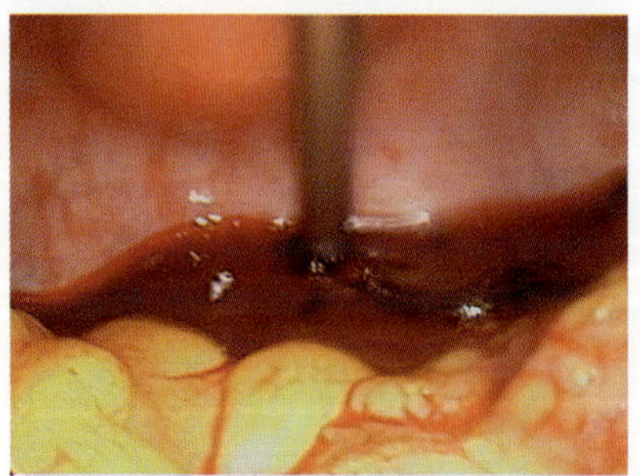 **Fig. 6:** Presence of clotted blood in the pouch of Douglas.	**Explanation:** The presence of free fluid in the POD in a patient with a suspected ectopic pregnancy is highly suggestive of a ruptured ectopic pregnancy. This fluid typically represents blood that has leaked into the abdominal cavity. Rupture of an ectopic pregnancy is a serious complication that can lead to significant hemorrhage and requires urgent medical intervention. Such patients may often show features of hypovolemic shock (hypotension, tachycardia, etc). **Potential questions:** There could be questions related to various locations, clinical presentation, diagnosis, management, and complications of ectopic pregnancy.

Question	Answer	Comment
Q7. A transvaginal Doppler ultrasound reveals a "ring of fire" sign around an adnexal mass in a patient presenting with lower abdominal pain and a positive pregnancy test. What is the most likely diagnosis? 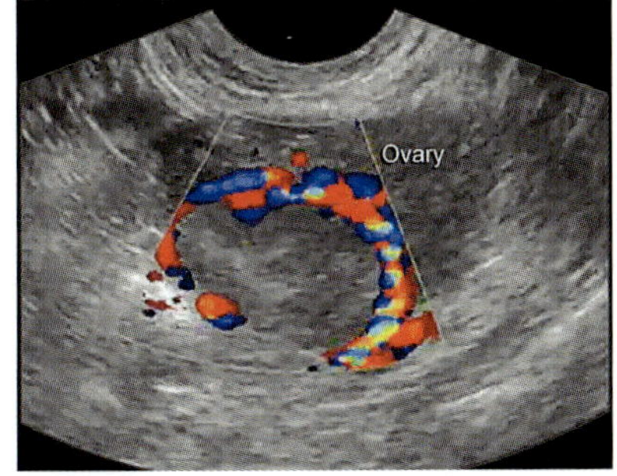 A. Ovarian cyst B. Pelvic inflammatory disease C. Ectopic pregnancy D. Uterine fibroid E. Normal intrauterine pregnancy	**Ans: C (Ectopic pregnancy)** In cases of suspicious adnexal masses, presence of gestational sac at any location is associated with increased vascularity, which may result in a "ring of fire" appearance on Doppler ultrasound (adjacent image). The laparoscopic finding in this case is demonstrated in **Figure 7**. 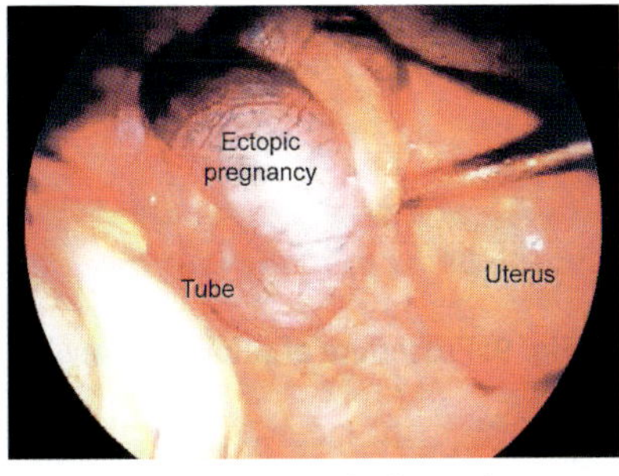 **Fig. 7:** Laparoscopic findings showing ectopic pregnancy in the right tube.	**Explanation:** The "ring of fire" sign on Doppler ultrasound is characterized by a hypervascular ring surrounding an adnexal mass, which indicates increased blood flow. This sign is most commonly associated with ectopic pregnancy, where the pregnancy is located at an extrauterine site. This finding is due to the trophoblastic activity of the ectopic pregnancy, making it a critical diagnostic feature in evaluating suspected ectopic pregnancies. **Potential questions:** There could be questions related to various locations, clinical presentation, diagnosis, management, and complications of ectopic pregnancy.
Q8. A 28-year-old woman comes in with lower abdominal pain, vaginal bleeding, and a positive pregnancy test. GPE reveals signs of hypovolemia. TVS is inconclusive, so a procedure involving blood aspiration is performed, as shown in the image. What is the name of this procedure? 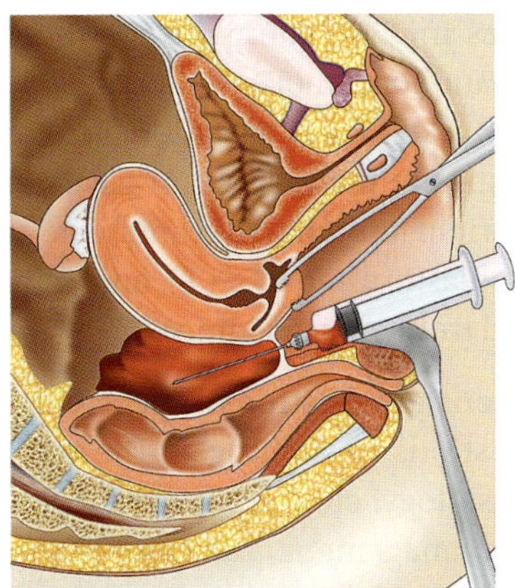 A. Culdoscopy B. Paracentesis C. Amniocentesis D. Culdocentesis E. Colpotomy	**Ans: D (Culdocentesis)** This image demonstrates the process of culdocentesis for diagnosis of ectopic pregnancy. This involves insertion of 18 gauge spinal needle, attached to 20 mL syringe through the posterior vaginal wall into the rectouterine pouch to aspirate fluid from cul-de-sac **(Fig. 8)**. The test is said to be positive when more than 2 mL of nonclotting blood is obtained. 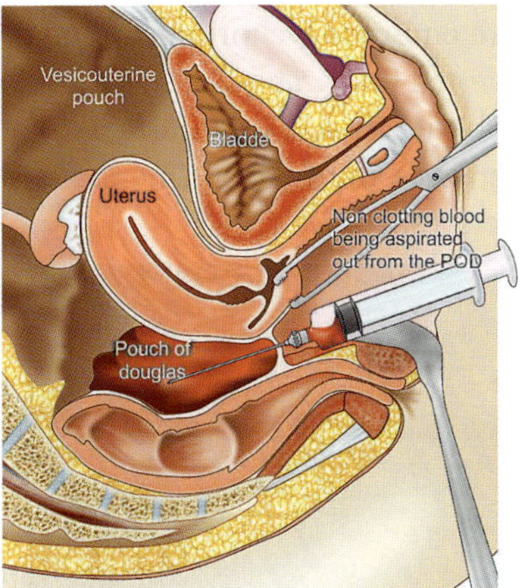 **Fig. 8:** Culdocentesis for the diagnosis of ectopic pregnancy.	**Explanation:** Culdocentesis can be performed to help diagnose blood in the cul-de-sac. Presence of nonclotted blood in the pouch of Douglas (POD) is diagnostic of chronic hemorrhage in the peritoneal cavity and is suggestive of a ruptured ectopic pregnancy. Before the widespread use of ultrasound, culdocentesis was commonly used as a diagnostic test for ectopic pregnancy. Even today, this method can be used in unstable patients where ultrasonography is not immediately available. **Potential questions:** There could be questions related to various locations, clinical presentation, diagnosis, management, and complications of ectopic pregnancy.

Question	Answer	Comment
Q9. What is the name of the surgical procedure (as shown in the image), performed to preserve the fallopian tube in a 30-year-old woman with an ectopic pregnancy, confirmed by TVS? 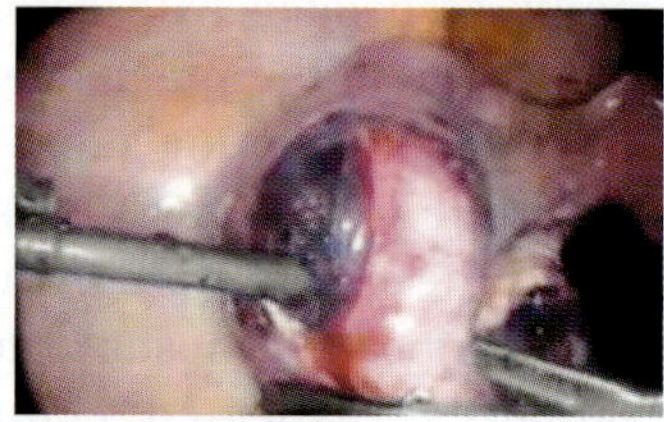 A. Colpotomy B. Salpingotomy C. Laparotomy D. Salpingectomy E. Oophorectomy	**Ans: B (Salpingotomy)** The procedure shown in the adjacent image is salpingotomy/salpingostomy. In the 21st century, treatment for ectopic pregnancy has shifted to MIS (salpingotomy and salpingostomy), replacing past methods like laparotomy and salpingectomy. 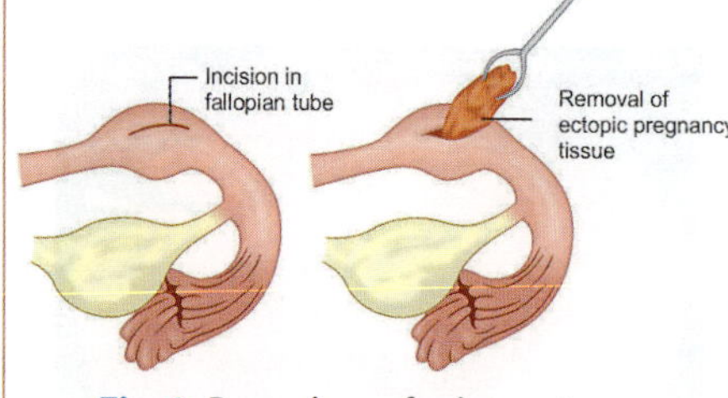 **Fig. 9:** Procedure of salpingotomy.	**Explanation:** Salpingotomy is a procedure where a small incision is made in the fallopian tube to remove the ectopic pregnancy while preserving the tube **(Fig. 9)**. This procedure is often chosen to maintain fertility. Unlike salpingectomy, which removes the entire tube, salpingotomy aims to conserve the reproductive organs. Its main drawback is the risk of persistent or recurrent ectopic pregnancy. **Potential questions:** There could be questions related to various locations, clinical presentation, diagnosis, management, and complications of ectopic pregnancy.

HYDATIDIFORM MOLE

Question	Answer	Comment
Q10. A 38-year-old woman underwent hysterectomy for second-trimester bleeding. Hysterectomy specimen is shown in the image below. HPE shows diffuse trophoblastic proliferation and hydropic villi. What is the most likely diagnosis? 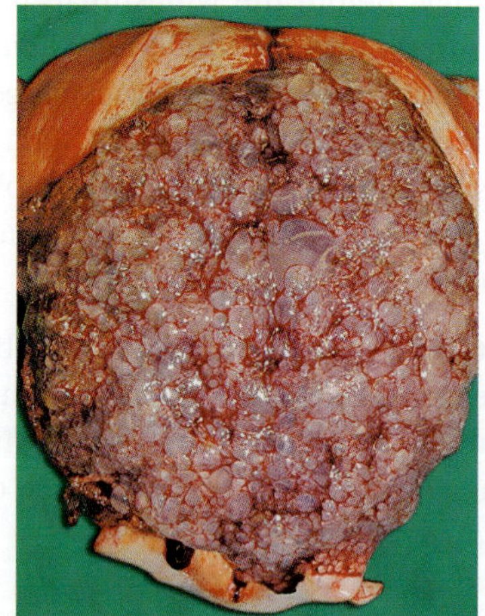 A. Complete hydatidiform mole B. Partial hydatidiform mole C. Choriocarcinoma D. Invasive mole E. PSTT	**Ans: A (Complete hydatidiform mole)** Hydatidiform mole (H. mole) belongs to a spectrum of disease known as gestational trophoblastic disease (GTD), resulting from overproduction of the chorionic tissue, which is normally supposed to develop into the placenta. **Figure 10** illustrates a magnified view showing vesicular grape-like structures. In this condition, the entire embryonic chorionic tissue gets converted into grape-like structures, in which each vesicle is connected to each other with the help of fine stalk-like structures. 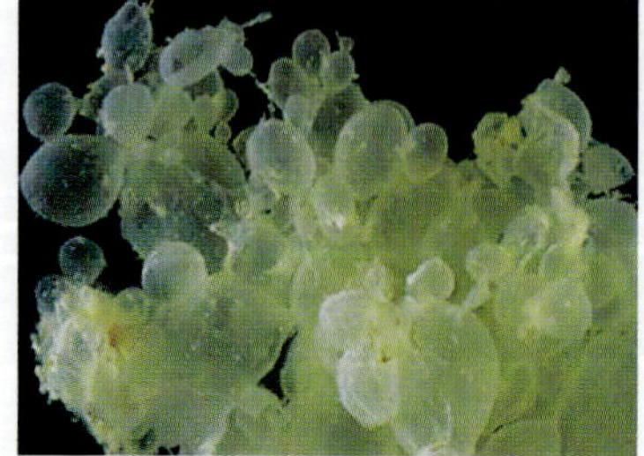 **Fig. 10:** Magnified view showing the vesicular structures.	**Explanation:** Histopathology of gestational trophoblastic disease shows diffuse trophoblastic proliferation and hydropic swelling of the villi, with complete moles lacking fetal tissue, while partial moles may have fetal tissue. It is classified into benign (90%) and malignant (10%) forms. Benign types include complete and partial hydatidiform moles, while malignant forms, known as gestational trophoblastic tumors, include invasive mole, choriocarcinoma, placental site trophoblastic tumor (PSTT), and epithelioid trophoblastic tumor. **Potential questions:** There can be questions pertaining to the pathophysiology, clinical features, diagnosis, management, and complications of both benign and malignant forms of GTD.

Question	Answer	Comment
Q11. What is the likely chromosomal configuration of a specimen of molar gestation shown in the below image? 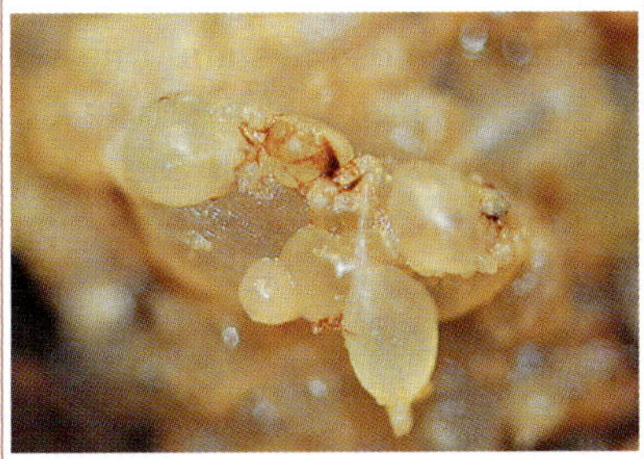 A. 46XY B. 46XX C. 69XXX D. 69XXY E. 69XYY	**Ans: B (46XX)** The adjacent image shows the specimen of a complete hydatidiform mole due to the complete absence of fetal tissue. The pathogenesis of a complete mole is demonstrated in **Figures 11A and B**. Both complete and partial hydatidiform moles are nonviable and genetically abnormal conceptions, showing excessive expression of paternal genes. Complete hydatidiform moles (CHMs) are usually diploid, with all chromosomes being derived from the father. 46XX karyotype is found in 90% of CHMs. A few cases may also have a 46XY karyotype. 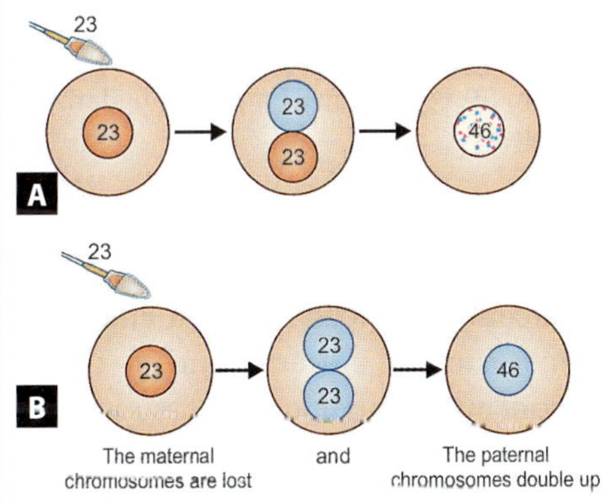 **Figs. 11A and B:** Pathogenesis of complete hydatidiform mole: (A) Normal process of fertilization; (B) Formation of a complete hydatidiform mole.	**Explanation:** In the normal process of fertilization, a sperm fertilizes an ovum resulting in the formation of a diploid zygote (containing 46 chromosomes). In a CHM, all chromosomes are derived from the father by means of either monospermic or dispermic fertilization. Monospermic fertilization results from fertilization of a sperm with an anucleate oocyte. The genetic material is duplicated, resulting in a 46XX karyotype. Rarely, CHM can also be produced due to dispermic fertilization in which there is fertilization of two different sperms with an anucleate oocyte. **Potential questions:** There can be questions pertaining to the pathophysiology, clinical features, diagnosis, management, and complications of both benign and malignant forms of gestational trophoblastic disease (GTD).

<table>
<tr><th>Question</th><th>Answer</th><th>Comment</th></tr>
<tr>
<td>Q12. What is the likely chromosomal configuration of a specimen of molar gestation shown in the image below?
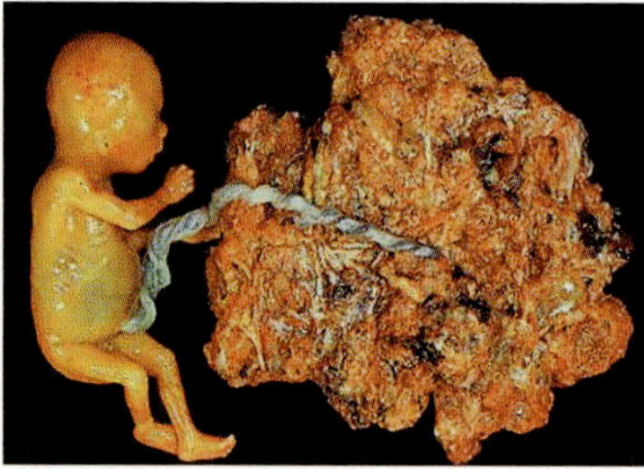
A. 46XY
B. 46XX
C. 69XXX
D. 69XXY
E. 69XYY</td>
<td>Ans: D (69XXY)
The adjacent image shows the specimen of partial mole, having chorionic vesicles along with the fetal tissue. Figure 12A shows the normal process of fertilization. Figure 12B shows the pathogenesis of partial hydatidiform mole (PHM).
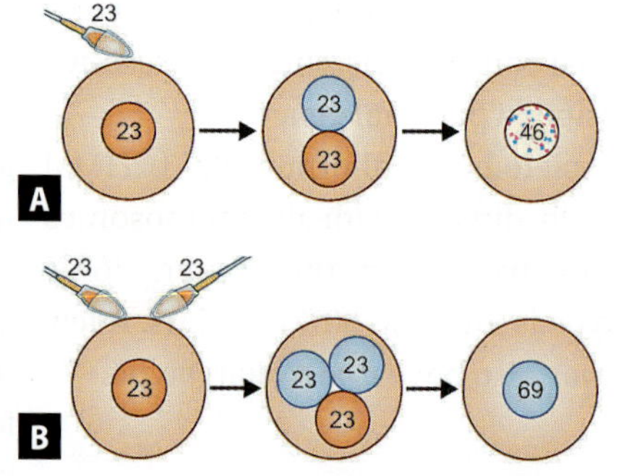

Figs. 12A and B: Pathogenesis of a partial hydatidiform mole: (A) Normal process of fertilization; (B) Formation of a partial hydatidiform mole.</td>
<td>Explanation: Partial hydatidiform moles are usually triploid, formed due to dispermic fertilization. In this case, two different sperms fertilize with an ovum, resulting in the formation of a triploid karyotype having two sets of paternal chromosomes and one set of maternal chromosomes (69XXX, 69XXY, or 69XYY,), with the most common chromosomal configuration being 69XXY.
About 10% of PHMs have tetraploid or higher karyotypes consisting of multiple sets of paternal chromosomes in combination with one set of maternal chromosomes.
Potential questions: There can be questions pertaining to the pathophysiology, clinical features, diagnosis, management, and complications of both benign and malignant forms of GTD.</td>
</tr>
<tr>
<td>Q13. A pregnant woman reports to the clinic at 13 weeks of gestation with a complaint of vaginal bleeding. Beta human chorionic gonadotropin (hCG) levels in the serum and urine are found to be elevated. The picture of the USG scan is shown below. What is the most likely diagnosis for this patient?
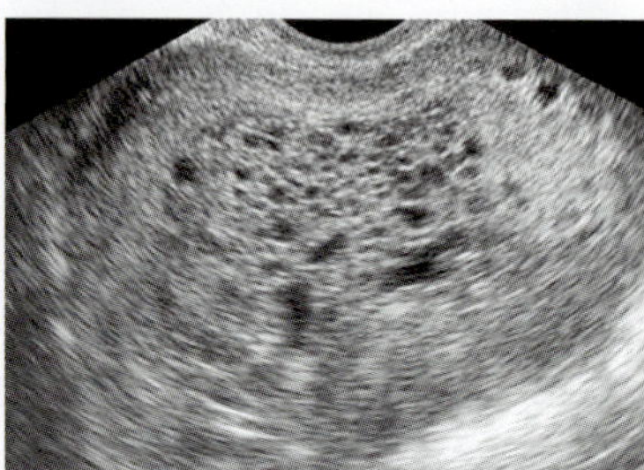
A. Abnormal villus morphology
B. Hydropic abortus
C. Early abortus with trophoblastic hyperplasia
D. Placental mesenchymal dysplasia
E. Hydatidiform mole</td>
<td>Ans: E (Hydatidiform mole)
The adjacent USG scan shows a characteristic vesicular pattern, due to the presence of numerous anechoic cysts with intervening hyperechoic material. This is also known as “snowstorm appearance” which is a characteristic feature of the hydatidiform mole (H. mole).
Though MRI examination is not required for diagnosis, Figure 13 demonstrates the appearance of a H. mole on MRI.
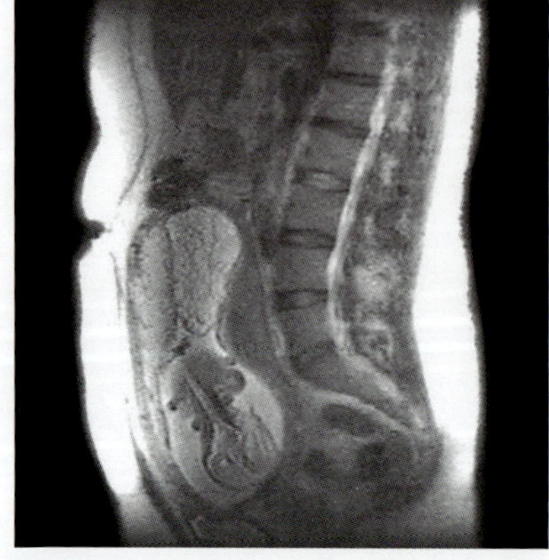
Fig. 13: MRI showing hydatidiform mole.</td>
<td>Explanation: H. mole can be considered an abnormal pregnancy in which placental villi become edematous (hydropic) and start proliferating, resulting in the development of cystic, grape-like structures filled with watery fluid. This results in characteristic “snowstorm” appearance.
Sonography is the imaging investigation of choice to confirm the diagnosis of H. mole. At present, pelvic MRI is not an essential investigation for the management of nonmetastatic molar gestation. However, it is beneficial in diagnosing the metastatic disease, for characterizing the degree of myometrial and/or parametrial invasion, and for assessing the response to chemotherapy.
Potential questions: There can be questions pertaining to the pathophysiology, clinical features, diagnosis, and management of H. mole and gestational trophoblastic neoplasia (GTN).</td>
</tr>
</table>

<table>
<tr><th>Question</th><th>Answer</th><th>Comment</th></tr>
<tr><td>

Q14. A 25-year-old woman presents with amenorrhea and vaginal bleeding. Ultrasound reveals an enlarged uterus with a "snowstorm" pattern and bilateral enlarged ovarian cysts as shown in the image below. What is the most likely diagnosis for enlarged ovaries in this case?

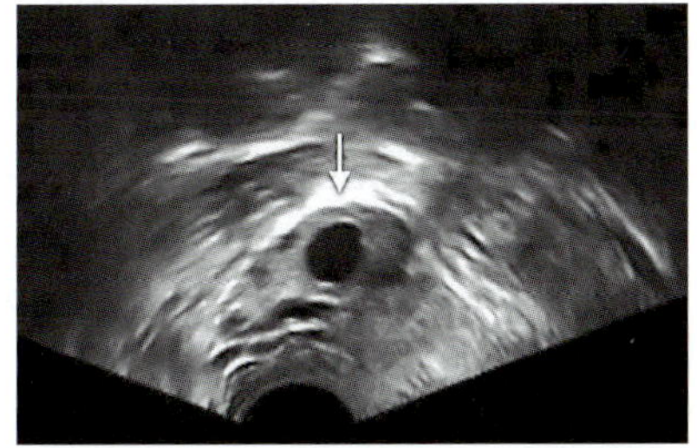

A. Ovarian hyperstimulation syndrome
B. Polycystic ovarian syndrome
C. Complete hydatidiform mole with theca lutein cysts
D. Ectopic pregnancy
E. Follicular cysts

</td><td>

Ans: C (Complete hydatidiform mole with theca lutein cysts)

Besides the characteristic snowstorm appearance, ultrasound may also show the presence of theca lutein cysts in the ovaries (as shown in **Fig. 14**). The presence of theca lutein cysts usually occurs in association with high serum β-hCG levels of >100,000 mIU/mL. High circulating levels of β-hCG associated with H. mole usually cause ovarian hyperstimulation, resulting in formation of these cysts.

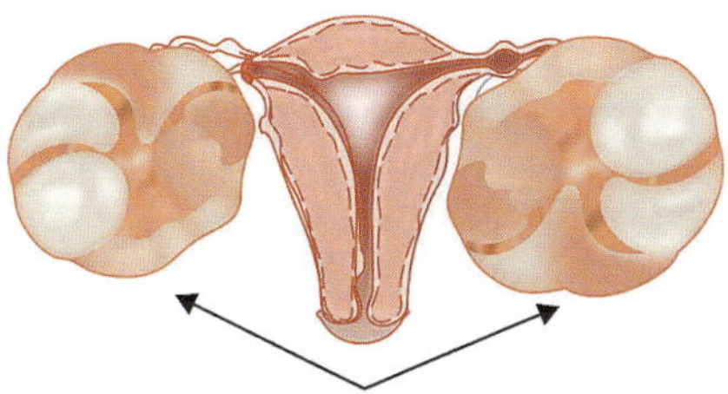

Fig. 14: Diagrammatic representation of theca lutein cyst.

</td><td>

Explanation: On sonograms, theca lutein cysts appear as large, septate, cystic ovarian lesions. They may be unilateral or bilateral and at times may be extremely large. In rare cases, theca lutein cysts may rupture, hemorrhage, or even cause ovarian torsion. However, before making the diagnosis of theca lutein cysts, the radiologist must exclude the possibility of a preexisting or concomitant cystic ovarian neoplasm.

A repeat sonographic evaluation must be done following suction evacuation after serum β-hCG levels have normalized. In most patients, no treatment is required because theca lutein cysts regress within 8–12 weeks after the evacuation of H. mole.

Potential questions: There can be questions pertaining to the pathophysiology, clinical features, diagnosis, and management of H. mole, and GTN.

</td></tr>
<tr><td>

Q15. On a chest X-ray as shown below, what is a characteristic feature of pulmonary metastasis in malignant GTD?

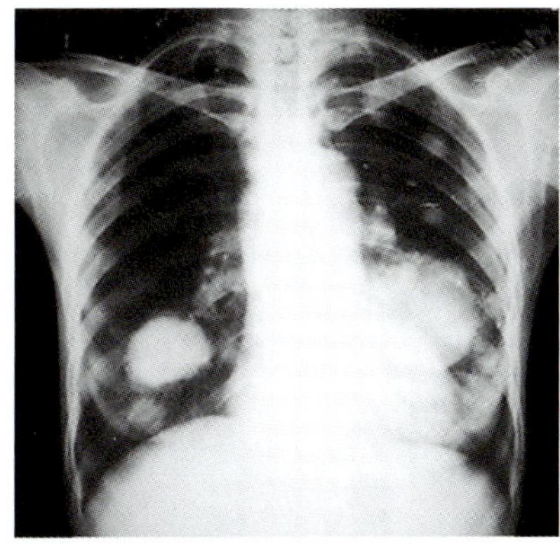

A. Single large pleural effusion
B. Cannonball appearance
C. Consolidation in the lower lobes
D. Ground-glass opacities in the upper lobes
E. Isolated cavitary lesion

</td><td>

Ans: B (Cannonball appearance)

The lungs are the most common site for metastasis in case of malignant GTD and may show the presence of distinct nodules or cannonball appearance. These lesions have been marked with red arrows in **Figure 15**.

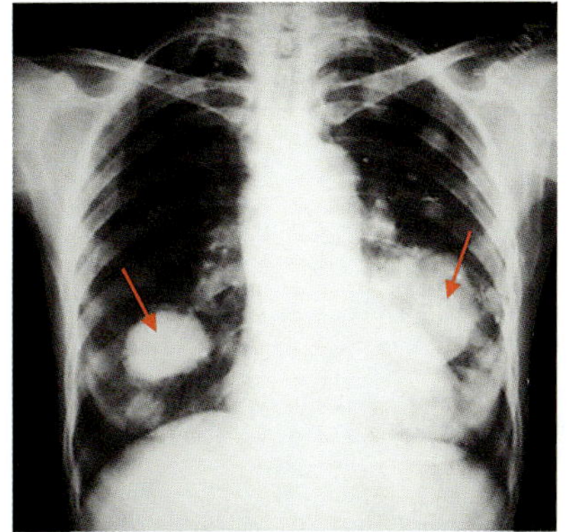

Fig. 15: X-ray showing cannonball appearance of pulmonary metastasis in cases of malignant GTN.

</td><td>

Explanation: The presence of these nodules is a result of hematogenous spread of the trophoblastic cells. This pattern is distinct and helps in differentiating GTD metastasis from other pulmonary conditions.

A suspicion of pulmonary metastasis on chest X-ray must be followed by a CT or MRI examination of both head and abdomen.

Potential questions: There can be questions pertaining to the pathophysiology, clinical features, diagnosis, and management of H. mole and GTN.

</td></tr>
</table>

MISCARRIAGE

Question	Answer	Comment
Q16. A 28-year-old woman at 10 weeks' gestation presents with vaginal bleeding and mild lower abdominal cramping. Ultrasound reveals a closed cervical os and a gestational sac with a fetal heartbeat, as depicted pictorially in the below image. What is the most likely diagnosis? 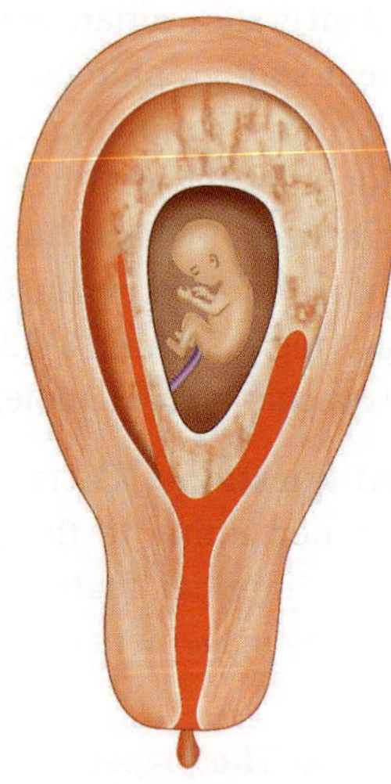 A. Inevitable miscarriage B. Complete miscarriage C. Threatened miscarriage D. Missed miscarriage E. Ectopic pregnancy	**Ans: C (Threatened miscarriage)** Ultrasound evaluation in these cases would help in assessing fetal viability, measuring fetal growth and development, identifying the cause of bleeding (e.g. subchorionic hematoma, etc.), **(Fig. 16)**. Some features suggestive of poor prognosis in these cases on ultrasound include early bradycardia, presence of large subchorionic hematoma, relative fetal inactivity, etc. 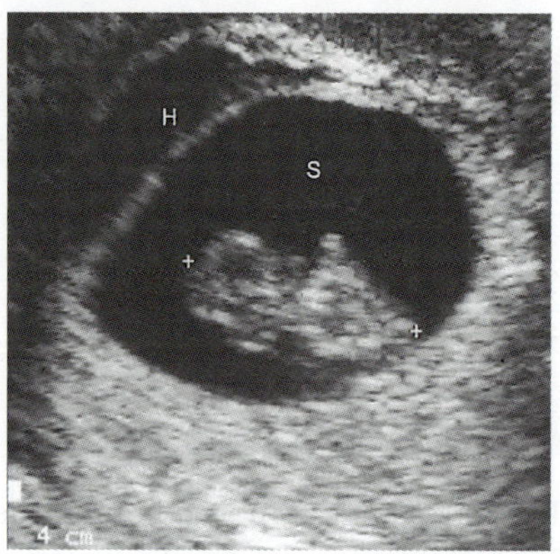 **Fig. 16:** Endovaginal ultrasound showing the presence of subchorionic hemorrhage (H) within the endometrial canal adjacent to the gestational sac (S).	**Explanation:** Threatened abortion is a type of abortion where the process of abortion has begun but has yet not progressed to a stage from where the recovery would be impossible. In case of threatened abortion, despite occurrence of bleeding or cervical discharge within the first 20 weeks of gestation, the cervical os remains closed. This feature distinguishes threatened miscarriage from other types of miscarriage where the cervix may be dilated or the pregnancy may be nonviable. In cases of threatened miscarriage, the fetal heart rate may be present and there may be normal intrauterine growth. The bleeding may sometimes stop on its own and pregnancy may continue normally. **Potential questions:** There can be potential questions related to etiology, diagnosis, and management of various types of miscarriage.

Question	Answer	Comment
Q17. A 35-year-old woman at 12 weeks gestation presents with heavy bleeding, severe cramping, and a partially dilated cervix. Intrauterine fetal tissue is observed near the cervical canal as depicted pictorially in the below image. What is the likely diagnosis? 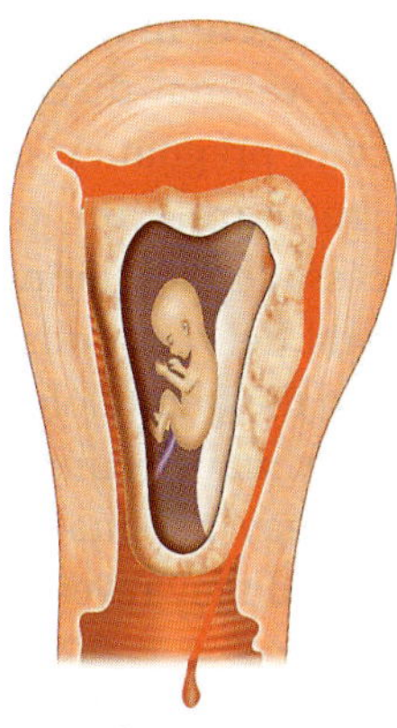 A. Threatened miscarriage B. Complete miscarriage C. Missed miscarriage D. Inevitable miscarriage E. Ectopic pregnancy	**Ans: D (Inevitable miscarriage)** Inevitable abortion occurs when pregnancy cannot continue, with an open cervical os. It may progress to either complete or incomplete miscarriage. 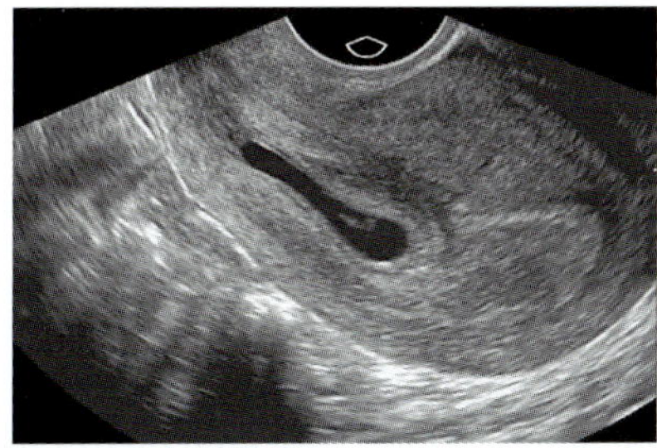 **Fig. 17:** Inevitable abortion. **Figure 17** shows ultrasound findings of inevitable abortion: a smaller gestational sac with loss of definition, absence of central echoes, no fetal cardiac activity, and the sac located in the lower uterine segment.	**Explanation:** Inevitable miscarriage involves heavy bleeding, cramping, and a dilated cervix with the pregnancy likely to be expelled. Unlike threatened miscarriage, the cervix is open. If bleeding is excessive, start an IV drip with 5% dextrose, arrange blood transfusion, and evacuate the uterus promptly. Suction evacuation is used if gestation is under 12 weeks, and oxytocin infusion can accelerate abortion if gestation exceeds 12 weeks. **Potential questions:** There can be potential questions related to etiology, diagnosis, and management of various types of miscarriage.
Q18. A 32-year-old woman at 9 weeks gestation presents with vaginal bleeding and cramping. Ultrasound shows RPCs with no fetal heartbeat. This is depicted pictorially in the below image. What is the likely diagnosis? 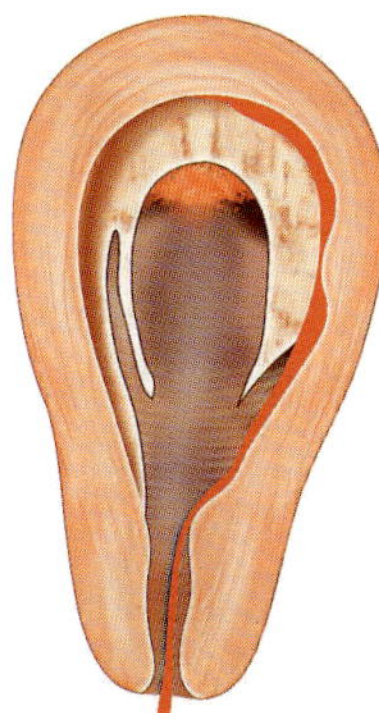 A. Missed miscarriage B. Complete miscarriage C. Incomplete miscarriage D. Threatened miscarriage E. Ectopic pregnancy	**Ans: C (Incomplete miscarriage)** The adjacent image shows an open cervical os with partial expulsion of fetal tissue, suggesting an incomplete miscarriage. **Figure 18** reveals an irregular, distorted gestational sac in the lower uterine segment with no yolk sac or embryo, confirming the diagnosis of incomplete miscarriage. 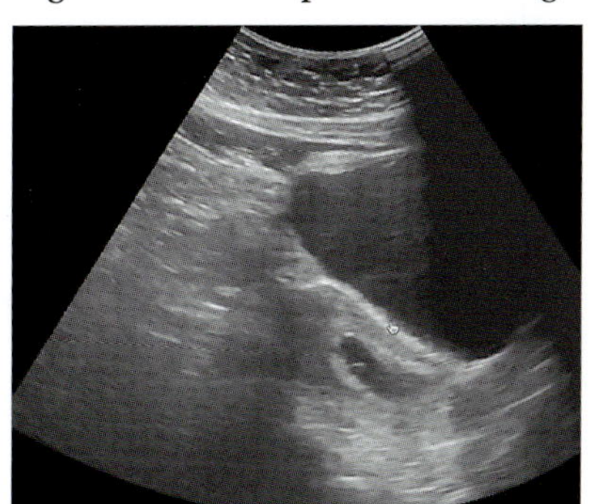 **Fig. 18:** Incomplete abortion.	**Explanation:** Incomplete abortion occurs when some fetal tissue is expelled while the rest remains in the uterus, causing pain and bleeding. The cervical os is open. Treatment is similar to inevitable abortion, and if the uterus is larger than 12 weeks, a single dose of 600 µg oral or 400 µg sublingual misoprostol can help complete the abortion. **Potential questions:** There can be potential questions related to etiology, diagnosis, and management of various types of miscarriage.

<table>
<tr><th>Question</th><th>Answer</th><th>Comment</th></tr>
<tr>
<td>Q19. A 28-year-old woman at 10 weeks gestation reports no cramping or bleeding. Ultrasound shows a fetus without a heartbeat, measuring 8–9 weeks. The diagrammatic representation of the same is shown below. What is the likely diagnosis?
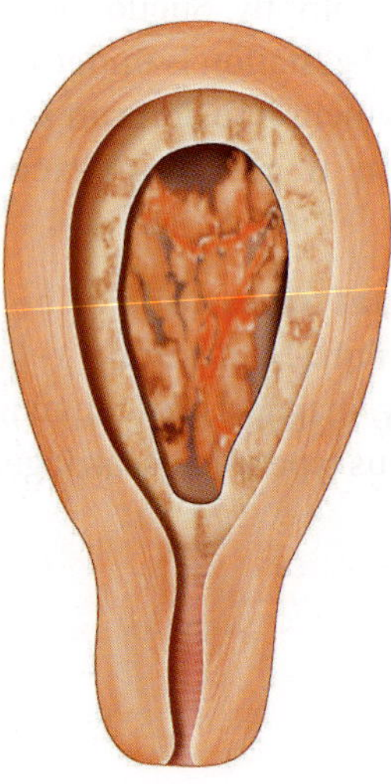
A. Threatened miscarriage
B. Complete miscarriage
C. Missed miscarriage
D. Inevitable miscarriage
E. Ectopic pregnancy</td>
<td>Ans: C (Missed miscarriage)
The adjacent image demonstrates missed miscarriage where the fetus is no longer viable, but the body has not yet recognized or expelled the pregnancy tissue.
Figure 19 demonstrates the ultrasound findings in case of missed abortion. There was absence of the growth of the fetal pole over the observation period of a week. The Doppler ultrasound revealed abnormal placental blood flow, pointing towards a non-viable pregnancy. The fetal heart rate was also absent, indicating that fetal demise occurred around 8–9 weeks, despite the woman not experiencing any miscarriage symptoms.
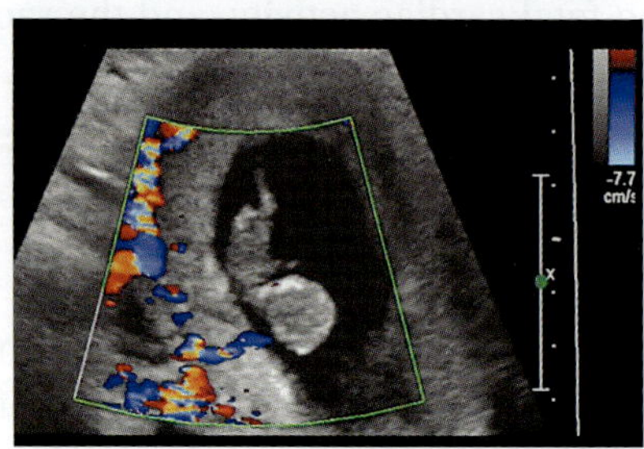

Fig. 19: Missed abortion.</td>
<td>Explanation: Missed abortion is a condition in which the fetus becomes dead and is retained inside the uterine cavity. Beyond 12 weeks of gestation, the liquor amnii gets absorbed and the placenta becomes papery, pale, and adherent. The patient is likely to present with features of threatened miscarriage. There may be presence of brownish vaginal discharge and subsidence of pregnancy symptoms such as retrogression of breast changes, cessation of uterine growth, etc. The fetal heart sounds may not be heard and the immunological tests for pregnancy may become negative. The uterus may be small for dates and ultrasound may reveal an empty gestational sac.
Before 12 weeks of pregnancy, the treatment comprises suction evacuation. Oxytocin can be used for inducing uterine contractions after 12 weeks of gestation. Misoprostol (single oral dose of 600 μg) can be used for inducing uterine contractions both before and after 12 weeks of gestation.</td>
</tr>
</table>

Question	Answer	Comment
Q20. A 36-year-old woman, gravida 4, para 1, with a history of 3 past miscarriages and multiple D&C procedures, presents with amenorrhea and infertility. Hysterosalpingography results are shown below. What is the likely diagnosis? 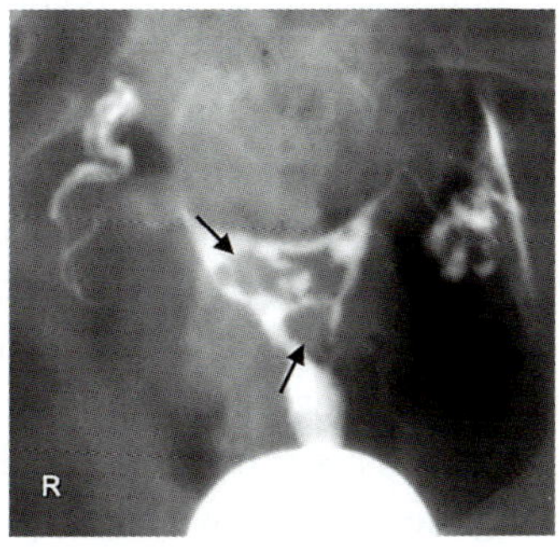 A. Endometriosis B. Asherman's syndrome C. Submucosal uterine fibroids D. Polycystic ovary syndrome (PCOS) E. Adenomyosis	**Ans: B (Asherman's syndrome)** The arrows in the adjacent image represent the presence of synechiae/adhesions. The clinical history and hysterosalpingography image point toward the diagnosis of Asherman's syndrome. Diagnosis of Asherman's syndrome can also be reached by doing tests like hysteroscopy, TVS, etc. Hysterosalpingogram revealing irregular filling defects in the endometrium is suggestive of endometrial adhesions. 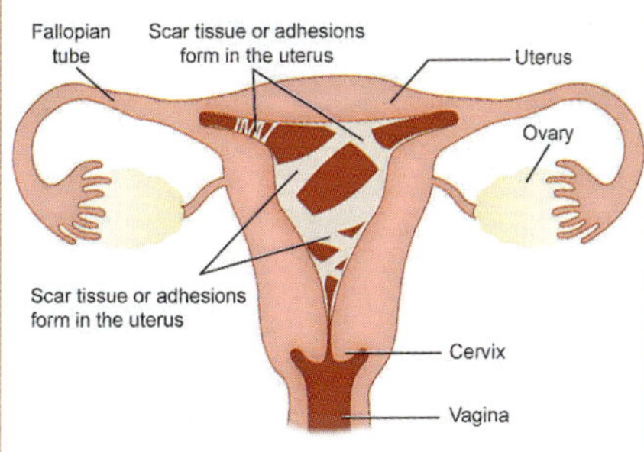 **Fig. 20:** Diagrammatic representation of Asherman's syndrome.	**Explanation:** Asherman's syndrome, or intrauterine adhesions, typically develops after a uterine surgery, such as D&C. It is characterized by the formation of scar tissue inside the uterine cavity **(Fig. 20)**, leading to symptoms like light or absent periods and infertility. The most accurate method of diagnosis of Asherman's syndrome is direct visualization via hysteroscopic assessment. These adhesions can also be removed on hysteroscopy. To prevent reformation of adhesions following surgery, prescription of estrogen supplementation or intrauterine placement of a splint, balloon, or copper device may prove useful. **Potential questions:** There can be potential questions related to etiology, diagnosis, and management of various causes of recurrent miscarriage.

Question	Answer	Comment
Q21. A 28-year-old woman presents with a history of three consecutive first-trimester miscarriages. Hysterosalpingogram (HSG) of the pelvis shows a uterus with two distinct endometrial cavities and a common cervical canal as shown below. What is the most likely cause of her recurrent miscarriages? 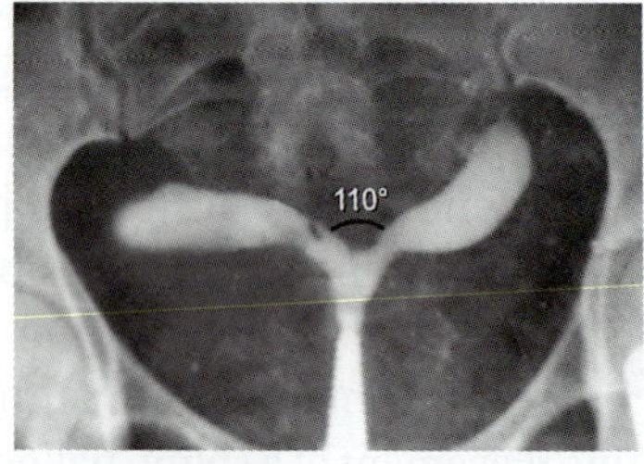 A. Septate uterus B. Bicornuate uterus C. Uterine fibroids D. Asherman's syndrome E. Cervical insufficiency	**Ans: B (Bicornuate uterus)** The adjacent image shows an HSG demonstrating a single cervical canal and a possible duplication of the uterine horns. In this case, it was difficult to differentiate between bicornuate uterus and septate uterus on ultrasound alone. Since an angle of >105° was found to be separating the two uterine horns on HSG, the diagnosis of a bicornuate uterus **(Fig. 21)**, rather than a septate uterus, was made. 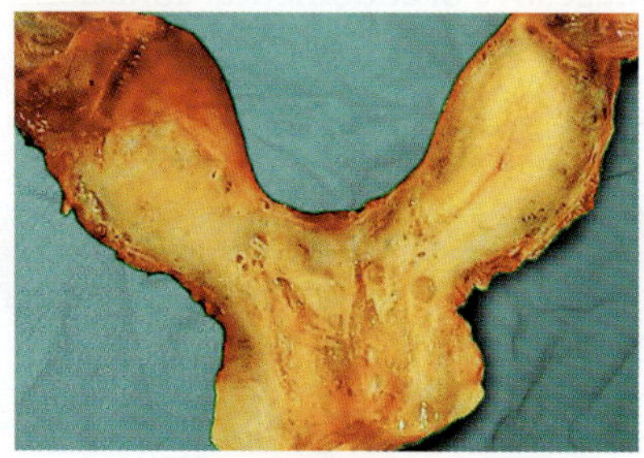 **Fig. 21:** Specimen showing cut section of a bicornuate uterus with a single cervix.	**Explanation:** A bicornuate uterus is a congenital uterine anomaly where the uterus is partially divided into two horns. This anomaly could be responsible for causing an abnormal or irregularly shaped uterus, which could result in improper implantation and/or growth of the embryo, thereby leading to recurrent miscarriages. If the patient is asymptomatic, often no treatment is necessary. For those experiencing recurrent pregnancy loss, preterm labor, or other complications, surgical correction (metroplasty) may be considered. This procedure involves unifying the uterine cavity to improve pregnancy outcomes. **Potential questions:** There can be potential questions related to etiology, diagnosis, and management of various causes of recurrent miscarriage.
Q22. A 30-year-old woman with a history of four consecutive first-trimester miscarriages undergoes HSG of the pelvis. The imaging results are shown below. What is the most likely cause of her recurrent miscarriages? 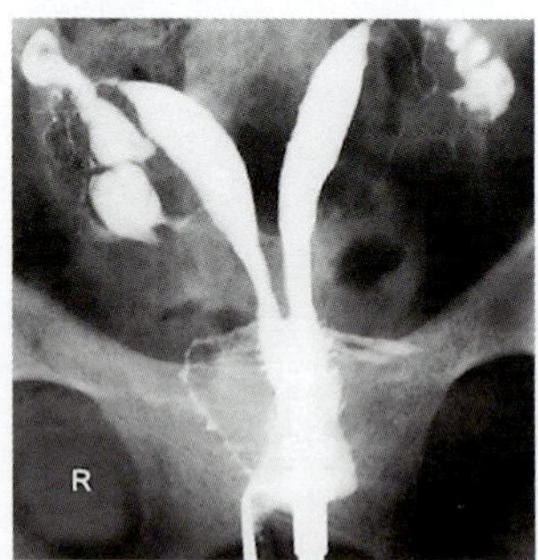 A. Bicornuate uterus B. Uterine septum C. Asherman's syndrome D. Uterine fibroids E. Cervical insufficiency	**Ans: B (Uterine septum)** The adjacent image demonstrates a HSG showing the presence of a uterine septum, which was confirmed on hysteroscopy. **Figure 22** illustrates hysteroscopic visualization of uterine septum. 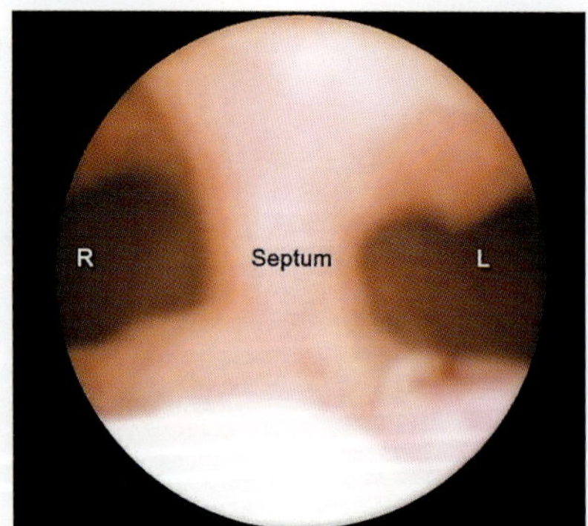 **Fig. 22:** Hysteroscopic examination showing the presence of uterine septum.	**Explanation:** A uterine septum is a congenital anomaly where a fibrous or muscular septum divides the uterine cavity. This condition is a significant cause of recurrent miscarriage, as the septum is poorly vascularized, leading to suboptimal implantation and an increased likelihood of miscarriage. Diagnosis is often confirmed through imaging techniques like MRI, 3D ultrasound, or hysteroscopy. **Potential questions:** There can be potential questions related to etiology, diagnosis, and management of various causes of recurrent miscarriage.

CERVICAL INCOMPETENCE

Question	Answer	Comment
Q23. A 28-year-old woman with a history of second-trimester miscarriage is at 14 weeks' gestation. Ultrasound shows cervical shortening, leading to a diagnosis of cervical incompetence. The below image depicts a surgical procedure where a suture is placed around the cervix to reinforce it. Which surgical procedure is being depicted? 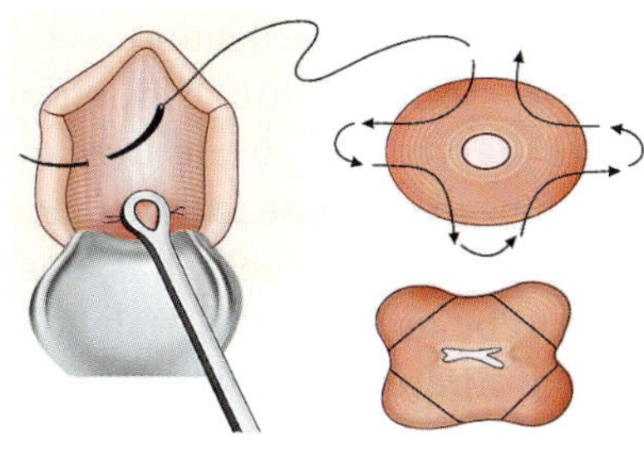 A. Hefner's cerclage B. McDonald's procedure C. Wurm's procedure D. Lash procedure E. Shirodkar's procedure	**Ans: B (McDonald's procedure)** The adjacent image shows McDonald's procedure for correcting cervical incompetence, where the cervix begins dilating and effacing between 16 to 28 weeks, unable to retain the pregnancy. **Figures 23A to D** illustrate the anatomical changes in the cervix due to this condition. 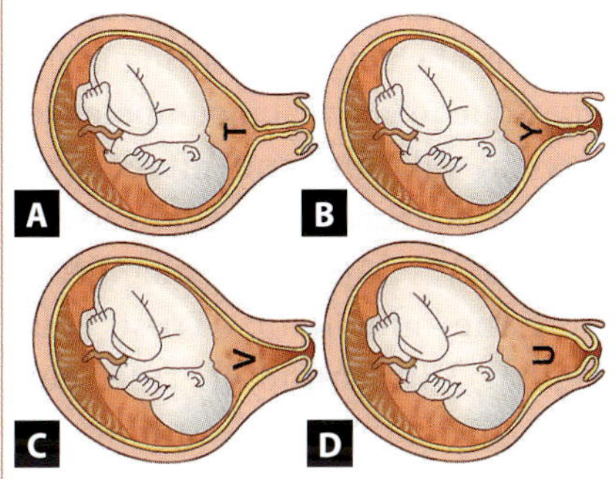 **Figs. 23A to D:** Anatomical changes occurring in cervix due to cervical incompetence.	**Explanation:** McDonald's procedure is a type of cervical cerclage performed to prevent preterm birth in women diagnosed with cervical incompetence. This procedure, which is performed vaginally, involves placement of a 5 mm band of permanent purse string suture around the ectocervix at the level of internal cervical os. This suture on approximation is likely to tighten the internal cervical os, thereby reducing the risk of miscarriage or premature delivery. This procedure is often done in cases where there is a history of second-trimester losses or early cervical dilation in current pregnancy. **Potential questions:** There could be questions related to indications, techniques, and complications of various surgical procedures performed for correction of cervical incompetence.
Q24. A 32-year-old woman with a history of recurrent second-trimester miscarriages is diagnosed with cervical incompetence at 13 weeks of pregnancy. She is scheduled for a cervical cerclage to provide additional support. Which surgical procedure is being depicted in this image? 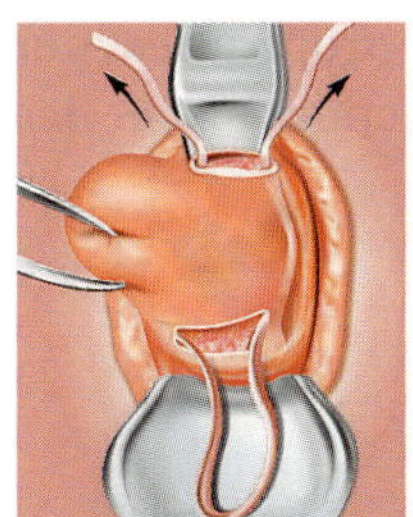 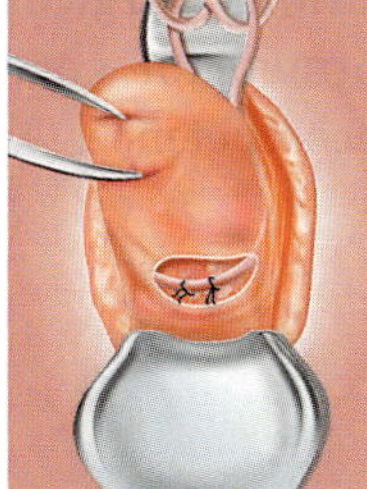 A. Hefner's cerclage B. McDonald's procedure C. Wurm's procedure D. Lash procedure E. Shirodkar's procedure	**Ans: E (Shirodkar's procedure)** In this procedure, a submucosal suture is placed near the internal os by making incisions on the anterior and posterior cervix, followed by dissection to separate the bladder and rectum. **Figure 24** shows the cervix after applying Shirodkar's stitch. 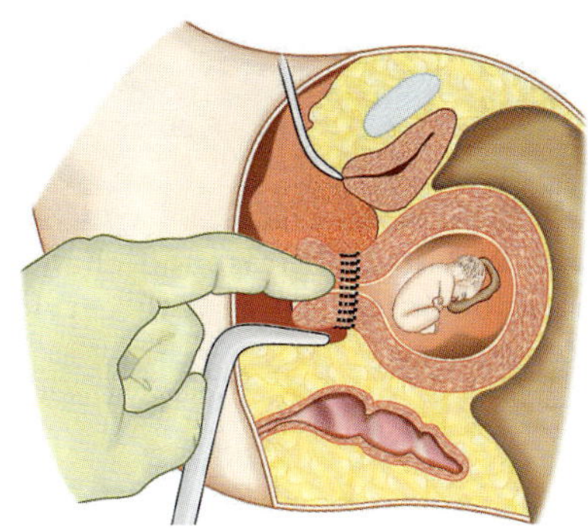 **Fig. 24:** Appearance of cervix after application of Shirodkar's stitch.	**Explanation:** Shirodkar's procedure is a type of cervical cerclage where a suture is placed high on the cervix, often requiring the bladder to be mobilized. It is used in patients with cervical incompetence to prevent second-trimester miscarriages and preterm birth. The procedure differs from McDonald's procedure in that it involves placing the suture higher on the cervix and is typically more secure, but also more invasive. Also, this suture, which is applied, would remain intact for life. Therefore, the patient has to be delivered by a cesarean section. **Potential questions:** There could be questions related to indications, techniques, and complications of various surgical procedures performed for correction of cervical incompetence.

Question	Answer	Comment
Q25. A 28-year-old woman with a history of second-trimester pregnancy losses is diagnosed with cervical incompetence and scheduled for a cervical cerclage to support the cervix. The image below depicts the technique of cervical reinforcement used in this procedure. Which surgical technique is shown in the image? 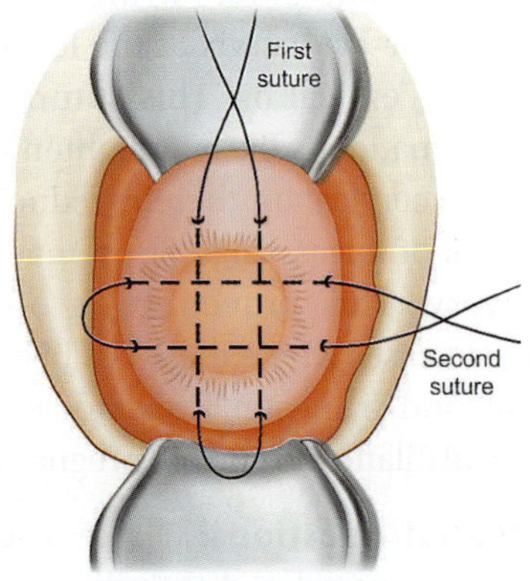 A. Beck's procedure B. McDonald's procedure C. Wurm's procedure D. Lash procedure E. Shirodkar's procedure	**Ans: C (Wurm's procedure)** Wurm's stitch, also known as Hefner's cerclage, is performed by application of U or mattress sutures. This is demonstrated in the adjacent image. This stitch appears to be most useful when minimal length of cervical canal has been left due to premature cervical effacement. **Figures 25A to D** illustrate ultrasound changes in response to various anatomical changes occurring in the cervix due to cervical incompetence. Cervical dilation and effacement produce changes in the cervix in the form of T, Y, V, U (can be remembered using the mnemonic "**T**rust **Y**our **V**aginal **U**ltrasound"). T-shaped cervix on ultrasound examination points toward a normal cervix. As the internal cervical os opens and the membranes start herniating into the upper part of endocervical canal, the cervical shape on ultrasound changes into a Y. With the further progression of the above-mentioned cervical changes, Y shape changes into V and then eventually into U. 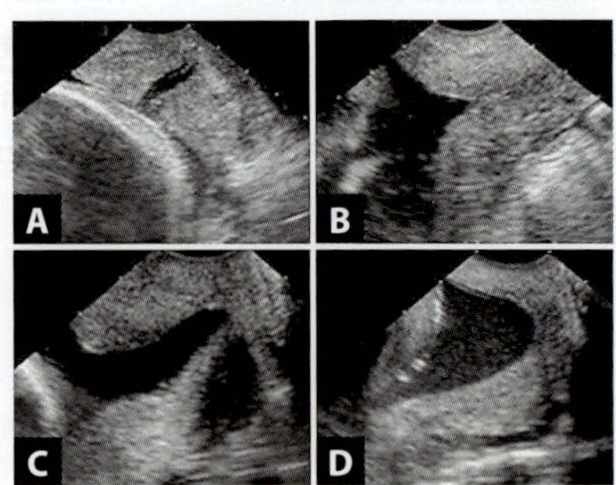 **Figs. 25A to D:** Ultrasound changes in endocervical canal with cervical incompetence.	**Explanation:** Wurm's stitch is a specific type of cervical cerclage that involves placing a suture at the level of the internal os to reinforce the cervix. This technique is particularly useful in cases of cervical incompetence, where the cervix dilates prematurely, leading to potential pregnancy loss or preterm birth. Unlike other cerclage techniques, Wurm's stitch focuses on applying the suture at a precise location for maximum effectiveness in preventing cervical dilation. Serial sonographic evaluation of the cervix for funneling and shortening in response to transfundal pressure every 2 weeks has been found to be useful in the evaluation of incompetent cervix. Besides changes in cervical shape observed on transvaginal ultrasound, other findings observed on ultrasound examination include the following: ▪ Cervical length < 25 mm ▪ *Funneling of cervix:* Funneling implies herniation of fetal membranes into the upper part of endocervical canal. ▪ Presence of the fetal parts in the cervix or vagina **Potential questions:** There could be questions related to indications, techniques, and complications of various surgical procedures performed for correction of cervical incompetence.

MEDICAL TERMINATION OF PREGNANCY

Question	Answer	Comment
Q26. A 30-year-old woman is scheduled for second-trimester pregnancy termination. The device shown in the image below is used for cervical dilation. Its primary action is: 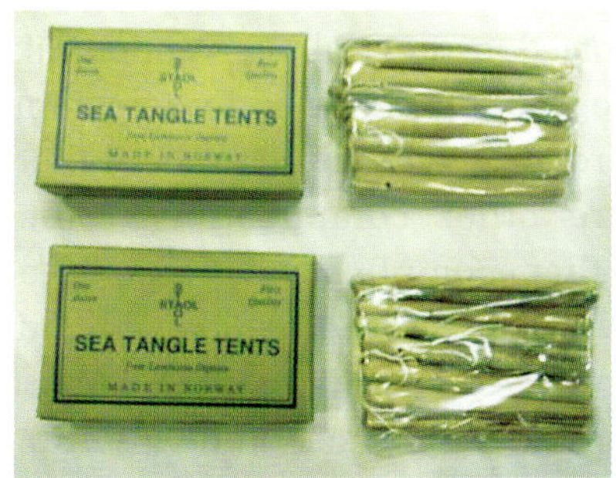 A. Chemical softening of the cervix B. Mechanical expansion by absorbing moisture C. Induction of uterine contractions D. Enzymatic collagen degradation E. Manual dilation by an operator	**Ans: B (Mechanical expansion by absorbing moisture)** The adjacent image shows laminaria tents, natural cervical ripening agents made from dried seaweed stems **(Fig. 26)**. They absorb cervical moisture, causing gradual mechanical expansion for gentle, controlled dilation before procedures like second-trimester termination or hysteroscopy. 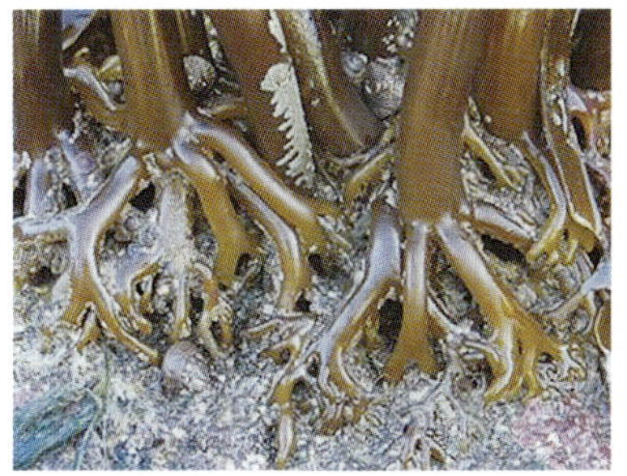 **Fig. 26:** Seaweed laminaria.	**Explanation:** Besides Hegar's dilators, other methods of cervical dilatation include osmotic dilatation using laminaria tents or pharmacological dilatation using medications such as misoprostol. Laminaria tents can also be used for cervical dilation to induce labor and delivery. Recently, there has been a decline in the use of laminaria tents due to an increased rate of infection as a result of ineffective sterilization techniques used on the plants prior to drying. **Potential questions:** There can be questions pertaining to the indications, prerequisites, equipment, technique, and complications associated with the procedure of MTP using vacuum aspiration, manual vacuum aspiration, and medical methods.
Q27. A 26-year-old woman at 8 weeks of gestation presents with incomplete miscarriage and mild vaginal bleeding. The image below shows the device used for uterine evacuation. What is the most likely complication associated with this procedure? 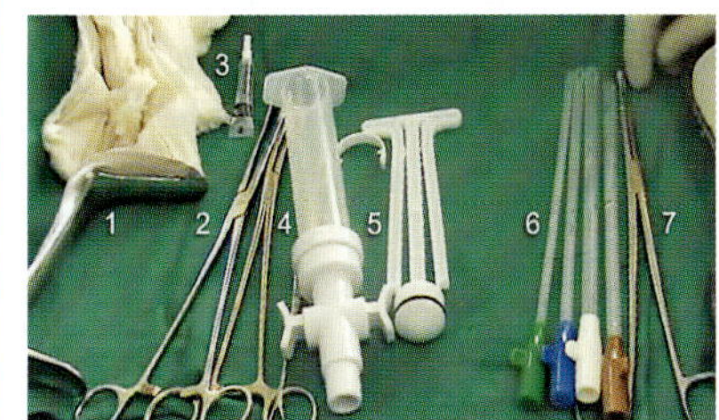 A. Uterine perforation B. Heavy bleeding C. Cervical laceration D. Infection E. Incomplete evacuation	**Ans: E (Incomplete evacuation)** The adjacent image shows equipment for MVA containing: (1) Sim's speculum, (2) vulsellum, (3) silicone gel, (4) syringe, (5) plunger, (6) suction cannula, and (7) sponge holder. The key component is the MVA syringe **(Figs. 27A and B)**, consisting of a syringe with valve/lock, plunger, and guard. 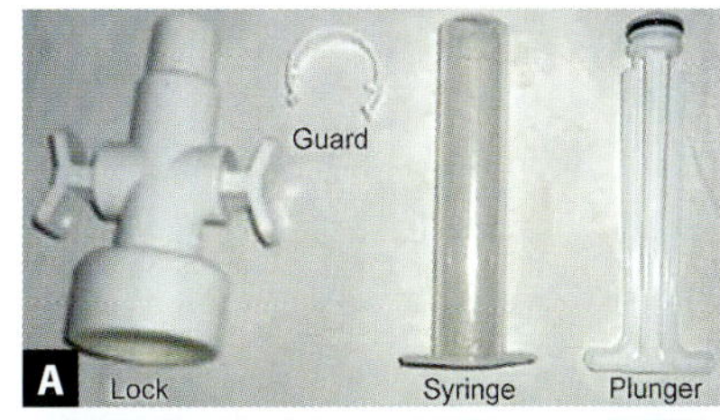 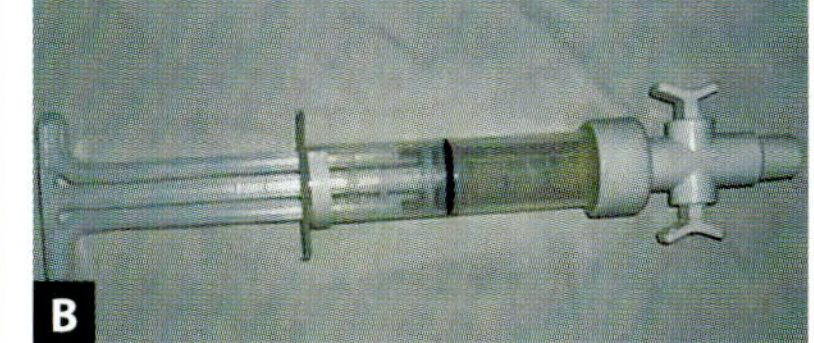 **Figs. 27A and B:** (A) Different parts of a vacuum aspirator syringe; (B) An assembled vacuum aspirator syringe.	**Explanation:** MVA (manual vacuum aspiration) is a safe, simple outpatient method for medical termination of pregnancy, ideally before 10 weeks and usable in uteri <6 weeks. It requires no cervical dilation, reducing complications like uterine perforation, though incomplete evacuation with retained tissue may occasionally occur. **Potential questions:** There can be questions pertaining to the indications, prerequisites, equipment, technique, and complications associated with the procedure of medical termination of pregnancy using vacuum aspiration, manual vacuum aspiration and medical methods.

Question	Answer	Comment
Q28. A 32-year-old woman at 10 weeks' gestation undergoes a procedure for MTP. The image below shows the procedure being performed. What is the most appropriate next step if the patient develops signs of endometritis post procedure? 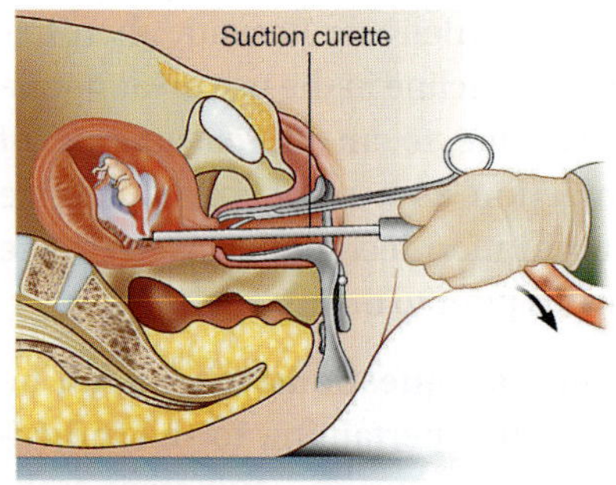 A. Repeat the procedure. B. Administer broad-spectrum antibiotics. C. Perform hysterectomy. D. Observe and manage expectantly. E. Initiate hormonal therapy.	**Ans: B (Administer broad-spectrum antibiotics)** The adjacent image shows the procedure of suction aspiration being performed for MTP. Surgical techniques in the first trimester practically comprise entirely of vacuum or suction techniques. The terms "vacuum curettage", "uterine aspiration", and "vacuum aspiration" are often used interchangeably. They all refer to evacuation of the uterus by suction, regardless of the source of suction. **Figure 28** shows the equipment used for performing this procedure. 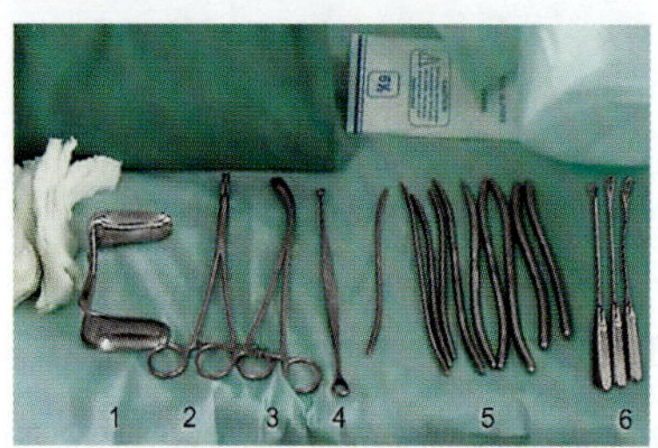 **Fig. 28:** Tray containing various equipment used for suction evacuation: (1) Sim's speculum, (2) sponge holder, (3) vulsellum, (4) anterior vaginal wall retractor, (5) Hegar's dilators of increasing sizes, (6) uterine curettes of varying sizes.	**Explanation:** Endometritis is a possible complication following suction aspiration and is characterized by fever, uterine tenderness, and foul-smelling discharge. The primary treatment is administration of broad-spectrum antibiotics to manage the infection. Surgical interventions like repeat aspiration or hysterectomy are rarely required unless there are other complications. Some other complications associated with the procedure may include minor complications such as post-operative nausea and vomiting, and hypotension, or more serious complications such as uterine perforation, incomplete evacuation, bleeding following and during the process, failure of the procedure, Asherman's syndrome, cervical lacerations, cervical incompetence, etc. **Potential questions:** There can be questions pertaining to the indications, prerequisites, equipment, technique, and complications associated with MTP using vacuum aspiration, manual vacuum aspiration, and medical methods.

MULTIFETAL GESTATION

Question	Answer	Comment
Q29. The ultrasound image below shows a twin pregnancy at 12 weeks of gestation. The fetuses have separate amniotic sacs and placentas. What is the most likely diagnosis for this twin pregnancy? 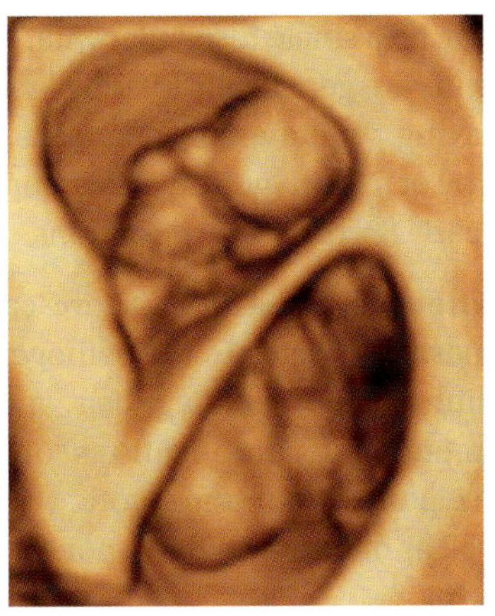 A. Monochorionic diamniotic twins B. Monoamniotic twins C. Conjoined twins D. Dizygotic twins E. Monochorionic monoamniotic twins	**Ans: D (Dizygotic twins)** The adjacent image demonstrates a three-dimensional ultrasound showing diamniotic dichorionic twins at 10-12 weeks of gestation. The intervening membrane between the two twins is composed of four layers: Two intervening layers of chorion surrounded by a layer of amnion on either side. The mode of development of dizygotic twins or nonidentical or fraternal twins is as demonstrated in **Figure 29**. 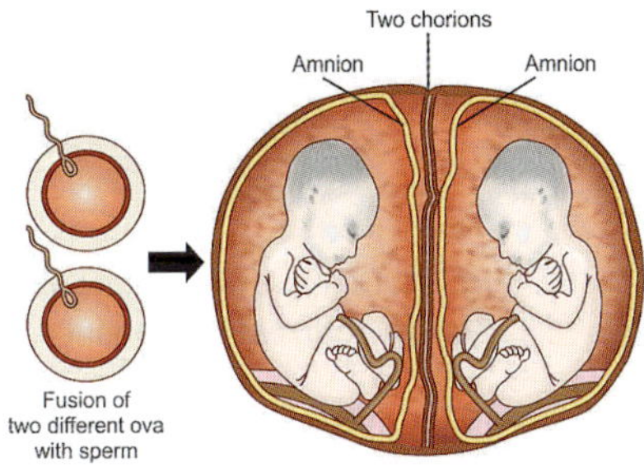 **Fig. 29:** Formation of dizygotic twins.	**Explanation:** When two or more ova are fertilized by two or more separate sperms, the result is development of dizygotic twins or nonidentical twins or fraternal twins. In dizygotic twins, the two embryos have separate placentae and there is no communication between fetal vessels of the two embryos. This is in contrast to monochorionic twins, which share a placenta. Dizygotic twins have different genetic makeup and gender, unlike monozygotic (identical) twins. Dizygotic twins comprise two-thirds of the total cases of twins. **Potential questions:** There can be questions related to pathogenesis, clinical features, diagnosis, management and complications of both dizygotic and monozygotic twins.
Q30. A 6-week scan shows two fetuses with separate amniotic sacs and a single fused placenta. The diagram below illustrates the mechanism of formation. The patient asks if these are identical or fraternal twins. What is the most likely explanation? 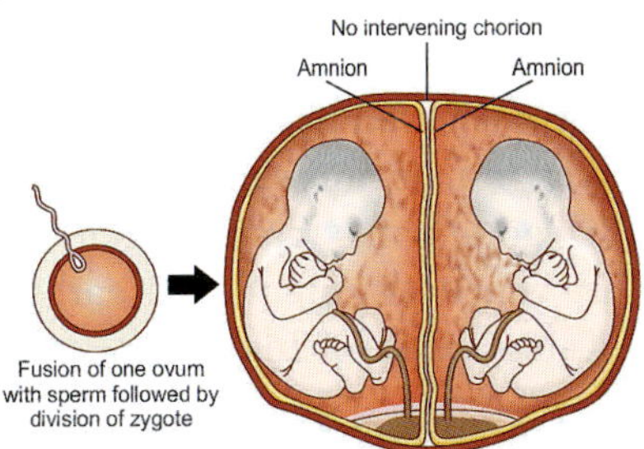 A. Monozygotic twins B. Dichorionic diamniotic dizygotic twins C. Monochorionic monoamniotic twins D. Dichorionic diamniotic monozygotic twins E. Fraternal twins	**Ans: A (Monozygotic twins)** The adjacent image shows the formation of monozygotic twins (of the type monochorionic diamniotic monozygotic twin) due to the division of a single fertilized egg. Different types of monozygotic twins can result depending on the timing of the division of the fertilized ovum **(Fig. 30)**. 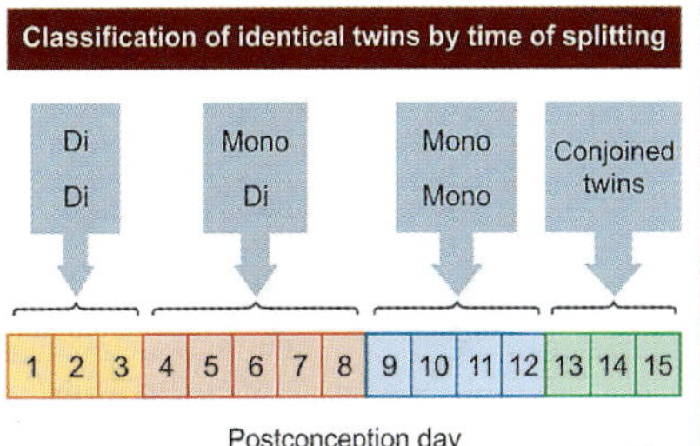 **Fig. 30:** Formation of monozygotic twins (Di Di: diamniotic dichorionic; Mono Di: monochorionic diamniotic; Mono Mono: monoamniotic Monochorionic)	**Explanation:** Monozygotic or identical twins are formed due to the division of a single fertilized egg into two distinct fetuses after a variable number of divisions. These twins will have the same gender and similar genetic constitution. These usually comprise one-third cases of twins. These twins usually share a single placenta. There can be communication between the fetal vessels. The composition of the intervening membrane between the twins varies with the type of monozygotic twin. **Potential questions:** There can be questions related to the pathogenesis, clinical features, diagnosis, management and complications of both dizygotic and monozygotic twins as well as different types of monozygotic twins.

<table>
<tr><th>Question</th><th>Answer</th><th>Comment</th></tr>
<tr><td>

Q31. An ultrasound image shows a pregnancy with two fetuses, each in separate amniotic sacs and with individual placentas. Given the genetic testing confirms monozygosity, what is the type of twin pregnancy depicted?

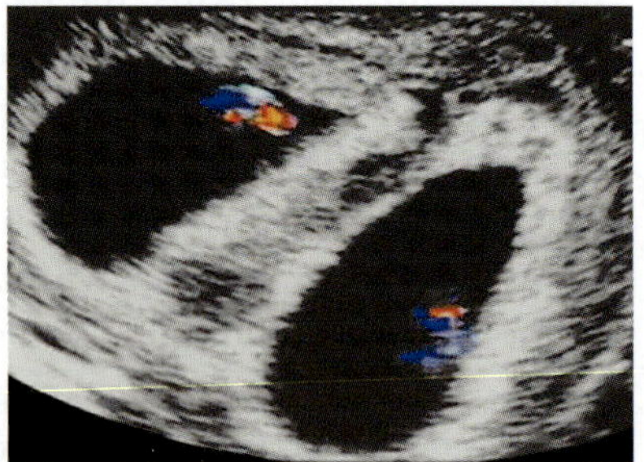

A. Monoamniotic monochorionic twins
B. Dichorionic diamniotic twins
C. Monochorionic diamniotic twins
D. Diamniotic dichorionic monozygotic twins
E. Dizygotic twins

</td><td>

Ans: B (Diamniotic dichorionic monozygotic twins)

The adjacent Doppler ultrasound image depicts diamniotic dichorionic twins at 7 weeks of gestation The intervening membrane between the twins is composed of four layers: Two layers of chorion in the middle surrounded by a layer of amnion on either side **(Fig. 31)**.

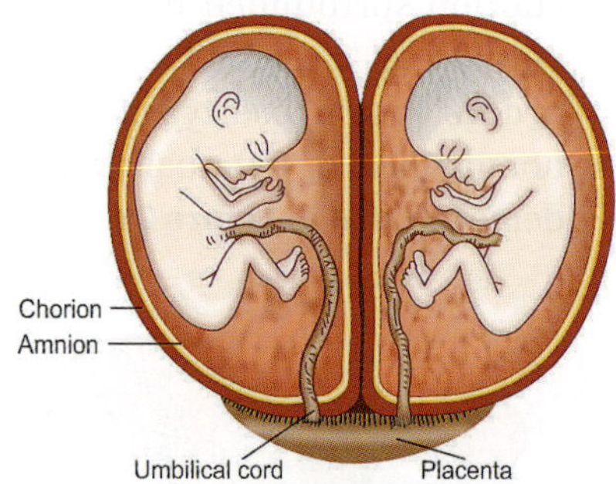

Fig. 31: Diamniotic dichorionic monozygotic twin pregnancy.

</td><td>

Explanation: Diamniotic dichorionic monozygotic twins result from the very early splitting of a single fertilized egg within the first 72 hours' postconception, leading to the formation of two separate placentas and amniotic sacs. In some cases, there may be a single fused placenta. These twins are genetically identical despite having separate amniotic sacs. This type of monozygotic twin accounts for nearly 8% of all twin gestations.

Potential questions: There can be questions related to the pathogenesis, clinical features, diagnosis, management and complications of both dizygotic and monozygotic twins as well as different types of monozygotic twins.

</td></tr>
<tr><td>

Q32. The ultrasound image below shows a twin pregnancy with a single shared placenta and two separate amniotic sacs. Based on these findings, what is the most likely diagnosis?

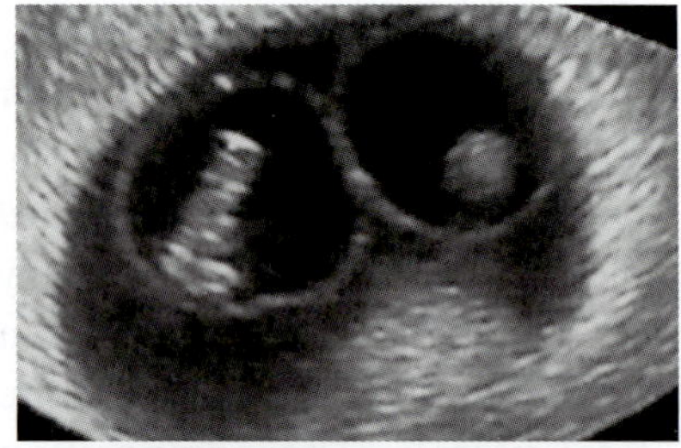

A. Dizygotic twins
B. Monochorionic diamniotic twins
C. Monoamniotic twins
D. Conjoined twins
E. Dichorionic diamniotic twins

</td><td>

Ans: B (Monochorionic diamniotic twins)

The adjacent image shows monochorionic diamniotic twins. Each embryo is surrounded by a separate amniotic sac. However, there is common chorionic sac which surrounds the two amniotic sacs. As a result, the intervening membrane between the two twins comprises two layers of amnion **(Fig. 32)**. Usually, there is a single fused placenta.

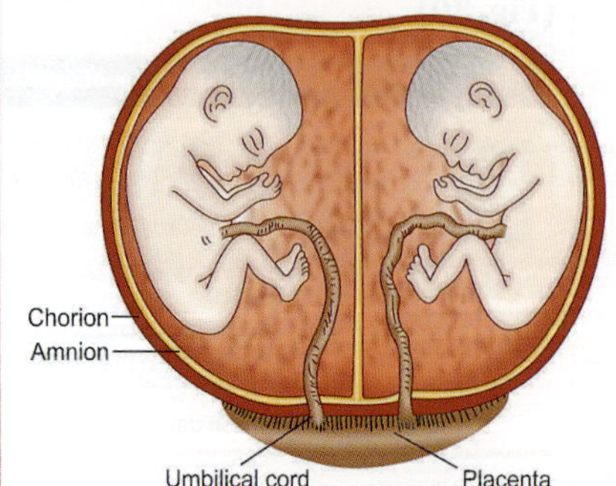

Fig. 32: Diagrammatic representation of diamniotic monochorionic monozygotic twins.

</td><td>

Explanation: Monozygotic (identical) twins result from the splitting of a single fertilized egg. In case of diamniotic monochorionic twins, the cleavage division is delayed until the formation of inner cell mass and the embryo splits between 4 and 7 days of gestation. As a result, these twins share a single placenta but have two separate amniotic sacs. This type of twin pregnancy is associated with increased risks such as twin-to-twin transfusion syndrome. Unlike dizygotic twins, monozygotic twins are genetically identical. Nearly 20% of all twins are of this type.

Potential questions: There can be questions related to pathogenesis, clinical features, diagnosis, management and complications of both dizygotic and monozygotic twins as well as different types of monozygotic twins.

</td></tr>
</table>

Question	Answer	Comment
Q33. The ultrasound image below shows a twin pregnancy with two fetuses sharing a single amniotic sac and a single placenta. What is the most likely diagnosis? 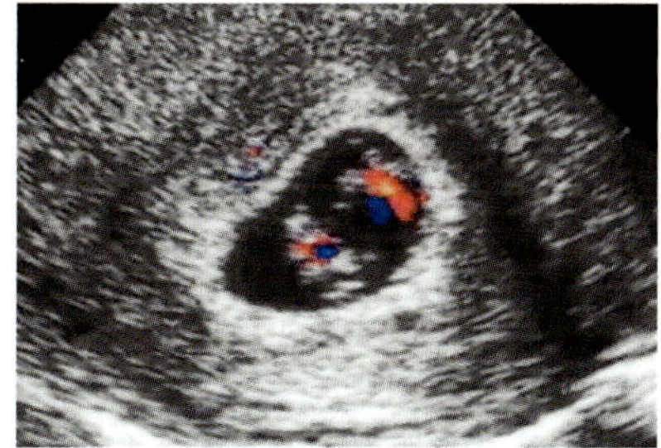 A. Monochorionic diamniotic twins B. Monoamniotic monochorionic twins C. Dichorionic diamniotic twins D. Monoamniotic dichorionic twins E. Conjoined twins	**Ans: B (Monoamniotic monochorionic twins)** The adjacent image shows monoamniotic monozygotic twins at 7 weeks of gestation. The two embryos are surrounded by a single amnion and a single chorion **(Fig. 33)**. As a result, there is no intervening membrane between the two fetuses. 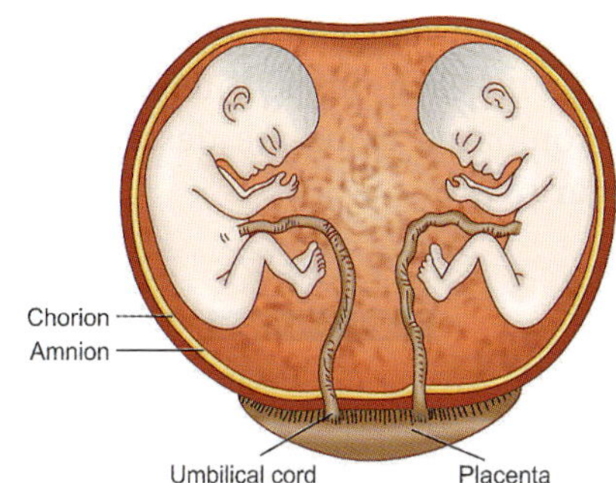 **Fig. 33:** Diagrammatic representation of monoamniotic monochorionic twins.	**Explanation:** Monoamniotic monochorionic twins occur when a single fertilized egg splits after the formation of both the chorion and the amnion, usually between days 8 and 13 after fertilization. These twins share both the placenta and the amniotic sac, which increases the risk of complications like cord entanglement and twin-to-twin transfusion syndrome. Such types of monozygotic twins are rare, accounting for less than 1% of all twin gestations. **Potential questions:** There can be questions related to pathogenesis, clinical features, diagnosis, management and complications of both dizygotic and monozygotic twins as well as different types of monozygotic twins.

Question	Answer	Comment
Q34. A dead neonate is born with a rare condition where two heads are joined at the skull and upper body, but have separate lower bodies. The autopsy picture is shown below. What is the most likely diagnosis? 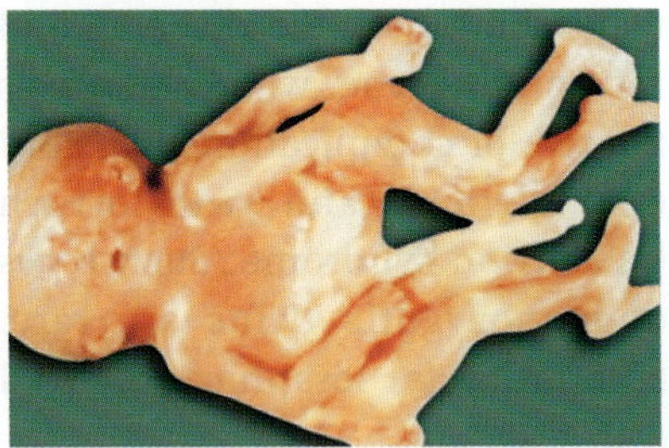 A. Thoracopagus conjoined twins B. Omphalopagus conjoined twins C. Craniopagus conjoined twins D. Pygopagus conjoined twins E. Cephalopagus conjoined twins	**Ans:** **E (Cephalopagus conjoined twins)** The adjacent image shows the autopsy specimen of cephalopagus twins, a rare type of conjoined twins where the twins are fused at the head, face, and upper body. Conjoined or Siamese twins are a type of monozygotic twins where the division of embryo occurs between 13 and 15 days after fertilization. In these cases, the twins share a particular body part with each other. Different types of conjoined twins are described in **Figure 34**. Ventral conjunctions Rostral Cephalopagus Thoracopagus Omphalopagus Caudal Ischiopagus Lateral Parapagus diprosopus Parapagus dicephalus Dorsal conjunctions Craniopagus Rachipagus Pygopagus **Fig. 34:** Different types of conjoined twins.	**Explanation:** The term "cephalopagus" refers to a more extensive fusion than other types, such as craniopagus twins, who are fused only at the skull. In cephalopagus twins, the fusion involves not only the skull but also parts of the face, such as the jaw, mouth, or even the forehead. Their facial structures may be partially or fully joined, which can lead to a shared mouth, nose, or eyes in some cases. They may also share chest or some part of the upper body. The cephalopagus twins may share parts of the brain or other cranial structures, making separation and survival more challenging. **Potential questions:** There can be questions related to pathogenesis, clinical features, diagnosis, management and complications of both dizygotic and monozygotic twins as well as different types of monozygotic twins including the conjoined twins.

<table>
<tr><th>Question</th><th>Answer</th><th>Comment</th></tr>
<tr><td>Q35. A set of conjoined twins are delivered with fusion at the chest. The twins died immediately at birth. Imaging done previously had revealed a shared pericardium and part of the liver, but they have separate digestive tracts and lungs. What type of surgery-related challenge is most likely to occur with these twins in case these were live?
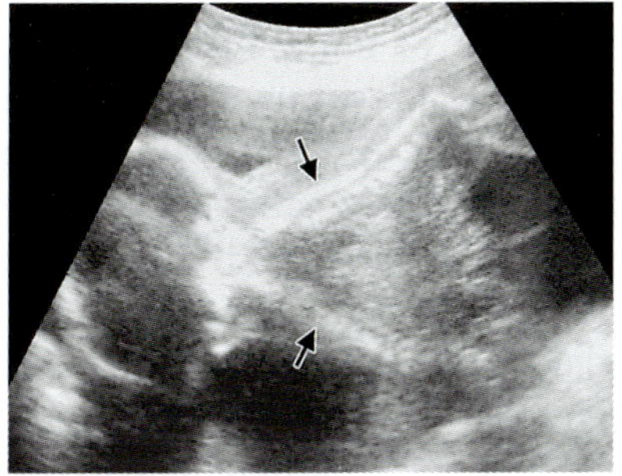
A. Complex cardiac separation
B. Respiratory system separation
C. Gastrointestinal tract separation
D. Neurological complications
E. Hepatic reconstruction</td><td>Ans: A (Complex cardiac separation)
The adjacent image shows the ultrasound appearance of twins fused in the region of anterior chest wall [thoracopagus twins, (Fig. 35)]. Both the twins appear to be facing one another, with their heads being at the same plane and level. Moreover, the thoracic cages of both the twins appear unusually close to one another.
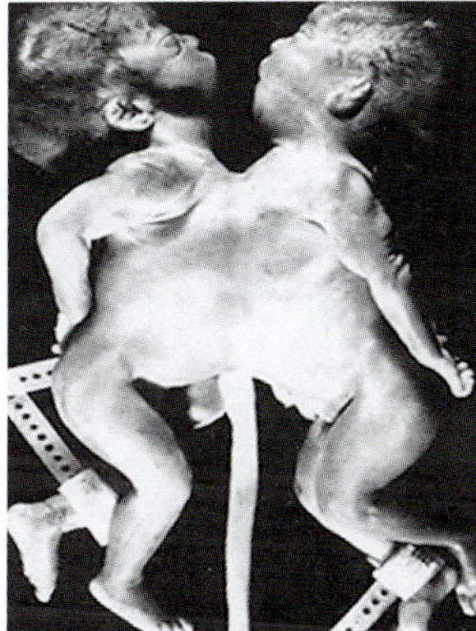
Fig. 35: Autopsy specimen of thoracopagus twins.</td><td>Explanation: In thoracopagus conjoined twins, the most challenging aspect of surgical separation is often the shared heart or pericardium. Cardiovascular complexity determines the feasibility and success of separation. Shared livers can often be successfully divided, but a shared heart presents serious life-threatening risks due to the intricate vascular structures involved.
Potential questions: There can be questions related to pathogenesis, clinical features, diagnosis, management and complications of both dizygotic and monozygotic twins as well as different types of monozygotic twins including the conjoined twins.</td></tr>
<tr><td>Q36. A 30-year-old primigravida at 20 weeks has an ultrasound showing twins in a single amniotic sac with conjoined bodies (image shown below). What is the diagnosis?
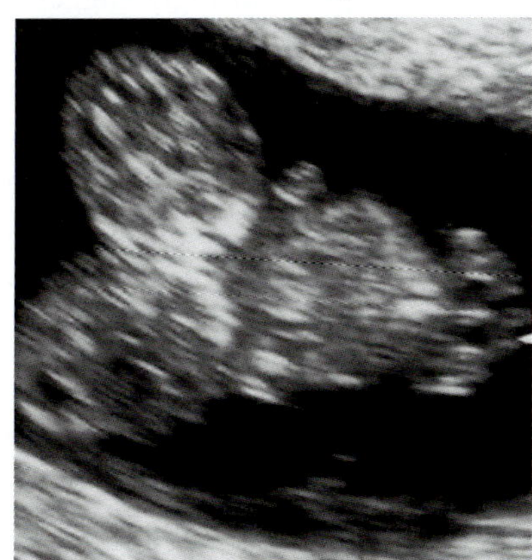
A. Thoracopagus conjoined twins
B. Craniopagus conjoined twins
C. Omphalopagus conjoined twins
D. Pygopagus conjoined twins
E. Parapagus conjoined twins</td><td>Ans: A (Thoracopagus conjoined twins)
The adjacent image shows thoracopagus conjoined twins fused at the thorax and abdomen, demonstrated here at 12 weeks and in live twins (Fig. 36).
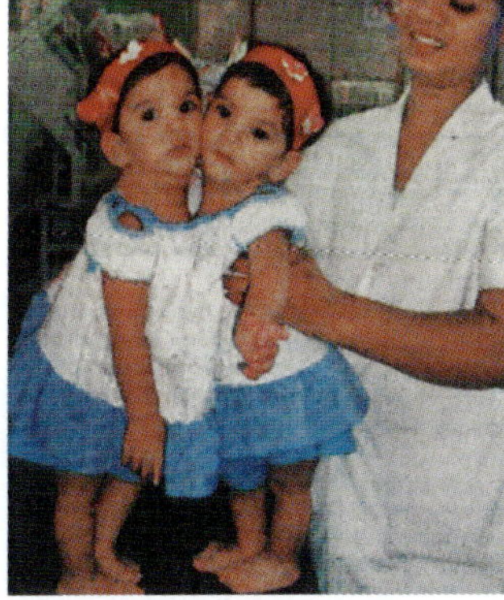
Fig. 36: Live thoracopagus twins, Aradhana and Stuti, were separated after a 12-hour surgery on June 20, 2012. Despite initial success, Aradhana died a month later due to two heart attacks. (Source: Navbharat Times)</td><td>Explanation: Thoracopagus twins are the most common (approximately 40%). Prenatal challenges include assessing the extent of organ sharing, separation feasibility, and obstetric risks. If pregnancy continues, cesarean delivery and postnatal surgical separation are preferred, though separation may be impossible when critical organs are shared
Potential questions: There can be questions related to pathogenesis, clinical features, diagnosis, management and complications of both dizygotic and monozygotic twins as well as different types of monozygotic twins including the conjoined twins.</td></tr>
</table>

Question	Answer	Comment
Q37. A 30-year-old woman presents at 7 weeks of gestation for an early ultrasound. The scan reveals two gestational sacs, each containing a fetal pole with a heartbeat as shown in the image below. What is the most likely diagnosis? 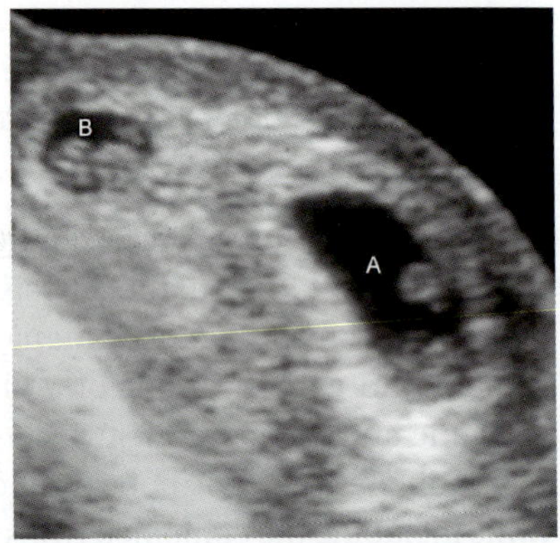 A. Dichorionic diamniotic twins B. Monochorionic monoamniotic twins C. Monochorionic diamniotic twins D. Singleton pregnancy with a vanishing twin E. Monozygotic twins with conjoined fetuses	**Ans: A (Dichorionic diamniotic twins)** Presence of multiple fetuses and/or multiple placentas on ultrasound examination is the most diagnostic feature of multifetal gestation. The adjacent image shows presence of two gestational sacs with A = 7.6 weeks and B = 5.7 weeks. In the same patient as shown in **Figure 37**, when an ultrasound examination was performed at 30 weeks of gestation, two fetal heads were identified. 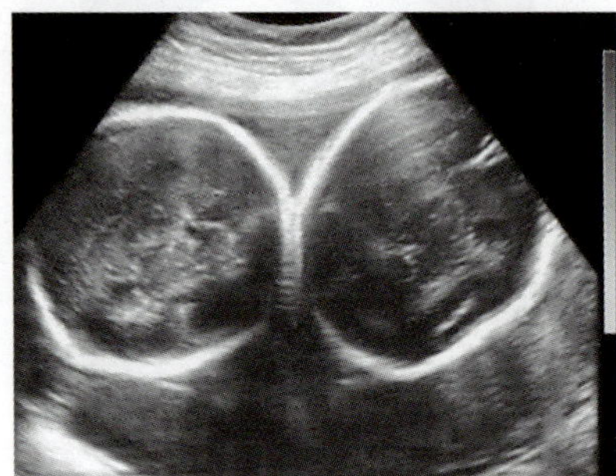 **Fig. 37:** Ultrasound of the same patient at 30 weeks, showing two fetal heads.	**Explanation:** At 7 weeks of gestation, the presence of two gestational sacs and fetal poles strongly suggests a dichorionic diamniotic twin pregnancy. This is the most common form of twin gestation, particularly in dizygotic (fraternal) twins, but it can also occur in monozygotic twins if the fertilized egg splits within the first 3 days after conception. Each fetus has its own amniotic sac and placenta. In case of multifetal gestation, there may be presence of two or more fetuses or gestational sacs on ultrasound examination. Also, there may be two placentas lying close to one another or presence of a single large placenta with a thick dividing membrane. This dividing layer could be composed of maximum up to four membranes (two layers of chorion fused in the middle, surrounded by amnion). **Potential questions:** There can be questions related to the different types of twin gestation, their pathogenesis, diagnosis, and management.
Q38. A 28-year-old primigravida at 7 weeks undergoes ultrasound (image shown below). What is the most likely type of multifetal pregnancy? 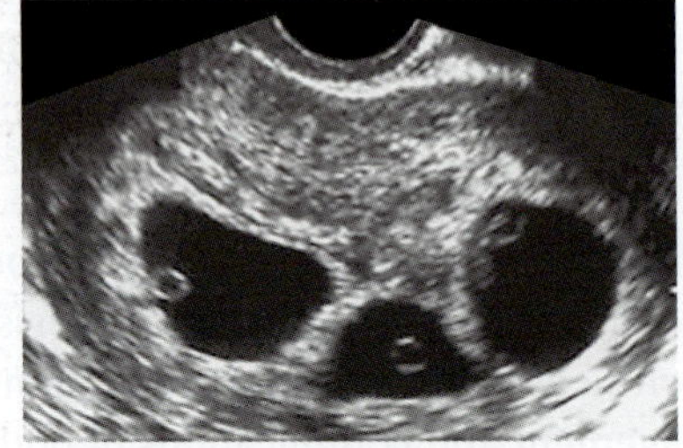 A. Monochorionic triamniotic triplets B. Dichorionic triamniotic triplets C. Monochorionic diamniotic triplets D. Monochorionic monoamniotic triplets E. Trichorionic triamniotic triplets	**Ans: E (Trichorionic triamniotic triplets)** The adjacent image shows triplets at 7 weeks of gestation. Three separate gestational sacs, each having an embryo, can be observed. Each fetus has its own separate placenta observed on Doppler ultrasound examination **(Fig. 38)**. 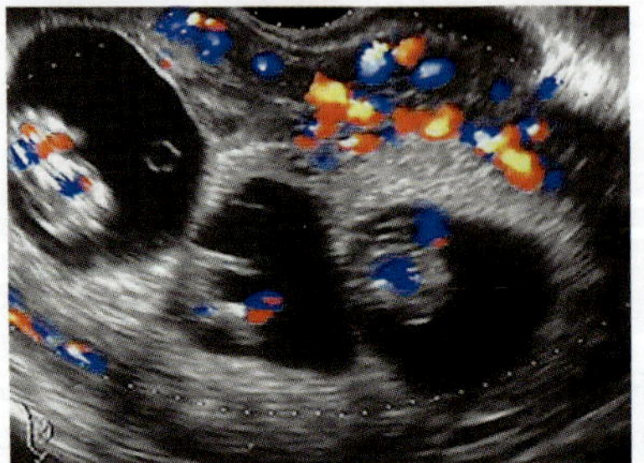 **Fig. 38:** Color Doppler ultrasound of the same patient.	**Explanation:** At 7 weeks, the finding of three gestational sacs, each with its own fetal pole, strongly suggests a trichorionic triamniotic triplet pregnancy. This is the most common configuration of triplet pregnancies, especially when caused by the fertilization of three separate eggs (trizygotic), resulting in each fetus having its own placenta and amniotic sac. **Potential questions:** There can be questions related to different types of multifetal gestation, their pathogenesis, diagnosis, and management.

Question	Answer	Comment
Q39. A 26-year-old woman at 16 weeks' gestation undergoes an ultrasound which reveals a twin pregnancy. The sonographer identifies a specific sign related to the presence of triangular projection of placental tissue at the intertwin membrane insertion as shown in the image below. What does this finding indicate about the type of twin gestation? 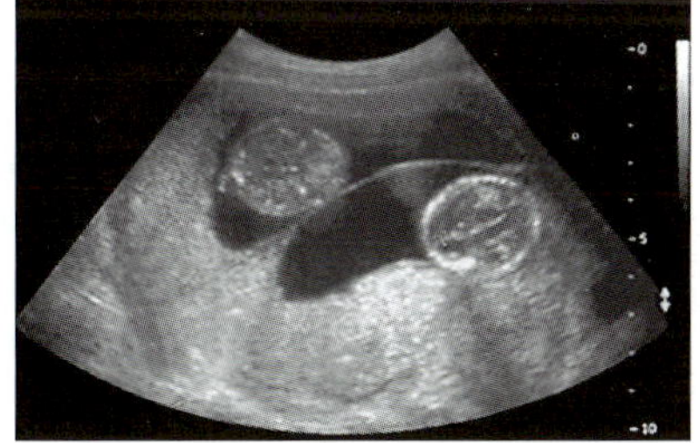 A. Monochorionic diamniotic twins B. Monochorionic monoamniotic twins C. Conjoined twins D. Dichorionic diamniotic twins E. Twin-to-twin transfusion syndrome	**Ans: D (Dichorionic diamniotic twins)** The lambda sign, also known as twin peak, refers to the triangular projection of placental tissue extending from the placental surface upward to a variable distance into the intertwin membrane, where it appears to be gradually tapering, resulting in the formation of triangular projection **(Fig. 39)**. 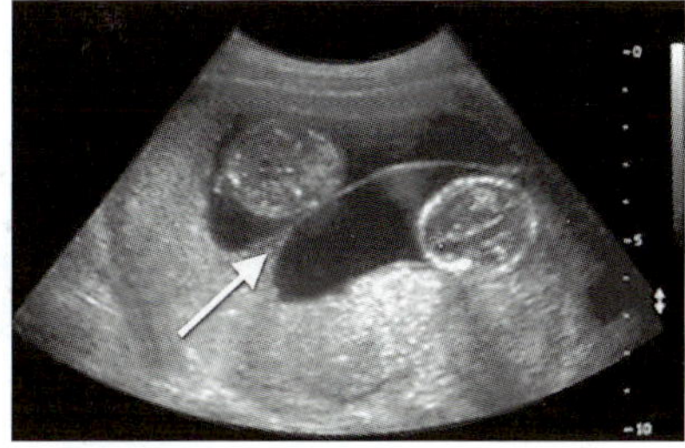 **Fig. 39:** Lambda sign (indicated by arrow).	**Explanation:** Presence of lambda sign on ultrasound scan is indicative of dichorionic diamniotic twin pregnancy. It is also indicative of extension of placental villi into the potential space formed as a result of reflection of apposed layers of amniotic and chorionic membranes from each fetus in case of dichorionic diamniotic twins. This occurs when the twins are either dizygotic (from two separate eggs) or, less commonly, monozygotic (from one egg that splits early enough to form two chorions). Monochorionic twins would not show this sign and instead present with a "T-sign" at the membrane insertion. **Potential questions:** There can be questions related to the types of twin gestation, their pathogenesis, diagnosis, management, and complications.
Q40. A 30-year-old pregnant woman undergoing an 11-week ultrasound shows a thin dividing membrane between twins with a T-shaped junction at the placenta, indicating a "T sign." What does this finding most likely indicate? 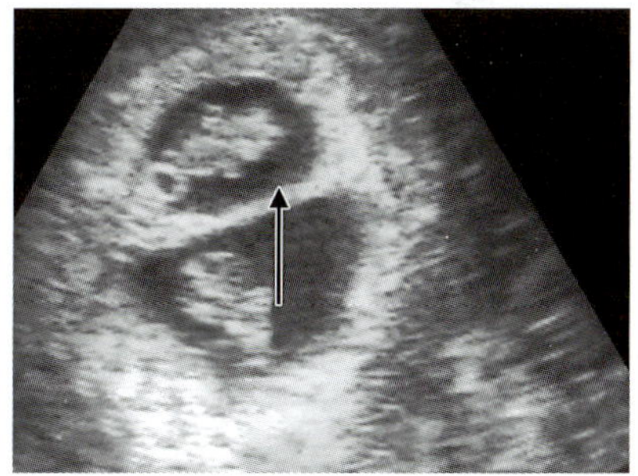 A. Monochorionic monoamniotic twins B. Monochorionic diamniotic twins C. Dichorionic diamniotic twins D. Conjoined twins E. Twin-to-twin transfusion syndrome	**Ans: B (Monochorionic diamniotic twins)** The adjacent image shows T sign on ultrasound (shown with the arrow), thereby indicating a monochorionic diamniotic twin pregnancy. This means that the twins share a single placenta (monochorionic), but each has its own amniotic sac (diamniotic). The pictorial representation of the lambda sign and the T sign is shown in **Figures 40A and B**. 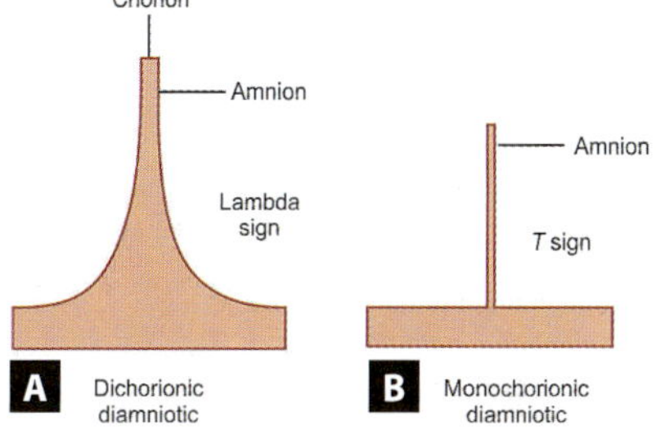 **Figs. 40A and B:** Pictorial representation of the lambda sign and T sign.	**Explanation:** The T sign represents the absence of chorion between the twins at the membrane insertion, contrasting with the lambda sign seen in dichorionic pregnancies. Identifying this is important, as monochorionic twins have a higher risk of complications like twin-to-twin transfusion syndrome (TTTS). Therefore, identification of this sign is important in the management of twin pregnancies because it helps in assessing the risk of twin-to-twin transfusion syndrome. This can help guide appropriate management and monitoring of pregnancy. **Potential questions:** There can be questions related to the types of twin gestation, their pathogenesis, diagnosis, management, and complications.

Question	Answer	Comment
Q41. At a routine 24-week gestation ultrasound, a 29-year-old woman, gravida 2, is found to have monochorionic twins with significant discordance in amniotic fluid volumes and fetal sizes. The obstetrician uses a schematic diagram as shown below to explain the diagnosis to the patient, while counseling her. What is the likely diagnosis in this case? 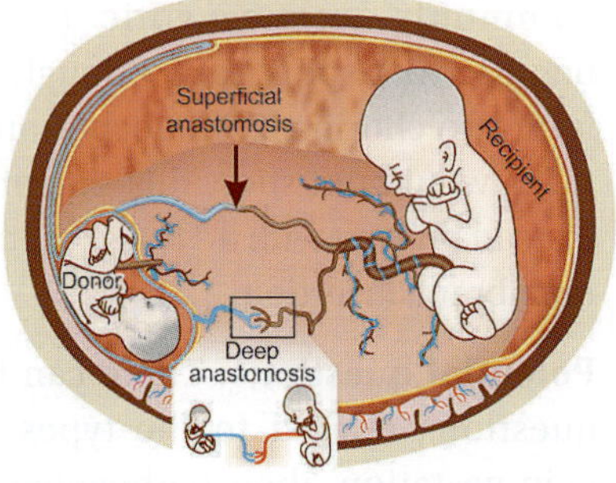 A. Selective intrauterine growth restriction (sIUGR) B. Monoamniotic twin gestation C. Twin-to-twin transfusion syndrome (TTTS) D. Fetal anemia E. Congenital anomalies in one twin	**Ans. C [Twin-to-Twin Transfusion Syndrome (TTTS)]** The adjacent image demonstrates the pathology of TTTS, which is a rare complication that can occur in monozygotic monochorionic twins. It causes the blood to pass from one twin to the other. As shown in **Figure 41**, the placental vascular anastomoses responsible for the development of TTTS could be from artery-to-artery (A-A), artery-to-vein (A-V), or vein-to-artery (V-A). 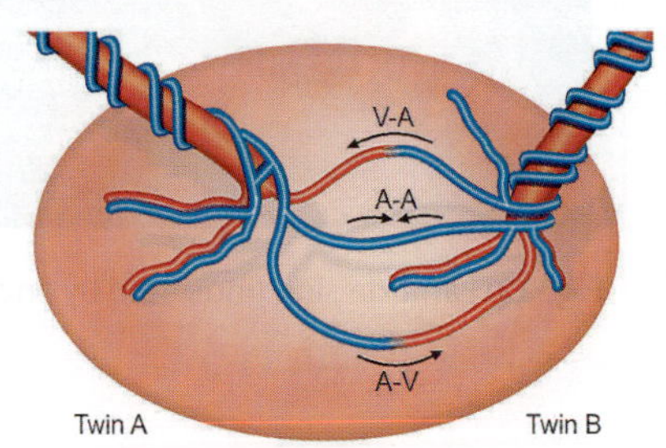 **Fig. 41:** Diagrammatic representation of placenta showing arteriovenous anastomosis.	**Explanation:** In TTTS, as a result of vascular communications, one of the twins, which donates blood (donor twin), becomes thin, pale, and undernourished, while the other twin who receives blood (recipient twin) grows at the expense of donor twin and becomes large and plethoric. Key findings on ultrasound include a significant difference in amniotic fluid volumes between the twins, with one twin in a polyhydramnios state and the other in oligohydramnios. Treatment options include amnioreduction, laser photocoagulation of the connecting blood vessels, and, in severe cases, selective reduction. **Potential questions:** There can be questions related to the types of twin gestation, their pathogenesis, diagnosis, management, and complications.

Question	Answer	Comment
Q42. An ultrasound of a monochorionic twin pregnancy at 18 weeks' gestation shows one normal twin and one acardiac twin without a functional heart. The normal twin demonstrates signs of high-output heart failure. The clinical image of the pathology involved is shown below. What is the most likely diagnosis? 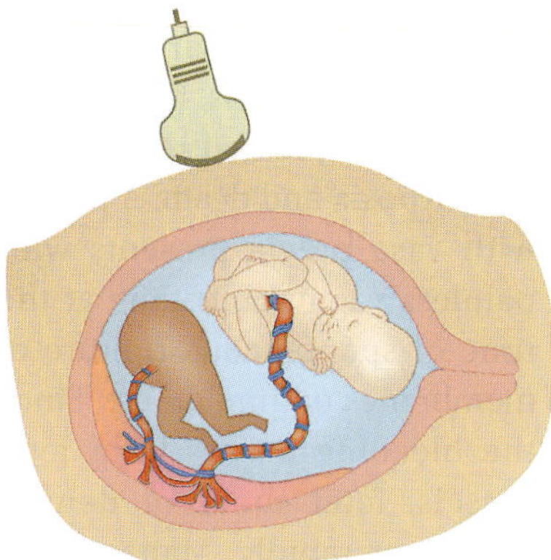 A. Selective intrauterine growth restriction (sIUGR) B. Twin-to-twin transfusion syndrome (TTTS) C. Twin reversed arterial perfusion (TRAP) syndrome D. Conjoined twins E. Fetal anemia	**Ans: C. [Twin reversed arterial perfusion (TRAP) syndrome]** The adjacent image is a diagrammatic representation of twin reversed arterial perfusion (TRAP) syndrome or acardiac twin. In these pregnancies, the umbilical cord from the acardiac twin branches directly from the umbilical cord of the normal twin **(Fig. 42)**. Thus, blood flow is reversed from the normal direction leading to the name for this condition—"twin reversed arterial perfusion syndrome". 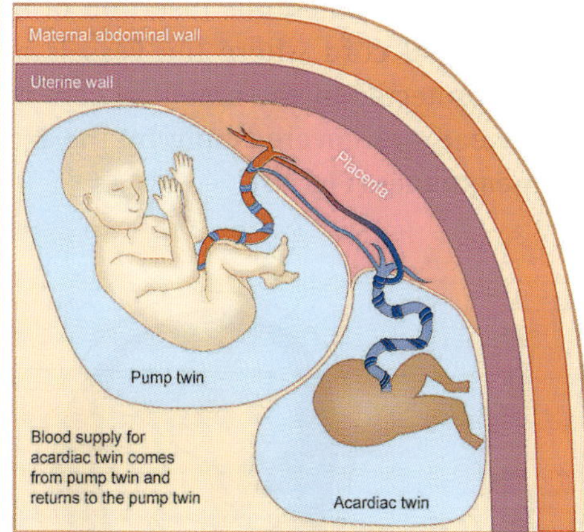 **Fig. 42:** Diagrammatic representation of TRAP (twin reversed arterial perfusion) syndrome.	**Explanation:** TRAP syndrome is a rare complication in monochorionic twin pregnancies where an acardiac twin (without a functioning heart) is supported by the normal (pump) twin via abnormal arterial connections. The pump twin supplies blood to both, leading to high-output cardiac stress and potentially heart failure. The acardiac twin lacks proper development, often with missing or malformed organs, especially the heart, head, and upper extremities. Perfusion of the malformed (acardiac) fetus occurs via A-A and V-V anastomoses between the fetuses. Deoxygenated umbilical arterial blood from the donor flows into the umbilical artery of the recipient, with its direction reversed. Doppler verification of reversed flow in the umbilical cord of the acardiac fetus helps in confirming the diagnosis. **Potential questions:** There can be questions related to the types of twin gestation, their pathogenesis, diagnosis, management, and complications.

ANTEPARTUM HEMORRHAGE

Question	Answer	Comment
Q43. A 32-year-old pregnant woman at 28 weeks' gestation undergoes a transvaginal ultrasound followed by Doppler ultrasound as shown in the images below. The sonographer identifies fetal blood vessels running across the internal cervical os without any placental tissue in that area. What is the most likely diagnosis? 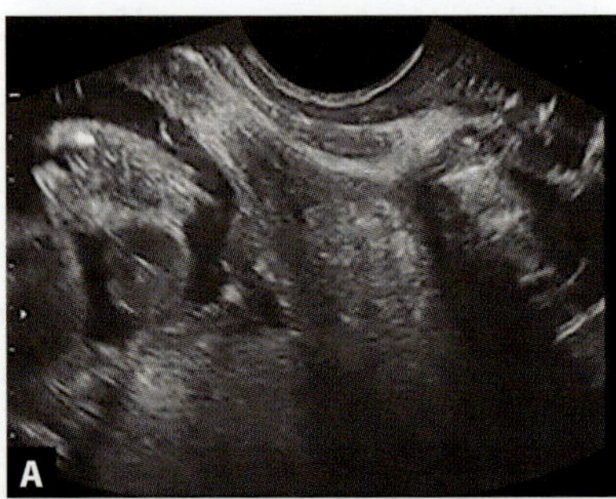 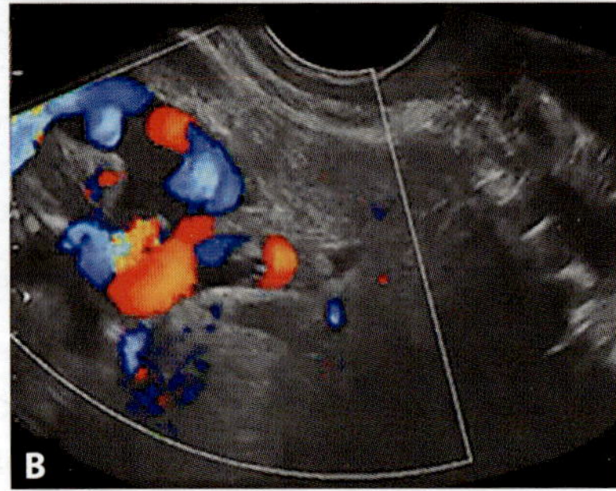 A. Placenta previa B. Vasa previa C. Velamentous cord insertion D. Placental abruption E. Uterine rupture	**Ans: B (Vasa previa)** Figure A in the adjacent column illustrates a transvaginal ultrasound image, whereas Figure B illustrates a Doppler ultrasound image in the same patient showing the presence of fetal vessels in front of the fetal presenting part. The diagnosis of vasa previa was established in this case. Vasa previa occurs when fetal blood vessels traverse the cervical os, often due to a velamentous insertion of the umbilical cord where the vessels are not protected by the umbilical cord but instead are covered only by the fetal membranes **(Fig. 43)**. 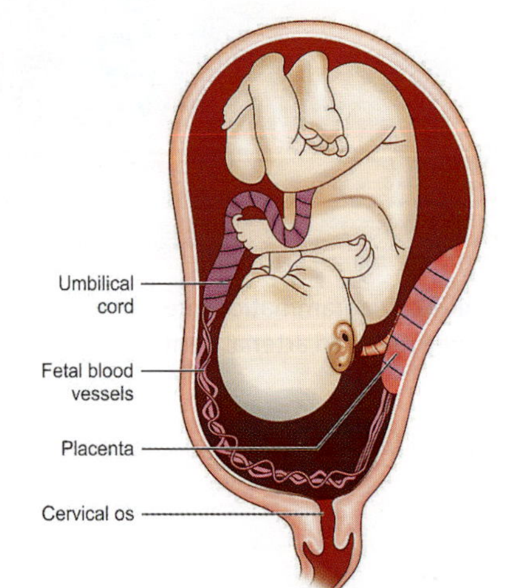 **Fig. 43:** Diagrammatic representation of vasa previa.	**Explanation:** Vasa previa is an uncommon obstetrical complication, which may be associated with a high risk of fetal demise, if it is not recognized before rupture of membranes. In vasa previa, umbilical vessels traverse the membranes in the lower uterine segment in front of the fetal presenting part. During uterine contractions, fetal vessels can get compressed resulting in fetal hypoxia and death. A patient with vasa previa presents with painless vaginal bleeding at the time of spontaneous rupture of membranes or amniotomy. Since the bleeding occurs from fetal vessels, fetal shock or demise can occur rapidly. Management involves planned cesarean delivery before the onset of labor to prevent vessel rupture and fetal hemorrhage. **Potential questions:** There can be questions related to various causes of antepartum hemorrhage, their etiology, pathogenesis, clinical presentation, diagnosis, management, and complications.

Question	Answer	Comment
Q44. A 29-year-old woman, 34 weeks pregnant, presents with sudden-onset severe abdominal pain, vaginal bleeding, and a tense, tender uterus. An ultrasound reveals a retroplacental clot as shown in the image below. 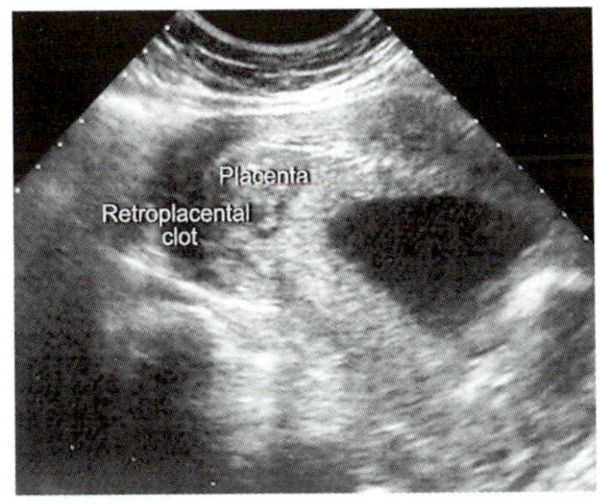 What is the most likely diagnosis? A. Placenta previa B. Uterine rupture C. Vasa previa D. Abruptio placentae E. Preterm labor	**Ans: D (Abruptio placentae)** The given case suggests antepartum hemorrhage. Ultrasound helps localize the placenta to confirm/exclude placenta previa, visualize a retroplacental clot (as shown in the adjacent image), confirming placental abruption, and assess fetal viability and presentation. Placental abruption (accidental hemorrhage) is the premature separation of a normally situated placenta, causing bleeding from uterine sinuses **(Figs. 44 A and B)** 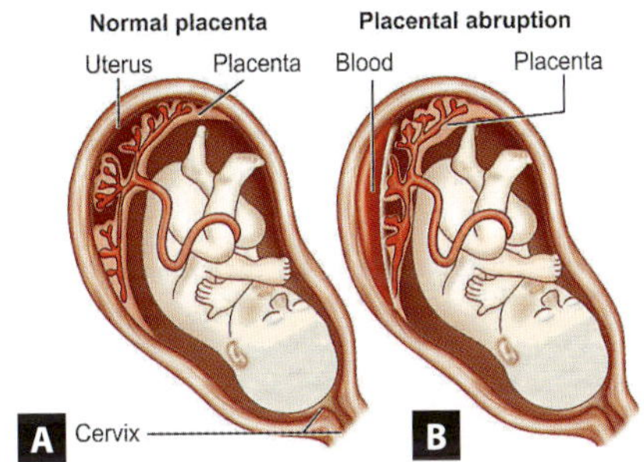 **Figs. 44A and B:** Placental abruption and its comparison with normal placenta.	**Explanation:** Abruptio placentae is the premature separation of a normally situated placenta, causing maternal and fetal complications like hemorrhage and preterm delivery. Blood collects in the decidua basalis, forming a retroplacental clot. Classic signs include vaginal bleeding, abdominal pain, uterine tenderness, fetal distress, and hypertonicity. Diagnosis is mainly clinical; ultrasound may show clots. Risk factors: trauma, hypertension, smoking. Management depends on gestational age and maternal–fetal stability. **Potential questions:** There can be questions related to various causes of antepartum hemorrhage, their etiology, pathogenesis, clinical presentation, diagnosis, management, and complications.
Q45. A 32-year-old third-trimester woman presents with severe abdominal pain, vaginal bleeding, and a rigid, tender uterus. During emergency cesarean, the uterus is discolored with blood infiltrating the muscle as shown in the below image. What is the likely diagnosis? 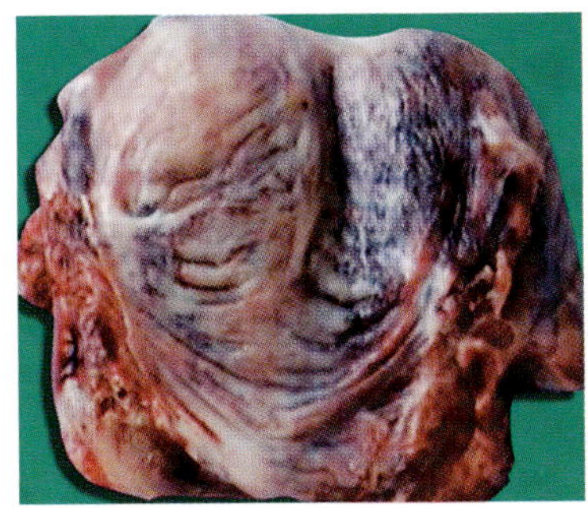 A. Uterine rupture B. Placenta accreta C. Couvelaire uterus D. Vasa previa E. Placenta previa	**Ans: C (Couvelaire uterus)** The adjacent image shows couvelaire uterus, characterised by massive blood infiltration into the uterine muscles up to the serosa, giving it a port-wine color **(Fig. 45)**. Blood between muscle fibers can impair contractions and increase the risk of severe postpartum hemorrhage. 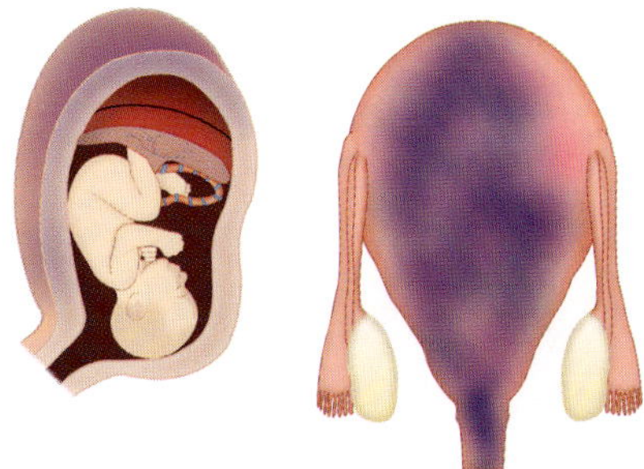 **Fig. 45:** Diagrammatic representation of Couvelaire uterus.	**Explanation:** Couvelaire uterus (uteroplacental apoplexy) is a rare severe placental abruption complication where blood infiltrates the myometrium, causing uterine discoloration and rigidity. Clinically, it presents with abdominal pain, uterine tenderness, and vaginal bleeding. Management focuses on stabilization of the patient and often emergency cesarean; hysterectomy is only needed for uncontrollable postpartum hemorrhage. **Potential questions:** There can be questions related to various causes of antepartum hemorrhage, their etiology, pathogenesis, clinical presentation, diagnosis, management, and complications.

Question	Answer	Comment
Q46. A 35-year-old pregnant woman at 36 weeks' gestation presents with severe abdominal pain, heavy vaginal bleeding, and hypotension. Ultrasound shows placental abruption. Following cesarean section, she develops widespread oozing from IV sites and surgical incisions. Laboratory results reveal thrombocytopenia, elevated D-dimer, and prolonged prothrombin time (PT) and activated partial thromboplastin time (aPTT). Findings of peripheral smear are shown below. What is the most likely diagnosis? 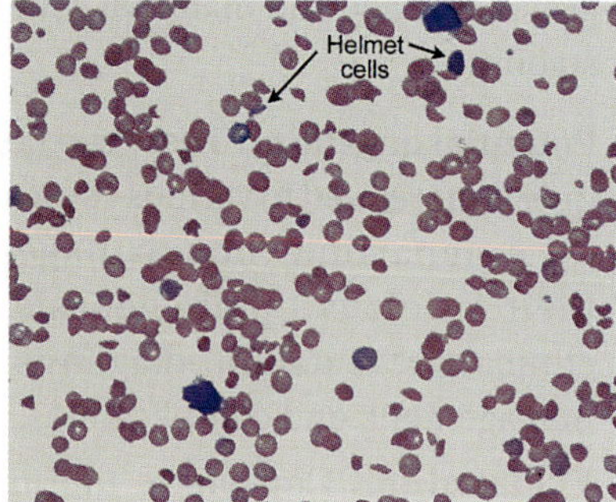 A. Hemorrhagic shock B. Amniotic fluid embolism C. Disseminated intravascular coagulation (DIC) D. HELLP syndrome E. Placenta accreta	**Ans: C [Disseminated intravascular coagulation (DIC)]** The diagnosis in the given case is disseminated intravascular coagulation (DIC), which is a known complication of severe placental abruption. The pathogenesis of DIC is described in **Figure 46**. Peripheral smear in a patient with DIC is suggestive of hemolytic anemia. The peripheral smear shows the presence of multiple helmet cells (as indicated by arrows in the adjacent image), fragmented RBCs, microspherocytes and schistocytes, and paucity of platelet cells. This is suggestive of microangiopathic hemolytic anemia. 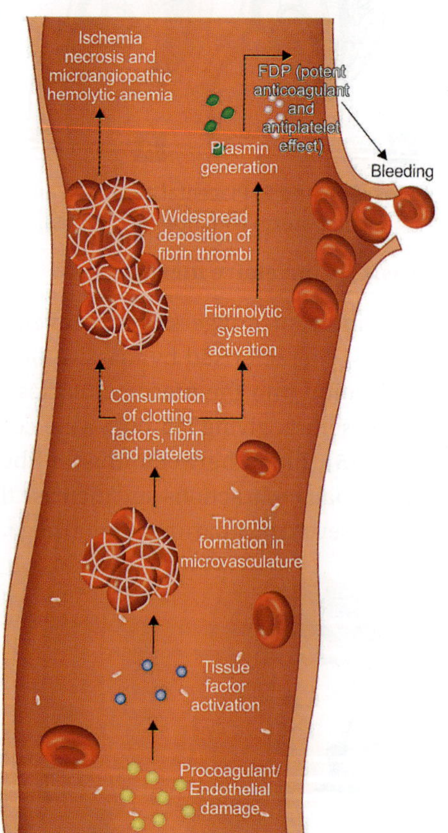 **Fig. 46:** Pathogenesis of disseminated intravascular coagulation (DIC). (FDP: fibrin degradation product)	**Explanation:** In DIC, initially there is activation of the coagulation pathways, both intrinsic and extrinsic due to thromboplastin, released from the decidual fragments and placental separation (in view of abruptio placentae). As the process of coagulation continues, it results in consumption of various clotting factors and widespread deposition of fibrin. This can result in development of hypoxia, widespread bleeding (oozing or frank bleeding), and ischemia and necrosis, which ultimately results in end-stage organ damage, especially renal and hepatic failure and hypovolemic shock. In the cases of DIC, fibrinogen levels are reduced; PT, aPTT, and thrombin time are prolonged; platelet levels are reduced; and levels of D-dimer and fibrinogen degradation products are increased. Immediate management focuses on treating the underlying cause, blood product replacement (especially with FFP or fresh frozen plasma), and stabilizing the patient.

Question	Answer	Comment
Q47. A 30-year-old woman at 32 weeks of gestation presents with painless vaginal bleeding. Ultrasound reveals a low-lying placenta. The placenta location in relation to cervical os is shown in the clinical image below. What is the most likely diagnosis? 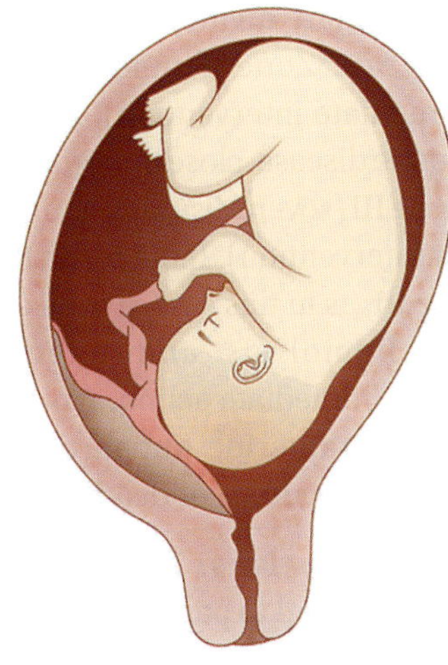 A. Type I placenta previa B. Type II placenta previa C. Type III placenta previa D. Type IV placenta previa E. Placental abruption	**Ans: B (Type II placenta previa)** Placenta previa occurs when the placenta is implanted in the lower uterine segment, partially or completely covering the internal cervical os. It presents with painless vaginal bleeding, usually in the third trimester. Ultrasound is the key diagnostic tool, showing the placenta's location over or near the cervical os. The grading system of placenta previa is demonstrated in **Figure 47**. 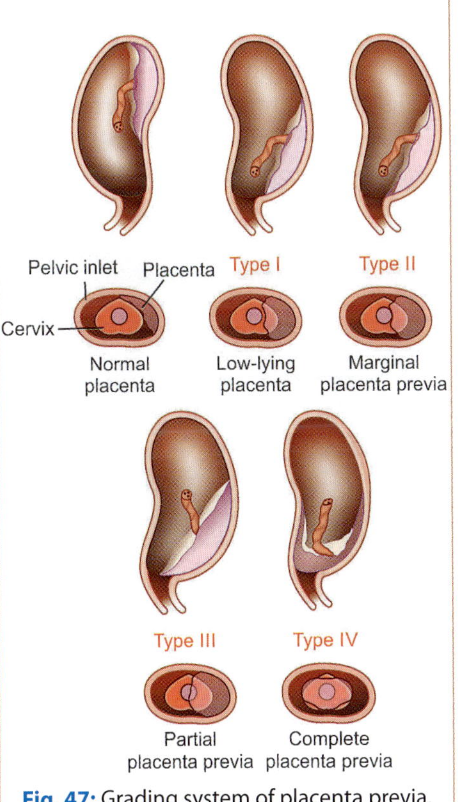 **Fig. 47:** Grading system of placenta previa.	**Explanation:** There are four distinct types of placenta previa based on the location of placenta in relation to the cervical os: *Type I (low lying)*: The placenta enters the lower uterine section and comes within 2-5 cm of the internal cervical os. *Type II (marginal)*: The placenta approaches but does not cover the cervical os. *Type III (partial)*: While the placenta covers the cervical os, the placental site is asymmetric, with the majority of the placenta towards one side of the os. *Type IV (complete)*: The placenta is situated in the center of the cervical os. **Potential questions:** There can be questions related to various causes of antepartum hemorrhage, their etiology, pathogenesis, clinical presentation, diagnosis, management, and complications.

Rh-NEGATIVE PREGNANCY

Question	Answer	Comment
Q48. A 28-year-old Rh-negative woman at 28 weeks' gestation presents for an evaluation due to a prior sensitization to Rh-positive blood. An amniocentesis reveals elevated bilirubin levels in the amniotic fluid. The results are plotted on a chart as shown below, and the reading falls in Zone III. What is the most likely course of action? 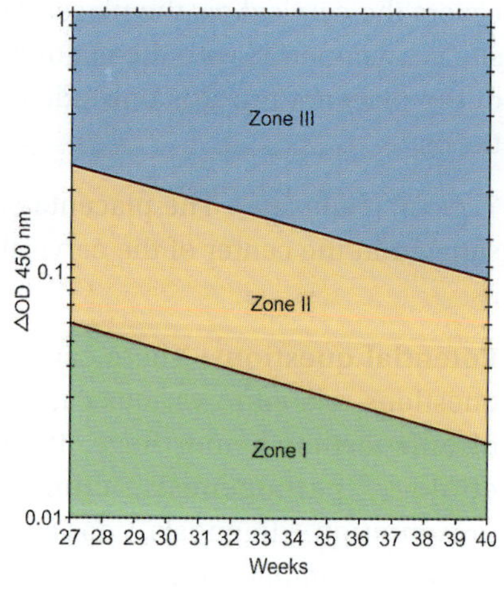 A. Perform intrauterine blood transfusion B. Schedule weekly amniocentesis for monitoring C. Expectant management and re-evaluate in 4 weeks D. Administer corticosteroids and plan delivery at term E. No intervention required, repeat the test in 2 weeks	**Ans: A (Perform intrauterine blood transfusion.)** The chart shown in the adjacent image is Liley's chart. Nowadays, previously used procedures such as serial amniocentesis for measuring delta OD 450 values and subsequently interpreting it with the help of Liley's or Queenan curve have largely become obsolete due to the use of noninvasive techniques involving measurement of MCA-PSV (middle cerebral artery-peak flow velocity) on Doppler ultrasound **(Fig. 48)**. There is a strong correlation between the high PSV in the MCA and the low levels of fetal hemoglobin. 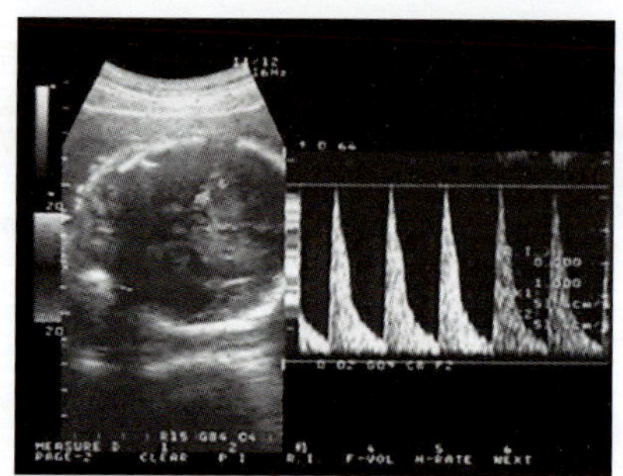 **Fig. 48:** MCA-PSV Doppler waveforms in a severely anemic fetus at 22 weeks' gestation.	**Explanation:** Liley's chart helps evaluate the severity of fetal anemia due to Rh sensitization by analyzing amniotic fluid bilirubin levels by calculating the ΔOD 450 values. These are then plotted over a standardized chart (Liley's chart or Queenan's chart). Liley's chart divides results into three zones: Zone I (mild disease, no immediate intervention), Zone II (moderate disease, close monitoring), and Zone III (severe disease, requiring urgent intervention). If the result falls in Zone III, as in this case, it indicates severe hemolysis and anemia, requiring immediate action, typically through intrauterine transfusion to prevent fetal hydrops or death. **Potential questions:** There can be questions related to pathophysiology, diagnosis, and management of complications associated with Rh alloimmunization.

Question	Answer	Comment
Q49. A 3-day-old baby with neonatal jaundice due to Rh alloimmunization is receiving phototherapy as shown in the image below. The baby's total serum bilirubin level is 20 mg/dL. What is the mechanism by which phototherapy reduces bilirubin levels? 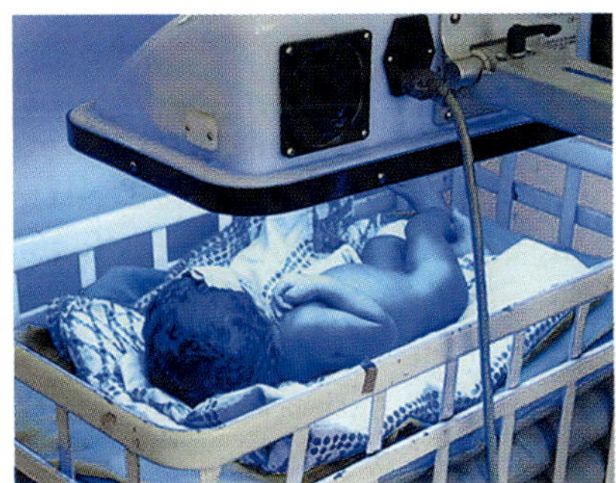 A. Converts bilirubin to lumirubin for bile excretion B. Promotes bilirubin conjugation in the liver C. Stimulates erythrocyte production, reducing hemolysis D. Decreases bilirubin reabsorption in intestines E. Enhances bilirubin breakdown by hepatic enzymes	**Ans: A (Converts bilirubin into lumirubin for bile excretion)** The adjacent image shows a baby receiving phototherapy for the treatment of neonatal jaundice caused by hyperbilirubinemia due to Rh alloimmunization. **Figure 49** shows a newborn baby with jaundice. Key considerations during phototherapy include monitoring bilirubin levels, ensuring adequate hydration of the baby, and protecting the baby's eyes and skin. 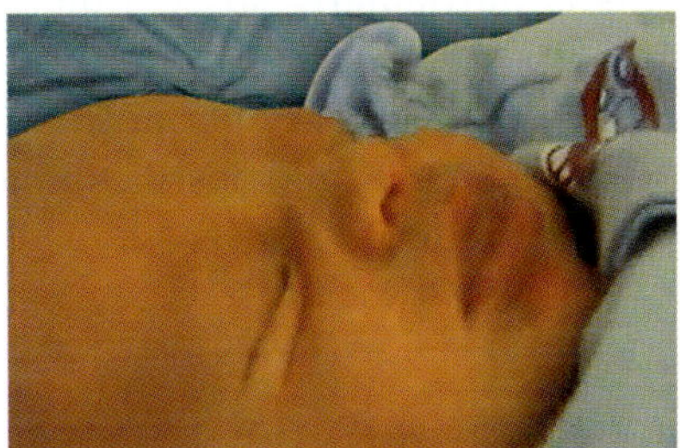 **Fig. 49:** Appearance of jaundice in the newborn baby.	**Explanation:** In cases of neonatal jaundice, particularly due to Rh alloimmunization, elevated levels of unconjugated bilirubin (>20 mg/dL) pose a risk to the baby by causing staining of the basal ganglia and hippocampus, resulting in kernicterus. Phototherapy works by converting bilirubin into water-soluble isomers, such as lumirubin, through a process called photoisomerization. This form of bilirubin can then be excreted via bile without requiring conjugation in the liver, rapidly reducing bilirubin levels and preventing neurological damage. **Potential questions:** There can be questions related to pathophysiology, diagnosis, and management of complications associated with Rh alloimmunization.

Question	Answer	Comment
Q50. A 32-year-old Rh-negative woman delivers a severely anemic newborn with generalized edema, ascites, and pleural effusions. The ultrasound during pregnancy had shown significant fetal edema. The baby was not able to survive at birth. The autopsy picture of the baby is shown below. What is the most likely cause of the newborn's condition? 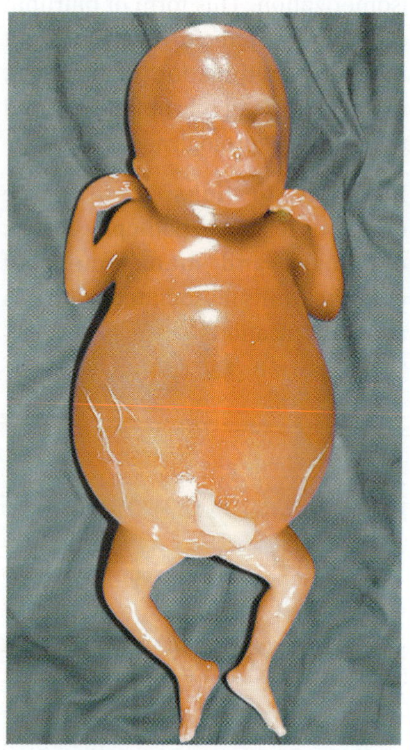 A. Congenital heart defect B. Fetal renal failure C. Rh alloimmunization leading to hemolytic disease of the fetus D. Twin-to-twin transfusion syndrome E. Parvovirus infection causing hydrops	**Ans: C (Rh alloimmunization leading to hemolytic disease of the fetus)** Hydrops fetalis is a condition, characterized by an accumulation of fluids within the baby's body, resulting in development of ascites, pleural effusion, pericardial effusion, skin edema, etc. **(Fig. 50)**. In many cases, it may also cause polyhydramnios and placental edema. Pleural effusion may interfere with the normal process of breathing, whereas pericardial effusion may be associated with congestive heart failure. The fetus is particularly susceptible to interstitial fluid accumulation due to increased capillary permeability, hypoproteinemia, and obstruction to lymphatic return. 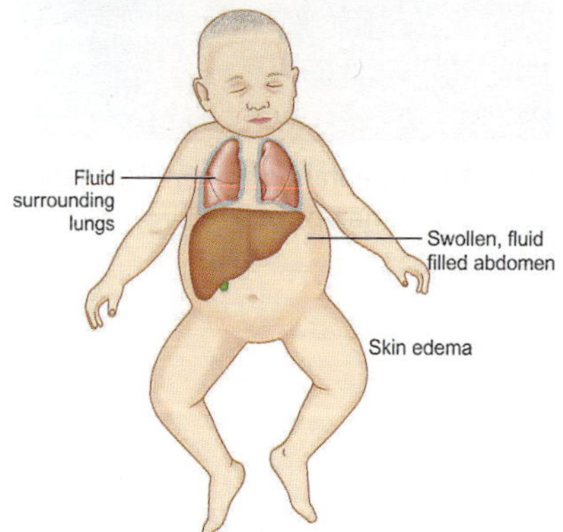 **Fig. 50:** Pathogenesis of immune fetal hydrops.	**Explanation:** Rh alloimmunization is a well-known cause of immune hydrops, especially in cases where the mother is sensitized. Hydrops fetalis in the context of Rh alloimmunization occurs when maternal Rh antibodies attack fetal red blood cells, leading to hemolysis, severe anemia, and subsequent heart failure, which causes fluid accumulation in various fetal compartments (edema, ascites, pleural effusions, etc.). Spontaneous remission of the condition has been reported in some cases. The following treatment strategies can be employed in cases of fetal hydrops: ▪ Maternal antiarrhythmic agents (e.g., digoxin) for the treatment of fetal arrhythmia ▪ Fetal intrauterine transfusion for the treatment of severe anemia ▪ In utero fetal surgery (fetal thoracocentesis, paracentesis, etc.) **Potential questions:** There can be questions related to pathophysiology, diagnosis, and management of complications associated with Rh alloimmunization.

AMNIOTIC FLUID AND ITS ABNORMALITIES

Question	Answer	Comment
Q51. A 32-year-old pregnant woman at 28 weeks' gestation undergoes a routine ultrasound. The sonographer notes an amniotic fluid index (AFI) of 28 cm. The fetus appears structurally normal. The ultrasound image is shown below. What is the most likely diagnosis? 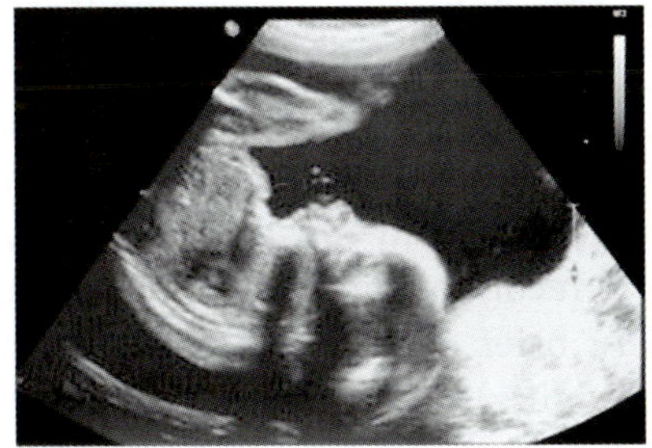 A. Oligohydramnios B. Polyhydramnios C. Preterm labor D. Intrauterine growth restriction (IUGR) E. Placental abruption	**Ans: B (Polyhydramnios)** The adjacent image shows ultrasound of a fetus with polyhydramnios. Polyhydramnios is diagnosed when there is an abnormally high volume of amniotic fluid, typically indicated by an AFI >25 cm or the depth of maximum vertical pocket of amniotic fluid >8 cm. Calculation of AFI is described in **Figure 51**. 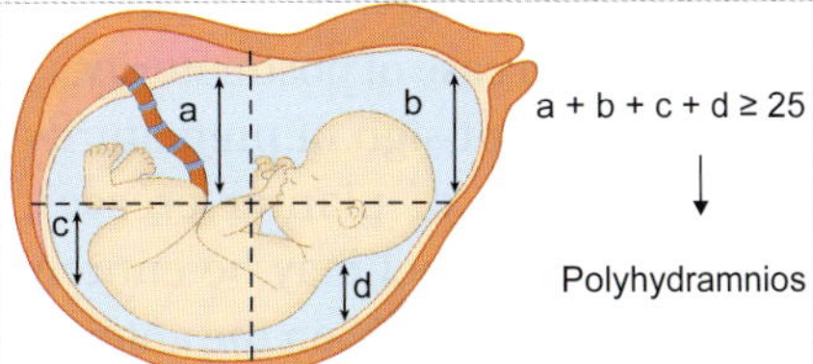 **Fig. 51:** Calculation of amniotic fluid index (AFI).	**Explanation:** Polyhydramnios can be associated with maternal diabetes, fetal anomalies (like gastrointestinal obstructions), or twin-to-twin transfusion syndrome in multiple pregnancies. Although the fetus in this case appears structurally normal, further investigations may be needed to rule out underlying conditions such as maternal diabetes or fetal anomalies. Management of polyhydramnios may include the following: Correction of the primary anomaly, decompression by amniocentesis, and treatment with indomethacin. **Potential questions:** There can be questions related to definition, etiology, diagnosis, management, and complications of polyhydramnios.
Q52. A 32-year-old pregnant woman at 28 weeks of gestation presents for a routine ultrasound. The results of the scan are shown in the image below. Which of the following is the most likely diagnosis based on the ultrasound findings shown below? 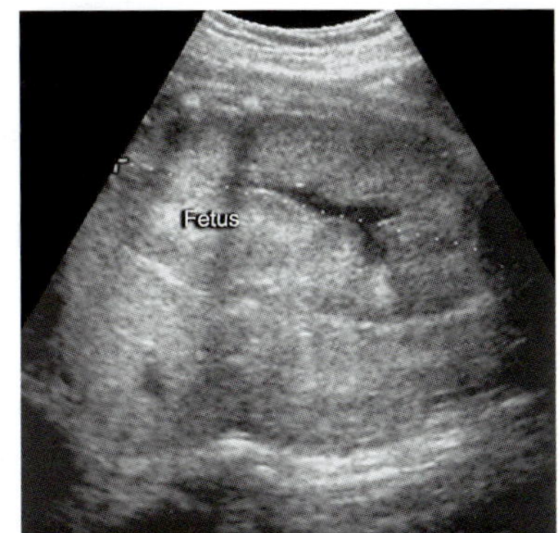 A. Placental abruption B. Preterm labor C. Oligohydramnios D. Fetal growth restriction E. Multiple gestation	**Ans: C (Oligohydramnios)** The adjacent ultrasound image shows oligohydramnios (reduced amniotic fluid) in a 26-week fetus. It can be associated with several complications (**Fig. 52**). In late pregnancy, it indicates fetal distress, often linked to IUGR, and increases the likelihood of cesarean delivery. 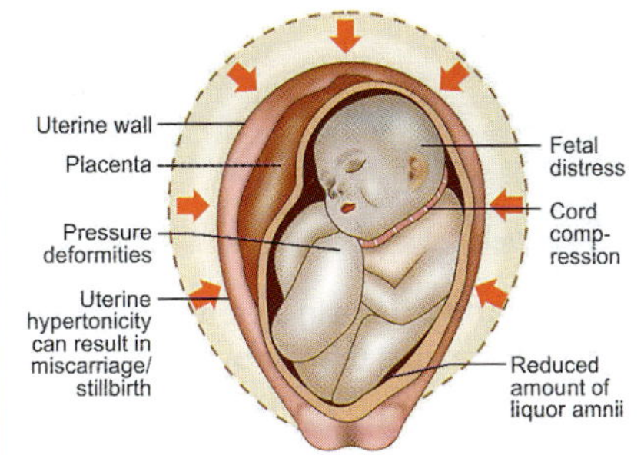 **Fig. 52:** Complications associated with oligohydramnios.	**Explanation:** Oligohydramnios is defined as a reduced amount of amniotic fluid (<200 mL), which can be identified on ultrasound as a decreased amniotic fluid index (AFI <5 cm) or a single deepest pocket (SDP ≤1 cm) of amniotic fluid. It is a condition that can be associated with several factors, including placental insufficiency, fetal anomalies, or rupture of membranes. **Potential questions:** There can be questions related to definition, management, and complications of oligohydramnios.

PRETERM BABY

Question

Q53. A newborn is assessed using the Dubowitz (Ballard) examination to determine gestational age. Which of the following findings would most likely indicate a preterm infant based on the Dubowitz (Ballard) assessment shown in the image below?

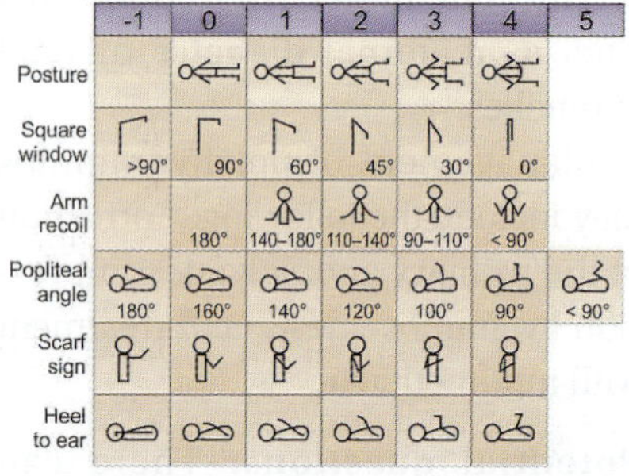

A. Opaque, thicker, and less transparent skin, with less visible veins
B. Well-developed ear cartilage with firm pinna
C. Presence of a prominent breast bud with well-defined areola
D. Minimal plantar creases on the soles
E. Larger testicular volume with pendulous scrotum

Answer

Ans: D (Minimal plantar creases on the soles)

The adjacent image shows Dubowitz (Ballard) examination, which is used for assessing fetal maturity based on the physical characteristics as well as the maturity of the neuromuscular system. Points are given for each parameter, which is assessed. Low scores (–1 or 0) are given in case of extreme prematurity. High scores (4, 5) are given in case of postmaturity.

An important sign of prematurity is the absence of plantar creases. Creases on the heel may be entirely absent or present only on the anterior one-third in the preterm babies **(Figs. 53A and B)**. The entire sole is covered with creases in case of a term child.

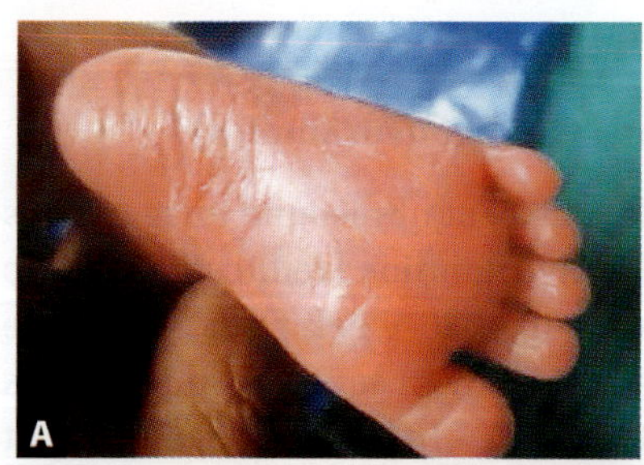

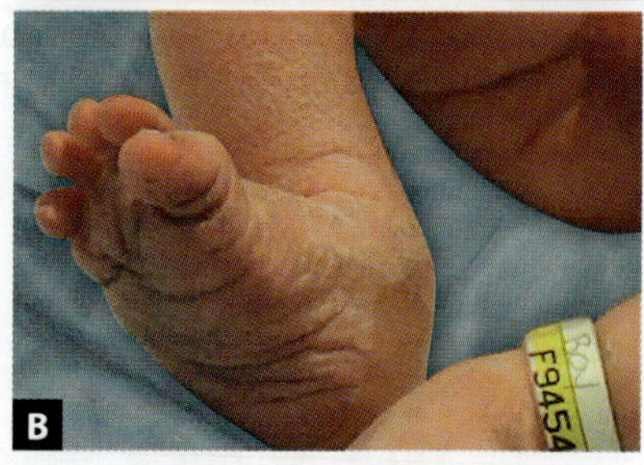

Figs. 53A and B: Heel in a preterm baby (A) in comparison to a term baby (B).

Comment

Explanation: The Dubowitz (Ballard) examination evaluates various physical and neurological characteristics to estimate gestational age. Physical characteristics, which are assessed, include parameters such as skin texture, lanugo hair, plantar creases, breasts, ears, and appearance of the genitalia. Assessment of neuromuscular maturity includes evaluation of parameters such as posture and square window (flexion of baby's hand toward the wrist), arm recoil (angle of recoil following very brief extension of the upper extremity), heel to ear movement (passive resistance to extension of posterior hip flexor muscles), popliteal angle (resistance of baby's knee to extension), and scarf sign (how far the elbow can be moved across the baby's chest). Key findings indicating prematurity on Dubowitz (Ballard) examination include:

- Minimal plantar creases on the soles
- Smooth, pink skin with visible veins
- Ear cartilage with flexible pinna: Ear cartilage is likely to become firm with increasing gestational age
- Absence of a prominent breast bud with well-defined areola
- Presence of small, less well-developed external genitalia

Potential questions: There could be questions related to various features and complications encountered in the premature infant.

Question	Answer	Comment
Q54. A premature infant born at 30 weeks of gestation is showing signs of respiratory distress shortly after birth. The chest X-ray reveals a "ground-glass" appearance and decreased lung volumes as shown below. Which of the following is the most likely diagnosis? 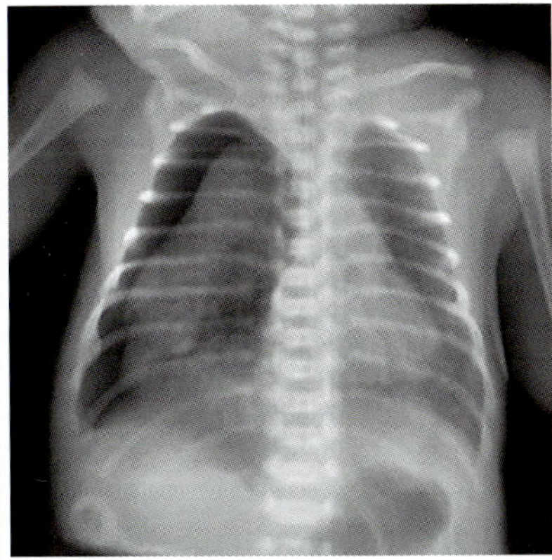 A. Transient tachypnea of the newborn (TTN) B. Respiratory distress syndrome (RDS) C. Meconium aspiration syndrome D. Pneumothorax E. Congenital pneumonia	**Ans: B [Respiratory distress syndrome (RDS)]** The adjacent X-ray image is of a newborn preterm baby, 2 days after birth. The image shows tension pneumothorax on the right side with collapsed lung. As a result, the mediastinum is pushed towards the left side. A nasogastric tube, which has been inserted in the esophagus, can also be visualized. Based on the findings of clinical examination and various investigations, diagnosis of respiratory distress syndrome (RDS) was made. Babies with RDS lack a protein surfactant, which normally prevents the lung alveoli from collapsing **(Figs. 54A and B)**. Administration of corticosteroids in cases of anticipated preterm delivery may help in promoting surfactant synthesis. 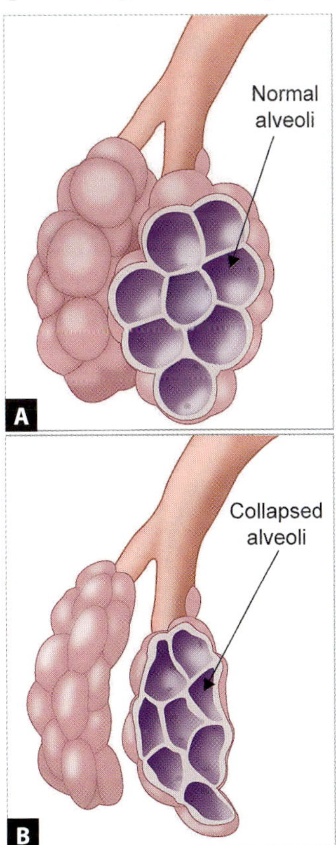 **Figs. 54A and B:** Presence of collapsed lungs in respiratory distress syndrome.)	**Explanation:** Respiratory distress syndrome is a common condition in premature infants due to surfactant deficiency. The typical findings on chest X-ray for RDS include: ▪ *"Ground-glass" appearance:* This is due to the presence of alveolar atelectasis and poor lung expansion, characteristic of surfactant deficiency. ▪ *Decreased lung volumes:* Reflects the inability of the alveoli to remain open and fully expand due to lack of surfactant. Management includes respiratory support with oxygen, continuous positive airway pressure (CPAP), or mechanical ventilation; administration of intravenous sodium bicarbonate for correction of acidosis, correction of hypovolemia and electrolyte imbalance; and administration of surfactant. **Potential questions:** There could be questions related to various complications encountered in the premature infant.

POST-TERM PREGNANCY

Question	Answer	Comment
Q55. A newborn is delivered with a birth weight of 4.5 Kg, as shown in the image below. The physical examination reveals a large infant with a prominent abdomen, and the mother had uncontrolled diabetes during pregnancy. Which of the following conditions is most likely associated with these findings? 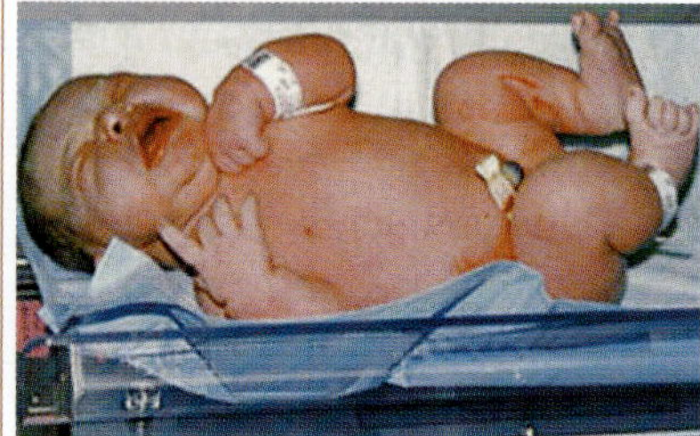 A. Large for gestational age (LGA) B. Macrosomia C. Polyhydramnios D. Fetal obesity E. Congenital anomaly	**Ans: B (Macrosomia)** The adjacent image shows a baby with macrosomia, a condition where a newborn has a birth weight significantly higher than the average for their gestational age, typically defined as greater than 4,000 g or the 90th percentile. One of the major obstetric complications which can be associated with macrosomia is shoulder dystocia. **Figure 55** shows "turtle sign", an important indicator of shoulder dystocia. 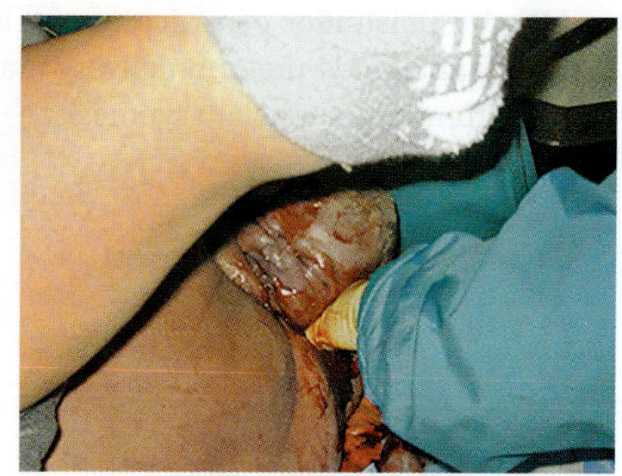 **Fig. 55:** Turtle sign: Neonatal face and head retracted up against the maternal perineum.	**Explanation:** Key features of macrosomia include large birth weight and prominent abdomen. The infant is notably larger than average. Postdated pregnancy is an important risk factor for macrosomia. Other risk factors for development of macrosomia include gestational diabetes mellitus, maternal obesity, excessive pregnancy weight gain, etc. Maternal diabetes is another major risk factor for macrosomia, as high blood sugar levels can lead to increased fetal growth. Presently, there is no method for predicting macrosomia. The woman must be posted for an elective cesarean delivery in case the expected fetal weight is >4,500 g in a diabetic mother and >5,000 g in a nondiabetic mother. Early induction has been tried in some cases. However, it is associated with an increased rate of failed induction. **Potential questions:** There can be questions related to various other complications of postdated pregnancy.

Question	Answer	Comment
Q56. A newborn delivered at 42 weeks' gestation has immediate respiratory distress and is noted to have meconium-stained amniotic fluid. The chest X-ray at 2 days is shown below. What is the most likely diagnosis? 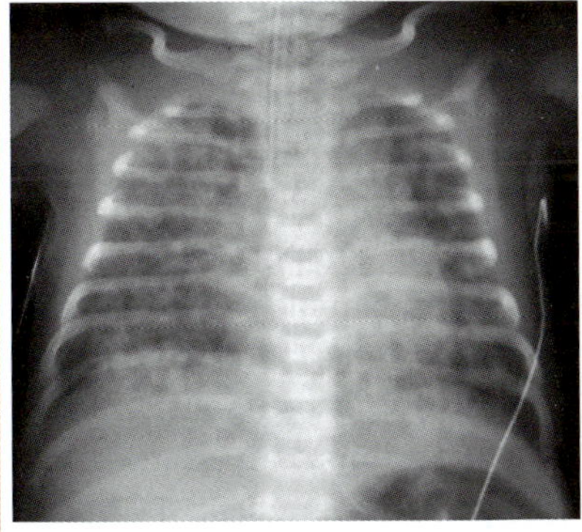 A. Respiratory distress syndrome (RDS) B. Meconium aspiration syndrome (MAS) C. Pneumothorax D. Transient tachypnea of the newborn (TTN) E. Congenital pneumonia	**Ans: B (Meconium aspiration syndrome)** The adjacent image shows the classic radiographic findings of meconium aspiration syndrome (MAS), namely atelectasis, pneumothorax, and hyperexpanded areas of the lung. In MAS, atelectasis appears as patchy, irregular white shadows with localized volume loss, occurring side-by-side with overinflated, darker regions of lung. MAS is an indicator of postmaturity and fetal distress or hypoxia. It is believed that hypoxia and acidemia stimulate the parasympathetic system. This causes the anal sphincter to relax whilst at the same time increasing the production of motilin, which promotes intestinal peristalsis resulting in passage of meconium into the amniotic cavity. 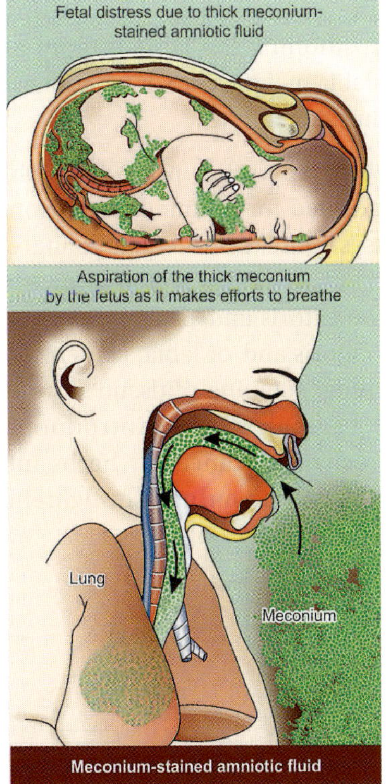 **Fig. 56:** Aspiration of meconium by the newborn baby as it makes efforts to breathe.	**Explanation:** Meconium aspiration syndrome is a disease of both term and post-term infants, and its severity is linked to coexisting fetal asphyxia. MAS occurs when a newborn inhales meconium-stained amniotic fluid into the lungs during or before delivery, leading to respiratory distress immediately after birth due to obstruction and chemical irritation from meconium in the airways **(Fig. 56)**. Complete obstruction of small airways with meconium can produce regional atelectasis and ventilation-perfusion mismatches. On the other hand, partial obstruction of airways can create a ball valve phenomenon, in which air flows past the meconium into the airways during inspiration. However, during expiration, this air gets trapped distally, leading to increase in expiratory lung resistance, functional residual capacity, and anterior posterior diameter of the chest. Air leaks can also develop leading to pneumothorax and pneumomediastinum. MAS may ultimately result in the development of hypoxia and respiratory failure. **Potential questions:** There can be questions related to various other complications of postdated pregnancy.

FEMALE GENITAL MUTILATION

Question	Answer	Comment
Q57. A woman at 10 weeks of gestation is seen at clinic. On examination, it was revealed that she had undergone female genital mutilation (FGM) when she was a child. The image below depicts the findings of clinical examination in her case. What is the likely diagnosis? 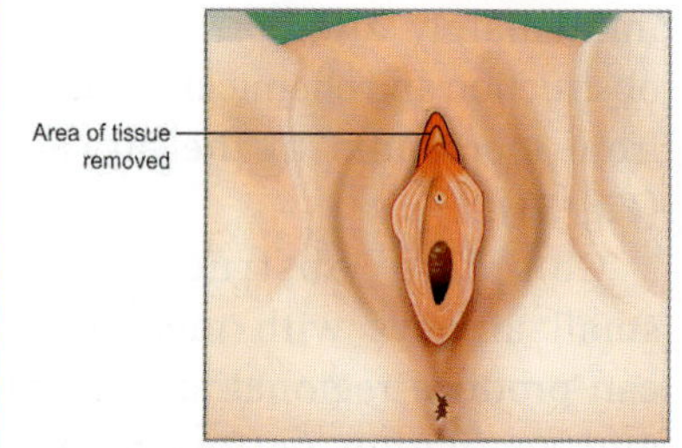 A. Type 1 FGM B. Type 2 FGM C. Type 3 FGM D. Type 4 FGM E. Female circumcision	**Ans: A (Type 1 FGM)** Female genital mutilation (FGM) refers to the partial or total removal of external female genitalia or other injury to the female genital organs for nonmedical reasons. The adjacent image shows type 1 FGM as there is partial excision of clitoris along with prepuce in the image. Classification of female genital mutilation as per the World Health Organization WHO (1995) is as follows **(Figs. 57A to D)**: *Type 1:* Partial or total excision of the clitoris and/or the prepuce (clitoridectomy). *Type 2:* Partial or total removal of the clitoris and the labia minora, with or without excision of the labia majora. *Type 3:* Infibulation or narrowing of the vaginal orifice by cutting and appositioning the labia minora and/or the labia majora, with or without excision of the clitoris. *Type 4:* Any other procedure which is performed for nonmedical reasons and causes injures to the female genital organs such as pricking, piercing, or incision of the clitoris and/or labia; stretching of the clitoris and/or labia; cauterization by burning; scraping of tissue surrounding the vaginal orifice; introduction of corrosive substances or herbs into the vagina for the purpose of tightening or narrowing it, etc. 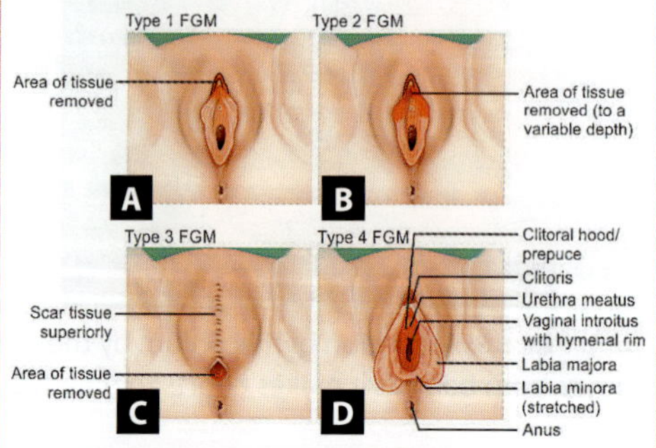 **Figs. 57A to D:** WHO classification of female genital mutilation (FGM).	**Explanation:** Female genital mutilation is often performed on girls between infancy and adolescence and is deeply rooted in cultural, religious, or social norms in certain communities, especially in East and Central Africa. FGM is recognized globally as a violation of human rights, causing severe physical and psychological harm. The practice can lead to complications such as infections, chronic pain, childbirth complications, and even death. Efforts by governments, health organizations, and advocacy groups aim to eradicate FGM and protect the rights and well-being of women and girls worldwide. FGM can be encountered in clinical practice in the UK due to the presence of several immigrant groups in the population. If the gynecologist encounters a patient with FGM, the police and social services must be immediately informed. **Potential questions:** There can be questions related to various types of FGM, based on the WHO classification system and their characteristics. This concept is especially important for the MRCOG exams.

CHAPTER 5

Medical Conditions During Pregnancy and Postpartum

MEDICAL CONDITIONS DURING PREGNANCY

ANEMIA IN PREGNANCY

Question	Answer	Comment
Q1. A 28-year-old pregnant woman at 24 weeks of gestation presents with fatigue and dizziness. Her hemoglobin level is 9.0 g/dL, and her serum ferritin is low. The picture of her peripheral smear is shown below. Based on the findings, what is the most appropriate management? 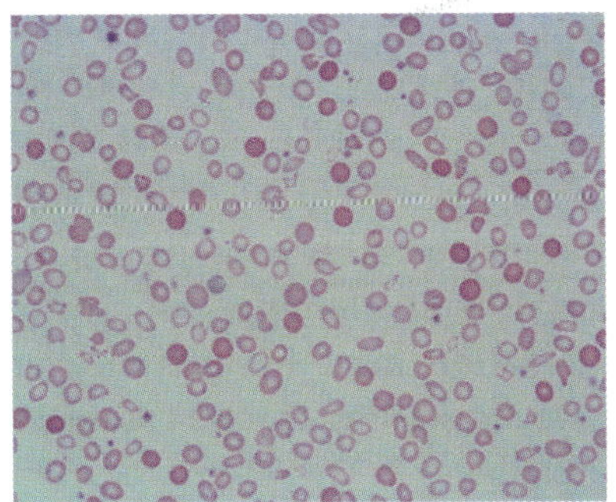 A. Treat with folic acid supplements B. Start oral iron supplementation C. Immediate blood transfusion is required D. Administer B12 injections. E. Start with parenteral iron therapy	**Ans: B (Start oral iron supplementation)** The patient's symptoms, low hemoglobin, and low serum ferritin indicate iron deficiency anemia. The adjacent image shows peripheral smear of blood with microcytic and hypochromic picture. There is presence of pale-looking RBCs with large central vacuoles (hypochromic RBCs). Iron deficiency anemia has a multifactorial etiology as shown in **Figure 1**. 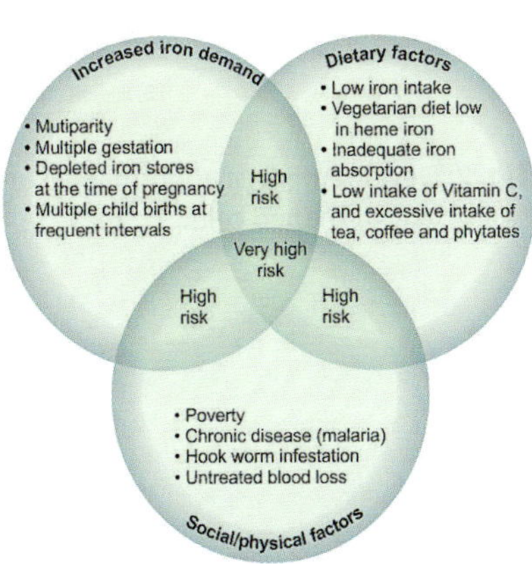 **Fig. 1:** Multifactorial etiology of iron deficiency anemia during pregnancy.	**Explanation:** Iron deficiency anemia can be considered as the most common type of anemia during pregnancy. Treatment typically includes oral iron supplements, with intravenous iron considered in severe cases or if oral iron is not tolerated. The peripheral smear in these cases show the following features: ▪ *Anisocytosis (abnormal size of cells):* The RBCs are small and deformed (microcytosis). ▪ *Poikilocytosis (abnormal shape of cells):* Presence of pencil cells and target cells. There is presence of ring or pessary cells with central hypochromia (large central vacuoles). **Potential questions:** There can be questions pertaining to the diagnosis and management of several types of anemia during pregnancy such as iron deficiency anemia, megaloblastic anemia, hemolytic anemia (e.g., sickle cell anemia and thalassemia), etc.

Question	Answer	Comment
Q2. A 26-year-old pregnant woman, with a known history of sickle cell anemia, presents at 22 weeks' gestation for a routine checkup. She reports episodes of joint pain and fatigue. A peripheral smear is done, and the result is shown in the image below. What is the most appropriate next step in managing this patient? 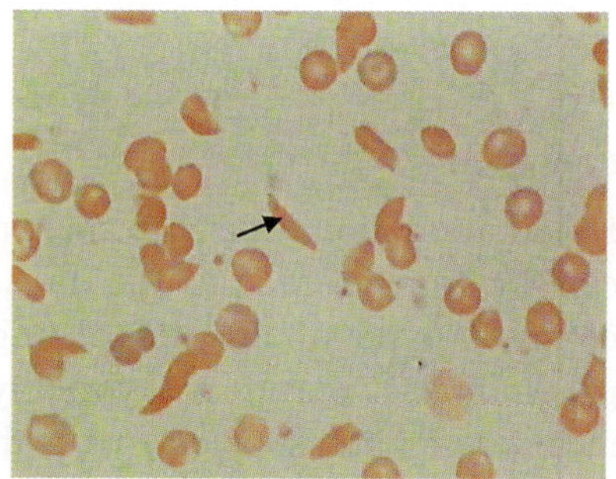 A. Start oral iron supplementation B. Prescribe hydroxyurea to reduce the frequency of crises C. Increase folic acid intake and provide pain management D. Perform an emergency blood transfusion E. Consider bone marrow transplant	**Ans: C (Increase folic acid intake and provide pain management)** The adjacent image shows peripheral smear in case of sickle cell anemia, with the arrow pointing toward a sickle-shaped-RBC, a hallmark of the disease. There can also be presence of crescent- shaped, long or target cells in these cases. If the patient is asplenic, there may be presence of RBCs containing nuclear material (Howell–Jolly bodies). Sickle cell disease belongs to a group of autosomal recessive disorders, which is associated with the mutation of hemoglobin gene. This causes the RBCs to take an abnormal sickle or crescent shape **(Fig. 2)**, thereby delivering reduced supply of oxygen to the tissues. Moreover, the sickle cells are fragile and more prone to rupture, resulting in anemia. 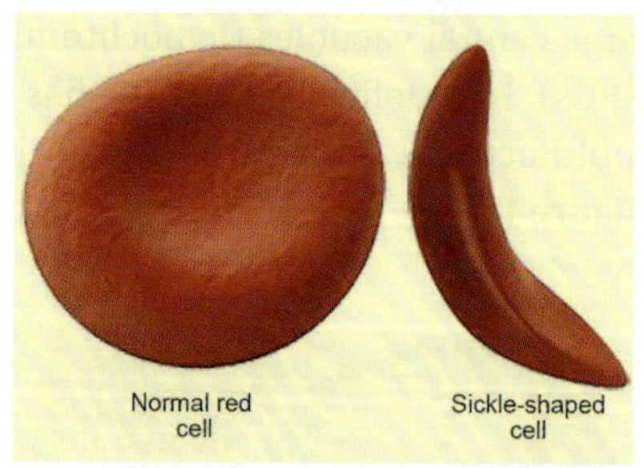 **Fig. 2:** Development of abnormal sickle-shaped cells.	**Explanation:** In pregnant patients with sickle cell anemia, management during pregnancy focuses on folic acid supplementation (to support increased red blood cell production), pain management, and prevention of vaso-occlusive crises. In case of acute painful crisis, the patient must be admitted to the hospital and given appropriate analgesia in the form of paracetamol or weak opioids. Pethidine should be preferably avoided due to an associated risk of seizures. Requirement for fluids and oxygen must be assessed, and they should be administered, if required. Hydroxyurea is generally avoided during pregnancy due to potential teratogenic effects. Blood transfusions are reserved for severe anemia or complications. Low-dose aspirin (75 mg) must be prescribed daily from 12 weeks of gestation to reduce the risk for developing preeclampsia. Women should receive prophylactic low molecular weight heparin (LMWH) during each hospital admission to prevent the risk of thromboembolism. Serial fetal biometry for growth evaluation must be offered every 4 weeks starting from 24 weeks of gestation. **Potential questions:** There can be questions pertaining to the diagnosis and management of several types of anemia during pregnancy such as iron deficiency anemia, megaloblastic anemia, hemolytic anemia (e.g., sickle cell anemia and thalassemia), etc.

<table>
<tr><th>Question</th><th>Answer</th><th>Comment</th></tr>
<tr>
<td>

Q3. A 30-year-old pregnant woman at 28 weeks' gestation presents with fatigue, pallor, and shortness of breath. Blood tests reveal macrocytic anemia, and a peripheral smear is obtained, which is shown in the image below. What is the most likely cause of her condition?

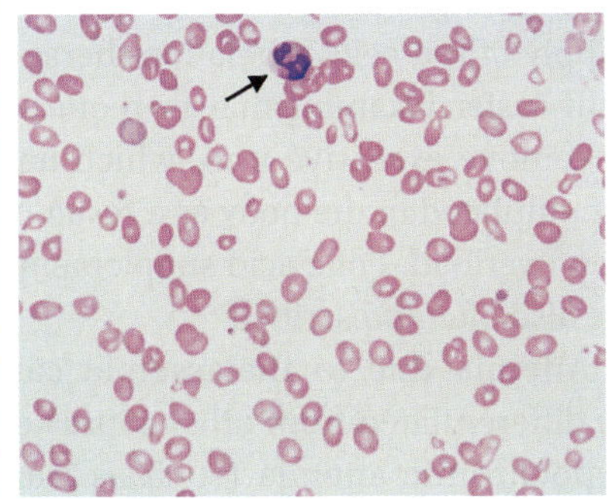

A. Iron deficiency anemia
B. Folate deficiency
C. Vitamin B12 deficiency
D. Hemolytic anemia
E. Sickle cell anemia

</td>
<td>

Ans: B (Folate deficiency)

The adjacent image shows peripheral smear in case of megaloblastic anemia, with the arrow pointing towards a hypersegmented neutrophil, which is a characteristic feature of megaloblastic anemia. **Figure 3** depicts a magnified image showing the same.

Other features which may be present on peripheral smear in case of megaloblastic anemia are:

- Presence of macrocytes and megaloblasts (cells larger than normal in size)
- Fully hemoglobinized RBCs

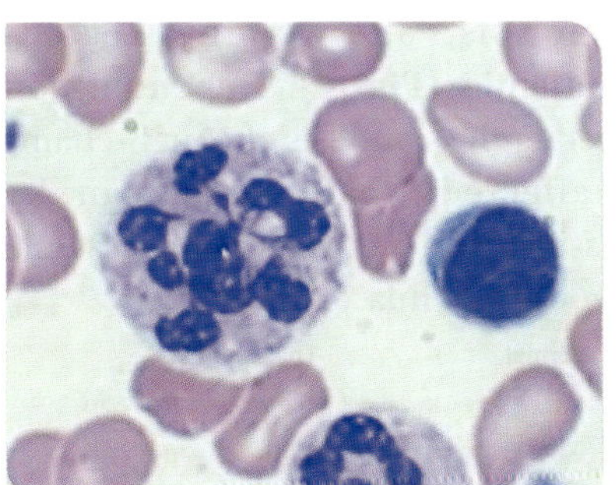

Fig. 3: Magnified view of the smear showing hypersegmented neutrophil.

Prevention of folate deficiency comprises prescribing a folate-rich diet (broccoli, asparagus, chickpeas, brussels sprouts, etc.). Oral folate supplements (400 μg daily) must be prescribed in the preconceptional as well as for the first 12 weeks of pregnancy.

</td>
<td>

Explanation: Megaloblastic anemia during pregnancy is most often caused by folate deficiency, as the demand for folic acid increases during pregnancy. Vitamin B12 deficiency can also cause megaloblastic anemia but is less common in pregnancy compared to folate deficiency. Iron deficiency and hemolytic anemia usually present with microcytic or normocytic cells. Sickle cell anemia shows sickle-shaped cells.

In megaloblastic anemia, similar to iron deficiency anemia, there is reduced heme production. The effect on the fetus in case of folate deficiency anemia in pregnancy can be in the form of neural tube defects and low birthweight babies.

Potential questions: There can be questions pertaining to the diagnosis and management of several types of anemia during pregnancy such as iron deficiency anemia, megaloblastic anemia, hemolytic anemia (e.g., sickle cell anemia and thalassemia), etc.

</td>
</tr>
</table>

Question

Q4. A 27-year-old pregnant woman at 20 weeks' gestation presents for routine follow-up. Blood work shows microcytic hypochromic anemia. Her hemoglobin level was found to be 10 g/dL. A peripheral smear reveals abnormal cells as shown in the image below. Hemoglobin electrophoresis reveals elevated HbA2 levels. What is the most likely diagnosis?

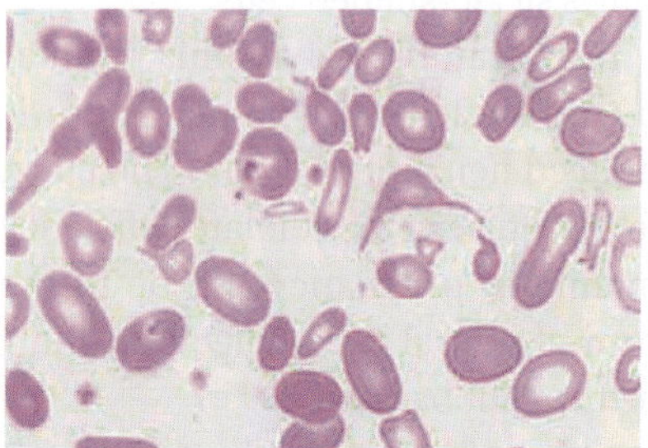

A. Iron deficiency anemia
B. Alpha-thalassemia minor
C. Beta-thalassemia minor
D. Sickle cell anemia
E. Beta-thalassemia major

Answer

Ans: C (Beta-thalassemia minor)

The adjacent image shows a peripheral smear in case of thalassemia. Peripheral smear in case of thalassemia shows microcytic hypochromic anemia, which is similar to that seen in iron deficiency anemia. Characteristic features which differentiate this from iron deficiency anemia include the presence of target cells and teardrop-shaped cells.

Thalassemia includes a group of genetically inherited disorders, which are characterized by impaired or defective production of one or more normal globin peptide chains. Abnormal synthesis of globin chains can result in ineffective erythropoiesis, hemolysis, and varying degrees of anemia **(Fig. 4)**. Depending on whether the synthesis of α- or β-chains is affected, thalassemia can be classified into two types: α-thalassemia or β-thalassemia.

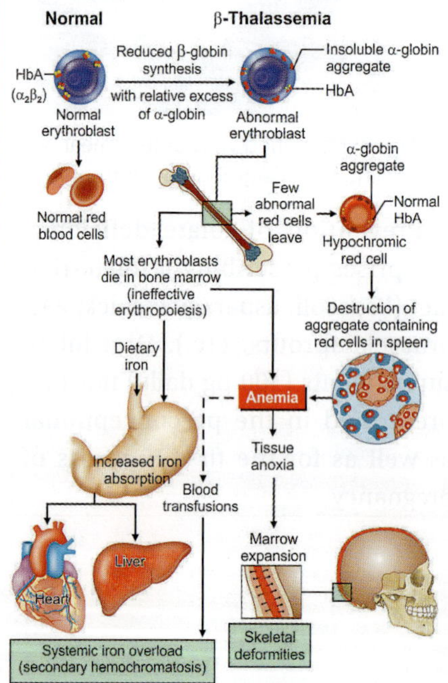

Fig. 4: Pathogenesis of β-thalassemia.

Comment

Explanation: Beta-thalassemia minor commonly presents with microcytic hypochromic anemia during pregnancy. The presence of target cells and elevated HbA2 on electrophoresis are characteristic findings.

Treatment of moderate-to-severe anemia comprises transfusion of red cells. Repeated blood transfusions may be required to maintain healthy supply of red cells. Chelation therapy with desferrioxamine may be required to remove excessive iron, which has accumulated in the body as a result of iron overload. Folic acid supplements are also often prescribed.

Anemia due to thalassemia can be differentiated from other causes of hypochromic anemia (such as iron deficiency anemia and anemia due to chronic disease) on the basis of various parameters. Although RBC indices, such as mean corpuscular volume (MCV), mean corpuscular hemoglobin (MCH), and mean corpuscular hemoglobin concentration (MCHC), are reduced in proportion to the severity of anemia in cases of iron deficiency, these indices may be reduced to very low values (disproportionate to the severity of anemia) in cases of thalassemia.

Serum iron concentration is usually normal or increased in thalassemic syndromes, while it is usually low in iron deficiency anemia.

Potential questions: There can be questions pertaining to the diagnosis and management of several types of anemia during pregnancy such as iron deficiency anemia, megaloblastic anemia, hemolytic anemia (e.g., sickle cell anemia and thalassemia), etc.

HYPERTENSIVE DISORDERS OF PREGNANCY

Question

Q5. A 28-year-old woman at 32 weeks of gestation presents with sudden onset of severe headache, blurred vision, and swelling in her hands and face. Blood pressure is 165/100 mm Hg. Urine dipstick shows significant proteinuria as shown in the image below. Which of the following mechanisms best explains the pathogenesis of preeclampsia?

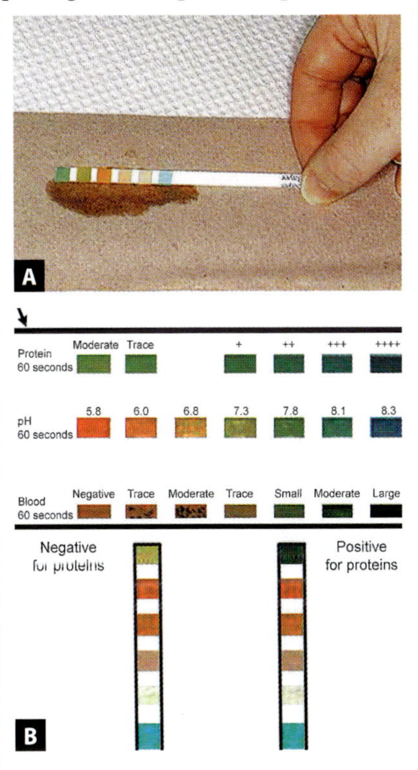

A. Failure of trophoblastic invasion of spiral arteries
B. Increased levels of prostacyclin and nitric oxide
C. Enhanced fetal blood flow through the placenta
D. Overproduction of aldosterone leading to fluid retention
E. Increased maternal immune tolerance to fetal antigen

Answer

Ans: A (Failure of trophoblastic invasion of spiral arteries)

The adjacent image demonstrates presence of proteinuria equivalent to 2+. The approximate equivalence of the dipstick result with the amount of proteinuria is as follows: 1+ = 0.3 g/L, 2+ = 1 g/L, 3+ = 3 g/L, and 4+ = 10 g/L. Proteinuria is defined as significant if the excretion of proteins exceeds 300 mg/24 hours or there is persistent presence of the protein (30 mg/dL or 1+ dipstick) in random urine sample in absence of any evidence of urinary tract infection.

The exact pathophysiology of preeclampsia is not yet understood. An important mechanism behind the development of preeclampsia is inadequate trophoblastic invasion of the spiral arterioles (as shown in **Figs. 5A and B**). Inadequate trophoblastic invasion of the maternal spiral vessels can interfere with normal villous development, resulting in placental insufficiency.

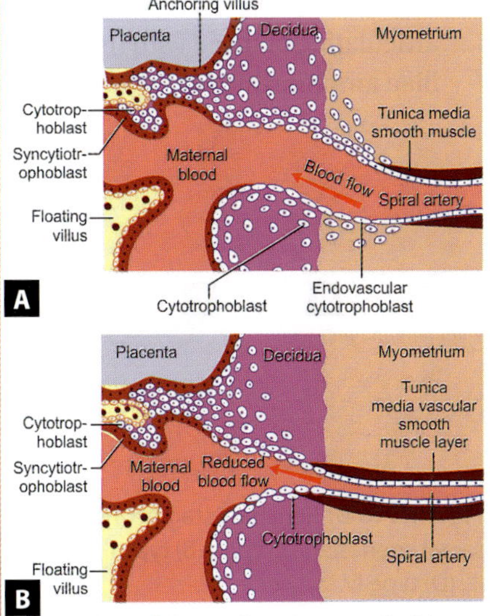

Figs. 5A and B: Inadequate trophoblastic invasion: (A) Trophoblastic invasion of spiral arterioles in normal pregnancy; (B) Reduced trophoblastic invasion of spiral vessels in preeclampsia.

Comment

Explanation: Preeclampsia can be defined as a pregnancy-specific, multifactorial disease, which presents as a syndrome of specific signs and symptoms. It is characterized by appearance of high BP (>140/90 mm Hg) for the first time during pregnancy after 20 weeks of gestation and presence of proteinuria ≥300 mg/24 hours or >1+ on the dipstick or urine protein to creatine ratio of ≥0.3).

or

In the absence of proteinuria, other symptoms suggestive of maternal end-organ dysfunction are neurological complications, pulmonary edema, hematological complications, renal insufficiency, and impaired liver function.

or

Uteroplacental dysfunction: Preeclampsia is characterized by abnormal placental development, specifically due to the failure of trophoblastic invasion of the spiral arteries. This results in inadequate blood flow to the placenta, leading to hypoxia and release of antiangiogenic factors. These factors cause endothelial dysfunction, hypertension, and proteinuria. Prostacyclin and nitric oxide levels are decreased, and not increased, in preeclampsia. The condition is not caused by increased fetal blood flow or aldosterone overproduction. Maternal immune tolerance to fetal antigens plays no significant role in preeclampsia.

Potential questions: There can be questions related to clinical manifestation, diagnosis, management, and complications of preeclampsia

GESTATIONAL DIABETES

Question	Answer	Comment
Q6. 25-year-old pregnant woman with uncontrolled diabetes undergoes a routine ultrasound at 22 weeks of gestation. The scan reveals absence of the lower spine and sacral region in the fetus, along with abnormal lower limb positioning. The X-ray image of this finding is shown below. What is the most likely diagnosis? 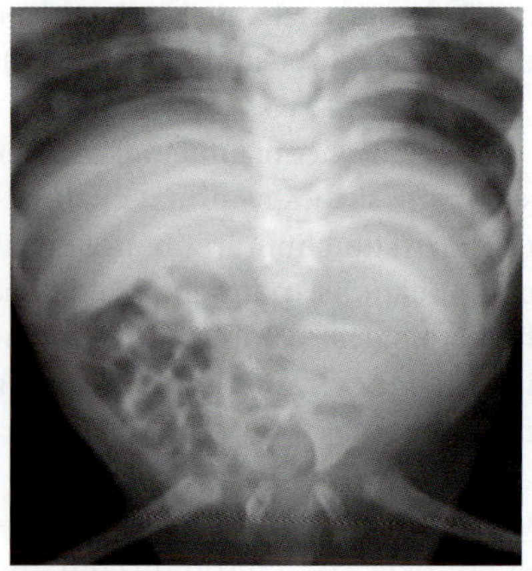 A. Spina bifida B. Caudal regression syndrome C. Meningocele D. Klippel-Feil syndrome E. Arnold-Chiari malformation	**Ans: B (Caudal regression syndrome)** The X-ray image in the adjacent picture depicts sacral agenesis, also known as caudal regression syndrome or sacral hypoplasia, and is associated with abnormal development of the sacral bone. It is usually diagnosed through prenatal ultrasound, often confirmed with MRI for detailed assessment. Renshaw (1978) classified sacral agenesis as follows **(Figs. 6A to D)**: ▪ *Type 1:* Unilateral sacral agenesis (partial or unilateral) ▪ *Type II:* Bilateral symmetrical partial sacral agenesis. The sacral vertebra may be normal or hypoplastic. There is stable articulation between the ilium and first sacral vertebra. ▪ *Type III:* There may be a variable amount of sacral agenesis. The ilia may be articulating with the sides of the lowest vertebra present. ▪ *Type IV:* There may be a variable amount of lumbar and total sacral agenesis with the caudal endplate of the lowest vertebra either articulating or fused with the ilia or iliac amphiarthrosis. 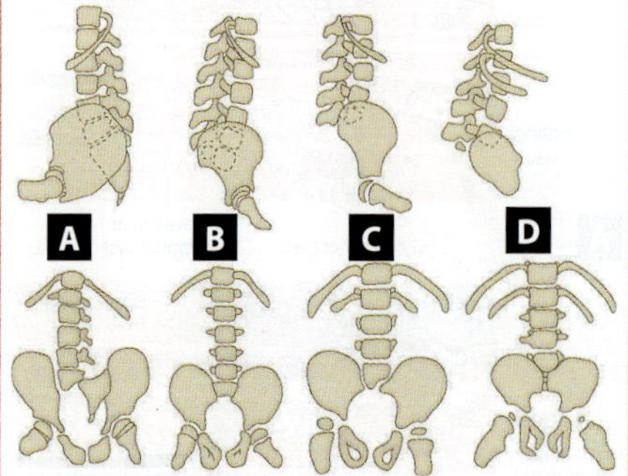 **Figs. 6A to D:** Renshaw staging system for sacral agenesis: (A) Type I, (B) type II, (C) type III, (D) type IV.	**Explanation:** Caudal regression syndrome is a congenital malformation often associated with maternal diabetes, characterized by partial or complete absence of the sacrum and sometimes lower lumbar vertebrae. The abnormal limb positioning also correlates with this condition. Minor abnormalities may not cause any deformity and hence do not require any correction. Severe cases may present with spinal-pelvic instability and/or severe knee contractures with popliteal webbing of the knees. Reconstruction of limbs may be required in type IV defects which may not be entirely successful. Bilateral subtrochanteric amputation may be done in some cases. Some surgeons have advocated spinal-pelvic fusion to protect the viscera from unphysiological compression and angulation. Knee flexion and foot deformities can be corrected at an early age using a combination of surgical release procedures, supracondylar femoral extension osteotomies, and serial casting. Implications of sacral agenesis for labor and delivery can include altered pelvic anatomy affecting the mode of delivery and potential neurological complications for the fetus. **Potential questions:** There can be questions related to clinical manifestation, diagnosis, management, and complications of gestational diabetes.

HEART DISEASE DURING PREGNANCY

Question	Answer	Comment
Q7. A 32-year-old pregnant woman at 34 weeks' gestation reports dizziness, light-headedness, and nausea while lying in a position shown in the image below during a routine checkup. Her blood pressure drops significantly. What is the most likely cause of these symptoms? 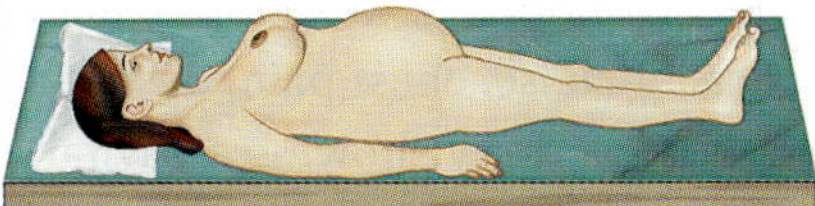 A. Preeclampsia B. Supine hypotension syndrome C. Orthostatic hypotension D. Vasovagal syncope E. Severe anemia	**Ans: B (Supine hypotension syndrome)** The adjacent image is showing a pregnant woman lying on her back or in a supine position. This position is likely to result in a condition called supine hypotension syndrome, also known as aortocaval compression. This refers to the development of sudden hypotension in a pregnant woman who lies flat on the bed or in supine position because during this position, uterine contents of the gravid uterus press upon the inferior vena cava and aorta, thereby partially occluding them **(Figs. 7A and B)**. 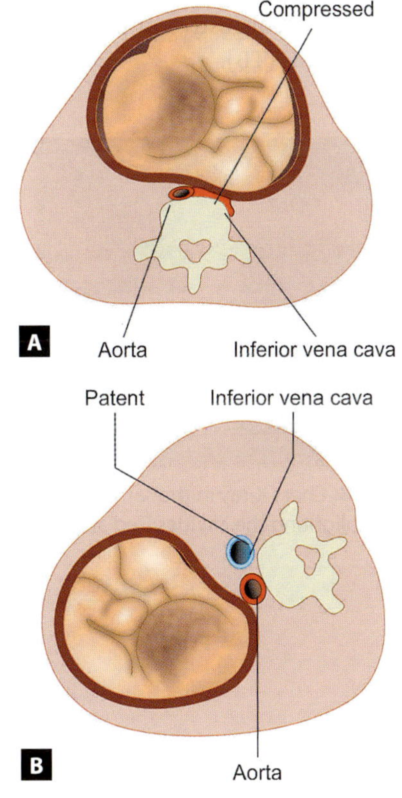 **Figs. 7A and B:** Pathogenesis of supine hypotension syndrome: (A) Supine position; (B) Left lateral position.	**Explanation:** Supine hypotension syndrome occurs when a pregnant woman lies flat on her back, leading to compression of the inferior vena cava by the enlarged uterus. This results in reduced venous return to the heart, causing a drop in cardiac output and blood pressure. This may result in the development of hypotension and symptoms such as pallor, reduced heart rate, sweating, dizziness, loss of consciousness, etc. The symptoms resolve when the woman changes position to the side. Supine hypotension syndrome can be prevented by advising the patient to assume a left lateral position while lying down rather than lying flat on a surface. **Potential questions:** There can be questions related to clinical presentation, diagnosis, management, and complications of various cardiac conditions during pregnancy.

CHEST INFECTION IN PREGNANCY

Question	Answer	Comment
Q8. A 28-year-old pregnant woman in her second trimester presents with persistent cough, night sweats, and weight loss. She belongs to Indian ethnicity and has migrated to UK a month back. Her chest X-ray is shown below. What is the most likely diagnosis? 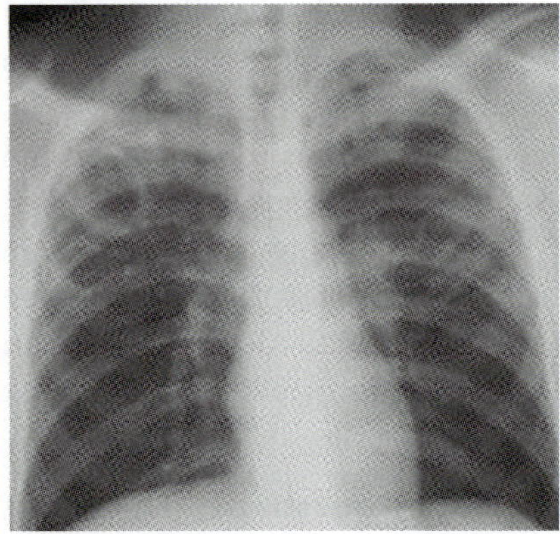 A. Bacterial pneumonia B. Tuberculosis C. Lung abscess D. Bronchiectasis E. Pneumothorax	**Ans: B (Tuberculosis)** The adjacent image shows the posterior–anterior view of chest X-ray. In this X-ray, there are two well-defined, thin-walled, air-filled cavities on the upper side of the right lung. One such similar cavity can be observed on the upper side of the left lung **(Fig. 8)**. Fibrosis can be observed on the upper side of both the lungs. There is no loss of lung volume. The costophrenic angles are clear. Therefore, there is no pleural effusion. Also, there is no peripheral or hilar lymphadenopathy. This is most likely suggestive of pulmonary tuberculosis (TB). 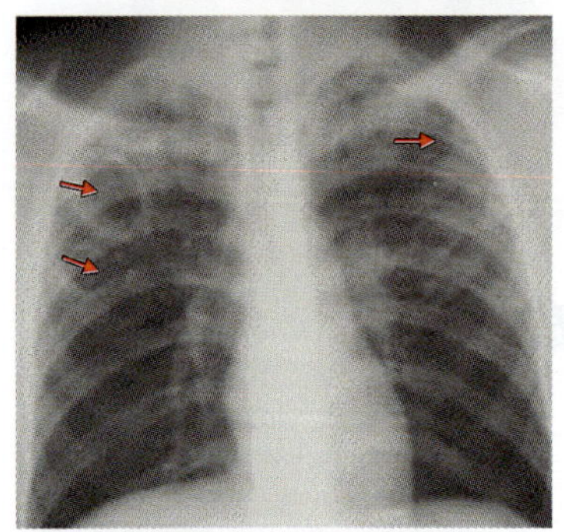 **Fig. 8:** Chest X-ray in the same patient highlighting the cavities (red arrows).	**Explanation:** The incidence of TB in the UK is higher among immigrant and ethnic minority groups (African and Indian ethnic groups, especially in the new immigrant population). TB in pregnancy may present with classic symptoms like low-grade fever (with late afternoon peak), persistent cough, hemoptysis, weight loss, night sweats, malaise, chest pain, dyspnea, etc. A chest X-ray showing a cavitary lesion and positive sputum for acid-fast bacilli are considered diagnostic for tuberculosis. Pregnancy does not have any adverse effect on the course of tuberculosis, nor does the disease have any adverse effect on the course of pregnancy. Untreated cases of tuberculosis during pregnancy may be associated with an increased incidence of complications such as preterm labor, intrauterine IUGR, increased perinatal mortality, etc. **Potential questions:** Since pulmonary tuberculosis may be encountered in the ethnic minority groups in the UK, questions related to diagnosis and management of TB are important for MRCOG exam.

MEDICAL CONDITIONS DURING THE POSTPARTUM PERIOD

ABNORMALITIES OF LACTATION

Question	Answer	Comment
Q9. A 30-year-old breastfeeding woman presents with a painful, erythematous area on her left breast, fever, and general malaise, nearly two weeks following a normal vaginal delivery. On examination, the affected area as shown in the image below is warm and tender to touch. What is the most likely diagnosis? 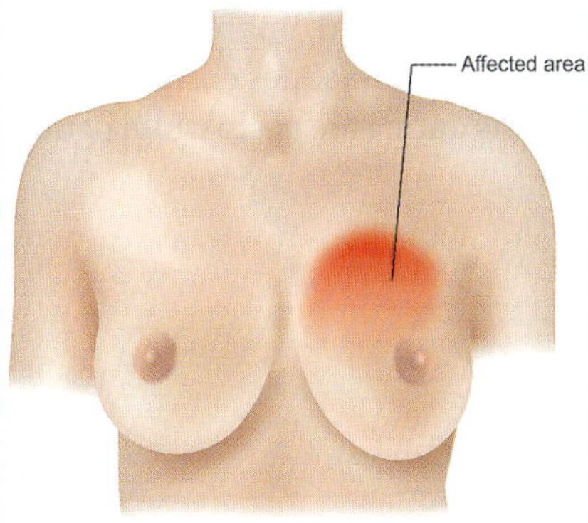 A. Breast abscess B. Mastitis C. Fibroadenoma D. Inflammatory breast cancer E. Galactocele	**Ans: B (Mastitis)** The area of inflammation shown in the adjacent image is due to mastitis. Mastitis can be defined as the parenchymatous infection of the mammary glands **(Fig. 9)**. The infection is usually unilateral, commonly occurs on the postpartum day 14, and is associated with marked swelling, inflammation, and redness of a single breast lobe. Fever may be present and is associated with chills or rigors. There may be hardening and reddening of the breast tissue and intense pain. 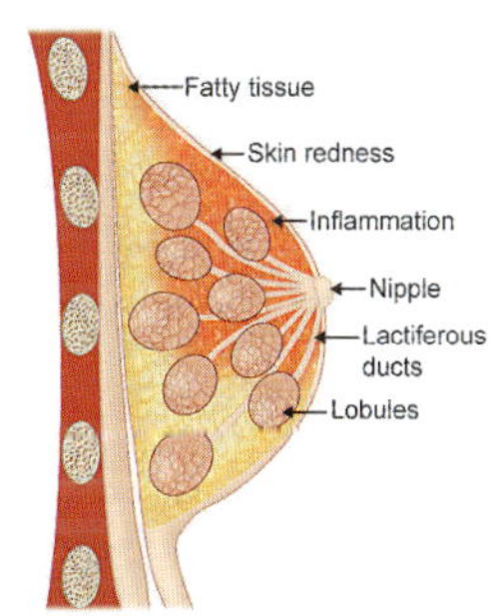 **Fig. 9:** Pathogenesis of mastitis.	**Explanation:** Mastitis is a common condition in breastfeeding women, often presenting with a painful, erythematous, and warm area on the breast, along with systemic symptoms like fever. The most important causative organism is *Staphylococcus aureus*, most commonly community-acquired methicillin-resistant *Staphylococcus aureus* (CA-MRSA). Treatment involves administration of antibiotics after bacterial identification and sensitivity. Infection usually resolves within 48 hours with treatment. Breastfeeding must be continued. Breast abscess may develop if untreated, but mastitis typically does not involve fluctuance, which would indicate abscess formation. **Potential questions:** There may be various questions related to etiology, diagnosis, and management of various abnormalities encountered in breasts during the postpartum period.

Question	Answer	Comment
Q10. A 28-year-old postpartum woman presents with swelling, pain, and redness in both breasts 3 days after delivery. On examination, the breasts are firm, warm, and swollen, as shown in the image below. On palpation, there are no discrete masses or signs of infection. What is the most likely diagnosis? 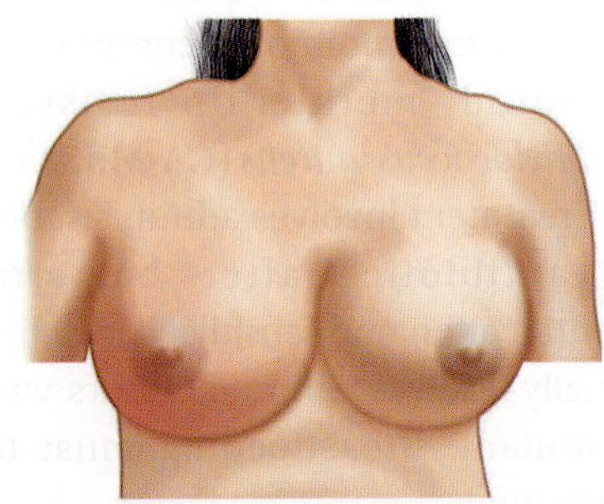 A. Breast abscess B. Mastitis C. Breast engorgement D. Fibrocystic changes E. Inverted nipple	**Ans: C (Breast engorgement)** The adjacent image and clinical presentation indicate breast engorgement. It presents with bilateral, diffuse swelling with pain and warmth due to excess milk accumulation, typically in the early postpartum period when milk ejection does not occur or is slower than production **(Figs. 10A and B)**. 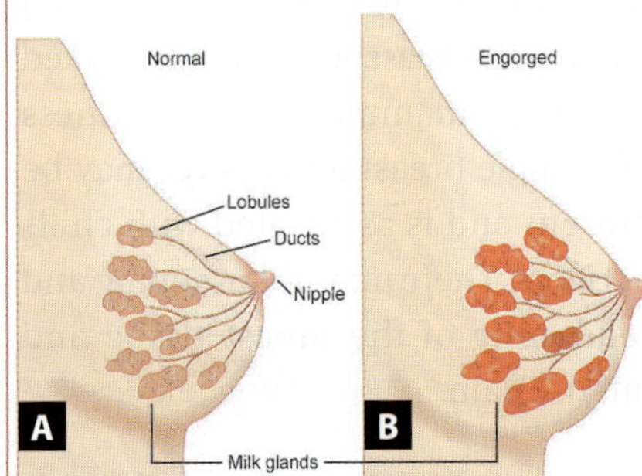 **Figs. 10A and B:** Pathogenesis of breast engorgement.	**Explanation:** Breast engorgement occurs when milk supply exceeds infant demand, often causing pain and fever around day 3 postpartum. Management includes using a supportive, well-fitting, feeding, brassiere, frequent 15–20-minute feeds every 2–3 hours, breast pumping, massage during feeds, avoiding nipple shields/pacifiers, and using paracetamol or ice packs for pain relief. **Potential questions:** There may be various questions related to etiology, diagnosis, and management of various abnormalities encountered in breasts during the postpartum period.

Question	Answer	Comment
Q11. A 32-year-old woman presents with a painful lump in her right breast. On examination, there is a fluctuating, tender mass in the upper outer quadrant of the breast as shown in the image below. Which of the following is the most likely diagnosis? 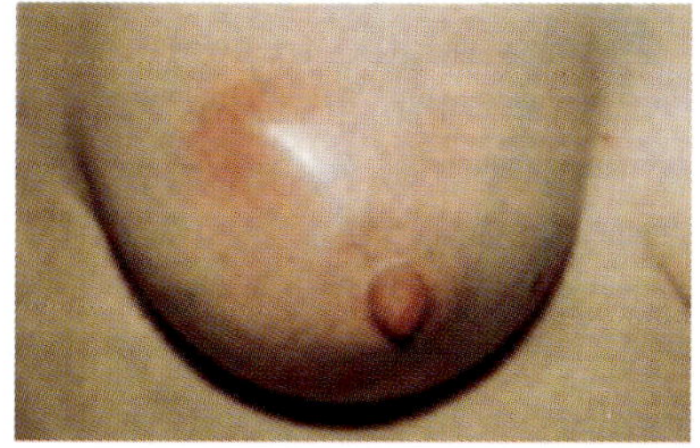 A. Fibroadenoma B. Breast cyst C. Breast abscess D. Phyllodes tumor E. Mastitis	**Ans: C (Breast abscess)** The patient's clinical presentation and the adjacent image are indicative of a breast abscess. It usually occurs due to severe mastitis and can commonly occur in women who breast-feed. The bacteria can commonly enter through a crack in nipples. The bacterium most commonly involved in the causation of breast abscess is *Staphylococcus aureus*. There is presence of a painful, fluctuant, pus-filled swelling in the breast tissue **(Figs. 11A and B)**. 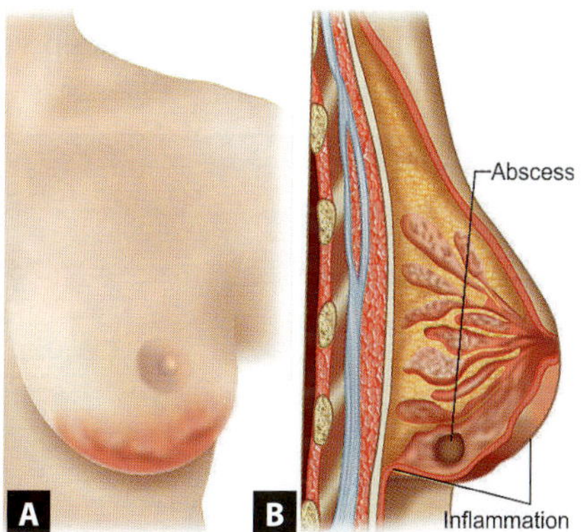 **Figs. 11A and B:** Pathogenesis of breast abscess.	**Explanation:** Breast abscess presents as a painful, tender mass with fluctuating characteristics on physical examination. There may be redness and warmth over the skin overlying the abscess, nipple discharge and tenderness, and fever. The lymph nodes of the affected side may also be tender and enlarged. The diagnosis can be confirmed on an ultrasound examination, which reveals a well-circumscribed fluid collection with internal echoes. The presence of internal echoes suggests pus or debris within the abscess cavity. Treatment with antibiotics and painkillers may be required. Though treatment with antibiotics is usually successful, surgical drainage is commonly required. Some commonly used antibiotics include nafcillin for treatment of penicillinase producing bacteria, vancomycin for treatment of bacteria resistant to nafcillin, clindamycin for treatment of both aerobic and anaerobic bacteria, etc. Breast-feeding should be continued even after drainage. **Potential questions:** There may be various questions related to etiology, diagnosis, and management of various abnormalities encountered in breasts during the postpartum period.

COMPLICATIONS OF PUERPERIUM

Question	Answer	Comment
Q12. A 34-year-old woman, 2 weeks postpartum, presents with unilateral leg swelling, pain, and tenderness in the left calf. She denies history of any recent trauma. What is the most likely diagnosis? 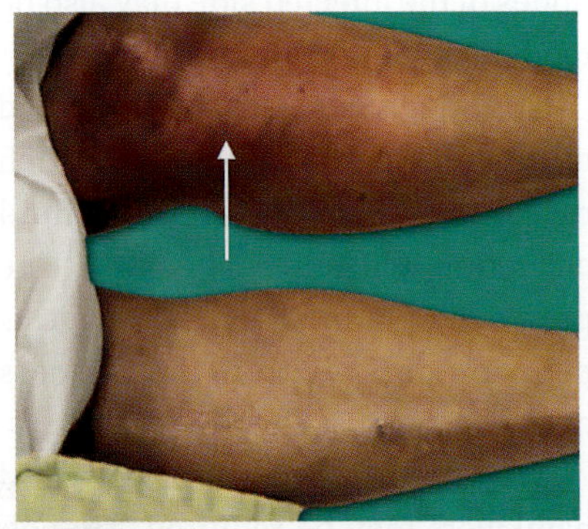 A. Superficial thrombophlebitis B. Cellulitis C. Deep vein thrombosis (DVT) D. Lymphedema E. Varicose veins	**Ans: C [Deep vein thrombosis (DVT)]** The adjacent image shows swelling, tenderness, and redness in the left calf (indicated by the arrow). On ultrasound, in this patient, there is an evidence of a thrombus within the left popliteal vein **(Fig. 12)**. This is indicative of deep vein thrombosis (DVT). DVT is a known risk in the postpartum period due to increased clotting tendency in the blood. This condition is characterized by unilateral leg swelling, pain, and the presence of a thrombus in a deep vein on ultrasound. 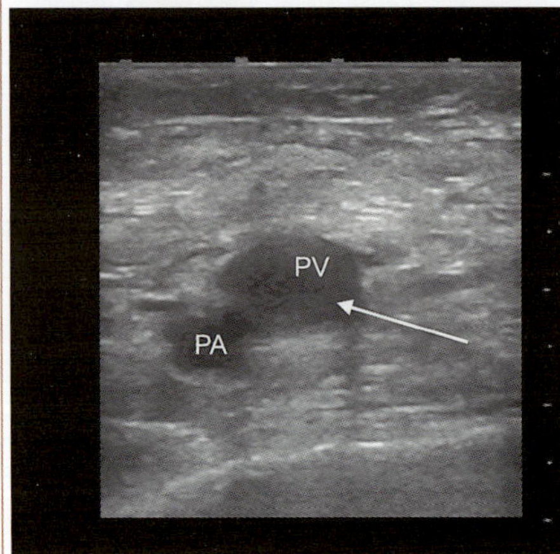 **Fig. 12:** Presence of clot in the popliteal vein on the ultrasound examination (indicated by the arrow) (PA: popliteal artery; PV: popliteal vein)	**Explanation:** Deep vein thrombosis is characterized by swelling, pain, and tenderness in the affected limb. Ultrasound examination is the investigation of choice in cases of DVT, which helps in detecting changes related to compression of the femoral veins. Filling defects in the vessels may occur due to an onsite or upstream flow obstruction. Also, there is a lack of compressibility of the vein when pressure is exerted by the ultrasound transducer. Management of cases of DVT comprises the following steps: ▪ Bed rest with foot elevation above the level of heart ▪ Analgesics can be used to provide pain relief ▪ Antimicrobial therapy must be started ▪ Anticoagulants, such as heparin, low molecular weight heparin and oral anticoagulants, such as warfarin, can also be used, but must be preferably avoided during pregnancy due to its teratogenic effects. ▪ Knee-length or thigh-length graduated elastic compression stockings help in reducing the risk of thrombosis Early ambulation helps in reducing the risk **Potential questions:** There may be various questions related to etiology, diagnosis, and management of various complications encountered by the woman during the postpartum period.

INJURIES TO THE BIRTH CANAL

Question	Answer	Comment
Q13. Examination of a 25-year-old woman after vaginal delivery, shows minimal tearing of vaginal mucosa but no involvement of underlying muscle. Clinical appearance of injury is shown in the image below. What is the most likely diagnosis? 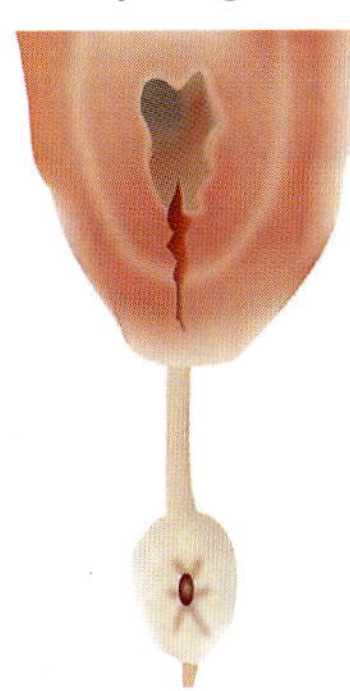 A. First-degree perineal tear B. Second-degree perineal tear C. Third-degree perineal tear D. Fourth-degree perineal tear E. Episiotomy	**Ans: A (First-degree perineal tear)** First-degree perineal tear as shown in the adjacent image involves only the vaginal mucosa and not the perineal muscles. **Figure 13** demonstrates the first-degree perineal tear. 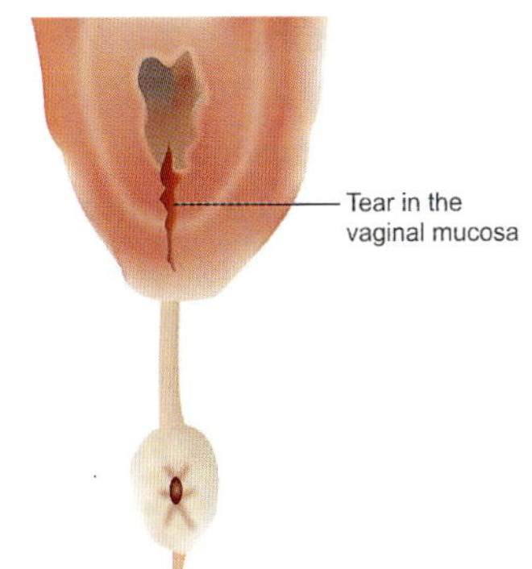 **Fig. 13:** First-degree perineal tear.	**Explanation:** First-degree perineal tear involves only the vaginal mucosa without any involvement of the underlying muscle. It is the least severe type of perineal tear and typically does not require extensive intervention. In case of presence of vaginal tears or lacerations, their repair is performed essentially in the same manner as that of the episiotomy to achieve hemostasis and to obliterate the dead space. When faced with: first-degree tear, the repair of mucosa is performed using continuous sutures with Vicryl (polyglycolic acid) 2-0 or 3-0. The first stitch must be taken 1 cm above the apex of tear in the vaginal mucosal tissues. **Potential questions:** There can be questions related to the diagnosis and management of different degrees of vaginal tears and lacerations.
Q14. A 30-year-old woman is evaluated following a vaginal delivery. She had refused an episiotomy. On examination, there is a tear, which does not involve the anal sphincter as shown in the image below. What is the most likely diagnosis? 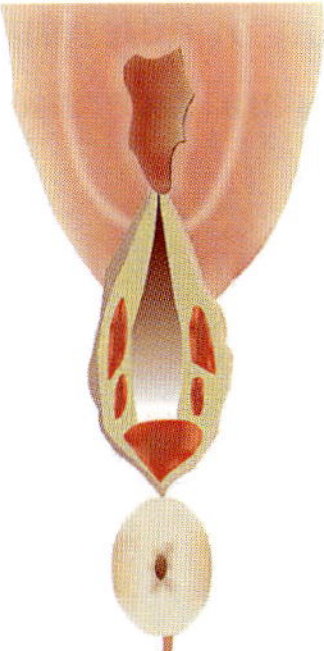 A. Second-degree perineal tear B. 3a third-degree perineal tear C. 3b third-degree perineal tear D. 3c third-degree perineal tear E. Fourth-degree perineal tear	**Ans: A (Second-degree perineal tear)** Second-degree perineal tear as shown in **Figure 14** involves the perineal muscles along with vaginal mucosa. However, the anal sphincters remain intact in these cases. 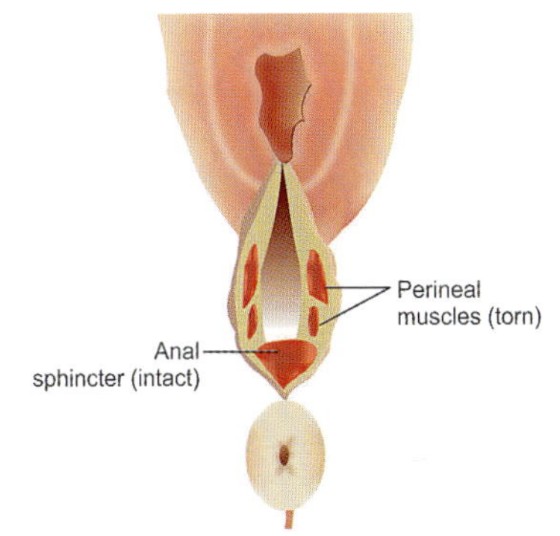 **Fig. 14:** Second-degree perineal tear involving the perineal muscles as well.	**Explanation:** Second-degree perineal tears extend through the vaginal mucosa and the perineal muscles but does not involve the anal sphincter. This type of tear requires repair but is not as extensive as third- or fourth-degree tears. While repairing the perineal tears, utmost importance must be given toward the maintenance of hemostasis and anatomical restoration without excessive suturing. The muscles are repaired with interrupted sutures using 2-0 Vicryl or polyglycolic acid. **Potential questions:** There can be questions related to the diagnosis and management of different degrees of vaginal tears and lacerations. There can also be questions related to the repair of cervical tear and technique of administration and repair of an episiotomy.

Question	Answer	Comment
Q15. A 29-year-old woman is examined after a vaginal delivery involving a difficult forceps application. She reports significant pain. The tear as visualized on examination is depicted in the image below. More than 50% of the external anal sphincter is involved. The internal anal sphincter, however, remains intact. What is the most likely diagnosis? 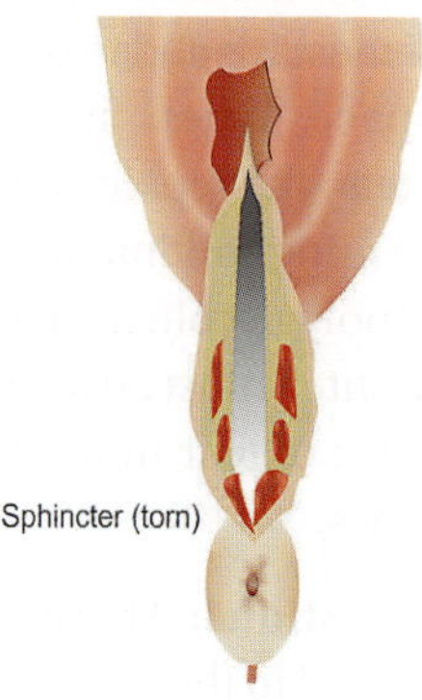 A. Second-degree perineal tear B. 3a third-degree perineal tear C. 3b third-degree perineal tear D. 3c third-degree perineal tear E. Fourth-degree perineal tear	**Ans: C (3b third-degree perineal tear)** The adjacent image depicts a third-degree perineal tear. As shown in **Figure 15**, the tear involves the anal sphincter complex. It can be further classified into three subtypes: 1. 3a: Less than 50% of external anal sphincter is torn. 2. 3b: More than 50% of external anal sphincter is torn. 3. 3c: Internal anal sphincter also gets involved. Since more than 50% of the external sphincter is involved and internal sphincter is intact, this is a 3b type of third-degree perineal tear. 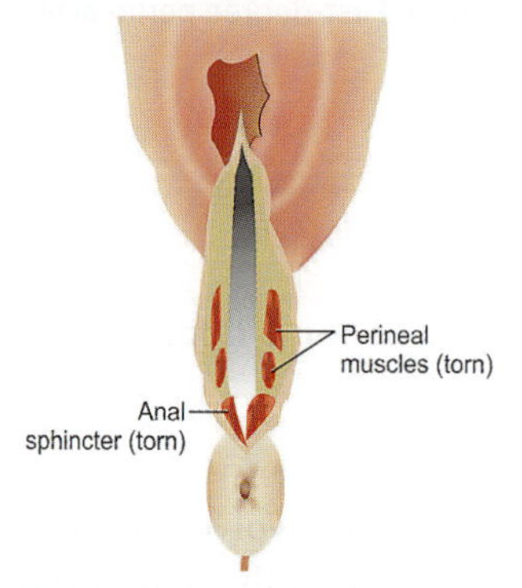 **Fig. 15:** Third-degree perineal tear.	**Explanation:** Third-degree perineal tear extends through the vaginal mucosa, perineal muscles, and involves the anal sphincter. At the time of repair, firstly the torn edges of the anal sphincter are isolated, approximated, and sutured together with three or four interrupted stitches using 3-0 Vicryl sutures. The internal anal sphincters need to be repaired in case of fourth-degree tears as well as some third-degree tears. The internal anal sphincter is identified as the thickening of circular smooth muscle layer at the distal 2–3 cm of the anal canal. It appears as the glistening white fibrous structure lying between the anal canal submucosa and the fibers of external anal sphincter. Following the repair of internal anal sphincters, the torn edges of external anal sphincters are identified and grasped with Allis clamp. The repair of these sphincters can be performed using either end-to-end repair or the overlap method. Rest of the repair is done as described before. **Potential questions:** There can be questions related to the diagnosis and management of different degrees of vaginal tears and lacerations.

Question	Answer	Comment
Q16. A 28-year-old woman experiences a traumatic vaginal delivery due to a large-sized baby. On inspection, a big tear is visualized. Its extent is depicted in the image below. What is the most appropriate diagnosis? 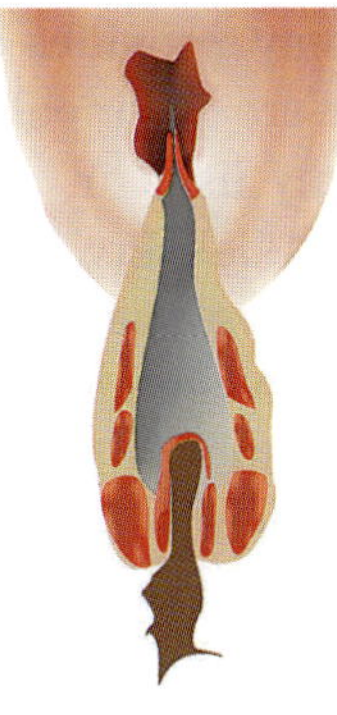 A. Second-degree perineal tear B. 3a third-degree perineal tear C. 3b third-degree perineal tear D. 3c third-degree perineal tear E. Fourth-degree perineal tear	**Ans: E (Fourth-degree perineal tear)** The adjacent image depicts a fourth-degree perineal tear. As shown in **Figure 16**, the tear also involves the rectal mucosa besides involving the anal sphincter. The key difference between third- and fourth-degree tears is the involvement of the rectal mucosa in the latter. 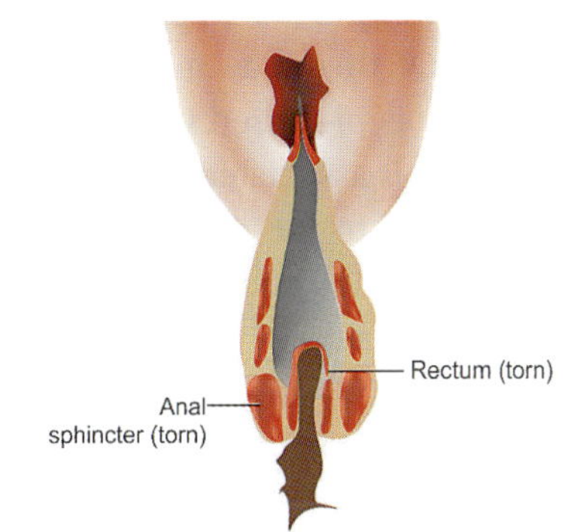 **Fig. 16:** Fourth-degree perineal tear.	**Explanation:** A fourth-degree perineal tear is the most severe type of obstetric injury, extending through the perineal muscles and anal sphincter into the rectal mucosa. It requires careful surgical repair to prevent complications like fecal incontinence. This tear requires careful surgical repair to prevent fecal incontinence in the following manner: ▪ *Anorectal mucosa and submucosa:* approximated with 3-0 or 4-0 chromic catgut/Vicryl (running suture). ▪ *Rectal muscularis:* Repaired with interrupted stitches. ▪ *Remaining perineal layers:* Repaired as usual. **Potential questions:** There can be questions related to the diagnosis and management of different degrees of vaginal tears and lacerations. There can also be questions related to the repair of cervical tears and technique of administration and repair of an episiotomy.

EPISIOTOMY

Question	Answer	Comment
Q17. A 28-year-old primigravida undergoes a vaginal delivery assisted by an episiotomy. The image below shows the incision site. What type of episiotomy is depicted in the image? 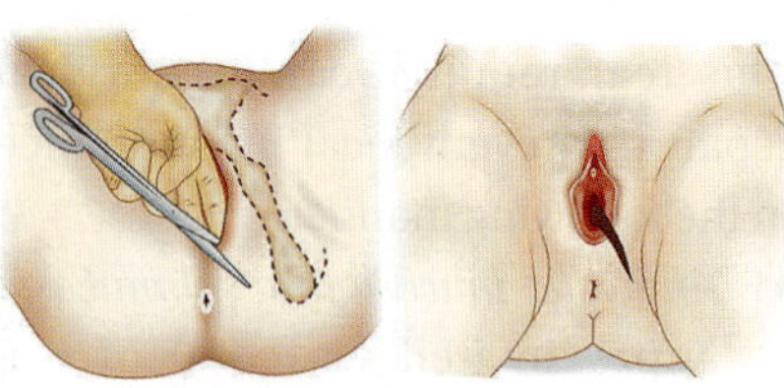 A. Midline episiotomy B. Mediolateral episiotomy C. Lateral episiotomy D. J-shaped episiotomy E. Anterior episiotomy	**Ans: B (Mediolateral episiotomy)** An episiotomy is a surgical incision given through the perineum to enlarge the vagina for assisting the process of childbirth. Episiotomy can be given in different directions as shown in **Figure 17**. Of the various incisions described, only mediolateral, median, or lateral episiotomies are commonly used in the clinical practice. Of these, a mediolateral episiotomy is preferred in India and Europe as it is associated with a lower risk of injury to the anal sphincters and rectum in comparison to a median approach. 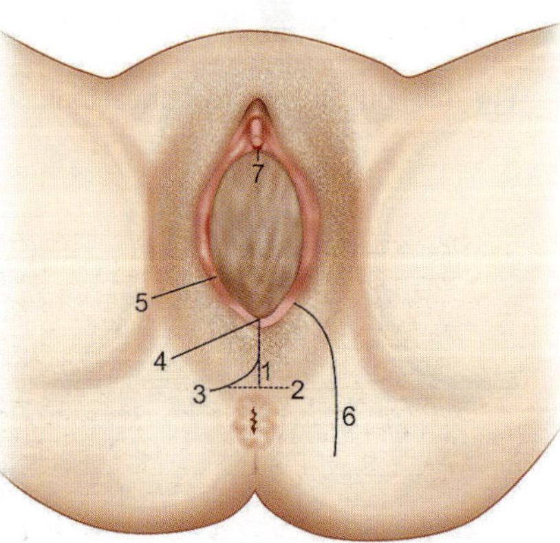 **Fig. 17:** Direction of giving different types of episiotomies: (1) Median episiotomy, (2) modified median episiotomy, (3) "J-shaped" episiotomy, (4) mediolateral episiotomy, (5) lateral episiotomy, (6) radical lateral (Schuchardt incision), (7) anterior episiotomy.	**Explanation:** A mediolateral episiotomy is characterized by an incision that starts at the midline of the lower edge of vaginal opening and extends laterally at a 45° angle, either toward right or toward left. Episiotomy provides protection against severe perineal tears and is commonly used in cases where instrumental delivery is anticipated or in cases where it becomes apparent that natural vaginal delivery may cause straining of the pelvic floor muscles, resulting in second-or third-degree tears. The repair of an episiotomy or vaginal lacerations (tears) is performed in three layers: The first layer comprising the vaginal mucosa and submucosal tissues (repaired using continuous sutures with 2-0 or 3-0 Vicryl), the second layer comprising the perineal muscles (repaired with interrupted sutures of 2-0 or 3-0 Vicryl), and the third layer comprising the skin and subcutaneous tissues (closed using interrupted stitches with silk or subcuticular stiches). **Potential questions:** There can be questions related to the indications, technique of administration, and repair of an episiotomy incision.

PLACENTA AND ITS ABNORMALITIES

Question	Answer	Comment
Q18. A 32-year-old woman presents on postpartum day 10 with heavy vaginal bleeding. She had a history of two prior cesarean deliveries. Since the ultrasound examination was nonconclusive, an MRI was performed, as shown below. Based on this MRI image, what is the most likely diagnosis? 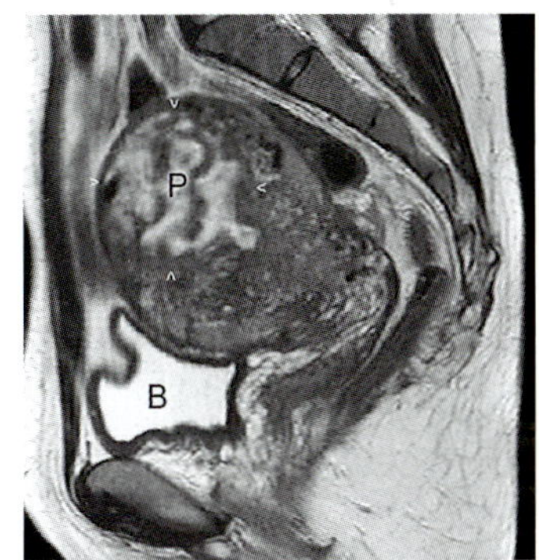 (B: bladder; P: placenta) A. Placenta previa B. Placenta accreta C. Placenta percreta D. Placenta increta E. Retained products of conception	**Ans: D (Placenta increta)** The adjacent image shows axial T2-weighted magnetic resonance image demonstrating a retained placental mass as well as focal thinning of the fundus. Since the placental mass was invading into the myometrium but not extending beyond the uterine wall, diagnosis of placenta increta was made. **Figure 18** shows histopathological appearance of placenta increta in the same patient. Placental villi can be observed on the right side. The myometrial tissue can be observed on the left side, and it can be noticed that it is being invaded by the placental tissue. The placental invasion is, however, confined only to the inner layers of myometrium and not the whole thickness of myometrium. 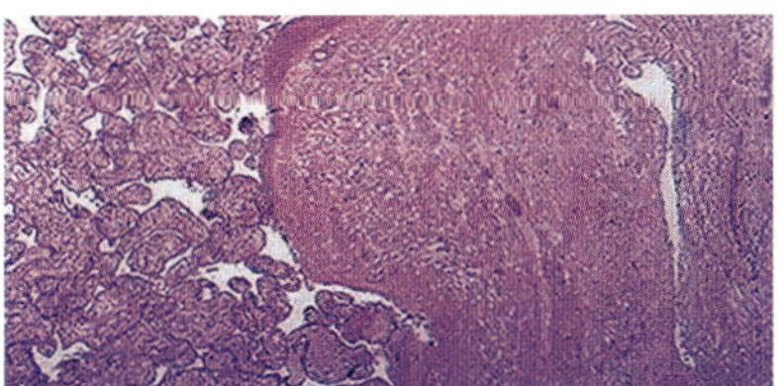 **Fig. 18:** Histological specimen showing placenta increta.	**Explanation:** Placenta increta is a condition where the placental villi invade into the myometrium but do not penetrate through it. This condition is part of the placenta accreta spectrum, which includes placenta accreta (villi attach to the myometrium), placenta increta (villi invade into the myometrium), and placenta percreta (villi penetrate through the myometrium into the serosa or beyond). The risk factors for placenta increta include previous cesarean sections, uterine surgeries, and placenta previa. Diagnosis is typically made via an ultrasound. Being a costly investigation, MRI is usually used as a supplementary diagnostic procedure in cases with an increased risk of abnormal placentation and where the placenta cannot adequately be assessed by sonography. **Potential questions:** There can be questions related to the definition, diagnosis, management, and complications of various conditions associated with placenta accreta spectrum.

Question	Answer	Comment
Q19. A 35-year-old woman with a history of three previous cesarean sections presents for a routine ultrasound at 28 weeks of gestation. Below is the ultrasound image showing the abnormal placental attachment. 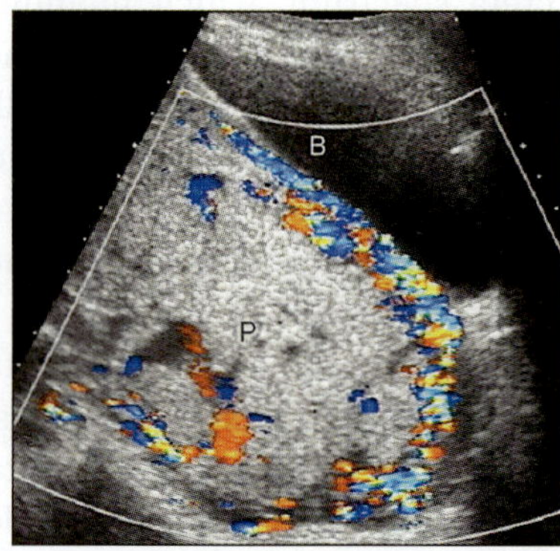 (B: bladder; P: placenta) What is the most likely diagnosis based on the ultrasound findings? A. Placenta accreta B. Placenta increta C. Placenta percreta D. Placenta previa E. Placental abruption	**Ans: C (Placenta percreta)** The adjacent image depicts color Doppler scanning at 27 weeks' gestation demonstrating prominent placental vessels extending across the myometrium into the bladder wall. This is likely to indicate placenta percreta. Doppler sonography has been found to be quite sensitive for the detection of morbidly adherent placenta. Ultrasonography, especially with color flow Doppler, serves as a useful investigation in establishing a prenatal diagnosis of morbidly adherent placenta because Doppler sonography can help in detection of abnormal vascularization of the myometrium. In case findings on ultrasound appear inconclusive, MRI may be used as an adjunct to sonography in cases with strong clinical suspicion of morbidly adherent placenta. **Figure 19** shows MRI imaging in the same patient showing placenta percreta. 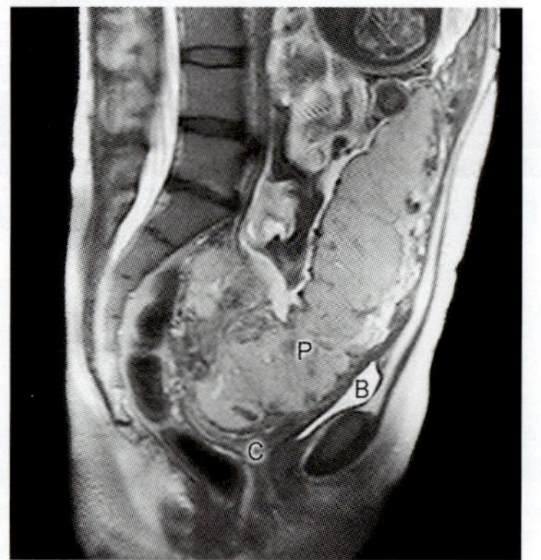 **Fig. 19:** Magnetic resonance imaging of the patient with placenta percreta in the same patient (B: bladder; C: cervix; P: placenta)	**Explanation:** Placenta percreta is the most severe form of the placenta accreta spectrum, where the placental villi penetrate through the entire myometrium and may also invade adjacent organs such as the bladder. This condition is associated with significant maternal morbidity and mortality due to the risk of massive hemorrhage. Risk factors include previous cesarean sections, uterine surgeries, and placenta previa. Diagnosis is typically made via ultrasound or MRI, which shows placental tissue extending beyond the uterine wall. The features on Doppler ultrasound which are highly predictive of myometrial invasion by the placenta are as follows: ▪ Distance of <1 mm between the interface of urinary bladder and uterine serosa ▪ Presence of large intraplacental lakes within the myometrium Management often involves planned delivery by cesarean section with preparations for potential massive hemorrhage and hysterectomy. **Potential questions:** There can be questions related to the definition, diagnosis, management, and complications of various conditions associated with placenta accreta spectrum.

UMBILICAL CORD

Question	Answer	Comment
Q20. Identify the structure pointed by the arrow in the given figure. 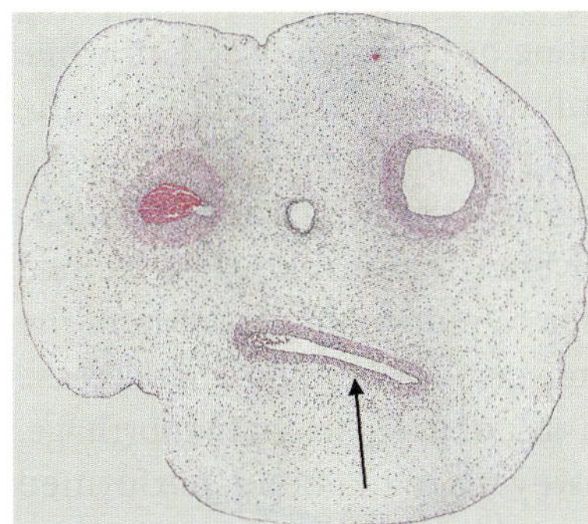 A. Allantoic duct B. Umbilical artery C. Umbilical vein D. Wharton's jelly E. Amniotic epithelium	**Ans: C (Umbilical vein)** The adjacent figure represents the cut section of the umbilical cord following parturition. The arrow shown in the figure represents the umbilical vein. **Figure 20** is a labeled image showing the actual location of the various vessels (umbilical arteries and vein) within the umbilical cord. 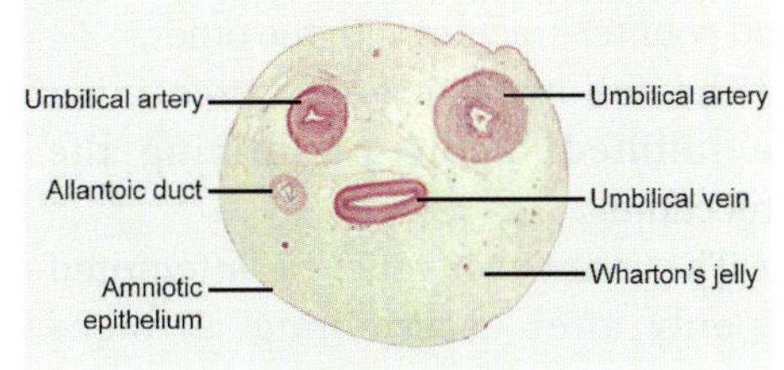 **Fig. 20:** Cut section of the umbilical cord.	**Explanation:** A normal umbilical cord has two umbilical arteries and one vein. Wharton's jelly is seen to be surrounding the umbilical vessels. Wharton's jelly, composed of mucopolysaccharides, fibroblasts, and macrophages, is derived from extraembryonic mesoderm and provides insulation to the umbilical vessels. There also may be presence of allantois. Allantois, on the other hand, is a tubular extension from the endoderm of yolk sac and plays an important role in the formation of umbilical cord and placenta in humans. **Potential questions:** Other structures in the umbilical cord could serve as potential questions.

POSTPARTUM HEMORRHAGE

Question	Answer	Comment
Q21. A 29-year-old woman undergoes a vaginal delivery. The image below shows a specific maneuver being performed during the third stage of labor. What is the primary purpose of controlled cord traction (CCT) in the management of the third stage of labor? 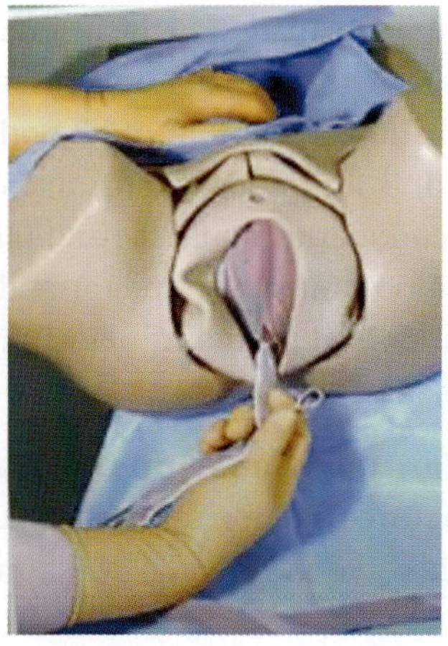 A. To reduce the risk of uterine inversion B. To expedite the delivery of the placenta C. To prevent postpartum hemorrhage D. To minimize the risk of cord rupture E. To ensure complete placental expulsion	**Ans: B (To expedite the delivery of the placenta)** The adjacent image demonstrates the maneuver, CCT or Brandt–Andrew's maneuver. The primary purpose of CCT is to aid in the delivery of the placenta while minimizing the risk of postpartum hemorrhage. The basic principle of this maneuver is application of traction with one hand and counter-traction with the other. The following prerequisites must be fulfilled before performing the procedure: ▪ The maneuver must be attempted only after ascertaining all signs of placental separation such as appearance of a suprapubic bulge due to hardening and contracting of uterus, sudden gush of blood, a rise in the height of the uterus (as observed over the abdomen) due to the passage of placenta to the lower uterine segment, and irreversible cord lengthening. ▪ Bladder must be empty before performing this procedure. Once one of the signs of placental separation occurs, the clinician must apply traction with their right hand and counter-traction with their left hand as shown in **Figure 21**. 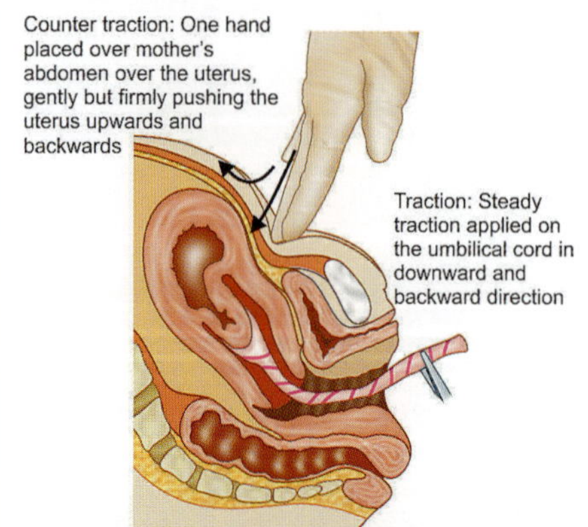 **Fig. 21:** Technique of controlled cord traction.	**Explanation:** Controlled cord traction is a technique used during the third stage of labor to facilitate the delivery of the placenta. By gently pulling on the umbilical cord while applying counterpressure to the uterus, the placenta is encouraged to separate from the uterine wall and be delivered more quickly. This method helps to reduce the duration of the third stage of labor and can decrease the risk of postpartum hemorrhage. However, it must be performed correctly to avoid complications such as uterine inversion or cord rupture. The following precautions must be observed: ▪ While applying CCT, the cord should never be pulled without applying counter-traction above the pubic bone. ▪ It should be performed with care to avoid excessive force, which can lead to uterine inversion or cord avulsion. ▪ As the placenta delivers, it should be held in two hands and gently turned, until the membranes are twisted and stripped off intact from the uterine wall. ▪ If the membranes tear, gentle examination of the upper vagina and cervix must be carried out to look for torn bits of membrane. These, if present, can be removed with the help of a sponge forceps. ▪ The entire placenta and membranes must be examined carefully to look for any missing lobe/membrane bit. **Potential questions:** There can be questions related to the principle, prerequisites, technique, and complications of this maneuver.

Question	Answer	Comment
Q22. A 33-year-old woman, gravida 3, para 2, experiences significant postpartum hemorrhage following vaginal delivery. The uterus is atonic. The obstetrician quickly initiates a manual technique to contract the uterus. This technique is depicted in the schematic diagram shown below. Which of the following steps is NOT part of the correct technique for bimanual uterine compression? 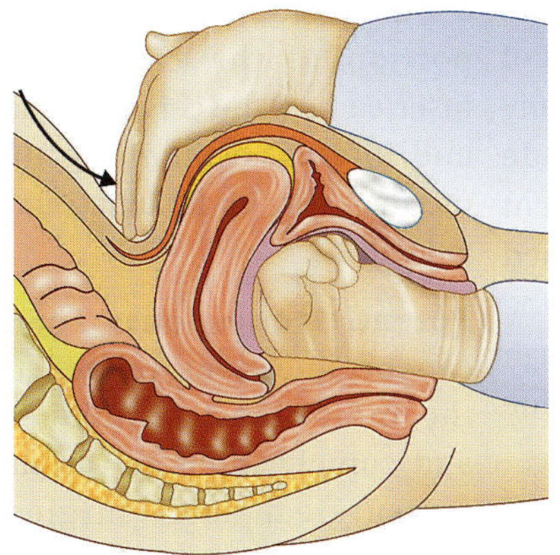 A. Insert one hand into the vagina and place it on the anterior fornix B. Place the other hand on the abdomen, over the uterine fundus C. Apply firm pressure with both hands to compress the uterus between them D. Massage the uterine fundus in a circular motion E. Maintain compression until bleeding is controlled or help arrives	**Ans: D (Massage the uterine fundus in a circular motion)** The maneuver demonstrated by the adjacent image is bimanual uterine compression. If the clinician finds the uterus to be soft/atonic upon bimanual examination, a bimanual uterine massage must be performed to contract the myometrial muscles. The maneuver involves the massage of the posterior aspect of the uterus with the abdominal hand and that of the anterior aspect of the uterus with the vaginal hand **(Fig. 22)**. 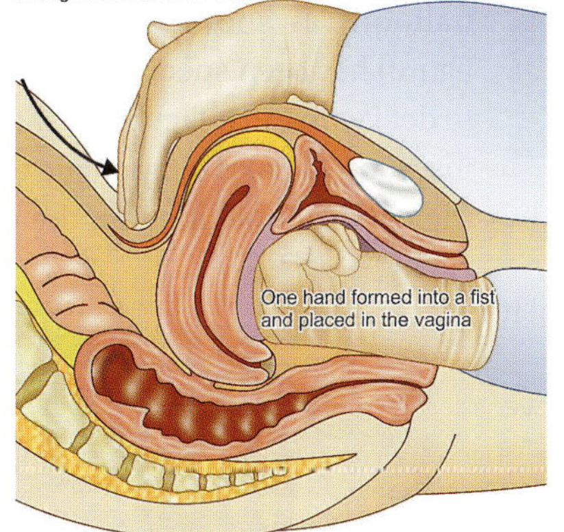 **Fig. 22:** Bimanual uterine compression.	**Explanation:** The procedure of bimanual uterine compression comprises the following steps: One of the clinician's hands is formed into a fist and placed inside the vagina, with the back of the hand directed posteriorly and knuckles in the anterior fornix so as to push against the body of the uterus. The other hand compresses the fundus from above through the abdominal wall. This maneuver involves compressing the uterus between the two hands to reduce cavity size and tamponade the bleeding vessels. It does not involve massaging the uterine fundus in circular motion. The uterus must be compressed every 15 minutes during the first 2 hours. If this maneuver controls the bleeding, the clinician must maintain this compression for at least 30 minutes. **Potential questions:** There can be questions related to the principle, prerequisites, technique, and complications of this maneuver.

Question	Answer	Comment
Q23. A 28-year-old woman presents with severe postpartum hemorrhage unresponsive to uterotonics. The attending physician decides to use a noninvasive method to help control the hemorrhage, using a device shown below. Which of the following steps is NOT part of the correct procedure for inserting the device as demonstrated in the image below? 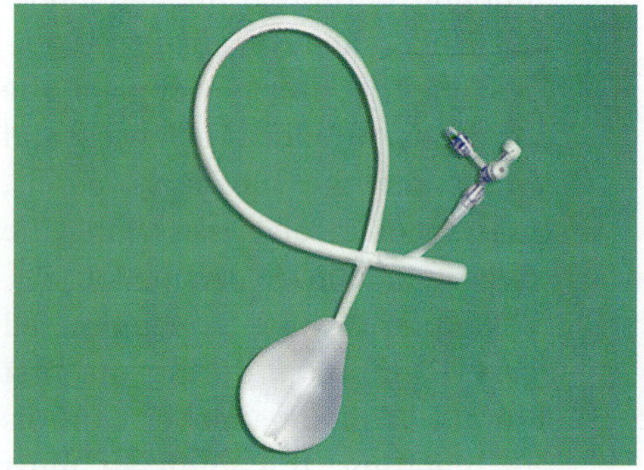 A. Insert the deflated balloon into the uterine cavity B. Fill the balloon with sterile saline until it fits snugly against the uterine walls C. Inflate the balloon with air to achieve tamponade D. Monitor for continued bleeding and adjust the balloon volume as needed E. Leave the balloon in place for 12–24 hours before gradual deflation and removal	**Ans: C (Inflate the balloon with air to achieve tamponade)** The device shown in the adjacent image is an SOS Bakri tamponade balloon. Balloon tamponade is a nonsurgical method to control PPH using a large bulb Foley's catheter, Sengstaken–Blakemore tube, or an SOS Bakri tamponade balloon. A Foley's catheter with a balloon of 30 mL (which may be inflated up to 100 mL) is quite effective in controlling postpartum bleeding. However, the shape of the balloon may not correspond to that of elongated uterine cavity. The recently available SOS Bakri tamponade balloon (as shown in the adjacent figure) has been specifically designed to deal with PPH. **Figure 23** shows the insertion of Bakri tamponade through the cervical opening into the uterine cavity. 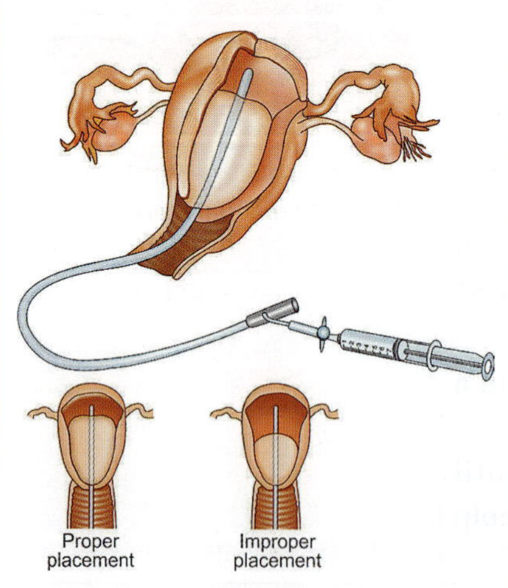 **Fig. 23:** Procedure of Bakri tamponade balloon.	**Explanation:** The Bakri tamponade balloon is specifically designed to be filled with sterile saline, not air. The balloon is inserted into the uterine cavity in a deflated state and then filled with sterile saline until it fits snugly against the uterine walls, providing pressure to control bleeding. The Bakri balloon catheter helps in temporary control of PPH, potentially avoiding a hysterectomy. The balloon portion of the catheter is inserted past the cervical canal and internal ostium into the uterine cavity under ultrasound guidance. **Potential questions:** There can be questions related to the indications, techniques, and complications of various nonsurgical and surgical methods for the control of PPH.

Question	Answer	Comment
Q24. A 30-year-old woman presents with severe postpartum hemorrhage (PPH) unresponsive to uterotonics. The attending physician decides to apply brace sutures as shown in the image below. Which of the following steps is NOT part of the correct technique for applying B-Lynch sutures? 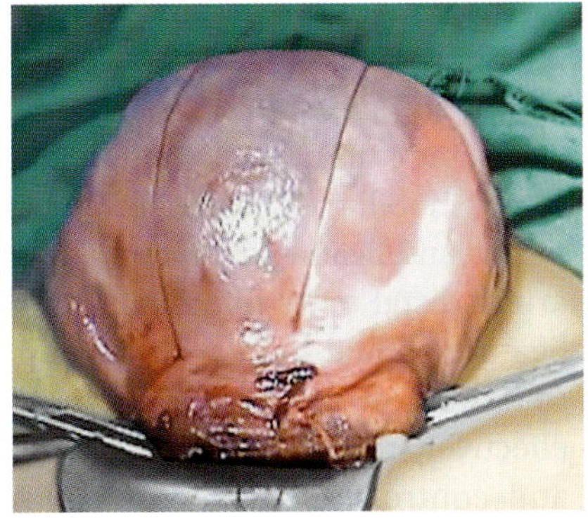 A. Exteriorize the uterus and identify the bleeding site B. Insert a large, curved needle with absorbable suture material through the lower uterine segment C. Pass the suture over the uterine fundus and back through the lower uterine segment D. Tie the suture tightly to compress the uterus and control bleeding E. Leave the suture ends long and untied for future adjustments	**Ans: E (Leave the suture ends long and untied for future adjustments)** The adjacent image shows a B-lynch brace suture which has been applied to the uterus. Compression sutures can be considered as the best form of surgical approach for controlling atonic PPH as they help in preserving the anatomical integrity of the uterus. The procedure for the application of B-Lynch sutures is demonstrated in **Figures 24A to C.** 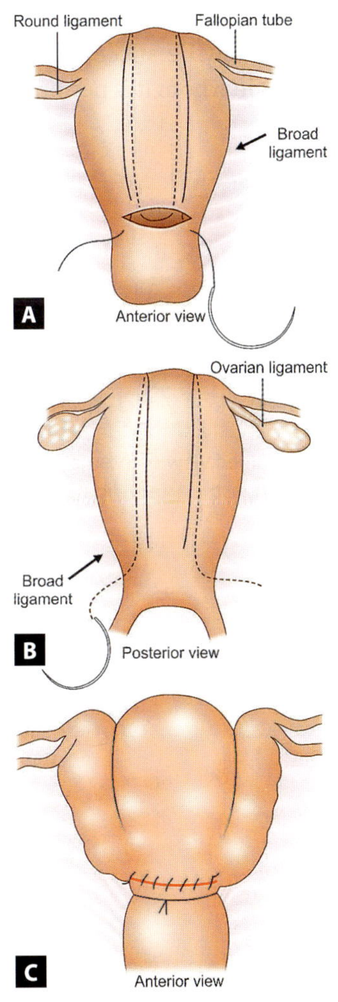 **Figs. 24A to C:** Diagrammatic representation of B-Lynch suture.	**Explanation:** The B-Lynch suture technique involves exteriorizing the uterus and identifying the bleeding site. A large, curved needle with absorbable suture material is inserted through the lower uterine segment, passed over the uterine fundus, and brought back through the lower uterine segment. The suture is then tied tightly to compress the uterus and control bleeding. After application of suture, when the sutures are in place, the assistant bimanually compresses the uterus while the chromic catgut sutures are pulled tightly by the surgeon. Thus, these sutures act as uterine bracing suture which when tightened and tied help in compressing the anterior and posterior uterine walls together. This technique is safe and effective and helps in retaining future fertility. Before using the B-Lynch suture, a bimanual compression must be performed to assess the effectiveness of these sutures. If the bleeding is controlled temporarily in this fashion, the application of B Lynch sutures is likely to be effective. **Potential questions:** There can be questions related to the indications, techniques, and complications of various nonsurgical and surgical methods for the control of PPH.

Question	Answer	Comment
Q25. A 35-year-old woman presents with severe PPH unresponsive to uterotonics and balloon tamponade. The attending physician decides to perform a ligation procedure as depicted in the image below. Which of the following steps is NOT part of the correct procedure? 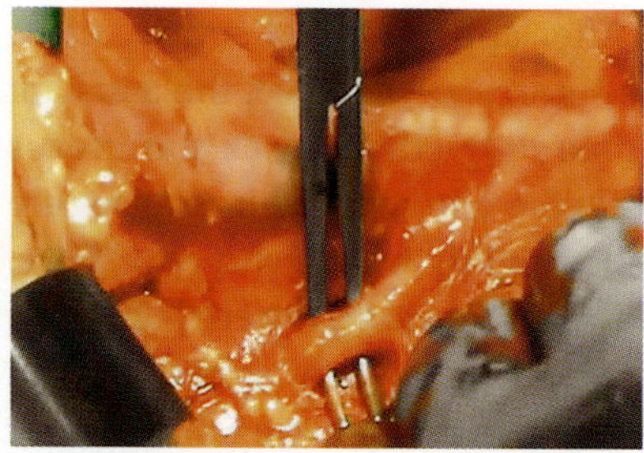 A. Identify the internal iliac artery by tracing it from the common iliac artery B. Mobilize the ureter to avoid injury during the procedure C. Ligate the internal iliac artery distal to its bifurcation D. Ensure that the ligature is placed proximal to the origin of the uterine artery E. Confirm hemostasis by checking for any residual bleeding	**Ans: D (Ensure that the ligature is placed proximal to the origin of the uterine artery)** The adjacent image shows the procedure of internal iliac artery ligation by placing Mixter's forceps around the internal iliac vessels. Bilateral ligation of internal iliac vessels was first performed by Kelly in 1894. Appreciable reduction in the amount of bleeding can be achieved by the ligation of internal iliac vessels **(Fig. 25)**. The procedure, however, is technically difficult and may be successful only in 50% of cases in whom it is performed. 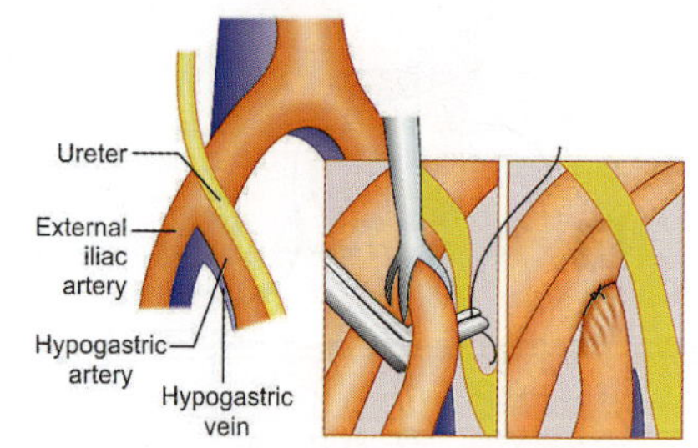 **Fig. 25:** Magnified view of internal iliac artery (hypogastric artery) ligation.	**Explanation:** Internal iliac artery ligation helps in accomplishing hemostasis via the process of simple clot formation and is a highly effective method, which is indicated in cases of PPH due to uterine atony, ruptured uterus, and placenta accreta. It also helps in preserving fertility of women desiring pregnancy in future. The correct technique for internal iliac artery ligation involves identifying the internal iliac artery by tracing it from the common iliac artery, mobilizing the ureter to avoid injury, and ligating the internal iliac artery distal to its bifurcation. The ligature should be placed distal to the origin of the uterine artery to effectively reduce pelvic blood flow and control hemorrhage. Placing the ligature proximal to the uterine artery would not achieve the desired hemostatic effect. **Potential questions:** There can be questions related to the indications, techniques, and complications of various nonsurgical and surgical methods for the control of PPH.

Question	Answer	Comment
Q26. A 34-year-old woman presents with severe PPH unresponsive to uterotonics and balloon tamponade. The attending physician decides to perform ligation of a major blood vessel as indicated by arrows in the below image. Which of the following steps is NOT part of the correct procedure for uterine artery ligation? 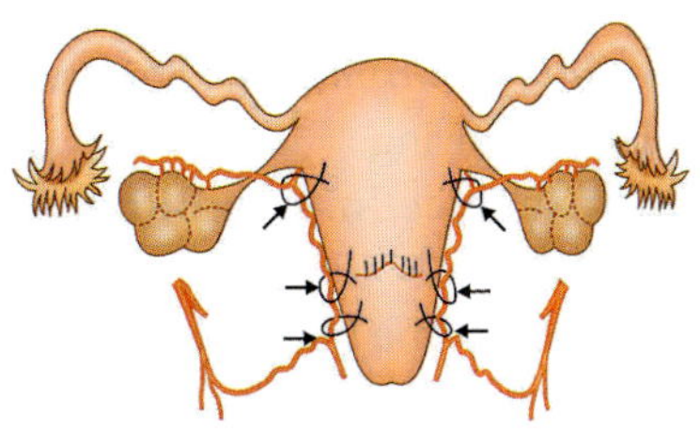 A. Trace the uterine artery from the internal iliac artery B. Mobilize the ureter to prevent injury C. Ligate the uterine artery at the lower uterine segment D. Place the ligature distal to the origin of ovarian artery E. Check for hemostasis and residual bleeding	**Ans: D (Place the ligature distal to the origin of ovarian artery)** The adjacent image depicts uterine artery ligation. The most common site of ligation of uterine artery is 2 cm below the level of transverse lower uterine incision site **(Fig. 26)**. The needle is then placed through an avascular portion of the broad ligament and tied anteriorly. Following the ligation of uterine artery, ligation of the cervical branch must also be performed. 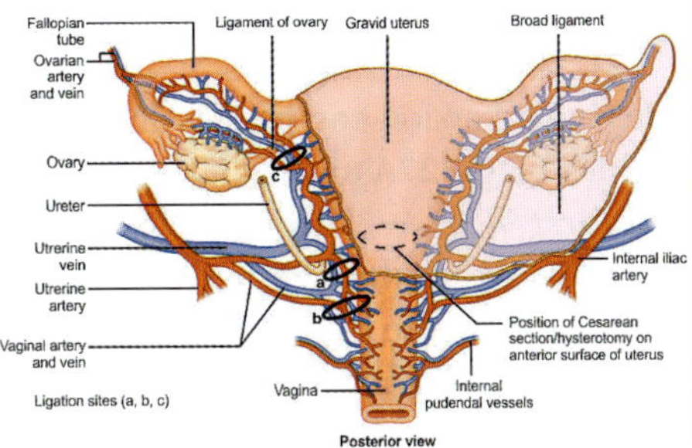 **Fig. 26:** Placement of ligatures in the process of stepwise devascularization. (a) Uterine vessel; (b) Low uterine vessel; (c) Utero-ovarian vessel.	**Explanation:** Since approximately 90% of the blood supply to the uterus is via the uterine artery, ligation of this vessel through the uterine wall at the level of uterine isthmus above the bladder flap is likely to control the amount of bleeding. If, despite bilateral ligation of uterine vessels, bleeding remains uncontrollable, ligation of utero-ovarian anastomosis is also done just below the ovarian ligament and not distal to the origin of ovarian artery. However, this method may not prove useful to control bleeding in case of placenta previa or ruptured uterus. Bilateral ligation of the uterine vessels has not been observed to interfere with future reproduction. **Potential questions:** There can be questions related to the indications, techniques, and complications of various nonsurgical and surgical methods for the control of PPH.

<table>
<tr><th>Question</th><th>Answer</th><th>Comment</th></tr>
<tr>
<td>

Q27. Shortly after spontaneous vaginal delivery, a 30-year-old woman, gravida 4, experiences sudden hemorrhage and shock. The obstetrician identifies a rare complication and uses a schematic diagram as shown below to explain the diagnosis to the patient while counseling her. What is the likely diagnosis in this case?

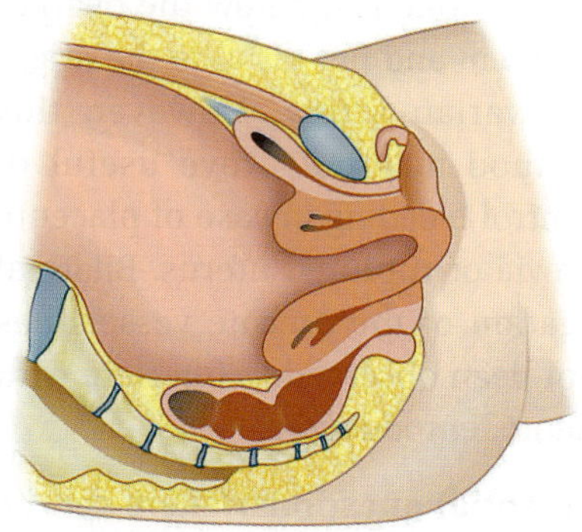

A. Cervical carcinoma
B. Uterocervical prolapse
C. Uterine inversion
D. Fibroid polyp
E. Endometrial carcinoma

</td>
<td>

Ans: C (Uterine inversion)

The adjacent image typically shows fundus of the uterus protruding through the cervix and lying outside the vagina. This is characteristic of uterine inversion, a condition in which the uterus is turned inside out either partially or completely. The uterine endometrium with or without attached placenta may be visible. Risk factors include excessive traction on the umbilical cord, fundal pressure before placental detachment, and conditions like placenta accreta or a relaxed uterus.

Uterine inversion can be classified as follows **(Figs. 27A to C)**:

- *First degree:* Dimpling of the uterine fundus, which remains well above the level of internal os
- *Second degree:* Uterine fundus passes through the cervix, but lies inside the vagina
- *Third degree (complete):* The uterus protrudes completely out of the vaginal introitus. The uterine endometrium with or without the attached placenta may be visible.

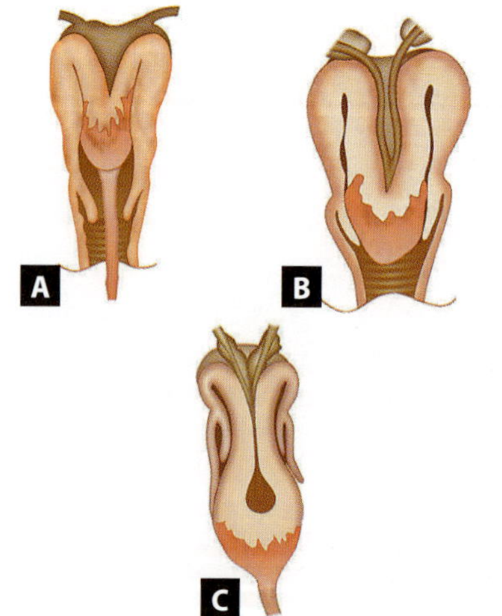

Figs. 27A to C: Degrees of uterine inversion: (A) First degree, (B) Second degree, (C) Third degree.

</td>
<td>

Explanation: Uterine inversion is a rare but life-threatening obstetric emergency that can lead to severe hemorrhage and shock if not promptly recognized and treated.

Diagnosis of uterine inversion is based on the following:

Abdominal examination: There is an absence of uterine fundus or presence of an obvious defect of the fundus upon abdominal palpation.

Bimanual examination: This may reveal the following:

- Profuse bleeding through the cervical os
- Palpation of the inverted fundus at the cervical os or vaginal introitus
- In cases of incomplete inversion, the fundal wall may be palpated in the lower uterine segment and cervix

Ultrasound: On transverse scans, a hyperechoic mass in the vagina with a central hypoechoic H-shaped cavity may be visualized. A depressed longitudinal groove, extending from the uterine fundus to the center of the inverted part, may be observed on the longitudinal scans.

Magnetic resonance imaging: Appearance of the uterus is similar to that found on sonographic imaging.

Management: The mainstay of treatment in these cases is urgent manual replacement of the uterus preferably under general anesthesia.

Potential questions: There can be questions related to risk factors, etiopathogenesis, clinical presentation (including the grading system), diagnosis, management, and complications in case of uterine inversion.

</td>
</tr>
</table>

NEWBORN INFANT AND ITS CARE

<table>
<tr><th>Question</th><th>Answer</th><th>Comment</th></tr>
<tr><td>

Q28. The image below shows a view obtained through a laryngoscope. What is the next most appropriate step in airway management?

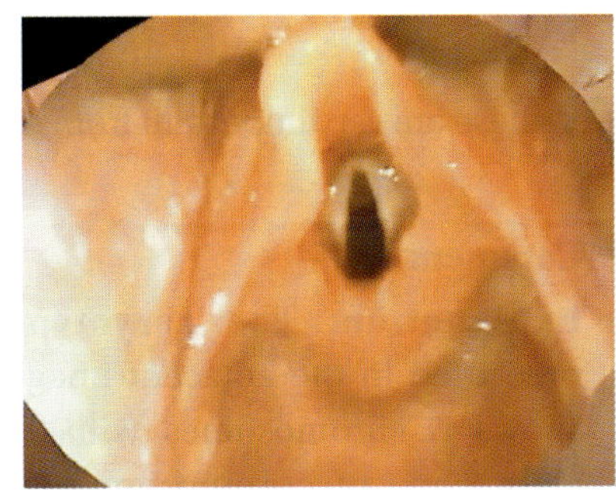

A. Perform tracheostomy
B. Insert nasogastric tube
C. Perform endotracheal intubation
D. Perform cricothyroidotomy
E. Laryngeal mask airway insertion

</td><td>

Ans: C (Perform endotracheal intubation)

The adjacent image illustrates the view observed through a laryngoscope, showing the vocal cords. The visualization of the vocal cords is essential to proceed with the procedure of endotracheal intubation. The endotracheal tube (ETT) is passed between the vocal cords as shown in **Figure 28**. This procedure is commonly used in emergency situations, during surgery, or in critical care settings to maintain airway patency and support breathing. This procedure is performed to ensure that the airway remains open and to facilitate ventilation of the lungs.

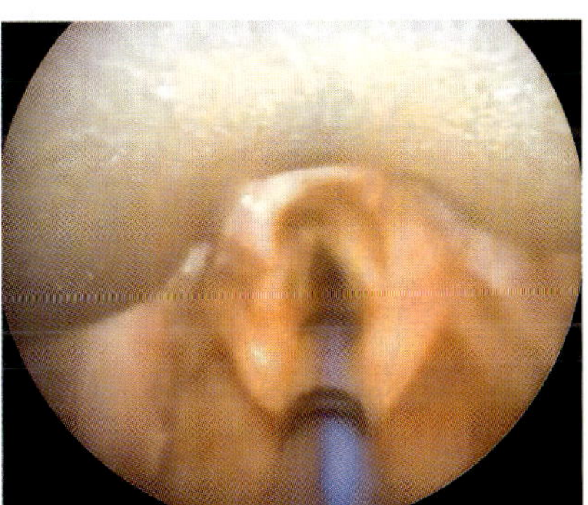

Fig. 28: Insertion of endotracheal tube through vocal cords.

</td><td>

Explanation: Endotracheal intubation involves the insertion of a tube through the mouth into the vocal cords and then into the trachea. For a newborn, correct ETT placement is crucial to prevent complications. On an X-ray, the tip of the ETT should be positioned 1–2 cm above the carina.

Some indications for endotracheal intubation in newborns are as follows:

- Ineffective ventilation with bag-mask
- Prolonged positive pressure ventilation
- Administration of medications (e.g. endotracheal drugs such as epinephrine, surfactant, etc.)
- Special clinical situations (e.g. congenital diaphragmatic hernia, anticipated difficult airway, etc.)
- Elective/planned indications (e.g. surfactant therapy in preterm infants with respiratory distress syndrome).

Potential questions: There can be questions related to the indication and technique of endotracheal intubation as well as neonatal resuscitation.

</td></tr>
</table>

CHAPTER

6 Genetics

Questions on genetics are usually not a part of the NMC course curriculum. However, these are very important from the perspective of MRCOG course curriculum. Therefore, these are covered here.

Question	Answer	Comment
Q1. A newborn girl is found to have multiple midline malformations. Her physician suspects a chromosomal disorder and orders a karyotype in the below figure. Which of the following is the most likely diagnosis? 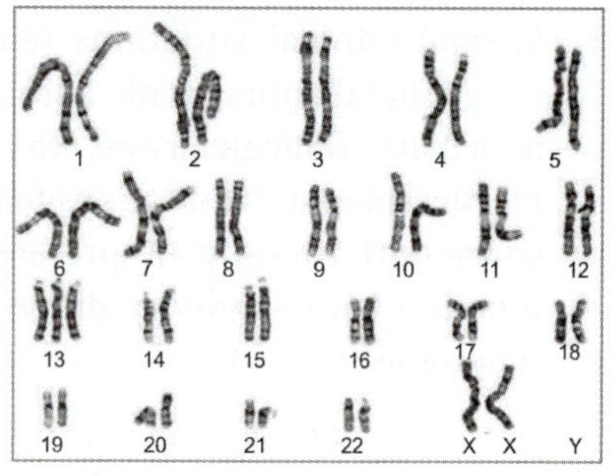 A. Cri-du-chat syndrome B. Down syndrome C. Turner syndrome D. Edwards syndrome E. Patau syndrome	**Ans: E (Patau syndrome)** There are three "chromosome 13" in the karyotype analysis shown in the adjacent figure. This is suggestive of Patau syndrome. The red arrow in **Figure 1** points out to the abnormality. 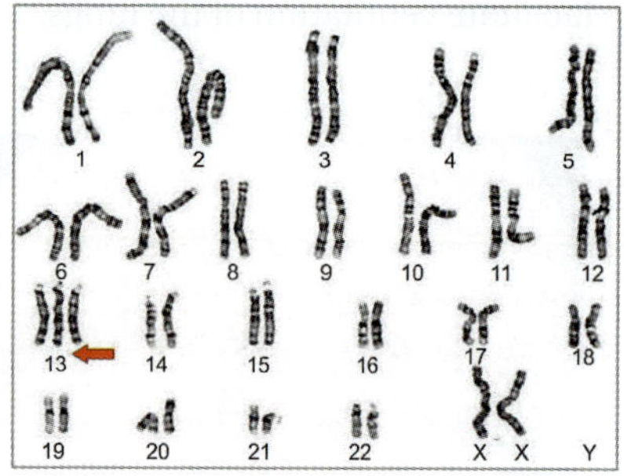 **Fig. 1:** Karyotype analysis in case of Patau syndrome.	**Explanation:** The karyotype presented in the adjacent image shows 47 chromosomes, with an extra copy of chromosome 13, indicating trisomy 13, also known as Patau syndrome. In a normal female karyotype, there would be 46 chromosomes, but in this case, the additional chromosome 13 causes a total of 47. This chromosomal abnormality is responsible for the severe congenital anomalies observed in affected infants, including craniofacial abnormalities (such as cleft lip/palate), cardiac defects (such as ventricular septal defects), polydactyly (extra fingers or toes), central nervous system anomalies, including holoprosencephaly, etc. **Potential questions:** There can be questions related to other trisomies such as trisomy 21 (Down syndrome) or trisomy 18 (Edwards syndrome).

Question	Answer	Comment
Q2. A 30-year-old male patient, born via vaginal birth after cesarean section, presents with infertility concerns. A karyotype analysis is performed, and the result is shown in the image below. Which of the following is the most likely diagnosis based on the karyotype? 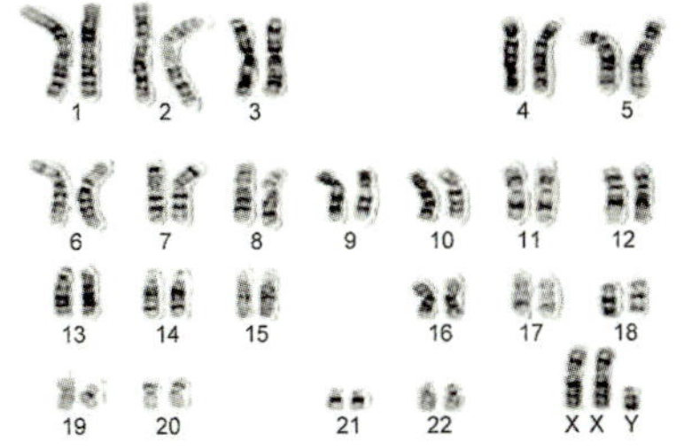 A. 46, XY normal male B. 45, XO Turner syndrome C. 47, XXY Klinefelter syndrome D. 47, XYY Sawyer syndrome E. Cri-du-chat syndrome	**Ans: C (47, XXY Klinefelter syndrome)** The karyotype in the adjacent figure shows two X chromosomes and one Y chromosome (47, XXY). Therefore, the figure is suggestive of Klinefelter syndrome. The red arrow in **Figure 2** points out to this abnormality. 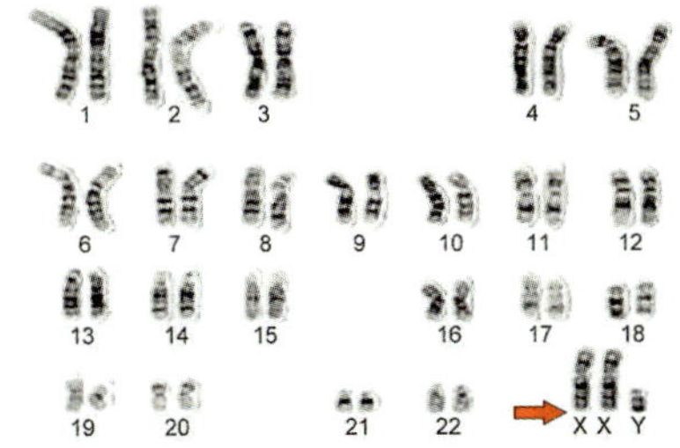 **Fig. 2:** Karyotype analysis in case of Klinefelter syndrome.	**Explanation:** The karyotype shown displays an extra X chromosome confirming the diagnosis of Klinefelter syndrome. Common clinical features include tall stature, gynecomastia, small testes, etc., which aligns with the patient's presentation of infertility. The karyotype shown displays an extra X chromosome confirming this diagnosis. **Potential questions:** There can be questions related to other genetic syndromes which may be associated with reduced fertility, e.g., Turner syndrome, triple X syndrome, androgen insensitivity syndrome, etc.
Q3. A mother of a 15-year-old girl with primary amenorrhea has come to you for diagnosis and treatment. On examination, you notice that the girl has short stature and wide shield-like chest and undeveloped nipples. You order a karyotype analysis which reveals the findings, shown in the image below. What does the karyotype analysis indicate? 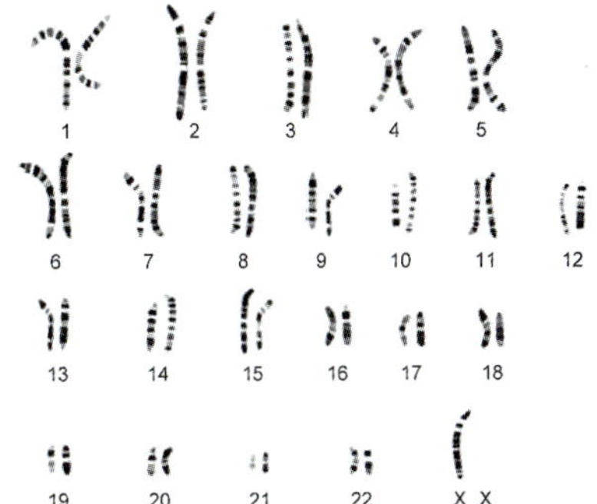 A. Noonan syndrome B. Marfan syndrome C. Turner syndrome D. Down syndrome E. Klinefelter syndrome	**Ans: C (Turner syndrome)** The adjacent karyotype image shows only one X chromosome. This is suggestive of Turner syndrome. The clinical picture is also suggestive of this syndrome. The red arrow in **Figure 3** points out to this abnormality. 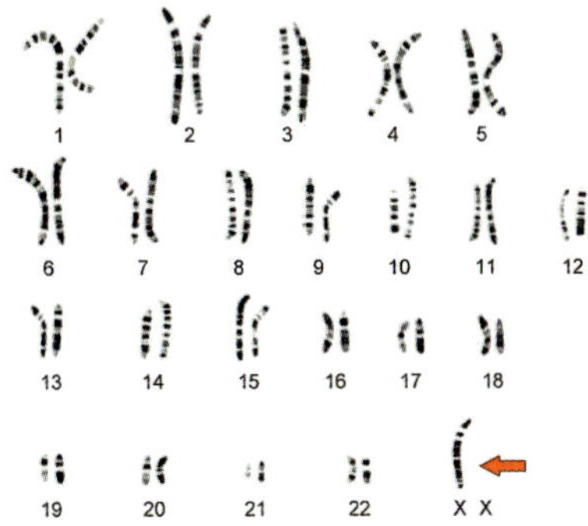 **Fig. 3:** Karyotype analysis in case of Turner syndrome.	**Explanation:** Turner syndrome is caused by the complete or partial absence of one X chromosome, resulting in a 45, XO karyotype. This condition primarily affects females and is associated with distinct physical characteristics such as short stature, webbed neck, and congenital lymphedema (swelling of the hands and feet). Turner syndrome significantly impacts fertility due to the high likelihood of premature ovarian insufficiency or ovarian failure. As a result, most women with Turner syndrome experience primary amenorrhea and infertility. **Potential questions:** There can be questions related to other genetic syndromes which may be associated with reduced fertility, e.g., Klinefelter syndrome, triple X syndrome, androgen insensitivity syndrome, etc.

<table>
<tr><th>Question</th><th>Answer</th><th>Comment</th></tr>
<tr>
<td>Q4. What does the below pedigree chart indicate?
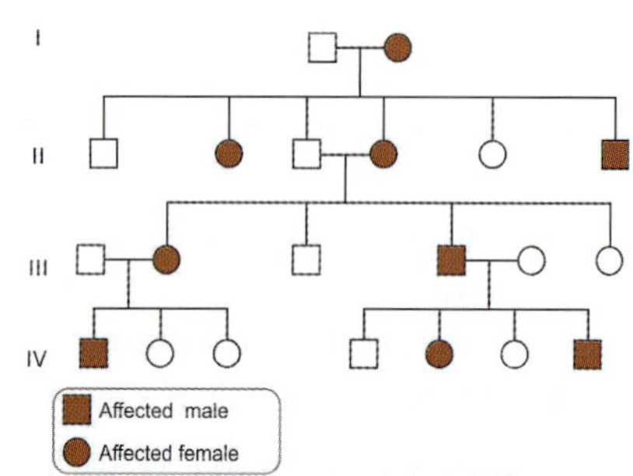

A. Autosomal recessive inheritance
B. Autosomal dominant inheritance
C. X-linked recessive inheritance
D. X-linked dominant inheritance
E. Multifactorial inheritance pattern</td>
<td>Ans: B (Autosomal dominant inheritance)
The adjacent figure is suggestive of an autosomal dominant trait. In case of autosomal dominant disorders, marriage between a normal male and an affected female is likely to result in a progeny having 50% chances of showing the manifest disease and 50% chances of being normal (Fig. 4).
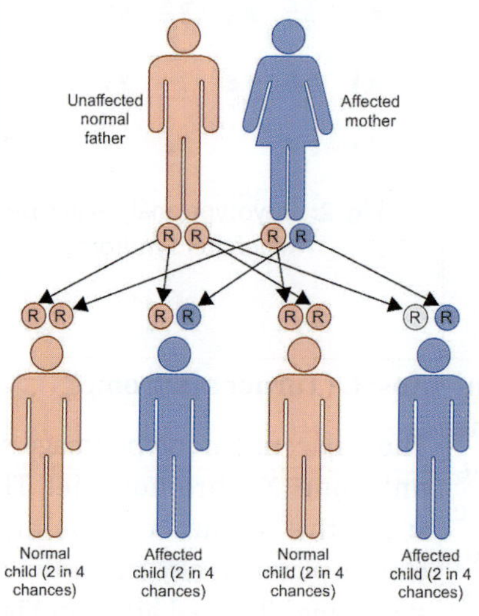

Fig. 4: Pattern of inheritance of an autosomal dominant disorder when an unaffected male marries an affected female.</td>
<td>Explanation: This figure is suggestive of an autosomal dominant trait. Dominant inheritance means that if an individual has even one abnormal gene, he/she gets the disease. Some of the features suggestive of an autosomal dominant trait include the following:
▪ Trait is common in pedigree.
▪ Trait is found in every generation.
▪ Affected individuals transmit the trait to half their children (regardless of sex).
▪ Both males and females may be affected.

Potential questions: There can be questions related to the pedigree analysis of various autosomal dominant conditions such as Marfan syndrome, achondroplasia, Huntington chorea, etc.</td>
</tr>
</table>

<table>
<tr><th>Question</th><th>Answer</th><th>Comment</th></tr>
<tr>
<td>

Q5. What does this pedigree chart based on the individual's phenotype indicate?

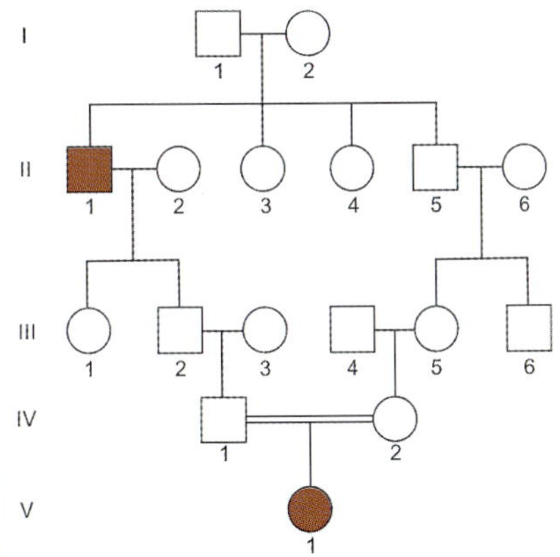

A. Autosomal recessive inheritance
B. Autosomal dominant inheritance
C. X-linked recessive inheritance
D. X-linked dominant inheritance
E. Multifactorial inheritance

</td>
<td>

Ans: A (Autosomal recessive inheritance)

The pedigree chart shown in this question is suggestive of autosomal recessive inheritance. **Figure 5** shows the pedigree chart similar to that given in the question, the only difference being that this chart is based on an individual's genotype, whereas the chart in the question is based on the individual's phenotype. In case of an autosomal recessive disorder, when an unaffected carrier female marries an unaffected carrier male, 50% of the progeny would be unaffected carrier, 25% would be normal and unaffected whereas 25% would be affected.

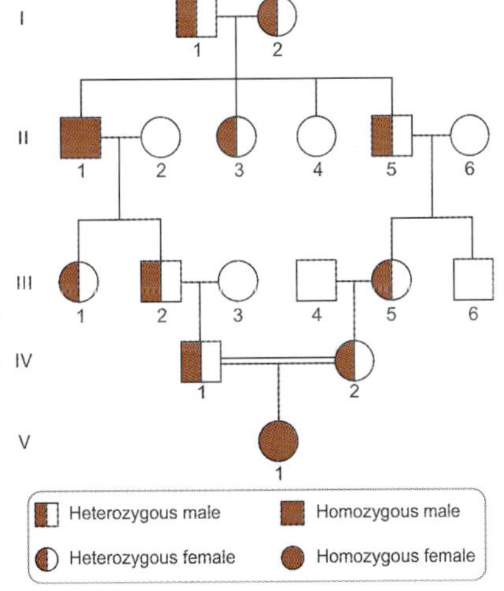

Fig. 5: Pedigree analysis based on the genotype of the individuals (both the parents are carriers).

</td>
<td>

Explanation: Autosomal recessive pattern of inheritance implies that an individual gets the disease, if he/she inherits two mutated genes, one from each parent. Features of autosomal recessive conditions include the following:

- Trait is rare in pedigree.
- Trait often skips generations (hidden heterozygous carriers).
- Trait affects males and females equally.
- Trait may especially become visible with consanguineous marriages.

Potential questions: There may be questions pertaining to the pedigree analysis of various autosomal recessive conditions, where one or both the parents could be carriers or one of the parents could be having a manifest disease and the other could be normal or a carrier.

</td>
</tr>
</table>

Question	Answer	Comment
Q6. What does the below pedigree chart indicate? 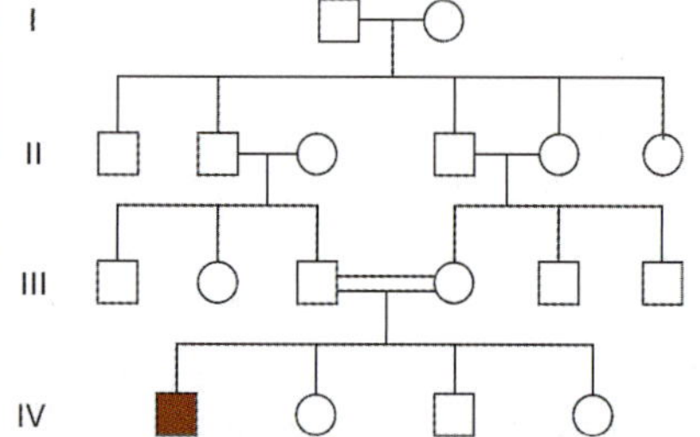 A. Autosomal recessive inheritance B. Autosomal dominant inheritance C. X-linked recessive inheritance D. X-linked dominant inheritance E. Multifactorial inheritance	**Ans: A (Autosomal recessive inheritance)** The adjacent pedigree chart depicts an autosomal recessive inheritance pattern where only one parent is a carrier. **Figure 6** shows the pedigree chart similar to that given in the adjacent question and is based on an individual's genotype, whereas the chart in the question is based on the individual's phenotype. 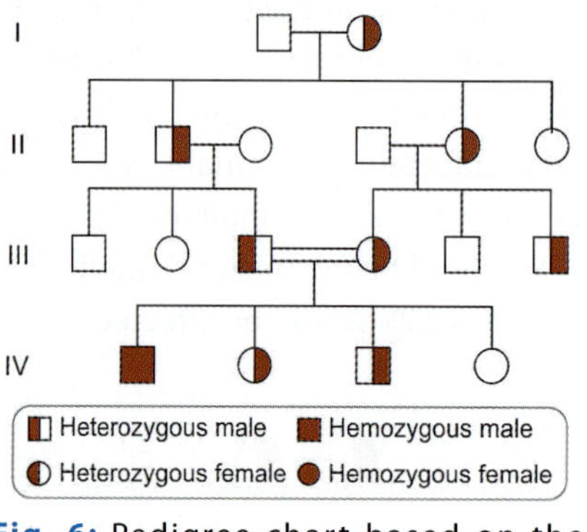 **Fig. 6:** Pedigree chart based on the genotype of the individuals (only one of the parents is a carrier).	**Explanation:** Features of autosomal recessive conditions have already been explained in Question 5. Marriage between an unaffected carrier of a recessive trait and a normal unaffected partner is likely to result in a progeny with 50% chances of being normal and unaffected and 50% chances of being a carrier. **Potential questions:** There may be questions pertaining to the pedigree analysis of various autosomal recessive conditions such as thalassemia, sickle cell disease, Tay-Sachs disease, cystic fibrosis, etc. There could be various scenarios such as one or both the parents could be carriers or one of the parents could be having a manifest disease and the other could be normal or a carrier.
Q7. What does the following pedigree analysis show? 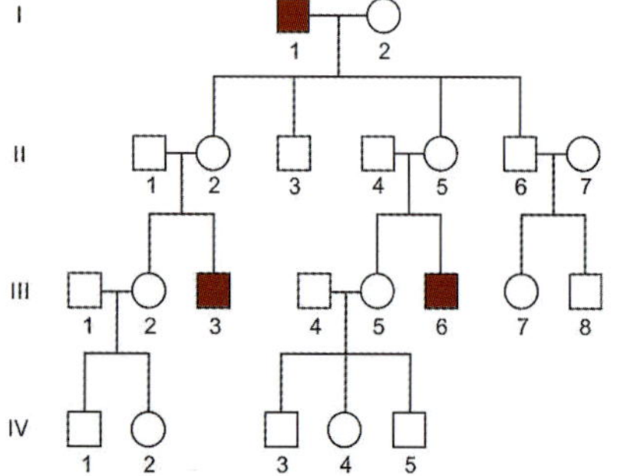 A. Autosomal recessive inheritance B. Autosomal dominant inheritance C. X-linked recessive inheritance D. X-linked dominant inheritance E. None of the above	**Ans: C (X-linked recessive inheritance)** The pedigree chart in the adjacent image is suggestive of X-linked recessive inheritance. **Figure 7** shows the pedigree chart of the adjacent question based on the genotype of the individuals. 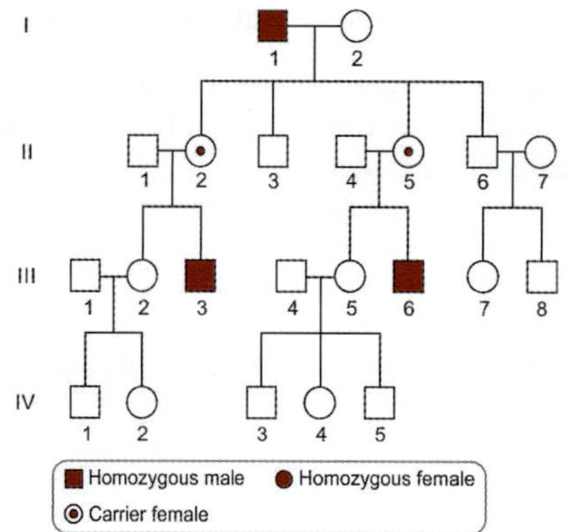 **Fig. 7:** Pedigree chart of the adjacent question based on the genotype of the individuals (father is suffering from the disease, whereas the mother is normal).	**Explanation:** X-linked recessive inheritance is a pattern of inheritance in which a mutant gene on X-chromosome causes the phenotype to be expressed in males because they have one X and one Y chromosome. On the other hand, the phenotype is expressed in only those females who are homozygous for the gene mutation. Features of X-linked recessive trait are as follows: ▪ Trait is rare in pedigree. ▪ Trait skips generation. ▪ Affected fathers DO not pass to their sons, but carrier mothers would pass the disease to their sons. ▪ Males are more commonly affected than females. **Potential questions:** There could be various pedigree scenarios in cases of diseases with X-linked recessive inheritance.

Question	Answer	Comment
Q8. Consider the pedigree described in the figure. A carrier mother married to a normal father has one affected son, two not affected children (one daughter and one son), and one carrier daughter. What is the likely mode of inheritance? 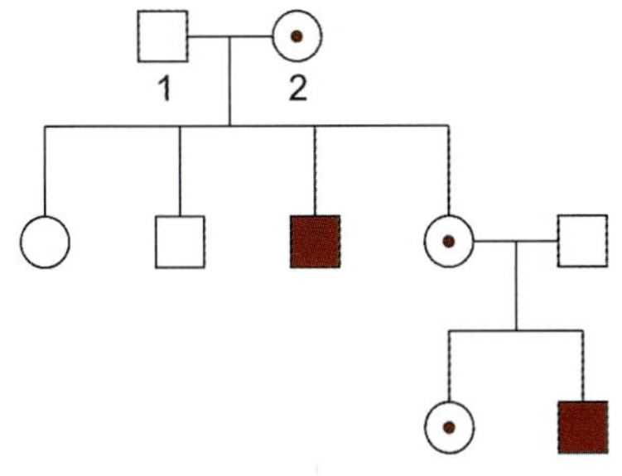 A. Autosomal dominant B. X-linked dominant C. Y-linked dominant D. Autosomal recessive E. X-linked recessive	**Ans: E (X-linked recessive inheritance)** The pedigree analysis in the adjacent image shows X-linked recessive inheritance. The pattern of inheritance of an X-linked recessive disorder when an unaffected carrier female marries an unaffected normal male is shown in **Figure 8**. 50% of her sons would be affected and 50% would be unaffected. On the other hand, 50% of the daughters would be carriers and 50% would be normal unaffected. 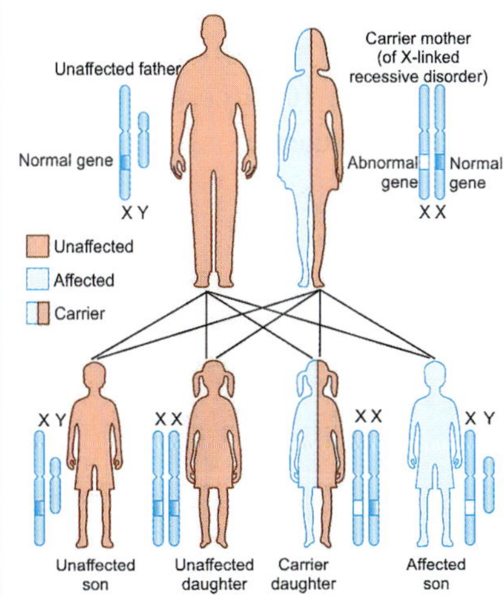 **Fig. 8:** Pattern of inheritance of an X-linked recessive disorder when an unaffected carrier female marries an unaffected normal male.	**Explanation:** Features of X-linked recessive trait have been explained in Question 7. As can be seen in **Figure 8**, the carrier mother transmits the disease to her son and not to her daughter. The daughter in this case is a carrier because she has mutation only on one X-chromosome. She would need the mutant gene to be present on both the X chromosomes to be able to manifest the disease. **Potential questions:** There may be questions pertaining to the pedigree analysis of various X-linked dominant conditions such as hemophilia A, glucose 6-phosphate dehydrogenase (G6PD) deficiency, color blindness, Duchenne's muscular dystrophy, etc. There could be pedigree analysis associated with various scenarios such as affected father and normal mother or carrier mother and unaffected father or affected mother and normal father.

Question	Answer	Comment
Q9. What does the following pedigree analysis show? 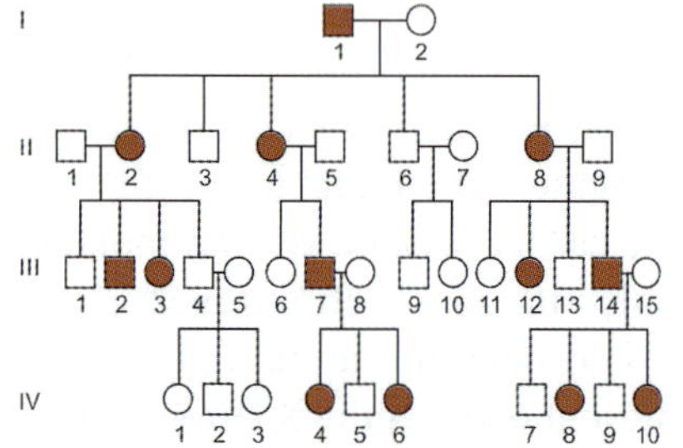 A. Autosomal recessive inheritance B. Autosomal dominant inheritance C. X-linked recessive inheritance D. X-linked dominant inheritance E. Multifactorial inheritance	**Ans: D (X-linked dominant inheritance)** The inheritance pattern in the adjacent pedigree chart is X-linked dominant. In case of X-linked dominant disorders, the pattern of inheritance is dependent on whether the mother or father is affected with this disorder. In case the father is affected, he is likely to pass the disorder to all his daughters **(Fig. 9)**, but none of his sons. In case the mother is affected, the chances of her son being affected with the disorder depend on whether she passes the normal X chromosome or the X chromosome with the mutant gene on to her son. In case the son is affected, it is 100% certain that the mother is affected. 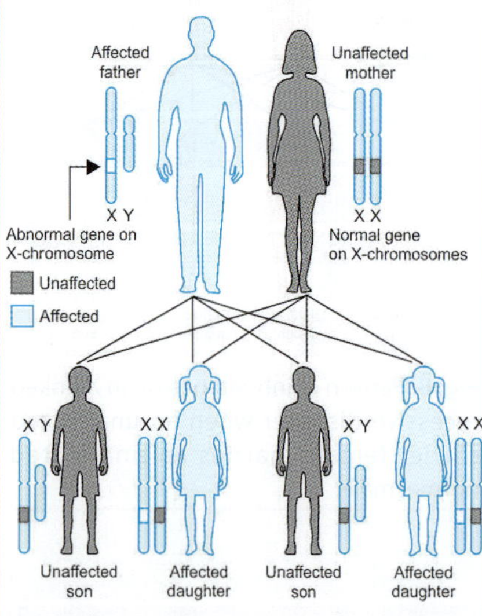 **Fig. 9:** Pattern of inheritance of an X-linked dominant disorder when the father is affected.	**Explanation:** Mutant gene on one X chromosome is likely to manifest the disease in case of diseases showing X-linked dominant mode of inheritance. Features of X-linked dominant inheritance pattern are as follows: ▪ X-linked dominant diseases are extremely unusual. ▪ Trait is common in pedigree. ▪ Affected fathers pass to ALL of their daughters. ▪ Males and females are equally likely to be affected. ▪ Often they are lethal (before birth) in males and only seen in females, e.g., incontinentia pigmenti (skin lesions) and X-linked rickets (bone lesions). **Potential questions:** There may be questions pertaining to the pedigree analysis of various X-linked dominant conditions such as fragile X syndrome, vitamin D-resistant rickets, etc. There could be pedigree analysis associated with various scenarios such as affected father and normal mother or affected mother and normal father.

Question	Answer	Comment
Q10. The following illustration describes a structural chromosomal abnormality. What does this structural chromosomal abnormality represent? 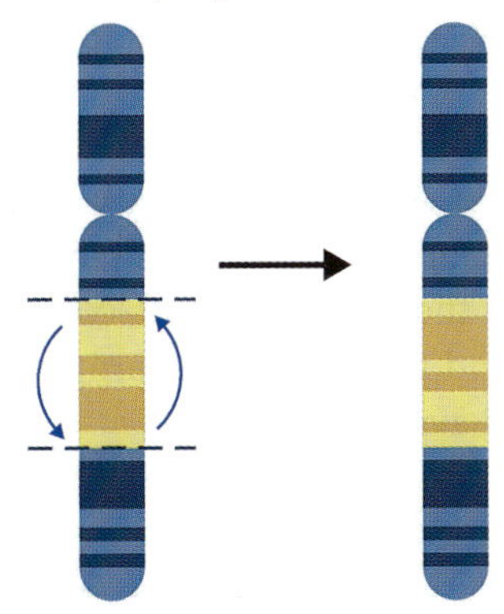 A. Insertion B. Inversion C. Deletion D. Duplication E. Translocation	**Ans: B (Inversion)** Various types of genetic aberrations which can occur are described in **Figures 10A to D**. 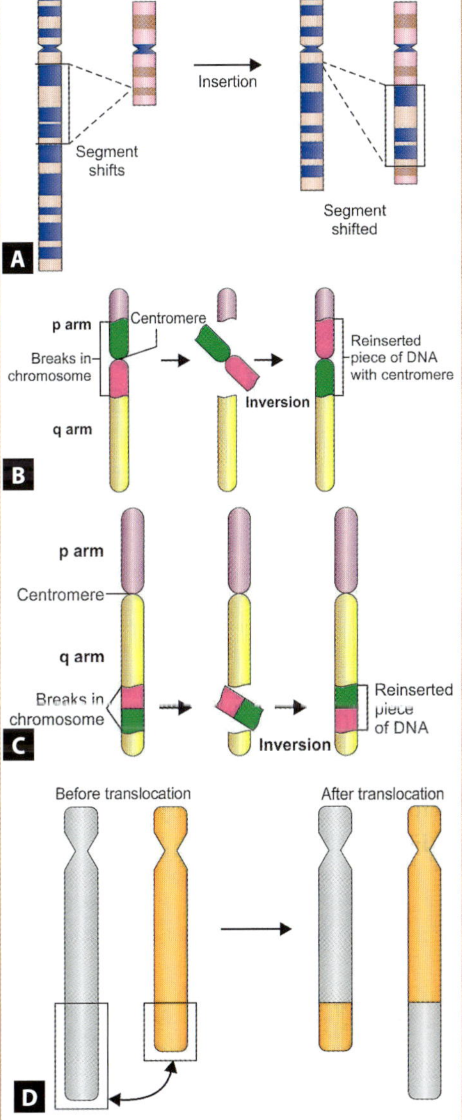 **Figs. 10A to D:** (A) Chromosomal insertion; (B) Pericentric inversion; (C) Paracentric inversion; (D) Chromosomal translocation.	**Explanation:** Some commonly encountered genetic aberrations are as follows: ▪ *Insertion:* This chromosomal mutation occurs when a portion of one chromosome has been deleted from its normal place and inserted into another chromosome **(Fig. 10A)**. ▪ *Inversion:* This type of chromosomal mutation occurs when two breaks occur in one chromosome, and the region between the breaks rotates 180° before rejoining with the two end fragments. Such an event creates a chromosomal mutation called an inversion. Unlike deletions and duplications, inversions do not change the overall amount of the genetic material. As a result, inversions are usually viable and are not associated with any particular abnormalities at the phenotypic level. Inversions can be of two types: Pericentric and paracentric. Pericentric inversion involves the centromere **(Fig. 10B)**, whereas paracentric inversion **(Fig. 10C)** does not involve the centromere. ▪ *Deletion:* Loss of chromosomal material ▪ *Duplication:* Presence of an additional chromosomal segment ▪ *Translocation:* This is a genetic abnormality involving the exchange of fragments of genetic material between two nonhomologous chromosomes **(Fig. 10D)**. **Potential questions:** There can be questions related to identification of different types of genetic aberrations described above.

Question	Answer	Comment
Q11. For karyotyping of human X chromosome with light microscopy after staining with Giemsa stain as shown in the below image, which of the following procedures is used as a standard technique? 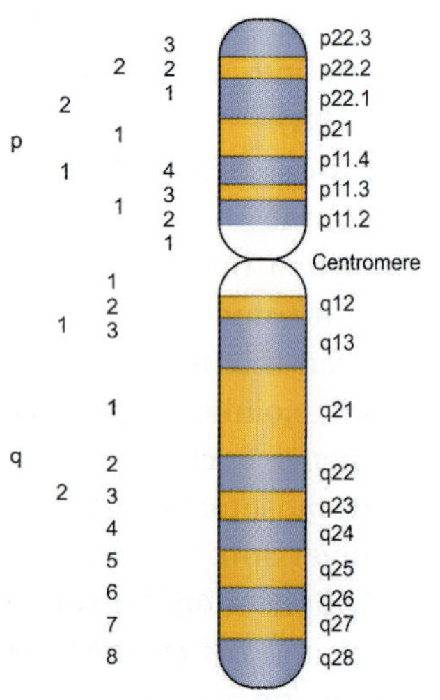 A. C-banding B. V-staining C. Q-banding D. G-banding E. None of the above	**Ans: D (G-banding)** The Giemsa dye produces chromosome-specific patterns known as G-bands. G-banding has been divided into regions, bands, and sub-bands. The adjacent figure shows a typical diagram of the bands of the human X chromosome on G-banding. The short arm is p and the long arm is q. Each arm is divided into larger regions that are further subdivided into smaller bands and interbands. Dark bands are AT (adenine-thymine) rich **(Fig. 11)**, while the light bands are GC (guanine-cytosine) rich. 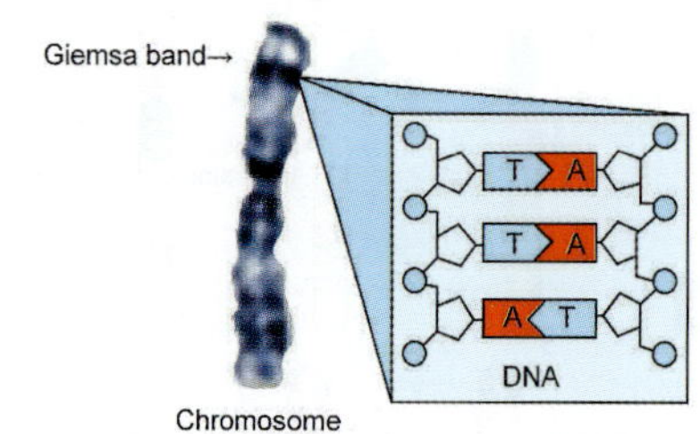 **Fig. 11:** Structure of dark bands on G-banding.	**Explanation:** Giemsa stain is the most widely used staining method for identifying each individual chromosome based on a distinct and consistent pattern of alternating light and dark bands running the length of the chromosome. Cells are stained with the dye Giemsa after arresting the cells at the metaphase with colcemid and treatment with proteolytic enzyme (trypsin). G- and R-banding (reverse of Giemsa staining) are the techniques most commonly used for identification of chromosome (karyotyping) and to elicit abnormalities related to chromosome number, size, shape, and aberrations. **Potential questions:** There can be different questions related to different banding techniques, especially G-banding and R-banding.
Q12. What type of structural chromosomal abnormality is depicted in the below image? 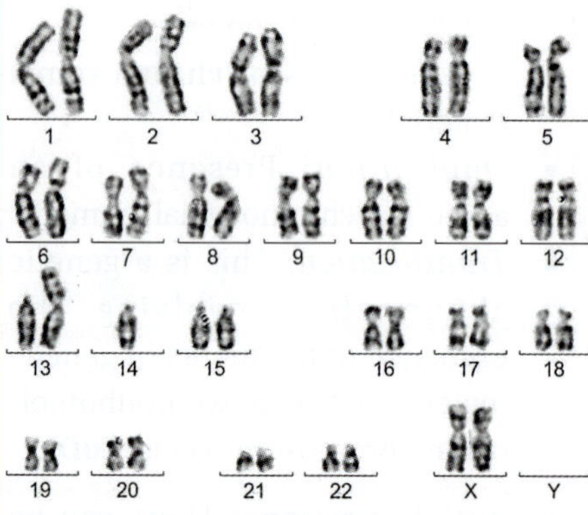 A. Reciprocal translocation B. Robertsonian translocation C. Insertion D. Deletion E. Pericentric inversion	**Ans: B (Robertsonian translocation)** There is presence of Robertsonian location, indicated by red arrow in **Figure 12.** 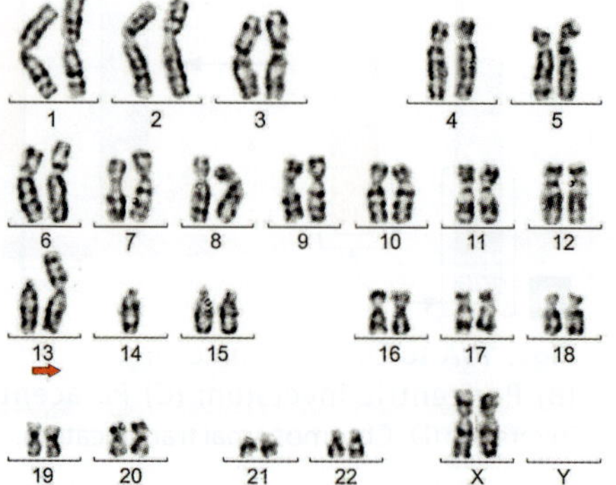 **Fig. 12:** Presence of Robertsonian location between chromosomes 13 and 14 (indicated by the arrow).	**Explanation:** Robertsonian translocation is a type of chromosomal rearrangement where two acrocentric chromosomes fuse at their centromeres, losing their short arms and forming a single larger chromosome. Commonly involves chromosomes 13, 14, 15, 21, and 22. Robertsonian (13;14) is the most frequent type (~75%), resulting in one fused chromosome 13 and loss of one chromosome 14. **Potential questions:** There can be different questions on Robertsonian translocations involving various acrocentric chromosomes such as 13, 14, 15, 21, and 22.

Question	Answer	Comment
Q13. In this pedigree, I-1 and II-2 have hemophilia. III-2 has cystic fibrosis, with an incidence being as high as 1 in 625 live births. The disease status for both hemophilia and cystic fibrosis is unknown for IV-1 and IV-2. What is the probability that III-3 is a carrier of hemophilia? 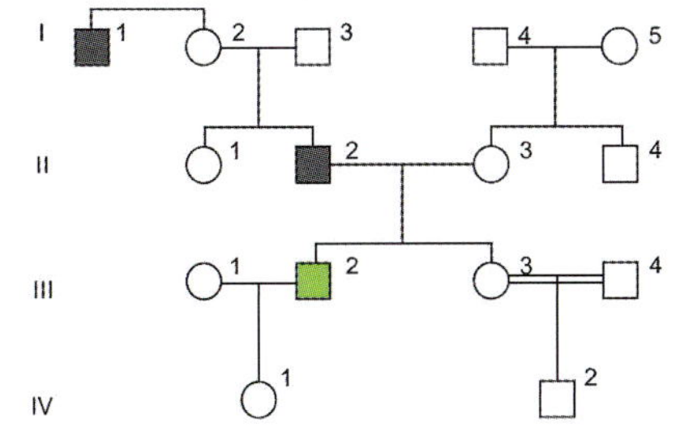 A. 50% B. 25% C. 66% D. 100% E. 0%	**Ans: D (100%)** The pedigree analysis in the adjacent image points to an X-linked recessive mode of inheritance. The pattern of inheritance of an X-linked recessive disorder when an affected male marries a normal woman is illustrated in **Figure 13**. 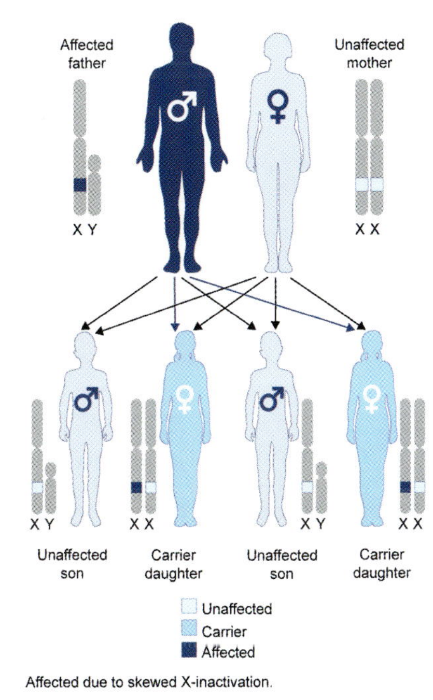 **Fig. 13:** Pattern of inheritance of an X-linked recessive disorder when an affected male marries a normal woman.	**Explanation:** X-linked recessive inheritance is a pattern of inheritance in which a mutant gene on X-chromosome causes the phenotype to be expressed in males because they have one X and one Y chromosome. On the other hand, the phenotype is expressed in only those females who are homozygous for the gene mutation. Since hemophilia is an X-linked recessive disorder, the daughter of an affected male is an obligatory carrier. In case of an affected man, all of his daughters would be carriers and none of his sons would be affected, implying that there is no male-to-male transmission. **Potential questions:** There could be questions pertaining to the pedigree analysis associated with various scenarios such as affected father and normal mother or carrier mother and unaffected father or affected mother and normal father in case of various X-linked recessive conditions.

Question	Answer	Comment
Q14. The below pedigree chart shows a family with a specific disease. Assuming no spontaneous mutations and full penetrance, identify the most probable mode of inheritance for this disease. *Note:* The individual marked with asterisk (*) does not carry any allele associated with the affected phenotype. 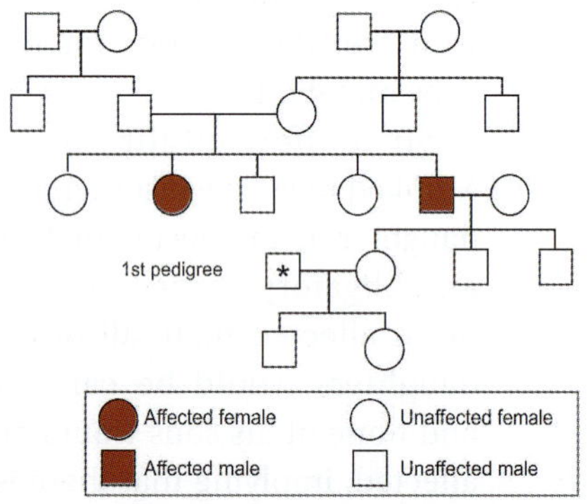 A. Autosomal dominant inheritance B. Autosomal recessive inheritance C. X-linked dominant inheritance D. X-linked recessive inheritance E. De novo mutation	**Ans: B (Autosomal recessive inheritance)** The pedigree shows autosomal recessive inheritance, affecting both sexes. **Figure 14** illustrates the pattern when two unaffected carriers marry. 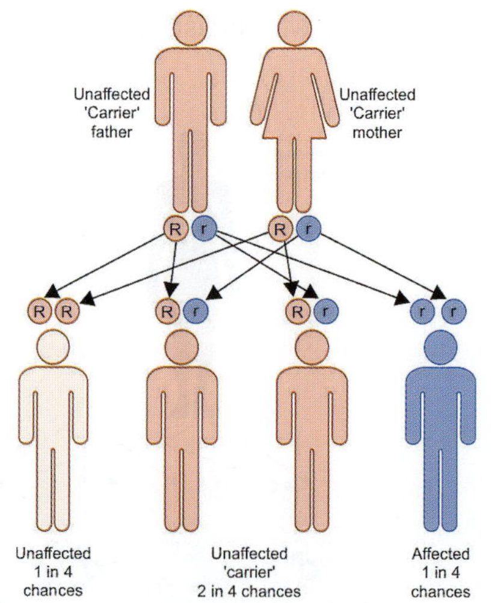 **Fig. 14:** Pattern of inheritance of an autosomal recessive disorder when an unaffected carrier female marries an unaffected carrier male.	**Explanation:** In autosomal recessive inheritance, disease appears only when both recessive alleles are inherited. Carriers have one allele. Males and females are equally affected, and generations may be skipped (horizontal transmission), allowing affected individuals to have unaffected children. **Potential questions:** There could be various pedigree scenarios in cases of diseases with autosomal recessive inheritance such as one or both the parents could be carriers or one of the parents could be having a manifest disease and the other could be normal or a carrier.
Q15. Mention the blood group of the offspring II-1 and offsprings III-2 and III-3. 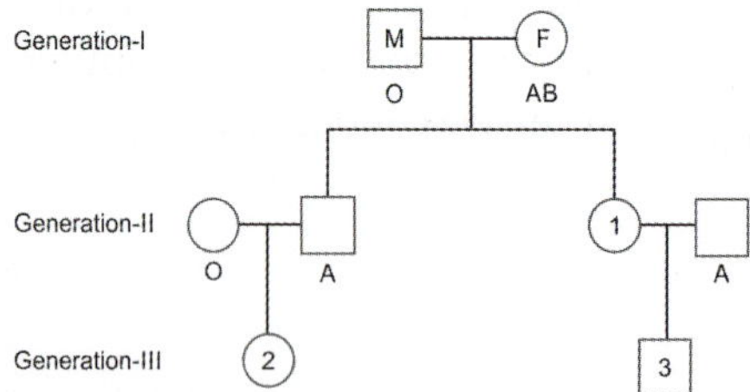 A. Blood group B, A, AB B. Blood group B, AB, AB C. Blood group O, A, B D. Blood group A, B, AB E. Blood group O, O, A	**Ans: A (Blood group B, A, AB)** The ABO blood group is controlled by the ABO gene on chromosome 9, with three alleles: A, B, and O **(Fig. 15)**. A and B are codominant, producing both antigens in AB individuals, while O is recessive and expressed only when inherited as OO, resulting in no antigen. 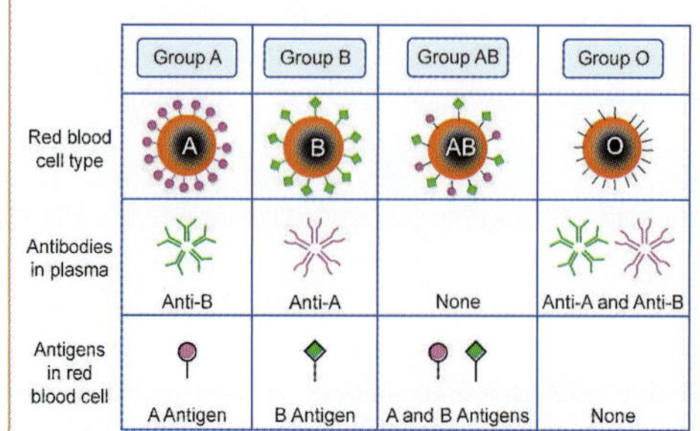 **Fig. 15:** Alleles expressed by various blood groups in the ABO system.	**Explanation:** The mode of inheritance of the ABO blood group system is autosomal codominant. A person with blood group A can have a heterozygous genotype of **IAi**. This means that they have one allele for blood type A (IA) and one allele for blood type O (i), where the A allele is dominant over the O allele ▪ *II-1:* Blood group = B; Genotype=IBi ▪ *III-2:* Blood group = A; Genotype = IAi ▪ *III-3:* Blood group = AB = IAIB **Potential questions:** Questions may involve parental ABO groups and require predicting the progeny's blood group.

SECTION 2

Gynecology

CHAPTER 7

Gynecological Anatomy and Physiology

GENERAL AND GYNECOLOGICAL ANATOMY

Question	Answer	Comment
Q1. During a laparoscopic examination, the following image shows the internal genitalia of a female patient. Identify the structure labeled A. 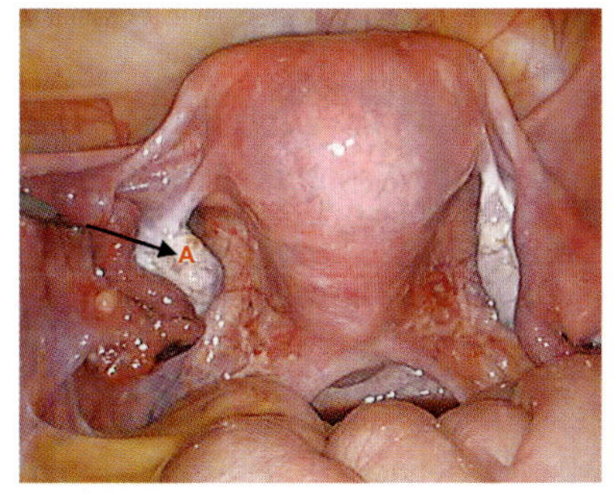 A. Uterus B. Ovary C. Fallopian tube D. Round ligament E. Broad ligament	**Ans: B (Ovary)** **Figure 1** shows a normal laparoscopic view of the pelvis demonstrating female internal genitalia present in the true pelvis. The female internal genitalia comprises a pear-shaped, muscular organ, the uterus, cervix, vagina, two fallopian tubes, emerging from the uterine cornu each, and two ovaries. 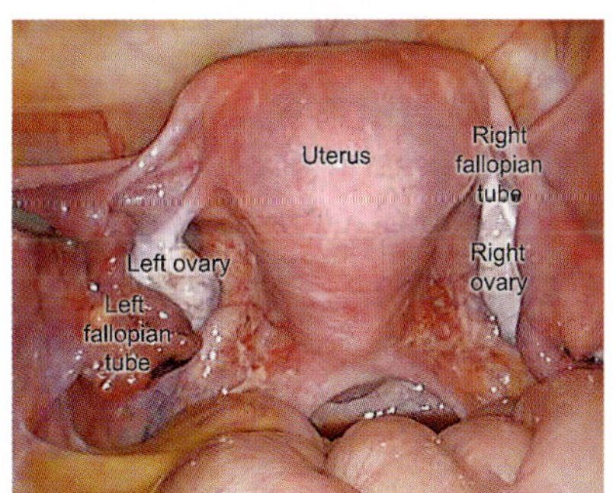 **Fig. 1:** Laparoscopic examination showing the female internal genitalia.	**Explanation:** The structure labeled A in the laparoscopic image is the ovary. The ovaries are paired almond-shaped structures located on either side of the uterus in the pelvic cavity. They are responsible for producing eggs (ova) and secreting hormones such as estrogen and progesterone. Identifying the ovaries is important for assessing ovarian health and diagnosing conditions such as ovarian cysts or tumors. **Potential questions:** There can be questions related to the identification of different structures of the female internal genitalia as well as different pelvic ligaments.

Question	Answer	Comment
Q2. During a laparoscopic examination, the following image shows the internal genitalia of a female patient. Identify the structure labeled B. 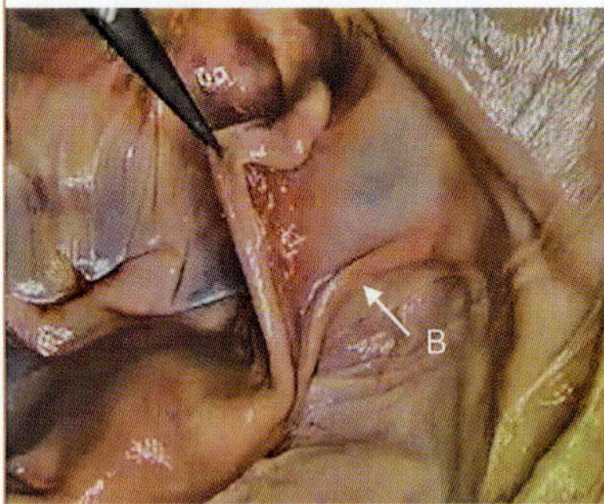 A. Uterus B. Ovary C. Fallopian tube D. Round ligament E. Broad ligament	**Ans: D (Round ligament)** The structure labeled B in the laparoscopic image is the round ligament. The round ligament is a remnant of the embryonic gubernaculum and originates at the uterine horns, where the fallopian tubes enter the uterus **(Fig. 2)**. Situated below the fallopian tubes, these ligaments are 10–12 cm long and extend from the lateral aspect of uterus, passing anteriorly between the layers of the broad ligament. They leave the pelvis through the deep inguinal ring by passing through the inguinal canal and eventually get inserted into the labia majora. 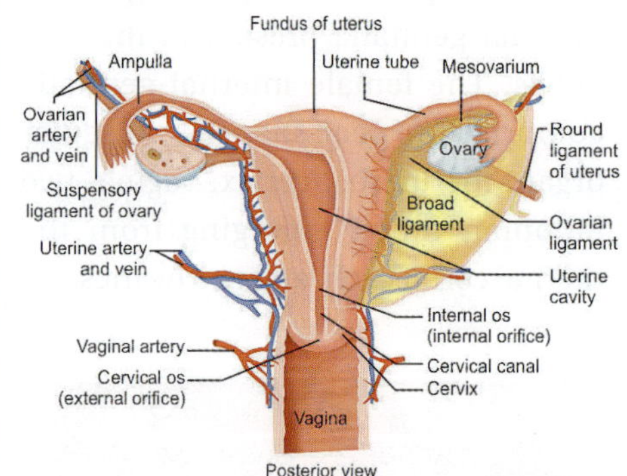 **Fig. 2:** Different ligaments of the uterus.	**Explanation:** The uterus is anchored by peritoneal folds, also known as the false ligaments, which primarily provide support and stabilization but not strong mechanical fixation. Besides the round ligament, some of these are as follows: *Ovarian ligament:* Also called the utero-ovarian ligament or proper ovarian ligament, this is a fibromuscular band of tissue that connects the ovary to the uterus. *Infundibulopelvic ligament:* Also known as the suspensory ligament of the ovary, this is a part of broad ligament which extends from the ovary to the pelvic side wall. It contains the ovarian vessels which enter the ovary at the hilum. *Broad ligament:* The largest peritoneal fold, this is a double layer of peritoneum that extends from the lateral border of the uterus to the lateral pelvic wall. The various parts of the broad ligament are as follows: ▪ *Mesometrium:* Lateral to uterus. ▪ *Mesosalpinx:* Around fallopian tube. ▪ *Mesovarium:* Attaches ovary to broad ligament. **Potential questions:** There can be questions related to the identification of different structures of the female internal genitalia as well as different ligaments.

Question	Answer	Comment
Q3. During a laparoscopic procedure, a structure is identified by an arrow in the image below. What is the primary function of this structure? 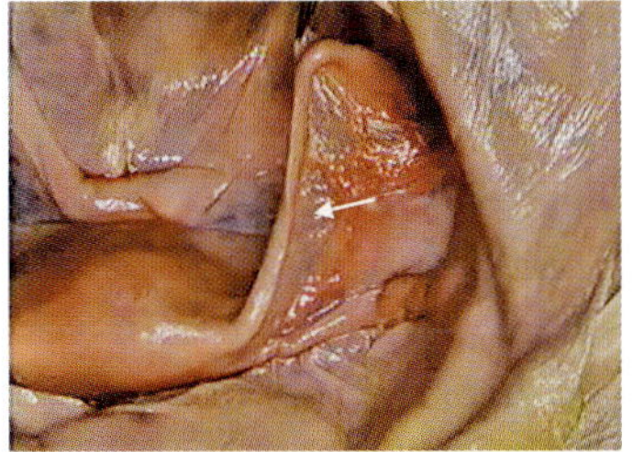 A. Connects ovaries to pelvic wall B. Supports the uterine tube C. Anchors uterus to bladder D. Supplies blood to fallopian tubes and ovaries E. Connects ovary to fimbriae of fallopian tube	**Ans: B (Supports the uterine tube)** The structure pointed by the arrow in the adjacent image is mesosalpinx. As shown in **Figure 3**, mesosalpinx can be considered as the portion of broad ligament which stretches from the ovary to the level of fallopian tube and encloses it. 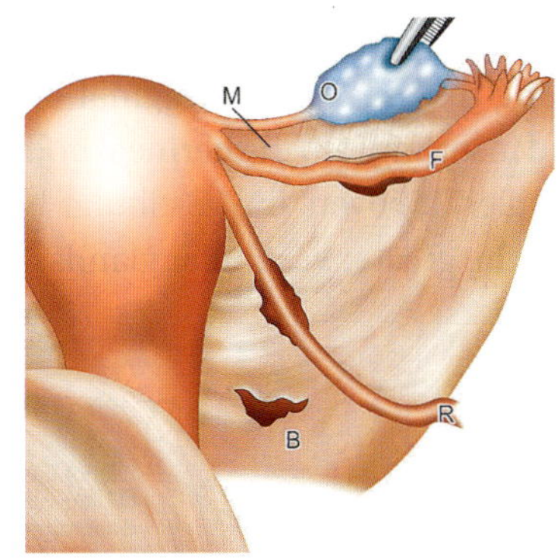 **Fig. 3:** Mesosalpinx. (B: broad ligament; F: fallopian tube; M: mesosalpinx; O: ovary; R: round ligament)	**Explanation:** The mesosalpinx is the part of the broad ligament that specifically surrounds and supports the fallopian tube. It helps in stabilizing the position of the fallopian tube while also serving as a conduit for blood vessels, lymphatics, and nerves that supply the uterine tubes. Since the mesosalpinx encloses the fallopian tubes, it also supports it. **Potential questions:** There can be questions related to the identification of different structures of the female internal genitalia as well as different ligaments.
Q4. A macroscopic specimen of the vagina and cervix shows a region of stratified squamous epithelium transitioning to columnar epithelium. In which anatomical region is this transition most likely to occur? 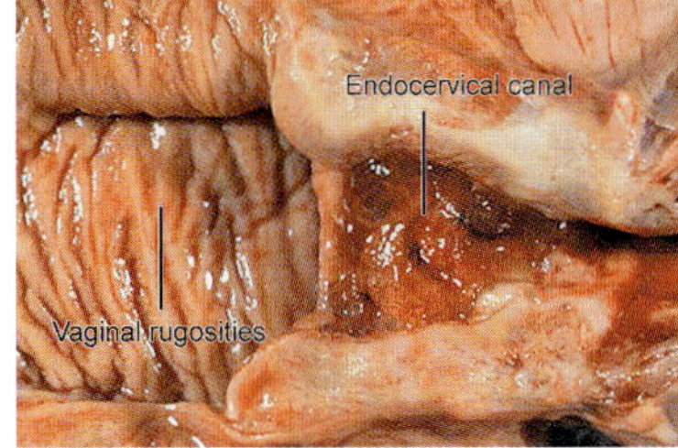 A. Internal os of the cervix B. Vaginal fornix C. Transformation zone D. External os of the cervix E. Upper third of the vagina	**Ans: C (Transformation zone)** The adjacent image demonstrates the macroscopic specimen of the cervix and vagina. The part of the cervix projecting into the vagina is known as portio vaginalis or ectocervix, whereas the region of the cervix opening into uterine cavity is known as endocervix. The opening of ectocervix inside vagina is known as external cervical os, while opening of cervix inside the uterine cavity is known as the internal cervical os. The endocervical canal extends between the internal and the external cervical os. 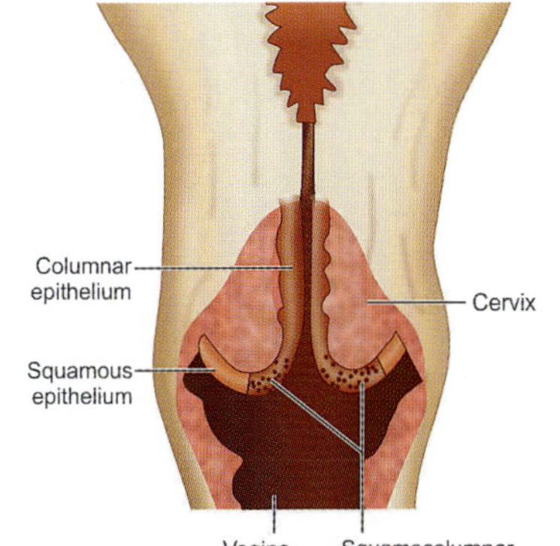 **Fig. 4:** Epithelium of the cervix.	**Explanation:** The vaginal canal is lined with nonkeratinized stratified squamous epithelium. On the other hand, the ectocervix is lined by squamous cells, while endocervical cells are mainly of the columnar type. The transformation zone lies at the junction of ectocervix and endocervix. Columnar cells are constantly changing into squamous cells in the transformation zone **(Fig. 4)**. Since cells in the transformation zone are constantly changing, this is the most common place for cervical dysplasia and malignancy to develop. This region serves as a key region for clinical evaluation, particularly at the time of Pap smears. **Potential questions:** There could be questions related to anatomical characteristics of cervix and vagina and types of epithelium present in various regions.

Question	Answer	Comment
Q5. Identify the structure labeled A in the below image of the female perineum. 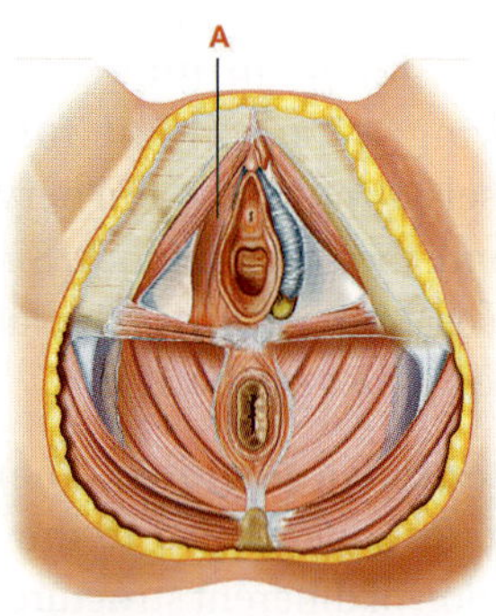 A. Ischiocavernosus muscle B. Bulbospongiosus muscle C. Superficial transverse perineal muscle D. External anal sphincter E. Perineal body	**Ans: B (Bulbospongiosus muscle)** **Figure 5** shows the diagram of female perineum demonstrating the three layers of pelvic muscles. The bulbospongiosus muscle is a paired superficial muscle of the perineum. The muscle is located anteriorly in the perineum, running along the sides of the vaginal orifice and inserting into the perineal body. In females, it covers the vestibular bulbs and the greater vestibular glands. 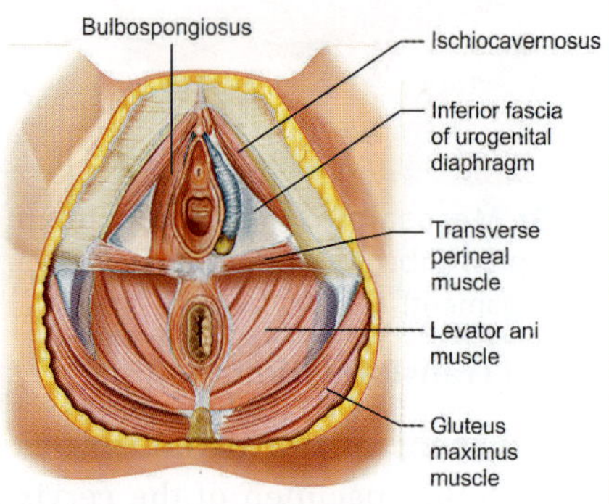 **Fig. 5:** Female perineum.	**Explanation:** There are three layers of pelvic muscles in the perineum, which are as follows: ▪ *Muscles of the pelvic diaphragm:* Levator ani muscle of both the sides. ▪ *Muscles of the urogenital diaphragm:* Deep transverse perineal muscle ▪ *Superficial muscles of the pelvic floor:* Superficial transverse perineal muscle, external anal sphincter, bulbospongiosus and ischiocavernosus. **Potential questions:** There can be different questions related to various muscles present in the perineum.

Question	Answer	Comment
Q6. What type of epithelium is depicted by X in the given figure? 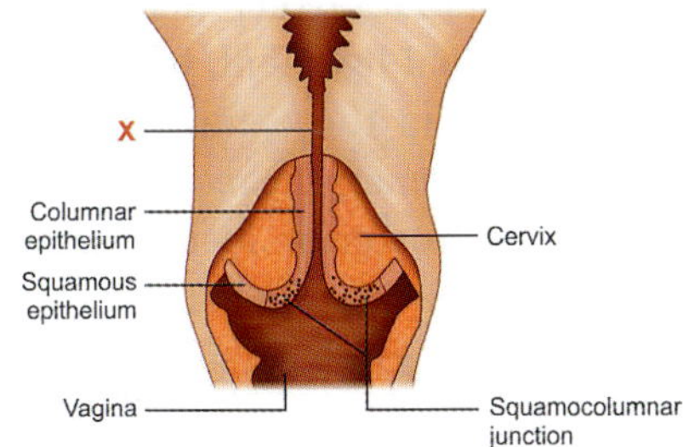 A. Simple columnar epithelium B. Simple cuboidal epithelium C. Simple squamous epithelium D. Stratified columnar epithelium E. Stratified squamous epithelium	**Ans: A (Simple columnar epithelium)** **Figure 6A** depicts magnified view of cervix showing the external cervical os. On the other hand, **Figure 6B** shows the squamocolumnar junction. 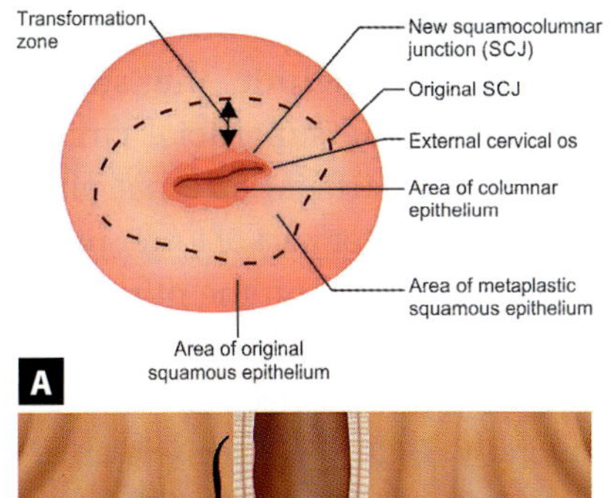 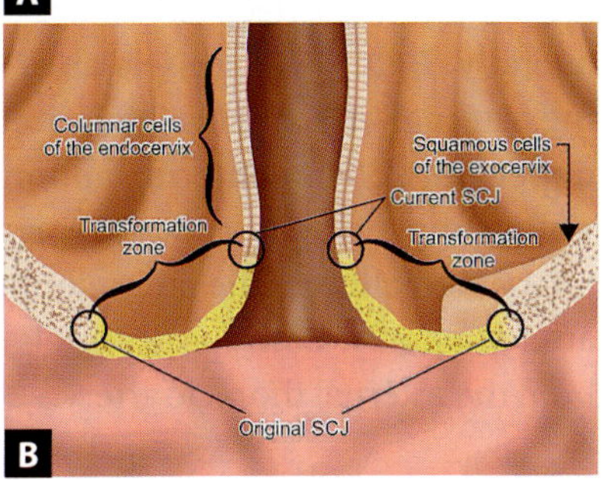 **Figs. 6A and B:** (A) Magnified view of the cervix showing external cervical os; (B) Magnified view of the squamocolumnar junction (SCJ).	**Explanation:** Cervix is the narrow, lower part of the uterus connecting to the vagina and is composed of: ▪ *Ectocervix (portio vaginalis):* Projects into the vagina; lined by nonkeratinizing stratified squamous epithelium; opens via external cervical os **(Fig. 6A)**. ▪ *Endocervix:* Opens into the uterine cavity via internal cervical os; lined by columnar epithelium **(Fig. 6B)**. The endocervical canal connects the two os. The transformation zone at the squamocolumnar junction lies at the junction of ectocervix and endocervix. Here, the columnar cells convert to squamous, and is a common site for cervical malignancy. **Potential questions:** There can be different questions related to the anatomy of cervix and squamocolumnar junction.
Q7. Identify the area represented by B in the figure shown below. 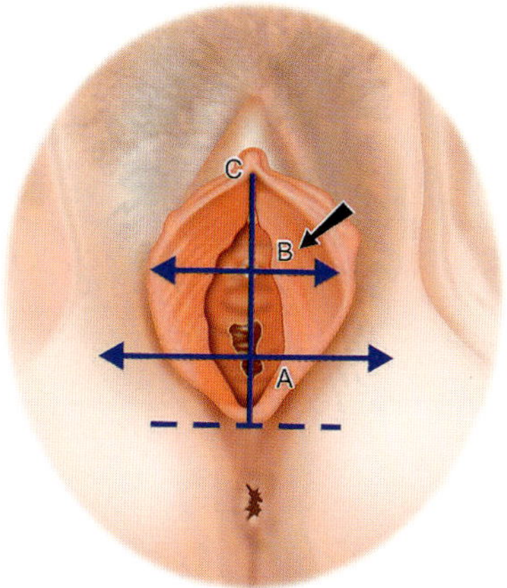 A. Pudendal cleft B. Vestibule C. Fourchette D. Fossa navicularis E. Labia minor	**Ans: B (Vestibule)** The external genital organs include the mons pubis, labia majora, labia minora, Bartholin's glands, and clitoris **(Fig. 7)**. An ill-defined area containing these external genital organs along with the perineum is known as the vulva. Anteriorly, the vulva is bound by mons pubis; posteriorly by the perineum; and on the two sides by the labia majora. 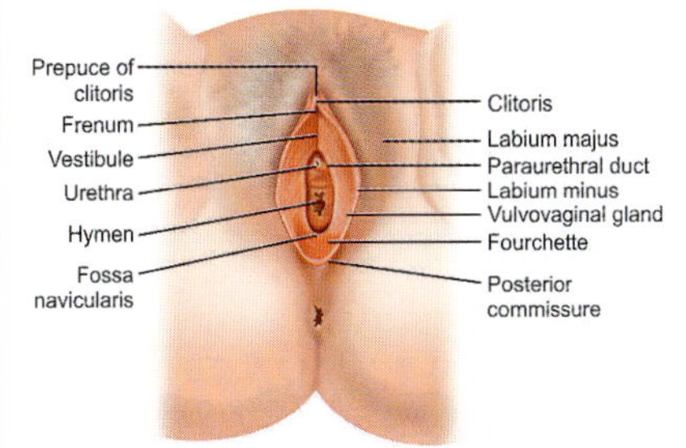 **Fig. 7:** Female external genitalia.	**Explanation:** Pudendal cleft can be described as a fissure between the two labia majora. Fourchette, also known as the posterior commissure of the labia minora, is a frenulum which represents the meeting point of two labia minora posteriorly. The vestibule is the part of the vulva lying between the two labia minora laterally and extends medially to the hymenal sulci. Fossa navicularis can be described as a boat-shaped depression formed by the fossa of vestibule in vagina. **Potential questions:** There can be different questions related to the location of various structures in the female external genitalia.

Question	Answer	Comment
Q8. Identify the artery labeled A in the provided image of the anterolateral abdominal wall. 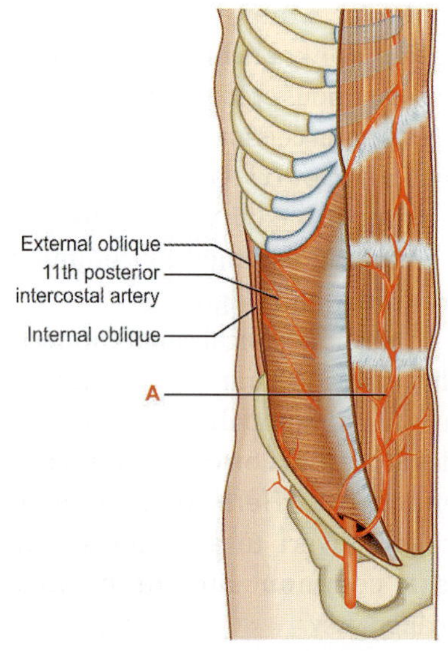 A. Superior epigastric artery B. Inferior epigastric artery C. Deep circumflex iliac artery D. Superficial circumflex iliac artery E. External iliac artery	**Ans: B (Inferior epigastric artery)** The primary blood supply to the abdominal wall is from the superficial and deep blood vessels, which is demonstrated in **Figure 8**. The superficial blood vessels originate from the femoral artery and include the superficial epigastric, the superficial circumflex, and the superficial external pudendal arteries. Deeper part of lower part of the abdominal wall, on the other hand, is supplied by the inferior epigastric artery medially, and the deep circumflex artery laterally. Both these vessels arise from the external iliac vessels. Moreover, the upper part of the anterior abdominal wall is supplied by the superior epigastric artery medially and the musculophrenic artery laterally. Both these vessels arise from the internal thoracic artery. 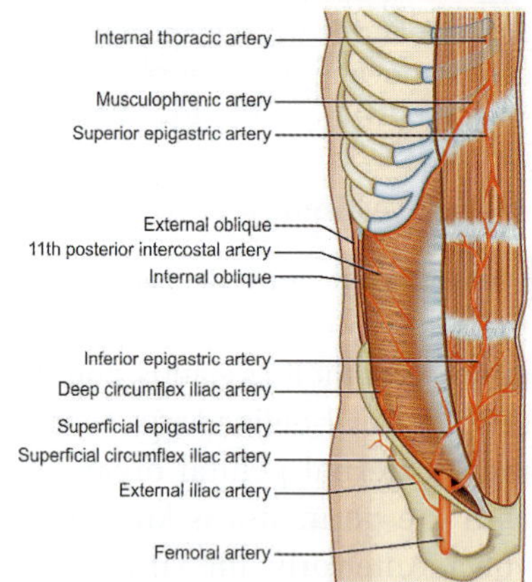 **Fig. 8:** Arteries of the anterolateral abdominal wall.	**Explanation:** The inferior epigastric artery arises from the external iliac artery just above the inguinal ligament. It ascends obliquely in the extraperitoneal tissue and enters the rectus sheath, running posterior to the rectus abdominis muscle. This artery supplies the lower part of the rectus abdominis and the overlying skin. It anastomoses with the superior epigastric artery, providing a collateral circulation between the subclavian and external iliac arteries. Anastomosis between the various vessels of abdominal wall helps in ensuring an excellent blood supply to all areas of the abdominal wall. **Potential questions:** There can be questions related to different blood vessels supplying various regions of the anterior abdominal wall. There can also be questions related to the origin of these vessels.

Question	Answer	Comment
Q9. Identify the structure labeled A in the below image of the rectus sheath. 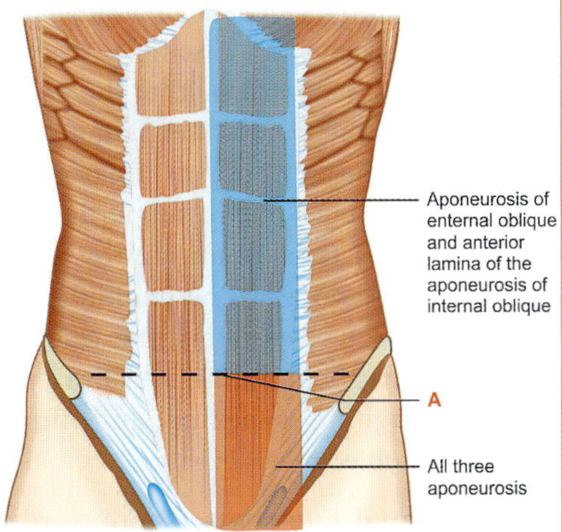 A. Dentate line B. Internal oblique aponeurosis C. Hilton line D. Linea alba E. Arcuate line	**Ans: E (Arcuate line)** The rectus sheath is a fibrous tissue layer covering and protecting the rectus abdominis muscle as shown in **Figures 9A and B** and is formed by the conjoined aponeuroses of the flat abdominal muscles. The arcuate line is a horizontal line that demarcates the lower limit of the posterior layer of the rectus sheath. The composition of the rectus sheath above and below the arcuate line is different and is shown by blue and red color, respectively, in the adjacent image. 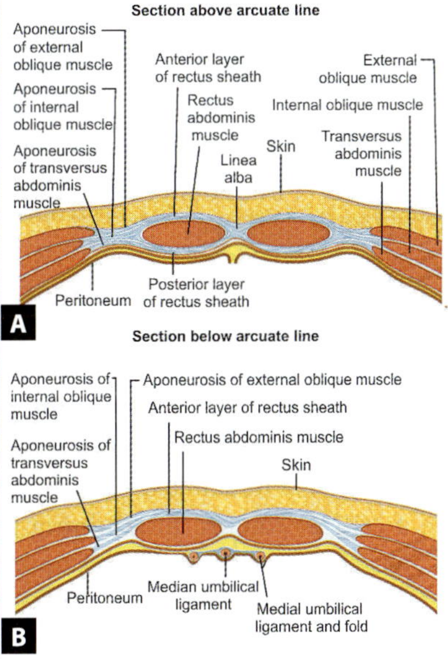 **Figs. 9A and B:** Composition of rectus sheath (A) above and (B) below the arcuate line.	**Explanation:** The arcuate line is located approximately midway between the umbilicus and the pubic symphysis. Above the arcuate line, the rectus abdominis muscle is enclosed by the anterior and posterior layers of the rectus sheath. Below this line, the rectus abdominis is in direct contact with the transversalis fascia, as the posterior layer of the sheath is absent. Above the arcuate line, the superior two thirds of the internal oblique aponeurosis splits into two layers (anterior and posterior) at the lateral border of rectus abdominis. The anterior and posterior lamina respectively join the aponeurosis of external oblique muscle, and internal oblique and transversus abdominis muscles to form the anterior and posterior layers of the rectus sheath. Below the arcuate line, the aponeuroses of the three flat muscles pass anterior to the rectus abdominis to form the anterior layer of the rectus sheath. The posterior layer of rectus sheath is formed by transversalis fascia. **Potential questions:** There can be questions related to the composition of rectus sheath both below and above the arcuate line.

<table>
<tr><th>Question</th><th>Answer</th><th>Comment</th></tr>
<tr><td>

Q10. Identify the muscle labeled A in the below image of the pelvic floor.

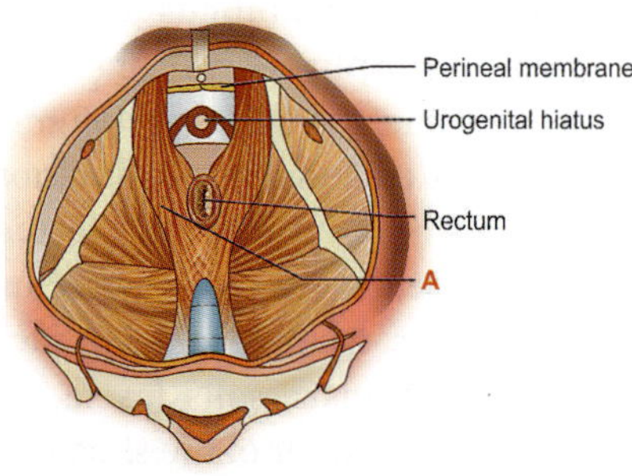

A. Pubococcygeus
B. Iliococcygeus
C. Coccygeus
D. Puborectalis
E. Obturator internus

</td><td>

Ans: A (Pubococcygeus)

Figure 10 illustrates the three layers of the muscles of pelvic floor: Muscles of the pelvic diaphragm (levator ani muscle), muscles of the urogenital diaphragm (deep transverse perineal muscle), and superficial muscles of the pelvic floor (superficial transverse perineal muscle, external anal sphincter, ischiocavernosus, and bulbospongiosus).

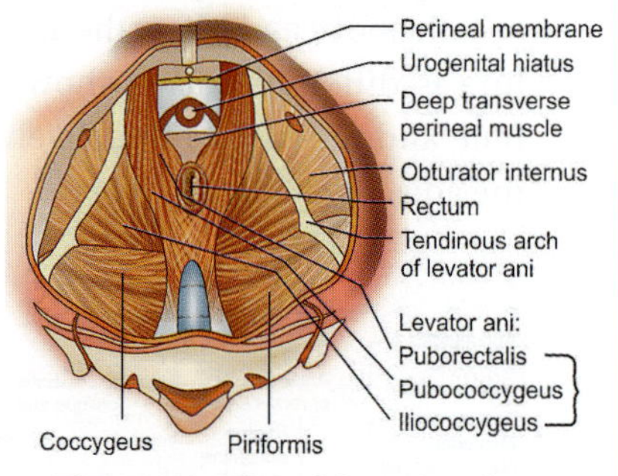

Fig. 10: Muscles of the pelvic floor.

</td><td>

Explanation: The pubococcygeus muscle is part of the levator ani group, which also includes the puborectalis, iliococcygeus, and ischiococcygeus muscles. It stretches from the pubic bone to the coccyx, forming a sling around the pelvic organs. This muscle plays a crucial role in supporting the pelvic viscera, maintaining continence, and assisting in childbirth. It is also involved in the contraction of the pelvic floor during activities such as coughing, sneezing, and lifting heavy objects

Potential questions: There can be different questions related to the various muscles of the pelvic floor.

</td></tr>
<tr><td>

Q11. The below clinical image shows a detailed view of the pelvic floor muscles. Which of the following muscles forms a supportive sling for the pelvic organs?

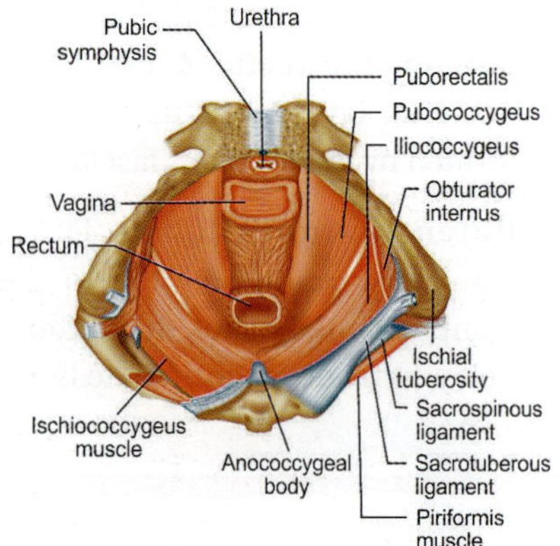

A. Ischiococcygeus muscle
B. Pubococcygeus and iliococcygeus muscles
C. Piriformis muscle
D. Pubococcygeus and ischiococcygeus muscles
E. Rectus abdominis muscle

</td><td>

Ans: B (Pubococcygeus and iliococcygeus muscles)

The levator ani group, comprising the pubococcygeus, iliococcygeus, and puborectalis muscles, helps form a supportive sling for the pelvic organs, such as the bladder, rectum, and uterus in females. This sling plays a critical role in maintaining pelvic organ support and aiding in urinary and fecal continence **(Fig. 11)**. Defects in these muscles can lead to conditions like pelvic organ prolapse.

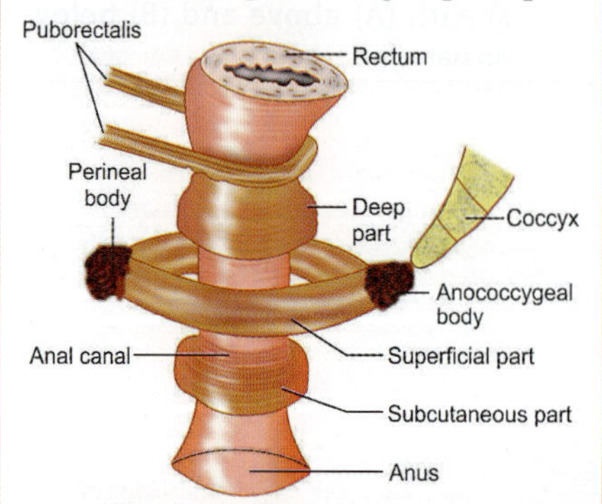

Fig. 11: Sling formed by levator ani muscles.

</td><td>

Explanation: The puborectalis muscle forms a sling around the rectum, creating the anorectal angle, which is important for maintaining fecal continence. It originates from the posterior surface of the pubic bones and wraps around the rectum, pulling it forward.

Some of the inner fibers of puborectalis fuse with the outer vaginal wall as they pass lateral to it. Other fibers decussate between the vagina and rectum in the region of perineal body. The decussating fibers divide the space between the two levator ani muscles into an anterior portion (hiatus urogenitalis), through which pass the urethra and vagina, and a posterior portion (hiatus rectalis), through which passes the rectum.

Potential questions: There can be questions related to different parts and functions of the levator ani muscle.

</td></tr>
</table>

<table>
<tr><th>Question</th><th>Answer</th><th>Comment</th></tr>
<tr>
<td>

Q12. Identify the ligament labeled A in the below image, which provides primary support to the uterus by extending from the lateral pelvic walls to the cervix.

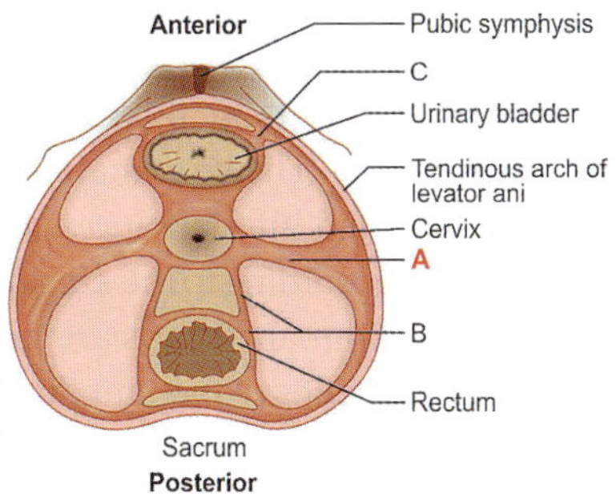

A. Broad ligament
B. Round ligament
C. Uterosacral ligament
D. Cardinal (transverse cervical) ligament
E. Pubocervical ligament

</td>
<td>

Ans: D [Cardinal (transverse cervical) ligament]

Figure 12 shows different ligamentous supports of the uterus, which include the cardinal ligaments, uterosacral ligaments, pubourethral ligaments, urethropelvic ligaments, and vesicopelvic ligaments. These ligaments play a significant role in maintaining the position of the uterus within the pelvic cavity and preventing uterine prolapse.

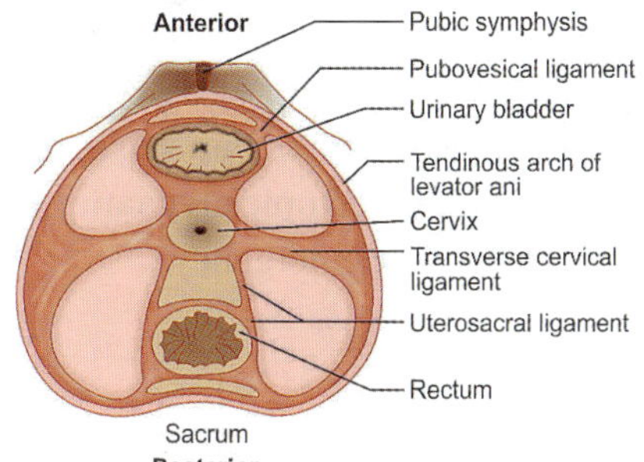

Fig. 12: Different ligamentous supports of the uterus.

</td>
<td>

Explanation: The cardinal (transverse cervical) ligament is a key structure in providing support to the uterus. It extends from the lateral pelvic walls to the cervix and the upper part of the vagina. This ligament contains the uterine artery and vein, which are crucial for the blood supply to the uterus.

The uterosacral ligaments provide attachment of the cervix to the bony sacrum at the level of S2 to S4. The pubourethral ligaments provide support to the middle portion of the urethra by anchoring it to the undersurface of the pubic bone. The urethropelvic ligaments are composed of the levator fascia. This ligament provides support to the urethra by helping in its attachment to the tendinous arc. On the other hand, the vesicopelvic ligament provides support to the bladder by facilitating its attachment to the tendinous arc.

Potential questions: There can be questions related to different supporting structures of the uterus.

</td>
</tr>
<tr>
<td>

Q13. Identify the structure labeled A in the image below, which serves as a central point of attachment for several perineal muscles.

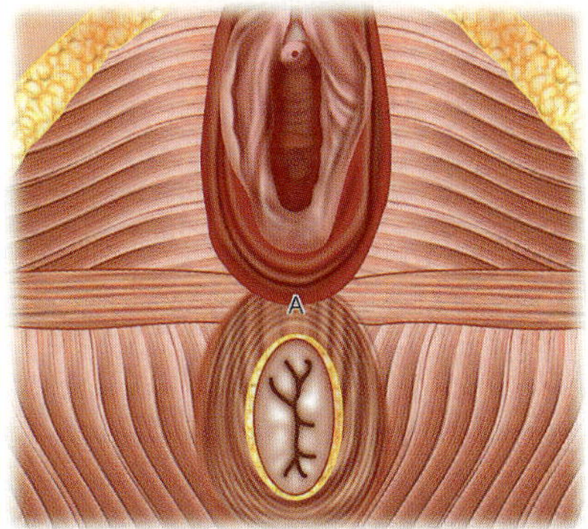

A. Ischiocavernosus muscle
B. Bulbospongiosus muscle
C. Perineal body
D. External anal sphincter
E. Internal anal sphincter

</td>
<td>

Ans: C (Perineal body)

The perineal body, also known as the central tendon of the perineum, is a pyramid-shaped fibromuscular mass located at the midpoint of the perineum, between the urogenital and anal triangles. It lies at the level of the junction between the middle third and lower one-third of the posterior vaginal wall.

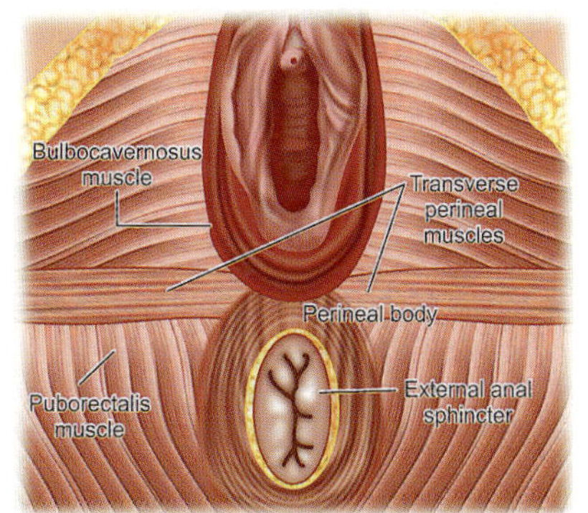

Fig. 13: Perineal body.

</td>
<td>

Explanation: Perineal body assumes importance in providing support to the pelvic organs as it provides attachment to the following eight muscles of the pelvic floor **(Fig. 13)**: Superficial and deep transverse perineal muscles and the levator ani muscles of both the sides, bulbocavernosus anteriorly, and the external anal sphincter posteriorly. Therefore, it plays a vital role in maintaining the integrity of the pelvic diaphragm and pelvic viscera.

Potential questions: There can be questions related to various muscles attached to the perineal body.

</td>
</tr>
</table>

GYNECOLOGICAL/GENERAL PHYSICAL EXAMINATION

Question	Answer	Comment
Q14. A patient presents with severe pain in the abdominal quadrant marked by letter A in the below image. Her pregnancy test is also positive. Which of the following conditions is most likely associated with this pain? 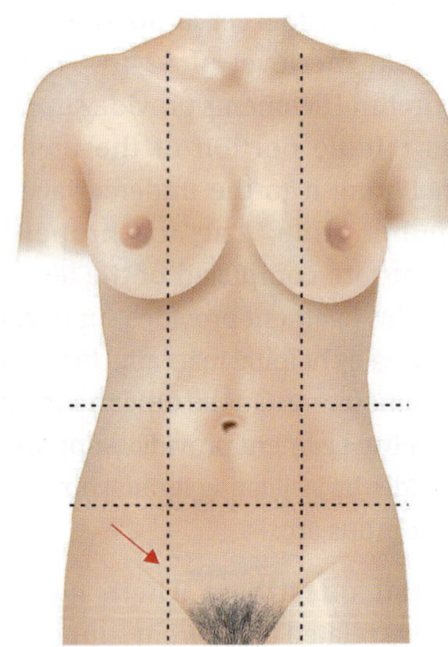 A. Cholecystitis B. Appendicitis C. Ectopic pregnancy D. Pancreatitis E. Splenic rupture	**Ans: C (Ectopic pregnancy)** The arrow in the adjacent image points toward the right iliac region. Nine abdominal quadrants which can be identified over the abdominal region are shown in **Figure 14**. Ectopic pregnancy can cause severe pain in the right iliac quadrant or left iliac quadrant of the abdomen, depending on the location of the ectopic implantation. A positive pregnancy test in conjunction with pain in the right iliac region raises a high suspicion for ectopic pregnancy, which is a medical emergency. 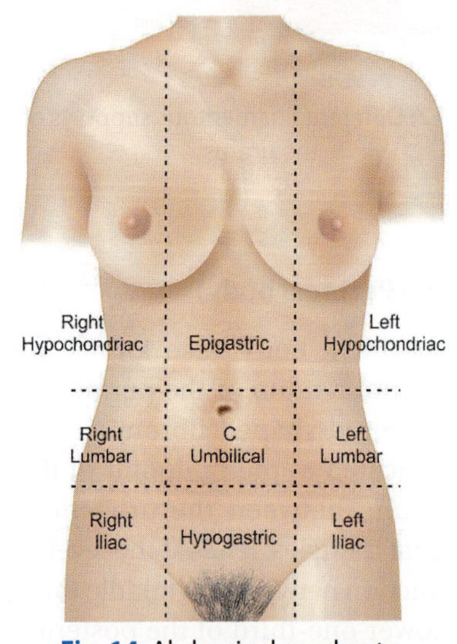 **Fig. 14:** Abdominal quadrants.	**Explanation:** The various abdominal quadrants are as follows: The umbilical region is around the umbilicus, the region above the umbilical region is epigastric region, and the region below the umbilical region is hypogastric region. The six remaining regions are divided into left and right and are named according to the area of the spine: The lumbar regions are on the left and right sides of the umbilical region. The regions on either side of the hypogastric are known as the left iliac and right iliac regions. The two regions on either side of the epigastric are termed the hypochondriac regions. **Potential questions:** There can be questions related to findings on abdominal examination of each of the quadrants.

Question	Answer	Comment
Q15. A gynecological examination reveals a cervix with a small, circular external os as shown in the image below. Which of the following best describes the patient's obstetric history? 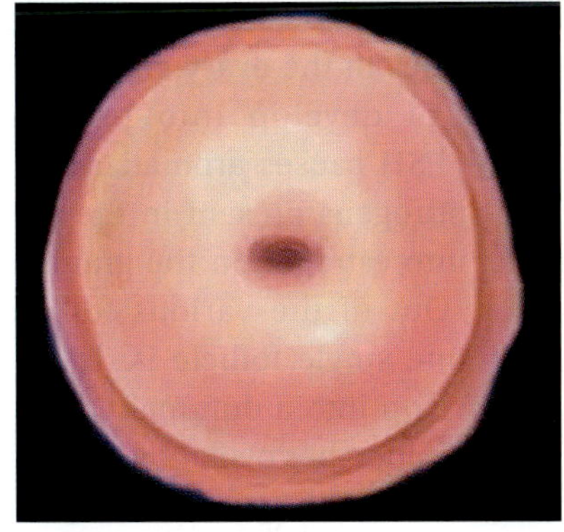 A. Multiparous woman B. Nulliparous woman C. Woman with a history of cervical surgery D. Postmenopausal woman E. Woman with a history of cervical cancer	**Ans: B (Nulliparous woman)** A nulliparous cervix appears to have a circular os as shown in the adjacent photograph. In this case, the nulliparous cervical os appears normal on per speculum examination and no further treatment is required. 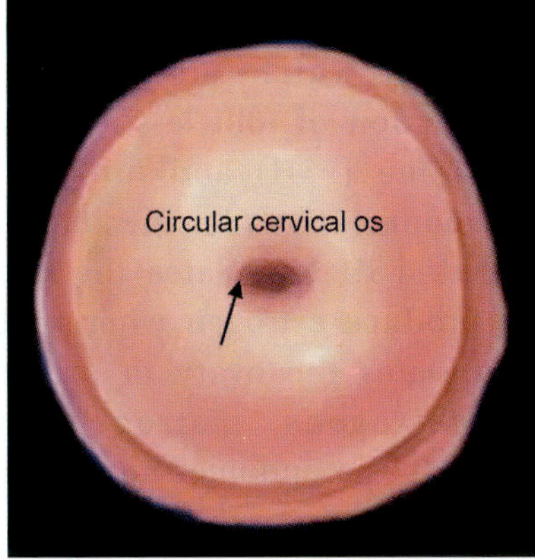 **Fig. 15:** Appearance of nulliparous cervical os.	**Explanation:** The appearance of the cervix can vary widely, depending on the age, parity, and estrogen status of the patient. The nulliparous cervical os is smooth and round, reflecting the lack of previous cervical dilation and stretching associated with labor and delivery **(Fig. 15)**. This characteristic appearance helps clinicians distinguish between nulliparous and multiparous women during a pelvic examination. **Potential questions:** There can be questions related to the appearance of cervix in various conditions: Physiological as well as pathological.
Q16. A gynecological examination reveals appearance of cervix as shown in the image below. Which of the following best describes the patient's obstetric history 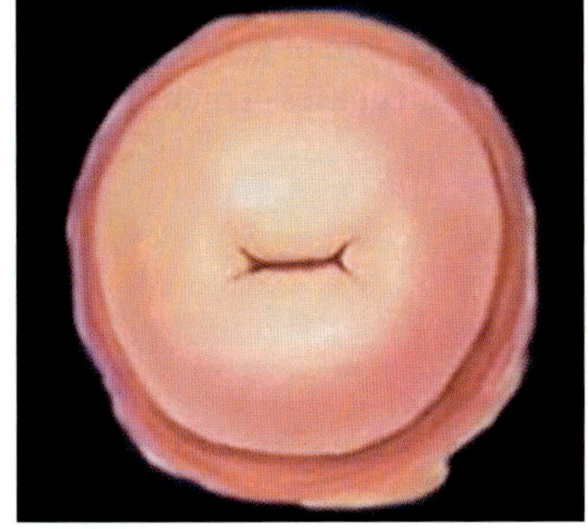 A. Nulliparous woman B. Multiparous woman C. Woman with a history of cervical surgery D. Postmenopausal woman E. Woman with a history of cervical cancer	**Ans: B (Multiparous woman)** A multiparous cervical os appears to have a transverse (horizontal) slit as shown in the adjacent figure. This appears to be a normal feature on per speculum examination and no further treatment is required. 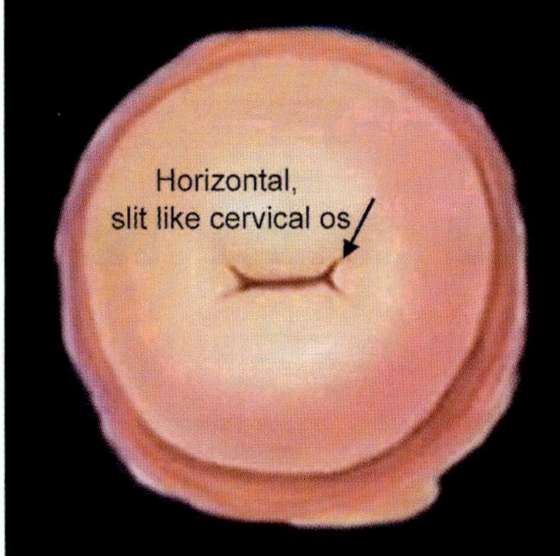 **Fig. 16:** Appearance of multiparous cervical os.	**Explanation:** Following childbirth, the outer appearance of external cervical os changes. It becomes wider and acquires a "fish-mouth" appearance **(Fig. 16)**. Moreover, the squamocolumnar junction can also be more easily visualized following normal vaginal delivery. This change occurs due to the stretching and dilation of the cervix during childbirth. This contrasts with the small, circular external os seen in nulliparous women. Recognizing these differences is important for clinicians during pelvic examinations to accurately assess a patient's obstetric history. **Potential questions:** There can be questions related to the appearance of cervix in various conditions: Physiological as well as pathological.

MENSTRUAL CYCLE

Question	Answer	Comment
Q17. The image below shows the interaction between hypothalamus and anterior pituitary gland. Identify the hormone depicted by the letter A in this image. 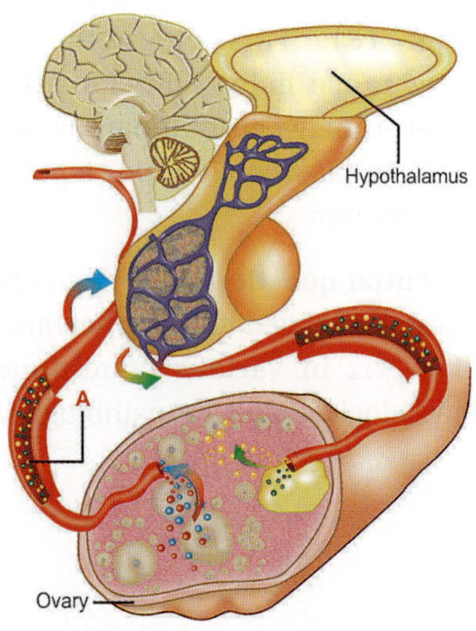 A. Follicle-stimulating hormone (FSH) and luteinizing hormone (LH) B. Estrogen and progesterone C. GnRH D. Options A + B E. Options A + C	**Ans: B (Estrogen and progesterone)** The adjacent image demonstrates the pathophysiology of menstruation, which is under the regulation of hormones produced by hypothalamus and pituitary gland. As shown in **Figure 17**, hypothalamus produces gonadotropins (GnRh), which stimulate the production of follicle-stimulating hormone (FSH) and luteinizing hormone (LH) from the pituitary gland. FSH stimulates the ovary to produce estrogen whereas LH stimulates the ovary to produce progestogens. Estrogen stimulates the endometrium to progress into the proliferative phase, whereas progestogens stimulate the endometrium to progress into the luteal phase. If pregnancy does not occur, the corpus luteum (CL) ceases to produce progestogens, which causes the spasm of arteriolar vessels, eventually resulting in menstrual flow and shedding of endometrium. 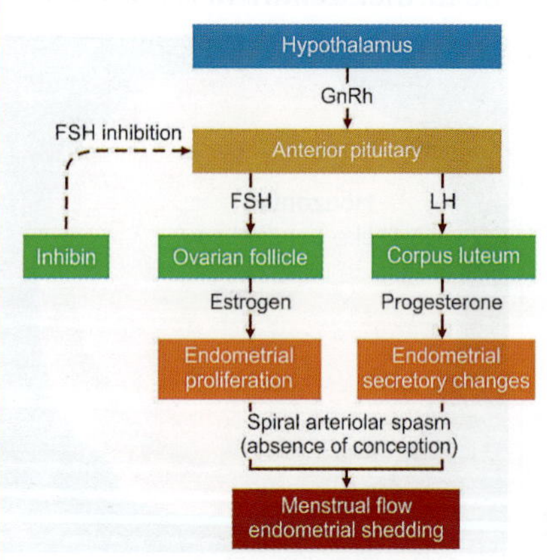 **Fig. 17:** Pathophysiology of menstruation.	**Explanation:** Initial follicular development is independent of hormonal influence. However, soon FSH, which is produced by pituitary, takes control and stimulates a cohort of follicles in the ovary encouraging them to develop into preantral stage. FSH causes aromatization of the androgens present in the theca cells into estrogen in the granulosa cells. Out of the various follicles, only one single follicle is destined to develop into a dominant follicle, which undergoes ovulation. With the progression of the proliferative phase, there is an increased production of estrogen. Besides causing a decline in FSH levels, the mid-follicular rise in estradiol levels also exerts a positive feedback influence on LH secretion. The presence of LH prior to ovulation is important for optimal follicular development, which ultimately results in the formation of a healthy oocyte. **Potential questions:** There can be different questions related to the pathophysiology of menstruation as well as the role of various hormones in different phases of menstruation.

Question	Answer	Comment
Q18. The image below shows histological changes in the endometrium across a particular phase of menstrual cycle. Based on the pathophysiology of the menstrual cycle, what is the predominant hormonal change during this phase? 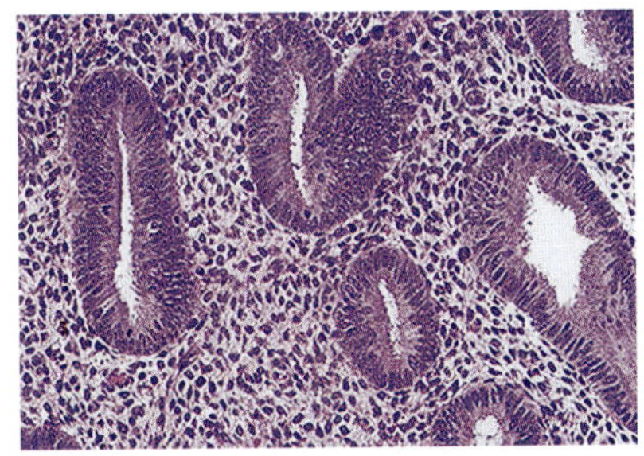 A. Decrease in follicle-stimulating hormone (FSH) levels B. Increase in estrogen levels C. Surge in luteinizing hormone (LH) D. Progesterone peak E. Endometrial shedding	**Ans: B (Increase in estrogen levels)** The adjacent image depicts the histological picture of the endometrium in the proliferative (follicular) phase, which extends from day 5 to day 14 of the typical cycle. In this phase, the endometrial proliferation occurs under estrogen stimulation. This phase ends as ovulation occurs. Various events occurring in a normal menstrual cycle are described in **Figure 18**. 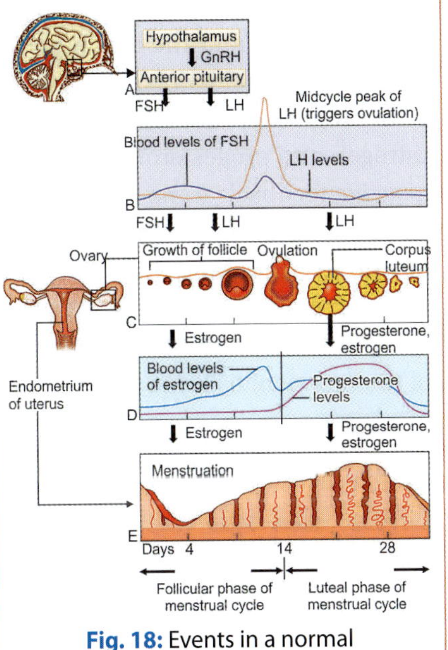 **Fig. 18:** Events in a normal menstrual cycle.	**Explanation:** During the follicular phase, which spans from the start of menstruation to ovulation, FSH promotes the maturation of ovarian follicles. The following changes take place during the proliferative phase: ▪ The functional and the basal layers of endometrium become well defined. The proliferation mainly occurs in the functional layer. ▪ The basal layer measures 1 mm in thickness, while the functional layer reaches a maximum thickness of about 3.5–5 mm by 14th day. ▪ There occurs marked cellular proliferation of the endometrium and an increase in the length and tortuosity of the spiral arteries. ▪ Endometrial glands develop and contain some glycogen. **Potential questions:** There can be different questions related to the pathophysiology of menstruation as well as the role of various hormones in different phases of menstruation.

<table>
<tr><th>Question</th><th>Answer</th><th>Comment</th></tr>
<tr>
<td>

Q19. The image below shows histological changes in the endometrium across a particular phase of menstrual cycle. Based on the pathophysiology of the menstrual cycle, what is the main event occurring during this phase?

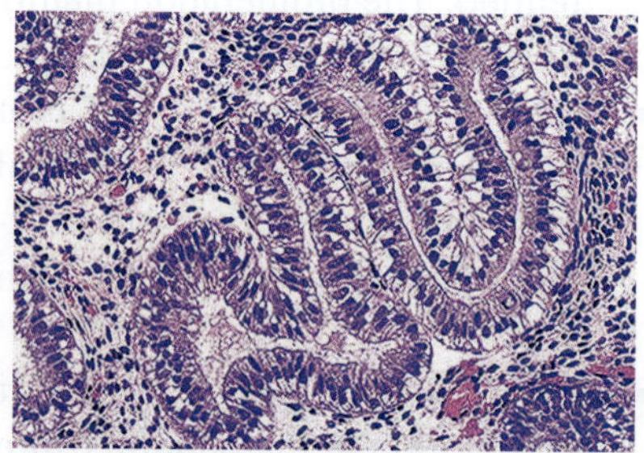

A. Proliferation of the endometrial lining
B. Increased glandular secretion and vascularization
C. Shedding of the functional layer of the endometrium
D. Decrease in estrogen levels
E. Ovulation triggered by luteinizing hormone (LH) surge

</td>
<td>

Ans: B (Increased glandular secretion and vascularization)

The adjacent image shows a histological picture of the endometrium in the secretory phase. The secretory phase is marked by production of progesterone and less potent estrogens by the corpus luteum (CL). It extends from day 15 to day 28 of the typical cycle. Various phases of menstrual cycle are described in **Figure 19**.

If pregnancy occurs, the placenta produces human chorionic gonadotropin (hCG) to replace progesterone, and the endometrium (and the accompanying pregnancy) is maintained.

If pregnancy does not occur, the estrogen and progesterone levels cause negative feedback at the hypothalamus, resulting in the fall in the levels of the hormones FSH and LH. The spiral arteries contract and have reduced blood flow. This causes disintegration of the functionalis layer and eventually menses.

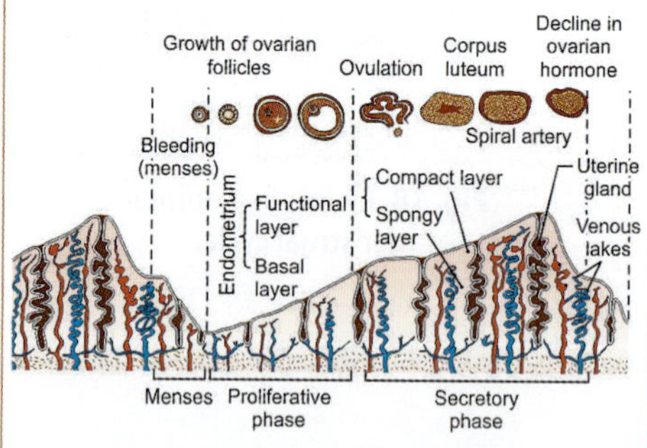

Fig. 19: Phases of endometrium.

</td>
<td>

Explanation: The endometrial features of the secretory phase include the following:

- The most characteristic feature of this phase is development of subnuclear vacuolation in the glandular epithelial cells. In this, the glycogen-filled vacuoles develop between the nuclei and the basement membrane (by the day 17–18).
- The endometrium measures about 8–10 mm in the secretory phase.
- The glands become crenated and tortuous to assume a characteristic corkscrew-shaped appearance. The corkscrew pattern of the glands becomes saw-toothed in the later part of the secretory phase.
- The stroma of the functional layer becomes edematous further.
- The functional layer of the endometrium can be divided into two layers: Superficial and deep.
- The spiral vessels become dense and deeply coiled.

Potential questions: There can be different questions related to the pathophysiology of menstruation as well as the role of various hormones in different phases of menstruation.

</td>
</tr>
</table>

<table>
<tr><th>Question</th><th>Answer</th><th>Comment</th></tr>
<tr>
<td>

Q20. The below image depicts hormone levels fluctuating during the menstrual cycle. What hormone levels are depicted by the letter B in the image?

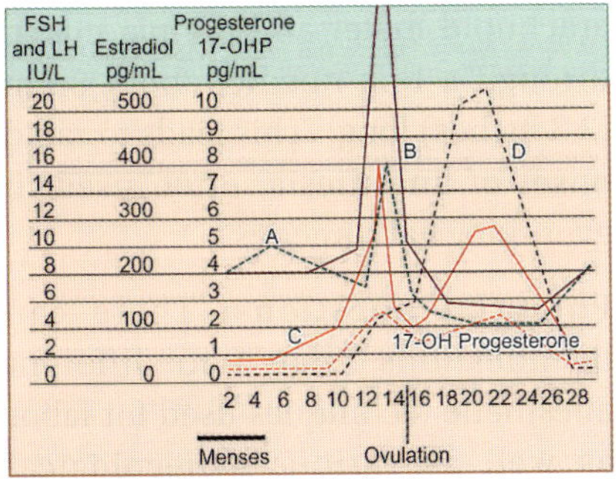

A. Estrogen
B. Progesterone
C. Luteinizing hormone (LH)
D. Follicle-stimulating hormone (FSH)
E. Inhibin

</td>
<td>

Ans: C (Luteinizing hormone)

Figure 20 illustrates changes in the levels of hormones during various phases of menstrual cycle. Increased levels of estrogen during the follicular phase exert a negative feedback effect on FSH production due to which growth of all the follicles except one, "the dominant follicle", is inhibited. A surge of luteinizing hormone (LH) takes place just prior to ovulation. This initiates luteinization and progesterone production in the granulosa layer. A preovulatory risein progesterone facilitates the positive feedback action of estrogen and may be required to induce the midcycle FSH peak.

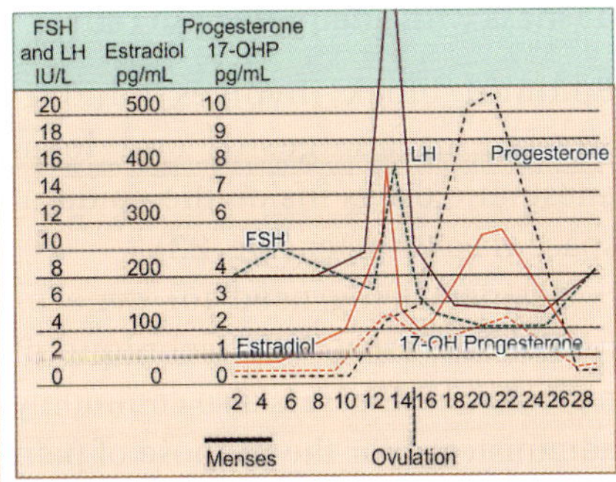

Fig. 20: Levels of various hormones during different phases of the menstrual cycle.

</td>
<td>

Explanation: Just before ovulation, there is a surge in LH levels, which is essential for triggering ovulation. This is known as the LH surge, and it is a key event in the menstrual cycle, marking the transition from the follicular phase to the luteal phase.

Estrogen levels peak before the LH surge, aiding in its stimulation but does not directly trigger ovulation.

Progesterone levels rise after ovulation, as it is secreted by the corpus luteum.

Ovulation occurs about 10–12 hours after the LH peak and 24–36 hours after the peak estradiol levels have been attained. The onset of LH surge is the most reliable indicator of impending ovulation.

Potential questions: There can be different questions related to the pathophysiology of menstruation as well as the role of various hormones in different phases of menstruation.

</td>
</tr>
</table>

PRINCIPLES OF SURGERY/ANESTHESIA

Question	Answer	Comment
Q21. The image below shows the administration of a spinal block for a gynecological procedure. Which anatomical space is targeted when performing a spinal block? 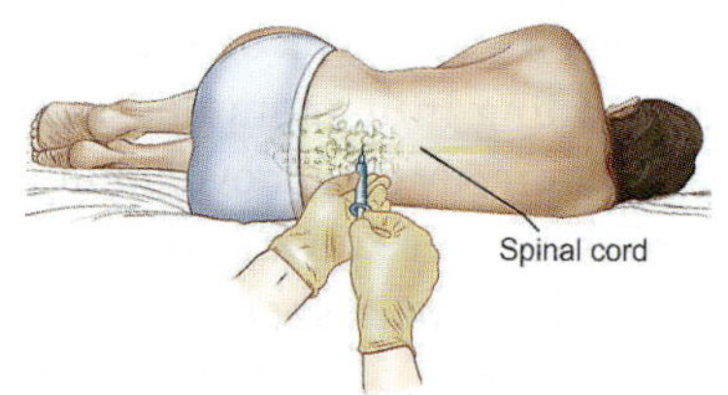 A. Epidural space B. Subarachnoid space C. Subdural space D. Intervertebral disc space E. Intravascular space	**Ans: B (Subarachnoid space)** Regional anesthesia has currently become the most effective means of providing analgesia during labor. The two most commonly used procedures for regional anesthesia are the spinal **(Fig. 21)** and epidural **(Fig. 22)** blocks. 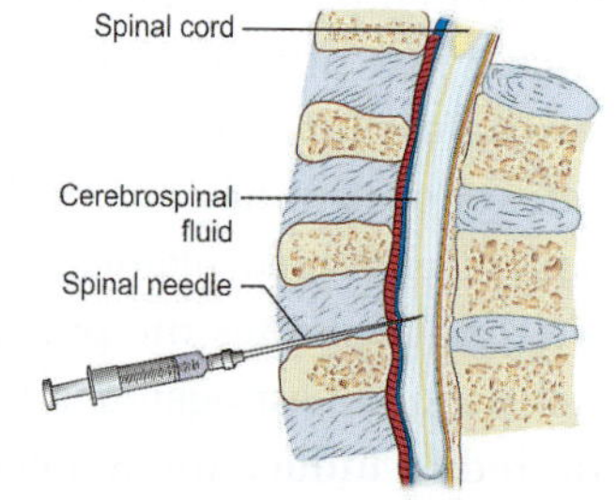 **Fig. 21:** Spinal block.	**Explanation:** The procedure of spinal anesthesia involves injection of a local anesthetic agent into the cerebrospinal fluid in the subarachnoid space [lying between the arachnoid mater and the pia mater, through a fine needle, about 9 cm (3.5 inches) long]. This leads to rapid onset of anesthesia, often used in gynecological surgeries. **Potential questions:** There can be questions related to different anesthetic techniques used for labor as well as various gynecological surgeries.
Q22. In the below image, an epidural block is being administered prior to gynecological surgery. What is the primary benefit of using an epidural block over general anesthesia in such surgeries? 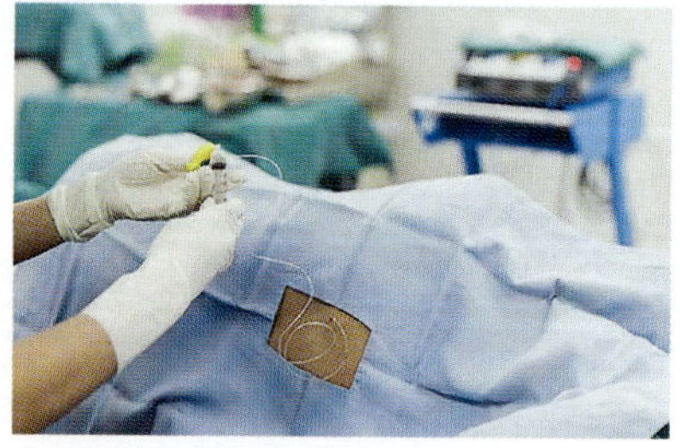 A. Faster recovery post surgery B. Complete loss of sensation in the whole body C. Preservation of consciousness with adequate pain relief D. Reduced risk of postoperative bleeding E. Full muscle paralysis during surgery	**Ans: C (Preservation of consciousness with adequate pain relief)** Epidural block involves administration of analgesics and local anesthetic drugs inside the epidural space via a catheter **(Fig. 22)**. Besides being used for gynecological surgeries, this technique of regional anesthesia is also commonly administered for the purpose of pain relief during labor. 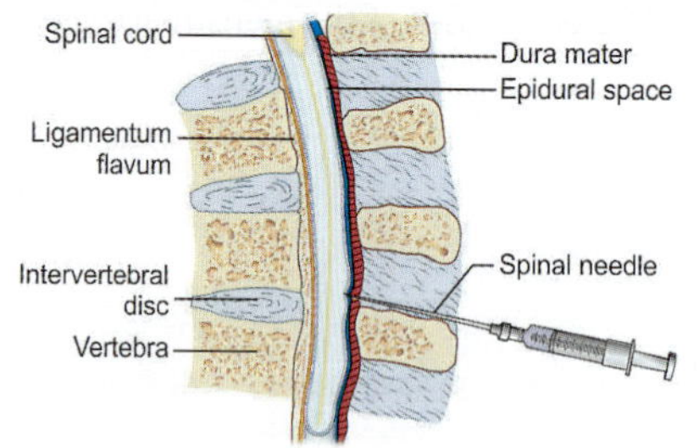 **Fig. 22:** Epidural block.	**Explanation:** An epidural block is often preferred in gynecological surgeries as it allows for significant pain relief while the patient remains conscious. This technique is effective at blocking pain in the lower abdomen and pelvic region, which is essential for many gynecological procedures. Unlike general anesthesia, it does not result in complete loss of consciousness and is associated with fewer postoperative side effects, such as nausea or delayed recovery. Moreover, it does not cause muscle paralysis like some general anesthetics, making it a safer option for many patients. **Potential questions:** There can be questions related to different anesthetic techniques used for labor as well as various gynecological surgeries.

Question	Answer	Comment
Q23. The image below depicts a type of nerve block procedure being performed transvaginally for the excision of Bartholin cyst. Which nerve function is blocked? 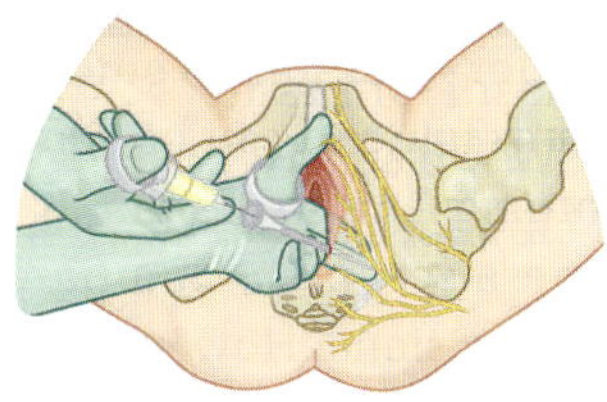 A. Innervation of the uterine smooth muscle B. Sensory supply to lower vagina and perineum C. Motor innervation to pelvic floor only D. The nerve controlling uterine blood supply E. Sensory innervation to ovaries	**Ans: B (Sensory supply to lower vagina and perineum)** The adjacent image depicts the procedure of pudendal nerve block, which blocks the pudendal nerve (S2–S4) using local anesthetic via a needle and guide. Injection is at the lesser sciatic foramen, ~1 cm inferior and medial to the attachment of sacrospinous ligament to the ischial spine **(Fig. 23)**. 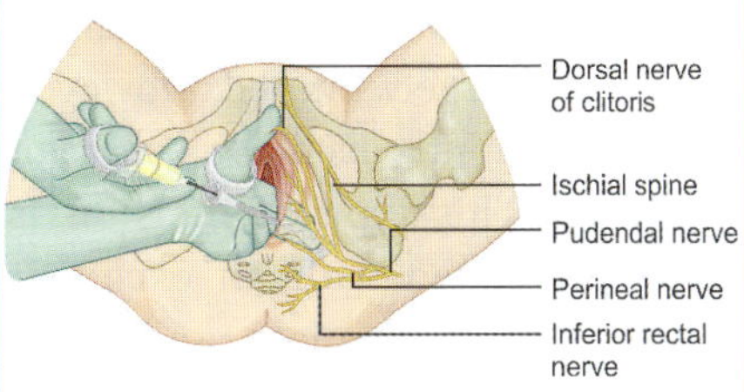 **Fig. 23:** Transvaginal pudendal nerve block.	**Explanation:** The pudendal nerve (S2–S4) supplies sensory and motor innervation to the lower vagina and perineum. Pudendal block is used during vaginal deliveries and gynecological procedures to provide anesthesia. While it also controls the external anal and part of the urethral sphincter, its main role here is pain relief in the lower vagina and perineum. **Potential questions:** There can be questions related to different anesthetic techniques used for labor as well as various gynecological surgeries.
Q24. Which landmarks best describe the nerve block shown in the image below: 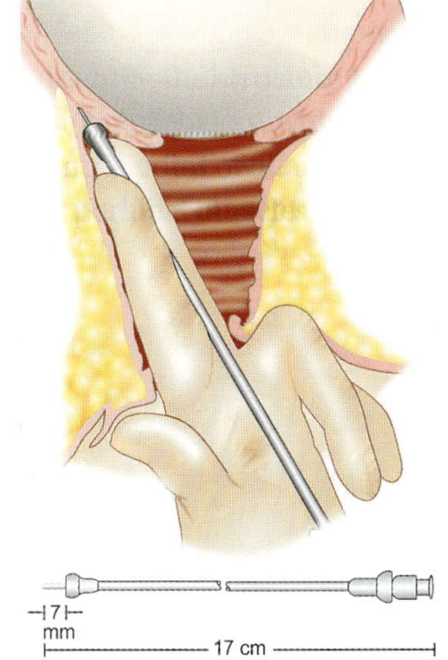 A. 2, 4, 8, 10 O'clock B. 12 & 6 O'clock C. 2 & 10 O'clock D. 4 & 10 O'clock E. 1 & 7 O'clock?	**Ans: A (Injection at 2, 4, 8, and 10 O'clock positions of the cervix)** The adjacent image shows administration of paracervical nerve block, an anesthetic procedure which involves injecting local anesthetic into the vaginal fornices along the cervix. It is simple, safe, and effective, ideal for dilatation and curettage, and can also be used for minor cervical procedures like cervical repair, conization, LEEP, or Shirodkar/Wurm operations. 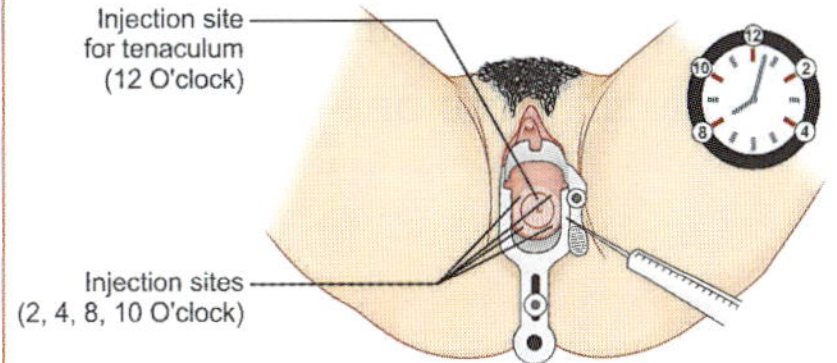 **Fig. 24:** Paracervical nerve block (sites of injection).	**Explanation:** Paracervical block involves injecting lidocaine at the cervicovaginal junctions (2, 4, 8, and 10 O'clock) after grasping the cervix at 12 O'clock. It targets the paracervical ganglia to provide anesthesia for cervical dilation or manipulation, with injections 3–7 mm deep into the fornices. A two-point technique (4 and 8 O'clock) may also be used. Maximum lidocaine dose: 4.5 mg/kg (200 mg). Its use has declined with the gaining popularity of epidural and spinal anesthesia. **Potential questions:** There can be questions related to different anesthetic techniques used for labor as well as various gynecological surgeries.

INCISIONS

<table>
<tr><th>Question</th><th>Answer</th><th>Comment</th></tr>
<tr><td>

Q25. A patient is undergoing a cesarean section, and the surgeon plans to use an incision as shown in the image below. Based on the below image, which of the following statements about this incision is most accurate?

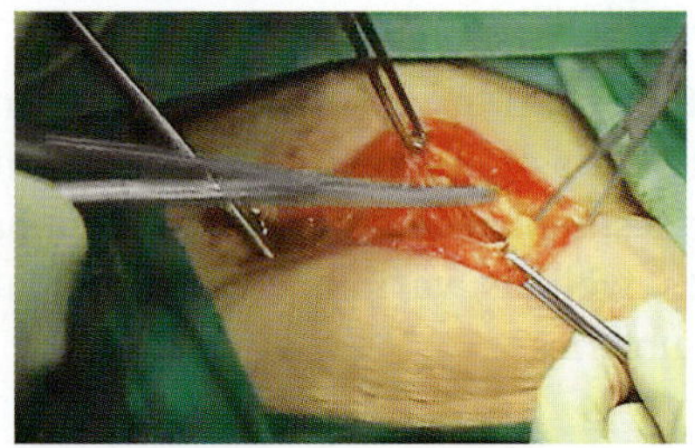

A. It is made transversely, just below the umbilicus
B. It is made transversely, just above the pubic symphysis
C. It provides the fastest access to the abdominal cavity
D. It results in higher postoperative pain than midline incisions
E. It is less cosmetically appealing compared to midline incisions.

</td><td>

Ans: B (It is made transversely, just above the pubic symphysis)

The abdominal incision shown in the adjacent image is the Pfannenstiel incision. The use of this incision is associated with good exposure to the central pelvis but limited exposure to the lateral pelvis and upper abdomen. As a result, the usefulness of this incision for gynecologic cancer surgery is largely limited. However, it is commonly used for cesarean delivery. This type of incision is also associated with an excellent postoperative strength and good cosmetic result.

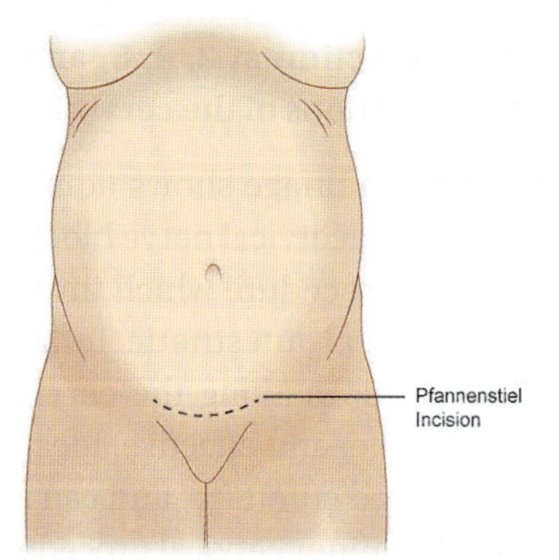

Fig. 25: Location of Pfannenstiel incision.

</td><td>

Explanation: The Pfannenstiel incision is a low transverse incision made just above the pubic symphysis **(Fig. 25)**. This type of incision is favored for its aesthetic outcome, as the scar is low and can be concealed by clothing. It also results in lower postoperative pain compared to vertical incisions. However, there is an increased risk of hematoma or seroma formation due to the large extent of dissection required and greater operating time.

Potential questions: There can be questions related to different types of incisions administered in the clinical gynecological surgical practice.

</td></tr>
</table>

Question	Answer	Comment
Q26. A gynecological surgeon is planning a surgery to remove a large fibroid. In order to gain wider access, she performs an incision as shown in the image below. Based on the below image, which of the following statements about this incision is correct? 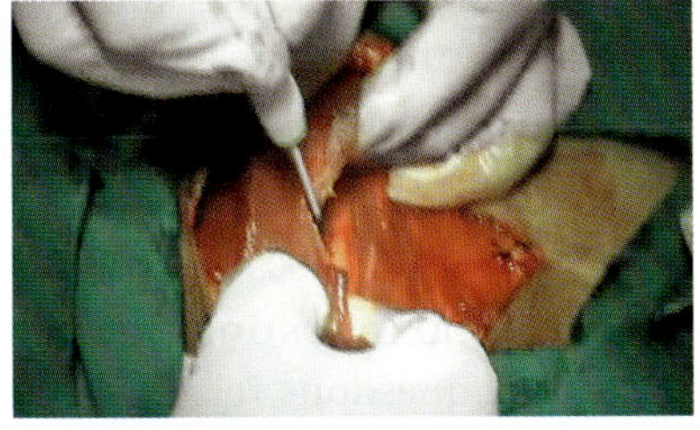 A. It is a vertical incision made along the midline of the abdomen B. It involves transection of the rectus abdominis muscles C. It is made just above the umbilicus. D. It does not require cutting through any muscle layers E. It provides faster abdominal access than the Pfannenstiel incision	**Ans: B (It involves transection of the rectus abdominis muscles)** The incision being shown in the adjacent image is Maylard's incision. It is different from Pfannenstiel incision in the sense that instead of separating the rectus muscles and fascia, the rectus muscles are cut transversely as shown in **Figure 26**. 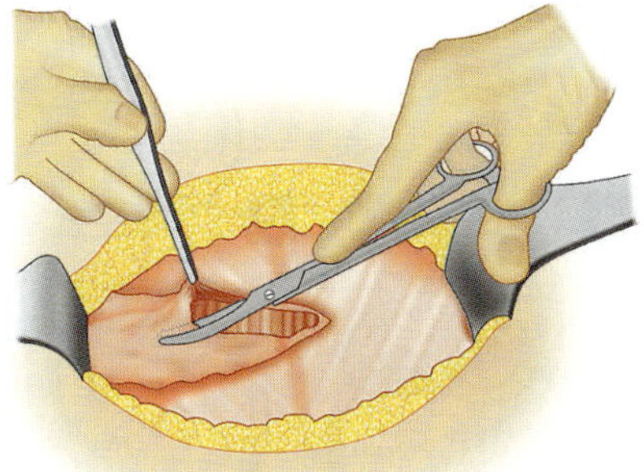 **Fig. 26:** Transection of rectus abdominis muscle (Maylard's incision).	**Explanation:** Maylard's incision requires transection of the rectus abdominis muscles. It is often used in cases requiring more extensive access than achieved via Pfannenstiel incision, such as large fibroid removal or other gynecological surgeries. However, it is associated with more postoperative pain and longer recovery period due to muscle transection. The disadvantage of using Maylard's incision is that this incision requires more time to accomplish and can be associated with potential blood loss in comparison to other incisions. **Potential questions:** There can be questions related to different types of incisions administered in the clinical gynecological surgical practice.
Q27. A surgeon is performing Cherney incision for a gynecological procedure. Based on the below image, which structure is being identified prior to its detachment? 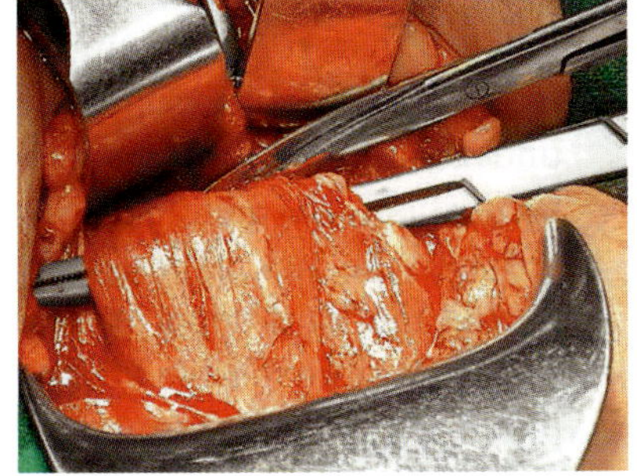 A. Rectus abdominis B. Pyramidalis C. Rectus sheath D. Internal oblique muscle E. External oblique muscle	**Ans: A (Rectus abdominis)** Cherney incision is similar to Pfannenstiel incision, except for the fact that in the Pfannenstiel incision the rectus muscles are separated, while in the Cherney incision, these muscles are detached from their insertion over the pubic bone (as shown in **Fig. 27**). 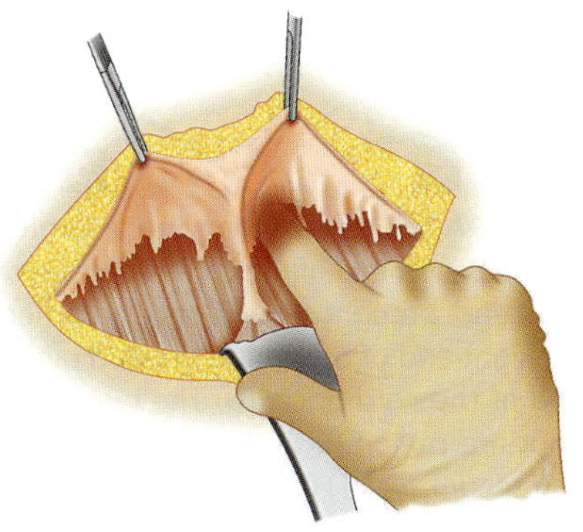 **Fig. 27:** Transection of the tendons of the rectus muscle.	**Explanation:** The Cherney incision is a transverse abdominal incision similar to the Pfannenstiel incision, but with one major difference: It involves the detachment of the rectus abdominis tendons from the pubic symphysis. This technique allows better access to the pelvic organs and is often used when deeper pelvic access is needed. The tendons are reattached after the surgery, which allows for greater exposure at the time of surgery while maintaining muscle function postoperatively. **Potential questions:** There can be questions related to different types of incisions administered in the clinical gynecological surgical practice.

SURGICAL KNOTS

Question	Answer	Comment
Q28. During a gynecological procedure, the surgeon is shown tying a knot, as demonstrated in the below image. Which of the following statements about this knot is correct? 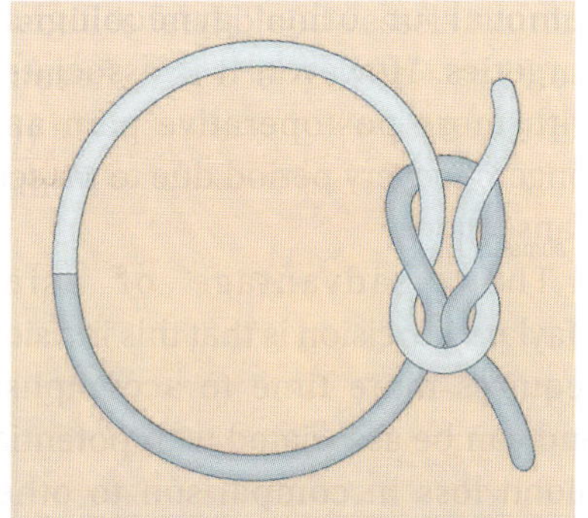 A. It requires two throws in the same direction B. It is less secure than a granny knot C. It requires alternating the direction of each throw D. It is used primarily for temporary suturing E. It is only used for deep tissue closure	**Ans: C (It requires alternating the direction of each throw)** The knot shown in the adjacent image is a square knot. A square knot can be considered as the most secure surgical knot commonly used in surgical procedures, including gynecological surgeries, for tying sutures. 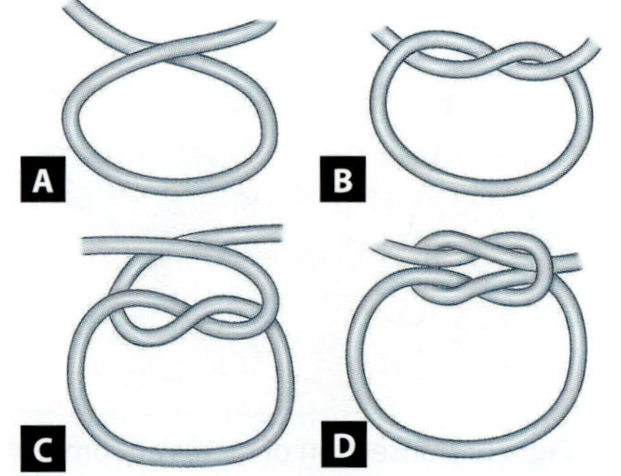 **Figs. 28A to D:** Steps for tying a square knot: (A and B) Right end of the cord is crossed over the left end and brought around once; (C) Left end of the cord is crossed over the right end of the cord once; (D) The two ends of the knot are pulled until the knot becomes tight and secure.	**Explanation:** A square knot is formed by making two throws, each in opposite directions (one clockwise and the other counterclockwise), ensuring that the knot stays tight and secure **(Figs. 28A to D)**. This technique helps in preventing slippage, making the square knot more secure than a granny knot, which involves throws in the same direction and is less stable. **Potential questions:** There can be questions related to the various types of knots used in the surgical practice.
Q29. In the image provided, which type of knot is shown? This knot is commonly used in gynecological surgeries to ensure secure tissue approximation, especially when handling slippery sutures or in areas of high tension.  A. Half hitch knot B. Square knot C. Surgeon's knot D. Granny knot E. Slip knot	**Ans: C (Surgeon's knot)** Surgeon's knot is the same as a square knot except that the first throw is a double one. The steps for tying a surgeon's knot are demonstrated in **Figures 29A to D**. 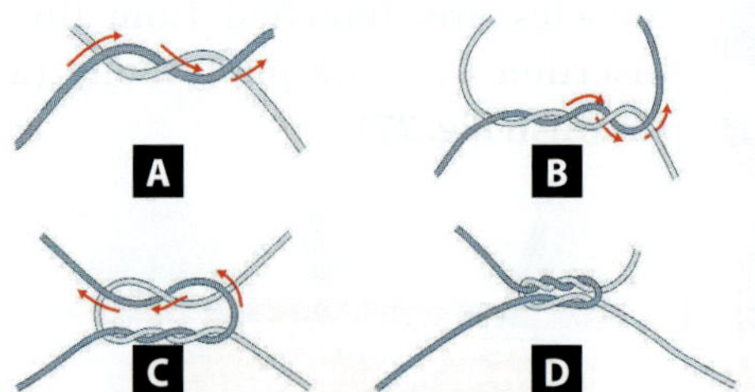 **Figs. 29A to D:** Steps for tying a surgical knot: (A and B) Left end of the cord is crossed over the right end, brought around once and then twice; (C) Right end of the cord is crossed over the left end of the cord once; (D) The two ends of the knot are pulled until the knot becomes tight and secure. (Take Figs. 5.14A to D tips and tricks, third edn)	**Explanation:** A surgeon's knot is a modification of a square knot that involves an additional twist on the first throw, providing extra friction. This makes it ideal in gynecological surgery where tissues may be slippery or under tension, ensuring a more secure hold. The additional twist reduces the risk of loosening during the knot-tying process, making it more reliable for deep tissue approximation compared to a square knot. **Potential questions:** There can be questions related to the various types of knots used in the surgical practice.

ADOLESCENT AND PEDIATRIC GYNECOLOGY

Question	Answer	Comment
Q30. Based on the image showing various stages of pubertal development in a female, which of the following represents the correct sequence of pubertal changes in women? 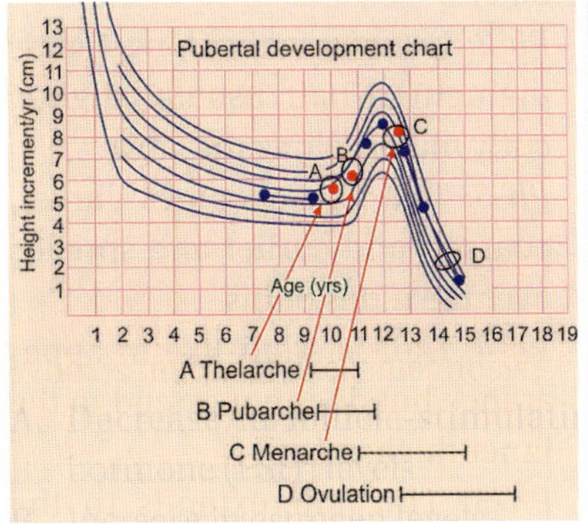 A. Menarche → Thelarche → Pubarche → Growth spurt B. Thelarche → Pubarche → Growth spurt → Menarche C. Pubarche → Thelarche → Menarche → Growth spurt D. Growth spurt → Pubarche → Menarche → Thelarche E. Thelarche → Menarche → Pubarche → Growth spurt	**Ans: B (Thelarche → Pubarche → Growth spurt → Menarche)** The correct sequence of pubertal changes in females typically starts with thelarche (development of breast tissue), followed by pubarche (development of pubic and axillary hair). The growth spurt occurs after the onset of pubarche, and menarche (the first menstrual period) typically follows later. This sequence is a hallmark of normal pubertal development in females. Various changes occurring during the normal pubertal development are described in **Figure 30**. 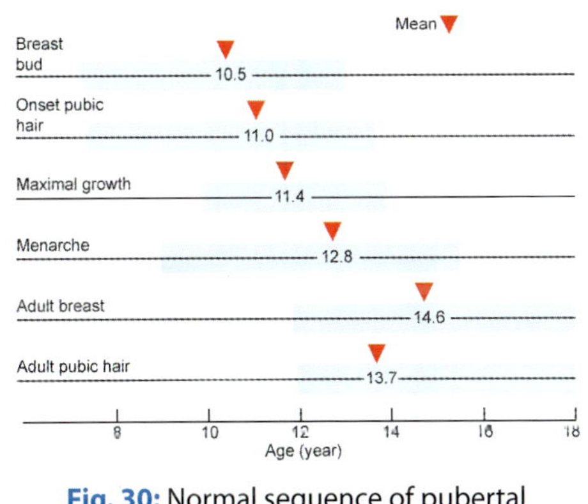 **Fig. 30:** Normal sequence of pubertal milestones.	**Explanation:** Various pubertal milestones can be described as follows: ▪ *Thelarche:* This refers to the breast development and occurs at the average age of 10.5 years. The first physical sign of puberty in girls is appearance of a firm, tender lump under center of the areola in one or both the breasts ▪ *Pubarche:* The next noticeable change of puberty is development of pubic and axillary hair, usually occurring within a few months of thelarche. ▪ *Growth spurt:* This refers to a rapid increase in height during mid-puberty. ▪ *Menarche:* This refers to the occurrence of first menstrual bleeding and typically occurs about 2 years after thelarche. **Potential questions:** There can be questions related to various pubertal milestones and their description.

Question	Answer	Comment
Q31. Based on the Tanner stages of breast development, which of the following Tanner stages corresponds to sparse, long, slightly pigmented hair along the labia in a female as shown in the image below? 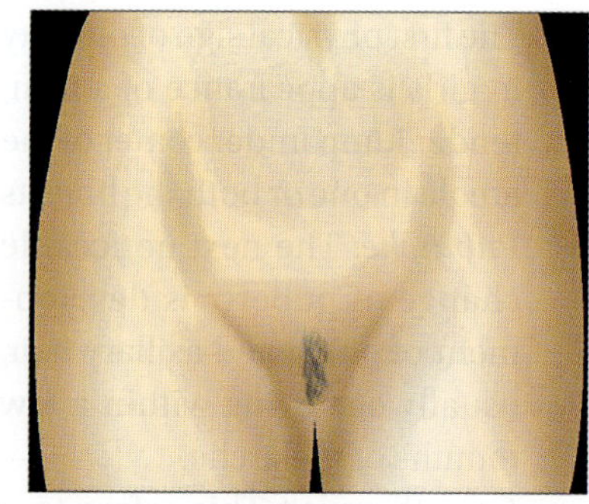 A. Tanner stage 1 B. Tanner stage 2 C. Tanner stage 3 D. Tanner stage 4 E. Tanner stage 5	**Ans: B (Tanner stage 2)** Tanner staging is used to describe the physical development of secondary sexual characteristics. The progression through the Tanner stages of pubic hair development continues with increased hair density, coarseness, and extension to the inner thighs in later stages. **Figure 31** describes the Tanner staging for the development of pubic hair in females. 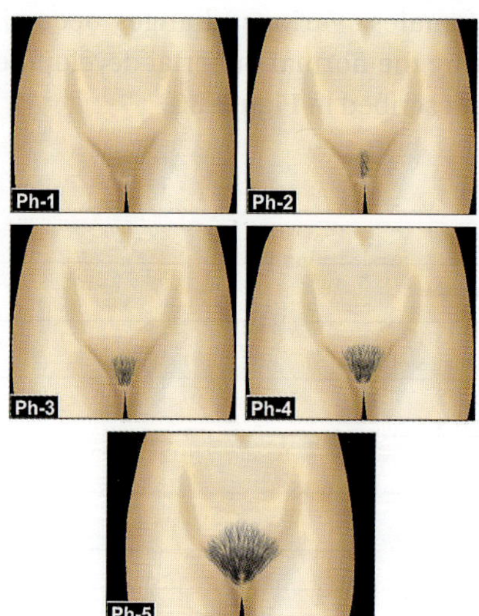 **Fig. 31:** Tanner staging for development of pubic hair in females.	**Explanation:** In Tanner stage 2, there is sparse growth of long, slightly pigmented, straight hair along the labia in females. This stage indicates the early onset of pubarche, marking the beginning of pubic hair development. Various Tanner stages can be described as follows: ▪ *Ph-1:* Prepubertal stage (no pubic hair) ▪ *Ph-2:* Sparse growth of long slightly pigmented hair usually slightly curly mainly along the labia ▪ *Ph-3:* The hair becomes darker, coarser, and curlier and spreads over the mons pubis ▪ *Ph-4:* Hair is adult-like in appearance but does not extend to the inner thighs. ▪ *Ph-5:* The hair extends to the medial surface of the thighs and is distributed as an inverse triangle. **Potential questions:** There can be questions related to various pubertal milestones and their description. There can also be questions related to Tanner staging of breast and pubic hair development.

Question	Answer	Comment
Q32. Based on the Tanner stages of breast development, which of the following Tanner stages corresponds to the formation of a secondary mound due to further enlargement of the areola and papilla as shown in the image below? 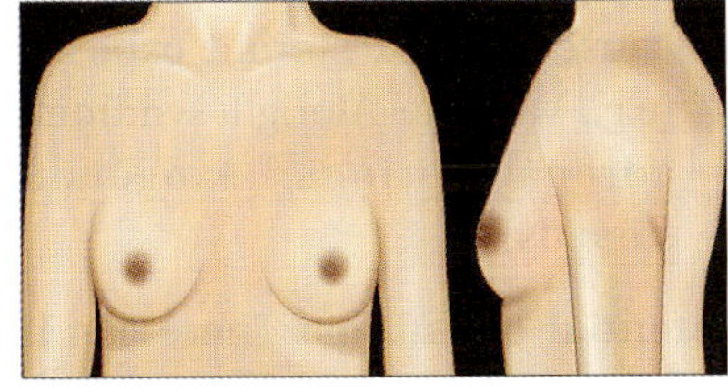 A. Tanner stage 1 B. Tanner stage 2 C. Tanner stage 3 D. Tanner stage 4 E. Tanner stage 5	**Ans: D (Tanner stage 4)** Tanner stages of breast development describe the various stages in development of breast tissues, which occur in a predictable sequence at the time of normal physical development in adolescents. **Figure 32** shows the Tanner stages of breast development. 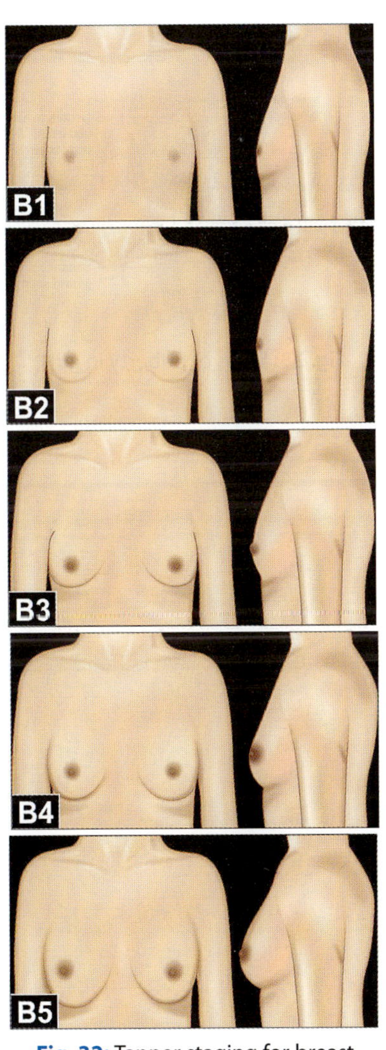 **Fig. 32:** Tanner staging for breast development.	**Explanation:** In Tanner stage 4, the areola and papilla (nipple) form a secondary mound above the level of the breast due to further growth, distinguishing this stage from the others. Various Tanner stages can be described as follows: ▪ *B1:* Prepubertal; no breast development ▪ *B2:* Development of breast bud; small mound forms as the breast and papilla enlarge ▪ *B3:* Enlargement of breast and areola with no separation of the breast contour ▪ *B4:* Projection of areola and papilla to form a secondary mound above the level of the breast ▪ *B5:* Recession of the areola to the general contour of the breast with projection of the papilla only; the secondary mound disappears; formation of mature adult breast; and the breast assumes its final shape. **Potential questions:** There can be questions related to various pubertal milestones and their description. There can also be questions related to Tanner staging of breast and pubic hair development.

Question	Answer	Comment
Q33. A 7-year-old girl shows Tanner stage 2 breast development as shown in the image below. Pubic hair growth is also observed. What is the most likely diagnosis? 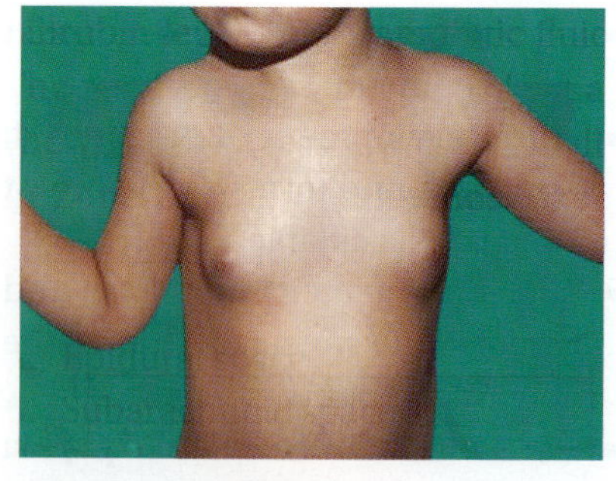 A. Normal puberty B. Precocious puberty C. Premature thelarche D. Adrenal hyperplasia E. Hypothyroidism	**Ans: B (Precocious puberty)** Precocious puberty is defined as development of secondary sexual characteristics (breast, pubic hair, or rapid growth) in girls before age 8 **(Fig. 33)**, or onset of menses before age 10. For boys, puberty before age 9 is considered precocious. 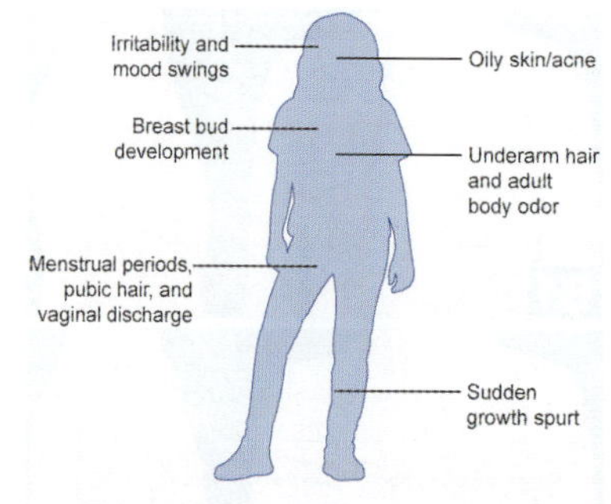 **Fig. 33:** Signs of puberty in girls.	**Explanation:** Signs of precocious puberty include early breast and pubic hair development. It can be: ▪ *Central precocious puberty (CPP) or constitutional/true/ complete precocious puberty:* Gonadotropin-dependent ▪ *Precocious pseudopuberty:* Gonadotropin-independent, caused by sex steroid exposure (e.g., McCune–Albright syndrome, adrenal lesions, exogenous steroids) **Potential questions:** There can be questions related to abnormalities in pubertal development (both delayed and precocious).

CHAPTER 8

Benign and Malignant Lesions of Genital Tract

FIBROIDS

Question	Answer	Comment
Q1. The clinical image below shows the macroscopic appearance of a well-circumscribed uterine tumor. What is the most likely diagnosis? 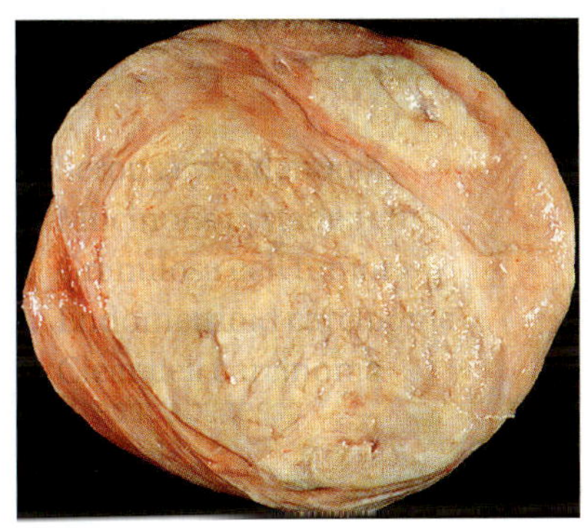 A. Adenomyosis B. Sarcoma C. Leiomyoma (fibroid) D. Ovarian cyst E. Polycystic ovary syndrome (PCOS)	**Ans: C [Leiomyoma (fibroid)]** Myomas (fibromyomas, leiomyomas, or fibroids) are well-circumscribed benign tumors developing from uterine myometrium, most commonly encountered among women of the reproductive age group (30–45 years), with their prevalence ranging between 20% to 40%. Different types of leiomyomas are shown in **Figure 1**. 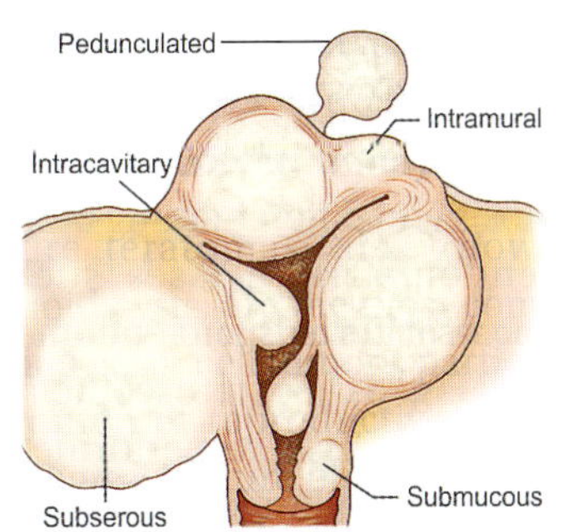 **Fig. 1:** Different types of leiomyomas.	**Explanation:** Leiomyomas appear as well-circumscribed, firm, and often multiple masses on gross examination. These tumors can vary in size and are typically white or tan in color. Fibroids are the most common benign tumors in women of reproductive age and can cause symptoms such as heavy menstrual bleeding, pelvic pain, and reproductive issues. Based on their location inside the uterus, the fibroids can be broadly classified into three types: Submucosal, intramural, and subserosal. Of the different types of fibroids, the most common are intramural (interstitial) fibroids, which are present in nearly 75% cases, followed by submucous (15%) and subserous (10%) fibroids. **Potential questions:** There can be questions related to etiology, histological appearance, clinical features and presentation, diagnosis, and management of cases of uterine fibroids.

<table>
<tr><th>Question</th><th>Answer</th><th>Comment</th></tr>
<tr>
<td>

Q2. The clinical image below shows the histological appearance of a uterine tumor. What is the most likely histological diagnosis?

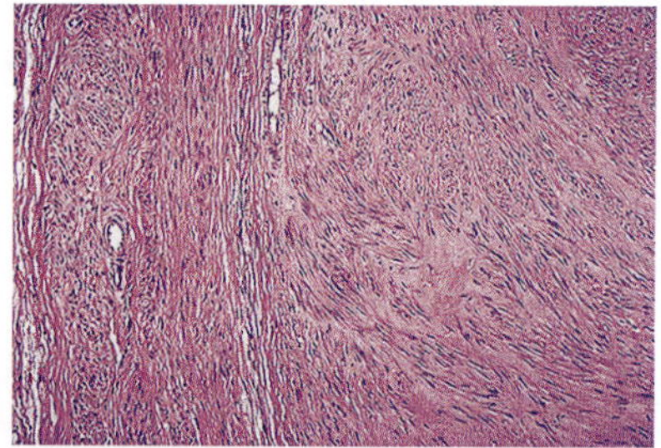

A. Adenomyosis
B. Endometrial carcinoma
C. Leiomyoma (fibroid)
D. Serous cystadenoma
E. Endometriosis

</td>
<td>

Ans: C: [Leiomyoma (fibroid)]

This well-circumscribed mass shows a whorled appearance on histopathological examination due to the presence of interlacing fibers of smooth myometrial muscle arranged in a whorled pattern, separated by varying amounts of connective tissue fibers **(Fig. 2)**. These cells are uniform in size and shape, with elongated nuclei and abundant eosinophilic cytoplasm.

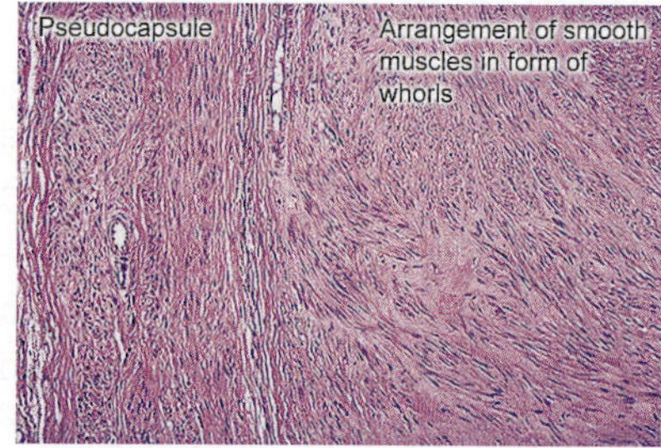

Fig. 2: Histological appearance of fibroid.

</td>
<td>

Explanation: The fibroid is surrounded by a pseudocapsule of compressed muscle fibers and connective tissue, which helps in fixing the tumor to the myometrium. This connective tissue capsule helps in forming a plane of cleavage along which the tumor can be easily enucleated at the time of surgery. The vessels supplying blood to the tumor lie in the capsule and send radial branches into the tumor. As a result, the central portion of the fibroid receives the least blood supply and is the first to undergo degeneration.

Potential questions: There can be questions related to etiology, histological appearance, clinical features and presentation, diagnosis, and management of cases of uterine fibroids.

</td>
</tr>
<tr>
<td>

Q3. A 35-year-old woman experiencing heavy menstrual periods and occasional pelvic pain undergoes an ultrasound examination as shown in the image below. Identify the type of fibroid shown in the image.

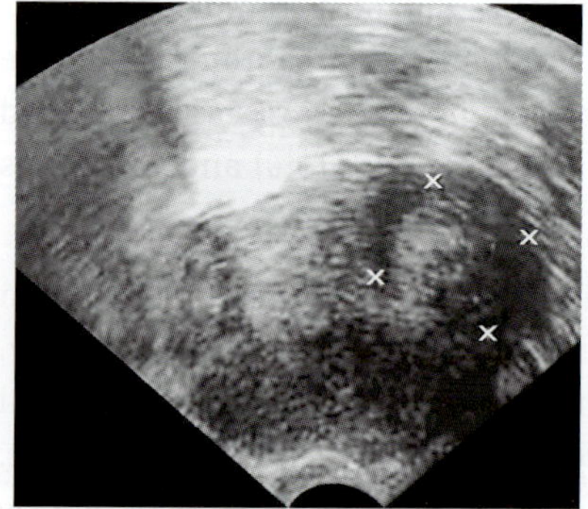

A. Submucosal fibroid
B. Intramural fibroid
C. Subserosal fibroid
D. Pedunculated fibroid
E. Cervical fibroid

</td>
<td>

Ans: A (Submucosal fibroid)

The adjacent ultrasound image depicts a submucous fibroid protruding inside the endometrial cavity.

Hysteroscopic examination in this case helps in confirming the diagnosis and differentiating between the endometrial masses such as submucosal fibroids and endometrial polyps **(Fig. 3)**. Hysteroscopic myomectomy can also be performed for surgical removal of myoma in these cases.

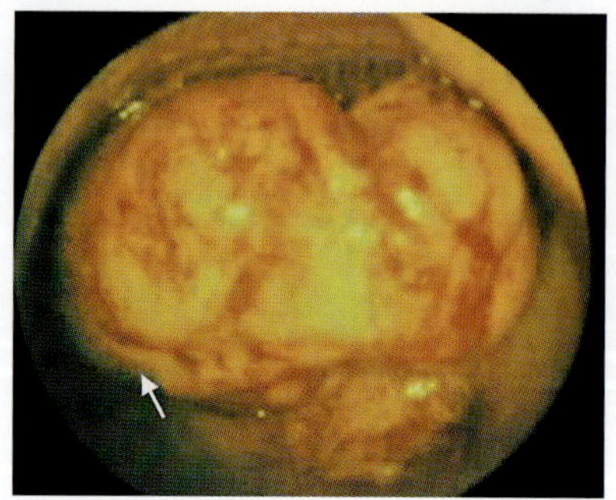

Fig. 3: Appearance of submucosal myoma on hysteroscopy (indicated by arrow).

</td>
<td>

Explanation: Nowadays, ultrasound examination (both transvaginal and transabdominal ultrasound) has become the investigation of choice for diagnosing myomas. Ultrasound examination helps in assessing the overall uterine shape, size, and contour; endometrial thickness; adnexal areas; and presence of hydronephrosis. It also helps in detection of small, focal, irregular, or eccentrically located endometrial lesions.

In this patient, transvaginal ultrasound examination reveals a well-defined hyperechoic area surrounded by an anechoic capsule, suggestive of a submucous fibroid, protruding inside the endometrial cavity.

Potential questions: There can be questions related to etiology, histological appearance, clinical features and presentation, diagnosis and management of cases of uterine fibroids.

</td>
</tr>
</table>

Question	Answer	Comment
Q4. A 40-year-old woman presented to the gynecology OPD with intermittent pelvic pain and a sensation of fullness in her abdomen. She reports irregular menstrual cycles with occasional heavy bleeding. During the pelvic examination, the gynecologist notes a mobile mass moving with the uterus. She then performs an ultrasound examination to explore the underlying cause of her symptoms. The ultrasound image is shown below. Which of the following complications is most commonly associated with this type of fibroid? 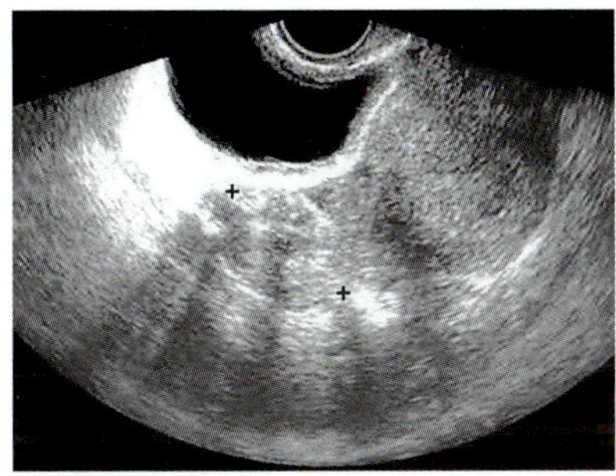 A. Uterine rupture B. Severe anemia C. Urinary frequency D. Endometrial hyperplasia E. Ovarian torsion	**Ans: C (Urinary frequency)** The adjacent transvaginal ultrasound shows a well-defined mass measuring about 3.74 cm in diameter. The mass is located separately from the uterine fundus and is connected with the help of a pedicle. As a result, diagnosis of a subserosal fibroid was made. Subserosal fibroids may sometimes develop a pedicle and extrude out from the serosal surface in the form of pedunculated fibroids. Both submucous and subserosal fibroids can be pedunculated. Long pedunculated fibroids may sometimes undergo torsion. **Figure 4** shows different locations of fibroids. 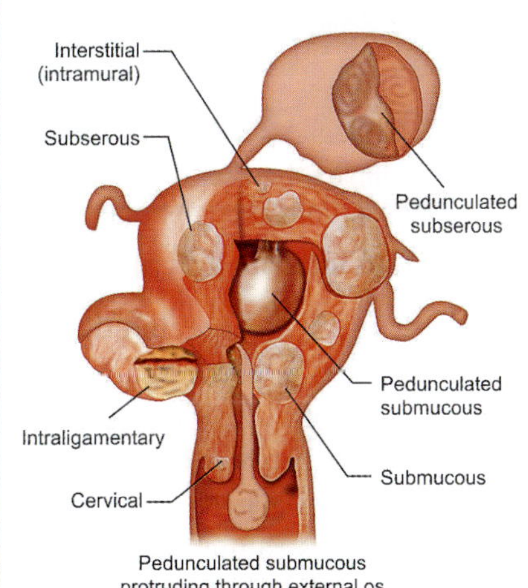 **Fig. 4:** Different locations at which fibroids may be present.	**Explanation:** Subserosal fibroids grow on the outer surface of the uterus and can become quite large. Due to their position, they often exert pressure on adjacent organs such as the bladder and rectum, resulting in symptoms like pelvic pain, a feeling of fullness, and pressure. Unlike submucosal fibroids, which are more likely to cause heavy menstrual bleeding and severe anemia, subserosal fibroids typically do not affect the endometrial cavity and thus are less likely to cause abnormal uterine bleeding. **Potential questions:** There can be questions related to etiology, histological appearance, clinical features and presentation, diagnosis. and management of cases of uterine fibroids.

Question	Answer	Comment
Q5. A 38-year-old woman presents with heavy menstrual bleeding and pelvic pain. A special type of transvaginal ultrasound is performed as shown in the image below. What is the most likely diagnosis suspected in this case? 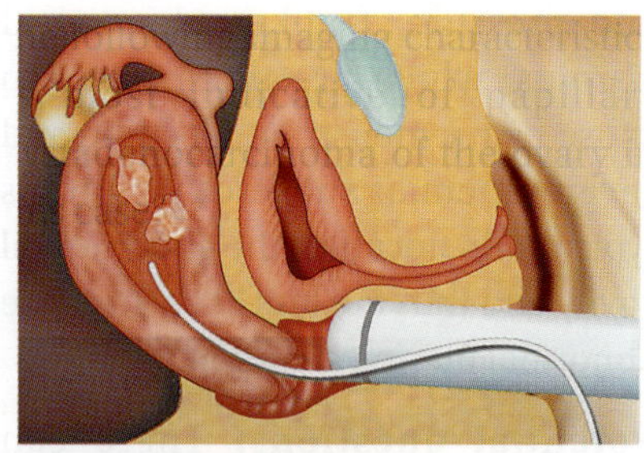 A. Submucosal fibroid B. Subserosal fibroid C. Intramural fibroid D. Endometrial polyp E. Adenomyosis	**Ans: A (Submucosal fibroid)** The adjacent image demonstrates the procedure of saline infusion sonography (SIS), a special type of TVS that outlines the uterine cavity using saline. To perform SIS, a small catheter is threaded through internal os into the endometrial cavity. Through this catheter, sterile saline is infused and the uterine cavity distended. In the adjacent case, infusion of saline inside the endometrial cavity caused uterine distension, illustrating numerous submucosal myomas **(Fig. 5)**. 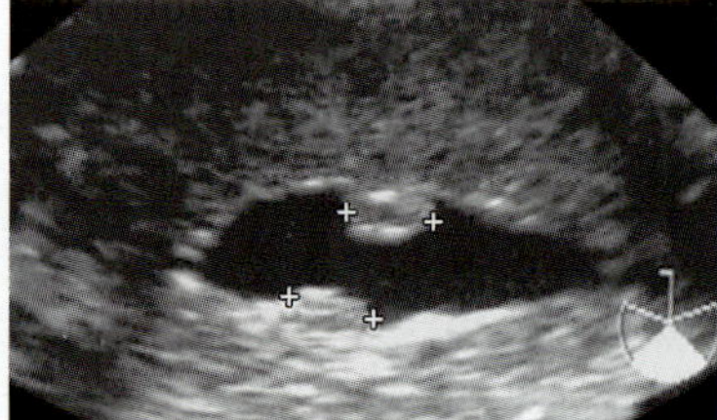 **Fig. 5:** Multiple submucosal myomas on saline infusion sonography (SIS).	**Explanation:** SIS may be sometimes required if no definitive diagnosis can be established on transvaginal sonography, especially in the presence of suspected endometrial pathology. The technique of SIS is particularly useful for identifying and characterizing uterine abnormalities such as submucous fibroids, endometrial polyps, synechiae, etc. SIS has been demonstrated to cause improved evaluation of the endometrial cavity and assessment of tubal patency. **Potential questions:** There can be questions related to etiology, histological appearance, clinical features and presentation, diagnosis, and management of cases of uterine fibroids.
Q6. A 47-year-old woman presents with intermenstrual spotting and a recent history of heavier menstrual periods. SIS is performed, and the image as shown below is obtained. What is the most likely diagnosis? 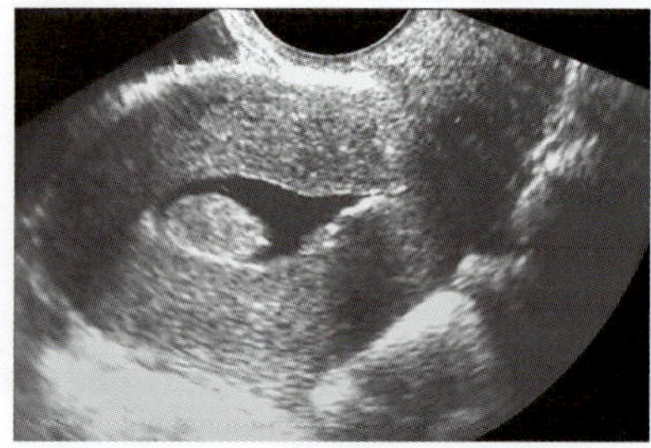 A. Submucosal fibroid B. Subserosal fibroid C. Intramural fibroid D. Endometrial polyp E. Adenomyosis	**Ans: D (Endometrial polyp)** Although TVS is associated with higher resolution in comparison to TAS, it may not always be useful in distinguishing between submucosal fibroid, endometrial polyp, and adenomyosis. SIS uses saline infusion into the endometrial cavity to enhance the detection of submucosal fibroids and polyps. The adjacent image shows SIS demonstrating a solitary endometrial polyp. **Figures 6A and B** compare an endometrial polyp with pedunculated submucosal fibroid. 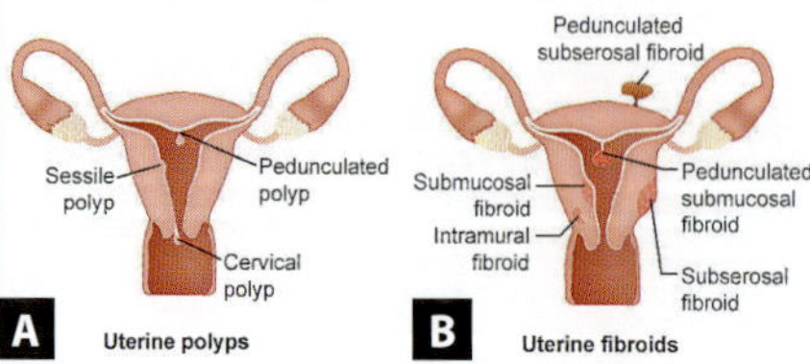 **Figs. 6A and B:** Comparison between (A) Uterine polyp and (B) Pedunculated submucosal fibroid.	**Explanation:** Endometrial polyps appear as focal masses within the endometrial cavity. On SIS, they are typically seen as well-defined, echogenic structures that may have a stalk attaching them to the endometrial lining. The saline infusion helps to outline these polyps clearly against the background of the fluid-filled uterine cavity. Treatment options include hysteroscopic polypectomy or medication to regulate hormone levels. **Potential questions:** There can be questions related to etiology, histological appearance, clinical features and presentation, diagnosis, and management of cases of uterine fibroids.

Question	Answer	Comment
Q7. A 42-year-old woman presents with pelvic pain and heavy menstrual bleeding. Since she was a research subject for an ongoing study, MRI of the pelvis was performed, which revealed a well-circumscribed, round mass within the uterus on T1-weighted imaging, as shown in the below image. 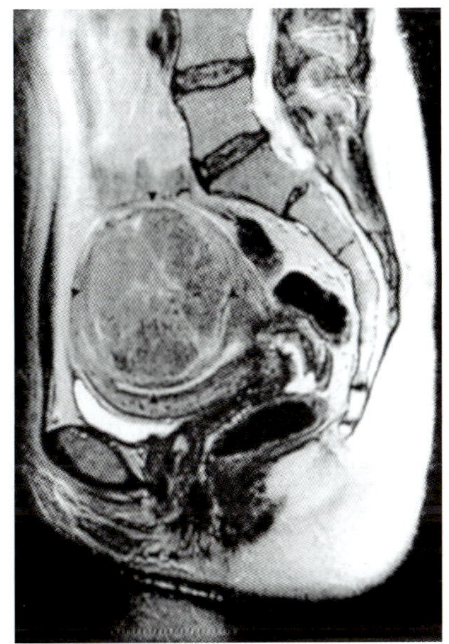 What is the most likely diagnosis? A. Submucosal fibroid B. Subserosal fibroid C. Intramural fibroid D. Endometrial polyp E. Adenomyosis	**Ans: C (Intramural fibroid)** The adjacent image is a T1-weighted magnetic resonance image showing an intramural fibroid. Presently, the ultrasound examination forms the most commonly used investigation modality for initial evaluation. **Figure 7** demonstrates the presence of a well-circumscribed mass within the uterine myometrium having homogeneous consistency in the same patient. 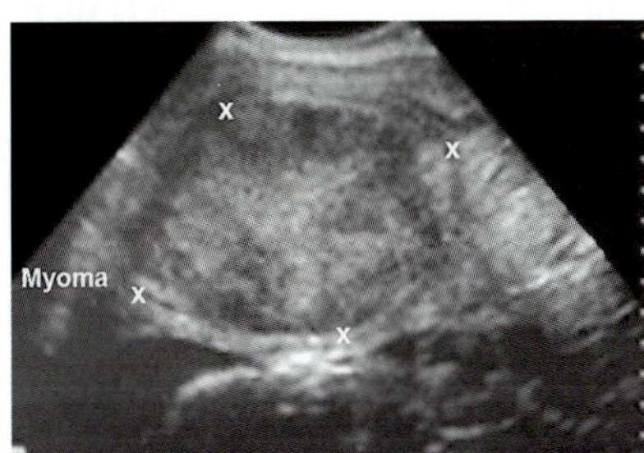 **Fig. 7:** Presence of a well-circumscribed lesion on ultrasound in the same patient.	**Explanation:** Although MRI is an investigation which helps in accurately establishing the definitive diagnosis of myomas, the high cost associated with its use prevents its widespread use in clinical practice. Therefore, it is not used as a modality of first choice for cases of fibroid uterus. MRI was performed in this patient in lieu of the study protocol because she was a research subject. On T1-weighted MRI, intramural fibroids typically appear as well-defined, homogeneously hypointense masses relative to the surrounding myometrium. Some masses may display heterogeneous signals due to degeneration or calcification. These characteristics help distinguish fibroids from other uterine or adnexal pathologies such as adenomyosis (which presents with diffuse thickening and high-signal intensity) and ovarian cysts (which show high intensity signals). **Potential questions:** There can be questions related to etiology, histological appearance, clinical features and presentation, diagnosis, and management of cases of uterine fibroids.

Question	Answer	Comment
Q8. A 35-year-old woman presents with abnormal uterine bleeding and pelvic pain. Findings on ultrasound scan were inconclusive. Therefore, an MRI scan was performed. The image on MRI scan is displayed below. What is the most appropriate next step in management? 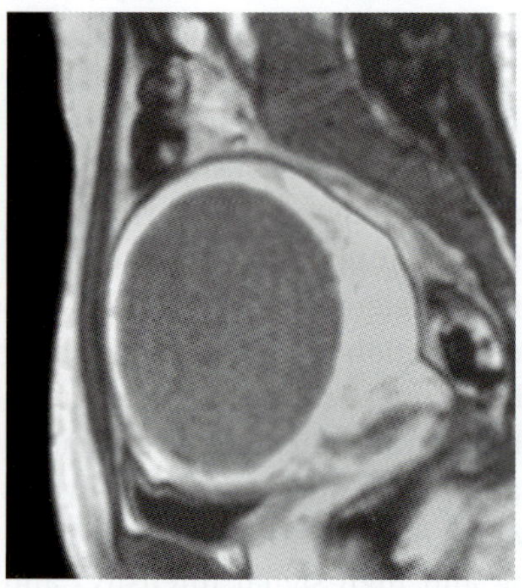 A. Laparoscopic myomectomy B. Hysteroscopic myomectomy C. Gonadotropin-releasing hormone (GnRH) therapy D. Uterine artery embolization (UAE) E. Hysterectomy	**Ans: B (Hysteroscopic myomectomy)** The adjacent image shows T1-weighted magnetic resonance image, depicting a submucosal fibroid with less than 50% invasion into the myometrium. In symptomatic patients, myomectomy is typically the treatment of choice, especially for those desiring future fertility. In this case due to the presence of submucosal myoma and less than 50% invasion into the myometrium, hysteroscopic myomectomy appears to be the treatment of choice **(Fig. 8)**. 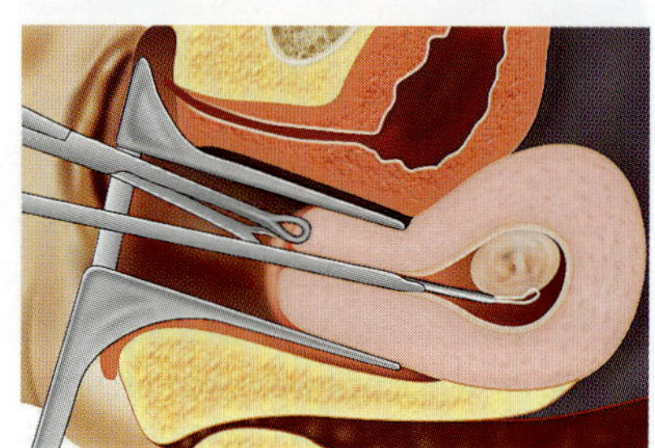 **Fig. 8:** Hysteroscopic resection of submucosal fibroids.	**Explanation:** Magnetic resonance images are able to clearly delineate the myometrium, junctional zone, and endometrium, allowing highly accurate mapping of the size, location, and degree of myometrial involvement of uterine leiomyomas. Though MRI gives images with better resolution, due to its high cost, MRI is usually reserved for only special cases. While the use of MRI is not routinely recommended, it is useful for mapping the size and location of leiomyomas and in accurately identifying adenomyosis if present. Other pelvic pathology such as ovarian neoplasms can also be identified on MRI. **Potential questions:** There can be questions related to etiology, histological appearance, clinical features and presentation, diagnosis, and management of cases of uterine fibroids.

Question	Answer	Comment
Q9. Identify the instrument marked by an arrow in the below image, used during myomectomy. 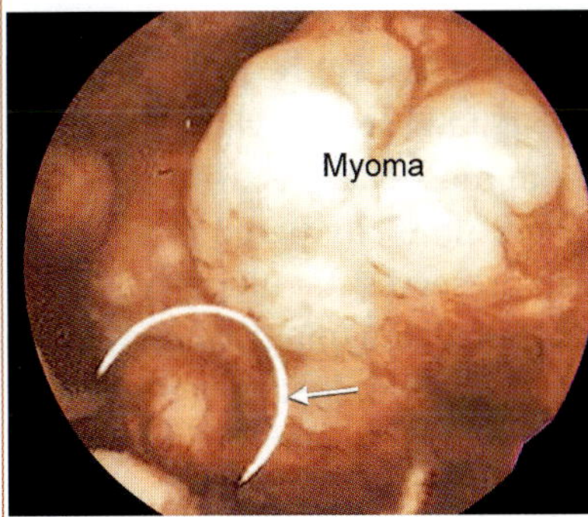 A. Laparoscope B. Resectoscope C. Hysteroscope D. Colposcope E. Cystoscope	**Ans: B (Resectoscope)** The instrument depicted by an arrow in the adjacent image is a resectoscope, used at the time of hysteroscopic myomectomy. The International Federation of Gynecology and Obstetrics (FIGO, 2018) system classifies fibroids based on their relationship to the endometrium and serosa. It uses numbers 0–8, plus hybrid categories and can be described as follows: ▪ *Submucosal fibroids:* These include: • *Type 0:* Pedunculated, entirely intracavitary. • *Type 1:* Less than 50% intramural extension. ▪ *Intramural:* These include: • *Type 2:* ≥50% intramural extension. • *Type 3:* Contacts endometrium, but 100% intramural. • *Type 4:* Completely intramural (no endometrial or serosal involvement). • *Type 5:* Subserosal, ≥50% intramural. ▪ *Subserosal:* These include: • *Type 6:* Subserosal, <50% intramural. • *Type 7:* Subserosal, pedunculated. • *Type 8:* Other (e.g., cervical, parasitic). ▪ *Hybrid types:* Two numbers are listed separated by a hyphen. By convention, the first refers to the relationship with the endometrium while the second refers to the relationship to the serosa. 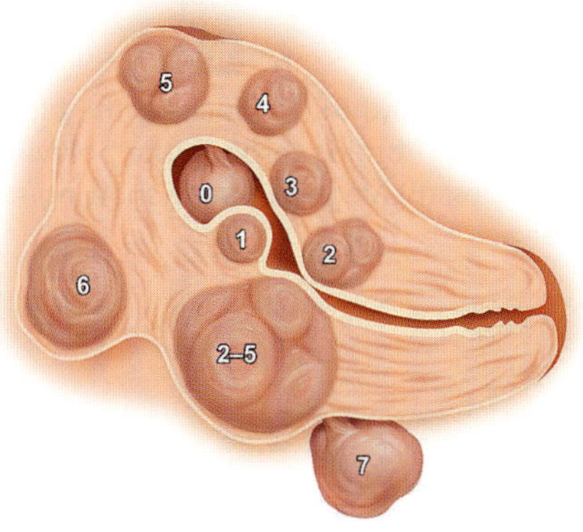 **Fig. 9:** FIGO classification of fibroids.	**Explanation:** FIGO Types 0, 1, and carefully selected Type 2 fibroids are the ones typically removed hysteroscopically. Hysteroscopic surgery may be technically more challenging in the type 2 fibroids. Type 3 to type 8 fibroids should preferably not be removed via a hysterescope. In these cases, laparoscopic, laparotomic, or combined approaches may be used depending on the fibroid size and symptoms. The resectoscope is a specialized hysteroscope equipped with a wire loop that uses high-frequency electrical energy to cut through fibroids during a hysteroscopic myomectomy. This instrument allows for precise removal of submucosal fibroids while minimizing damage to the surrounding uterine tissue. **Potential questions:** There can be questions related to etiology, histological appearance, clinical features and presentation, diagnosis, and management of cases of uterine fibroids.

Question	Answer	Comment
Q10. A 42-year-old woman presents with heavy menstrual bleeding and pelvic pressure. An ultrasound reveals multiple uterine fibroids. She desires to avoid surgery and preserve her uterus. A procedure as depicted in the image below was performed. What is the most appropriate minimally invasive treatment 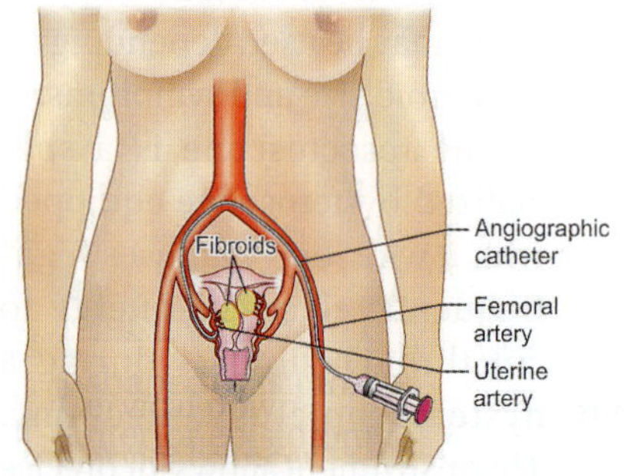 A. Hormonal therapy B. Myomectomy C. Uterine artery embolization (UAE) D. Hysterectomy E. Endometrial ablation	**Ans: C [Uterine artery embolization (UAE)]** The procedure depicted in the adjacent image is uterine artery embolization (UAE), which is a minimally invasive procedure used for treating symptomatic fibroids by cutting off their blood supply, leading to shrinkage. The interventional radiologist introduces and manipulates a catheter through the femoral artery into the internal iliac and uterine arteries. Introduction of an embolizing agent [gelatin microspheres (trisacryl gelatin) or polyvinyl alcohol] through the catheter inside the femoral vessels helps in reducing blood supply to the fibroids **(Figs. 10A and B)**. This helps in blocking both the uterine arteries, thereby cutting off blood supply to the fibroids. 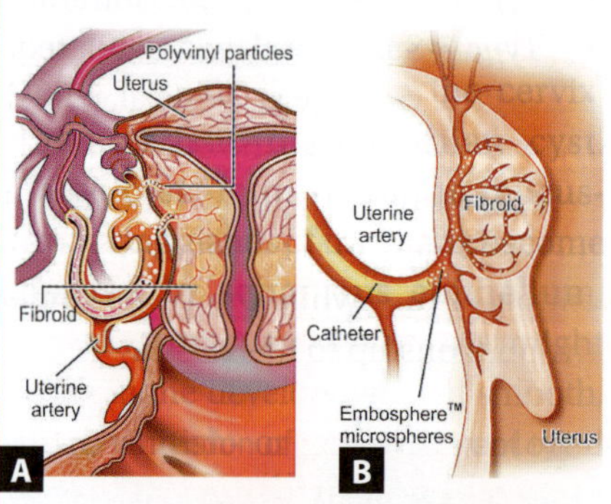 **Figs. 10A and B:** (A) Blocking the blood supply of fibroids through the polyvinyl particles; (B) Magnified view showing the same.	**Explanation:** Uterine artery embolization is an effective option for women who want to avoid surgery but still experience significant symptoms from fibroids. This procedure is image-guided and provides symptom relief in most patients, with minimal recovery time compared to surgery. It also preserves the uterus, which is important for women who wish to retain their reproductive organs. In UAE due to lack of sufficient blood supply, the fibroids become avascular and shrink, ultimately resulting in cell death, their degeneration, and eventual absorption by the myometrium. This occurs because in comparison to the normal uterine cells, fibroid cells are much more sensitive to low oxygen saturation. The normal myometrium, on the other hand, receives new blood supply from vaginal and ovarian vasculature. **Potential questions:** There can be questions related to etiology, histological appearance, clinical features and presentation, diagnosis, and management of cases of uterine fibroids.

OVARIAN LESIONS

Question	Answer	Comment
Q11. A 55-year-old postmenopausal woman presents with abdominal distension and irregular vaginal bleeding. An ultrasound reveals a large ovarian mass and the gynecologist orders a series of tests, including a biopsy, to determine the nature of the mass. The histopathological findings are shown in the image below. What is the most likely diagnosis? 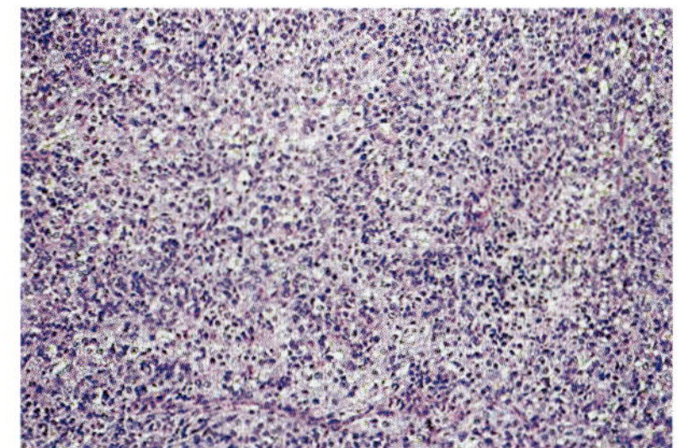 A. Serous cystadenoma B. Mucinous cystadenoma C. Granulosa cell tumor D. Endometrioid carcinoma E. Clear cell carcinoma	**Ans: C (Granulosa cell tumor)** The adjacent histopathological image is suggestive of granulosa cell tumors (GCTs), a type of sex cord-stromal tumor of the ovary, accounting for about 2–5% of all ovarian neoplasms. It can occur at any age and is composed of cells, which are identical to the granulosa cells of the Graafian follicle. The HPE may show Call–Exner bodies, which can be considered as primitive follicles comprising granulosa cells arranged haphazardly around a space containing eosinophilic fluid **(Fig. 11)**. 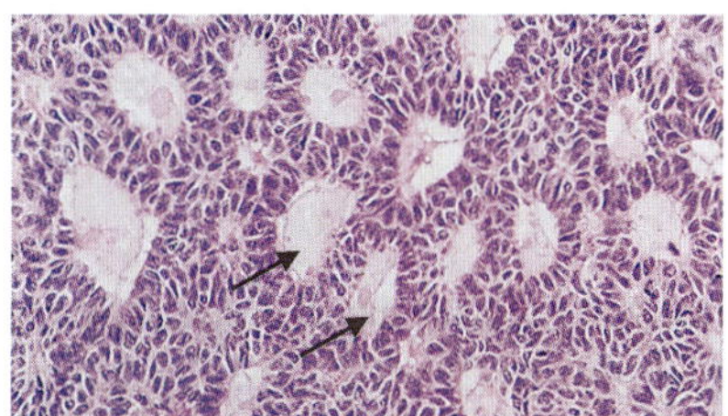 **Fig. 11:** Magnified view showing the presence of Call–Exner bodies.	**Explanation:** Functionally active granulosa cell tumors are responsible for producing estrogen. This can cause precocious sexual development in young girls. In adult women, this can cause endometrial hyperplasia, fibrocystic disease of the breast, endometrial carcinoma, etc. In postmenopausal women, this tumor can cause postmenopausal bleeding. The diagnosis is typically confirmed through histopathological examination and imaging studies. Measurement of serum inhibin levels is helpful in the diagnosis of granulosa cell tumors and for monitoring the disease following treatment. The most common treatment modality for these patients is surgery. **Potential questions:** There can be questions related to the characteristic features, presentation, diagnosis, and management of various ovarian neoplasms, including ovarian cancer.
Q12. A 22-year-old woman experiences intermittent pelvic pain. An ultrasound reveals a complex ovarian mass with solid and cystic components. HPE shows cystic structure with hair and sebaceous material. What is the most likely diagnosis? 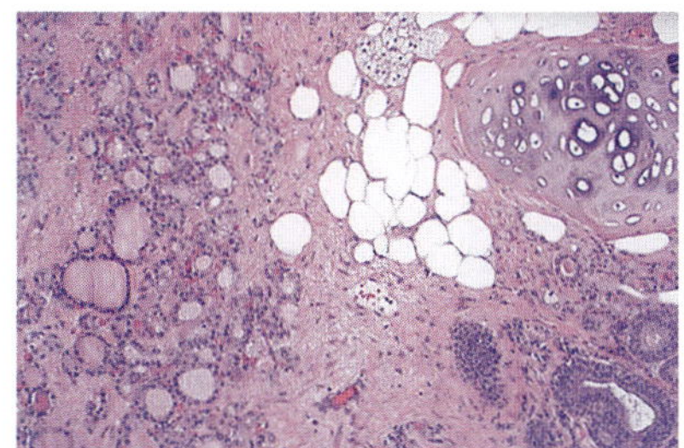 A. Serous cystadenoma B. Mucinous cystadenoma C. Mature teratoma D. Endometrioma E. Fibroma	**Ans: C (Mature teratoma)** Mature teratomas, also known as dermoid cysts, are the most common ovarian germ cell tumors, particularly in women of reproductive age. The histological picture of a mature cystic teratoma showing the presence of diverse tissues is shown in **Figure 12**. 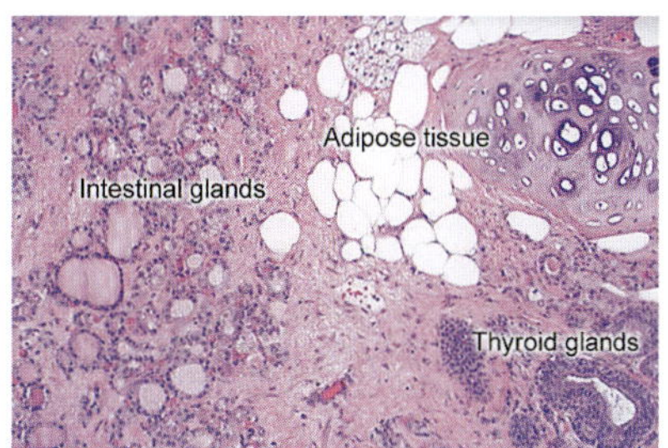 **Fig. 12:** Histological picture of a mature teratoma showing adipose tissue and intestinal glands at the right and thyroid tissue on the left.	**Explanation:** Mature teratomas are composed of well-differentiated tissues from at least two of the three germ cell layers. The presence of hair, sebaceous material, and sometimes teeth or bone within the cyst is characteristic. These tumors are usually benign but can cause symptoms due to their size or complications like torsion. These tumors may be associated with elevated levels of AFP and β-hCG. The diagnosis is made by imaging studies and management usually involves surgical removal. **Potential questions:** There can be questions related to the characteristic features, presentation, diagnosis, and management of various ovarian neoplasms, including ovarian cancer.

Question	Answer	Comment
Q13. A 45-year-old woman presents with abdominal distension and discomfort. An ultrasound reveals a large, multiloculated ovarian cyst as shown in the image below. The histopathological image shows cysts lined by mucin-producing columnar epithelium. What is the most likely diagnosis? 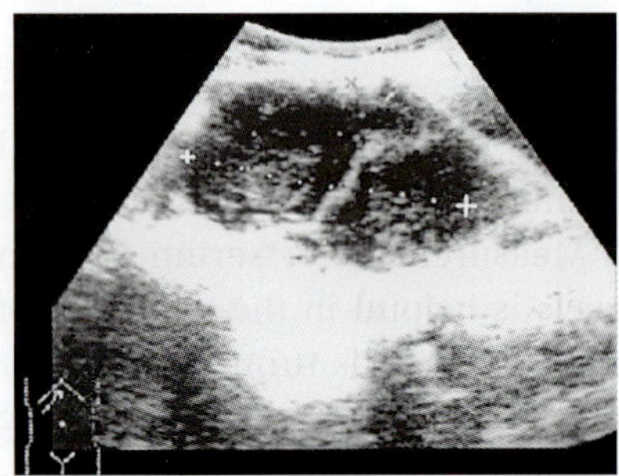 A. Serous cystadenoma B. Mucinous cystadenoma C. Endometrioma D. Fibroma E. Mucinous cystadenocarcinoma	**Ans: B (Mucinous cystadenoma)** The adjacent image is a transabdominal sonograph showing a multiloculated mass with presence of cystic areas along with a few brightly echogenic areas. In this case, differential diagnosis of mucinous cystadenoma and dermoid cyst was established based on the findings of sonography. Laparoscopic examination and histopathology confirmed the diagnosis of a mucinous cystadenoma. **Figure 13** depicts the specimen, showing presence of several septa within the mass, which give it a multiloculated appearance. Some of the loculi appear to be filled with a thick, viscid, straw-colored, mucin-like material. 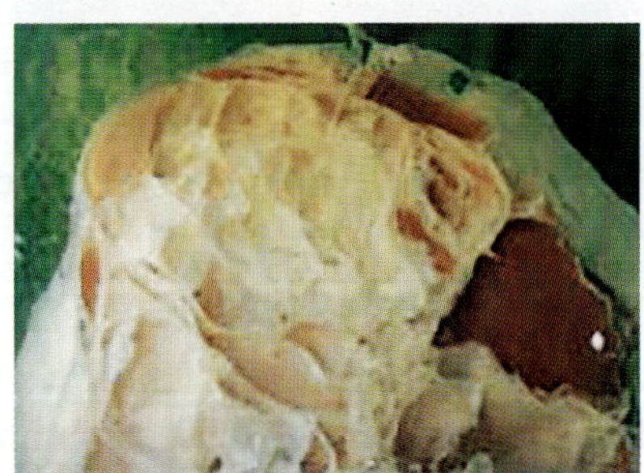 **Fig. 13:** Specimen showing mucinous cystadenoma of ovary.	**Explanation:** Mucinous cystadenomas are benign epithelial ovarian tumors characterized by large, multiloculated cystic masses lined by mucin-producing columnar epithelium. They are typically unilateral and can grow to a significant size, causing symptoms like abdominal distension and discomfort. Unlike their malignant counterparts, these tumors lack architectural complexity and cytologic atypia. Imaging often shows a multiloculated cystic appearance with thin septations. Ultrasonography (both transabdominal and transvaginal) is accurate in differentiating tumors of the ovary from other types of tumors of the pelvis, in more than 90% of the patients. **Potential questions:** There can be questions related to the characteristic features, presentation, diagnosis, and management of various ovarian neoplasms, including ovarian cancer.

Question	Answer	Comment
Q14. During a pelvic ultrasound for routine health screening, a 30-year-old woman is found to have a well-circumscribed, anechoic mass with smooth, thin walls and posterior acoustic enhancement in one ovary as shown in the image below. What is the most likely diagnosis? 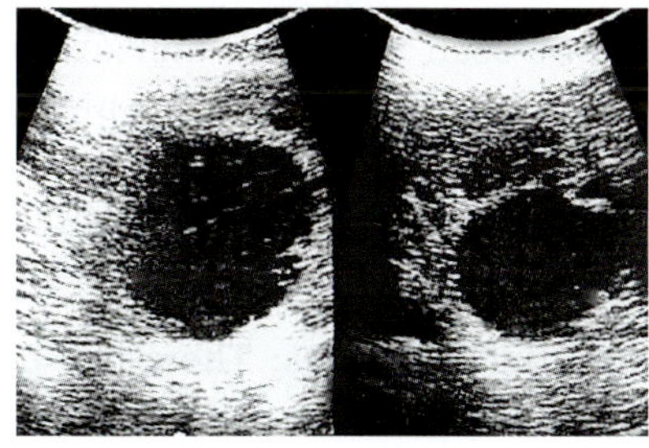 A. Serous cystadenoma B. Mucinous cystadenoma C. Simple ovarian cyst D. Endometrioma E. Dermoid cyst	**Ans: C (Simple ovarian cyst)** The adjacent image is a transvaginal sonograph revealing the presence of an ovarian cyst (with multiple internal echoes) on the right side. On the left side, the ovary is normal with the presence of a dominant follicle This was a small cyst, which was <5 cm in diameter and diagnosed as a functional, follicular cyst **(Fig. 14)**. Functional cysts usually appear as anechoic, small masses on ultrasound examination. The mass was found to be decreasing in size on repeated sonographic examination. It eventually disappeared on its own within 3–4 months' time. 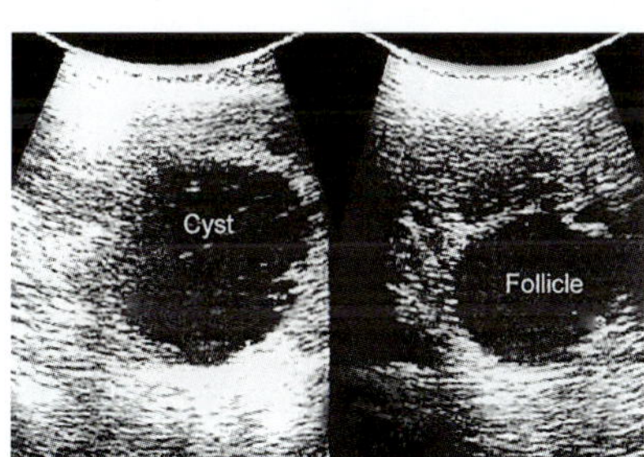 **Fig. 14:** Presence of a simple ovarian cyst in the right ovary.	**Explanation:** A simple ovarian cyst/follicular cyst is a fluid-filled sac within the ovary that is typically benign and often asymptomatic. These cysts are characterized by their unilocular, anechoic appearance on ultrasound, with a thin wall and posterior acoustic enhancement. They are common in women of reproductive age and usually resolve spontaneously. Management often involves observation and follow-up ultrasounds to ensure resolution. Discrimination between benign and malignant lesions of the ovary can be made on the basis of ultrasonic patterns. Though sonography cannot definitely rule out malignancy, anechoic or almost anechoic lesions have a high likelihood of being benign. As the percentage of echogenic material in the cysts increases, the likelihood of malignancy also increases. **Potential questions:** There can be questions related to the characteristic features, presentation, diagnosis, and management of various ovarian neoplasms, including ovarian cancer.

Question	Answer	Comment
Q15. A 50-year-old woman presents with abdominal bloating and pelvic discomfort. Clinical examination revealed a solid mass with irregular margins. Ultrasound reveals a large, multiloculated cystic ovarian mass as shown in the image below. Which of the following imaging characteristics is most indicative of papillary cystadenocarcinoma of the ovary in this case? 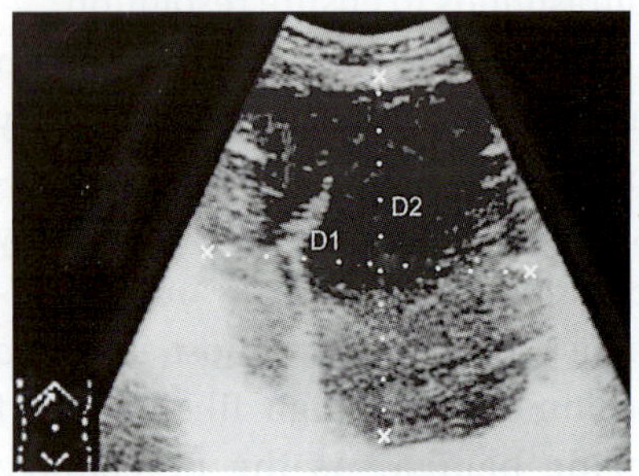 A. Unilocular cyst, thin walls, no solid components B. Multiloculated cyst, thin septa, no papillary projections C. Multiloculated cyst, solid components, and papillary projections D. Homogeneous cystic mass, no vascularization E. Well-circumscribed unilocular cyst, homogenous fluid	**Ans: C (Multiloculated cyst, solid components, and papillary projections)** The adjacent image of transabdominal sonograph shows presence of a large multiloculated cystic mass with solid components, papillary projections with multiple septa, and numerous internal echoes. The ultrasound features as well as the findings on clinical examination point towards malignancy in this case. The suspicion of malignancy was confirmed on biopsy, which revealed the diagnosis of serous cystadenocarcinoma **(Fig. 15)**. 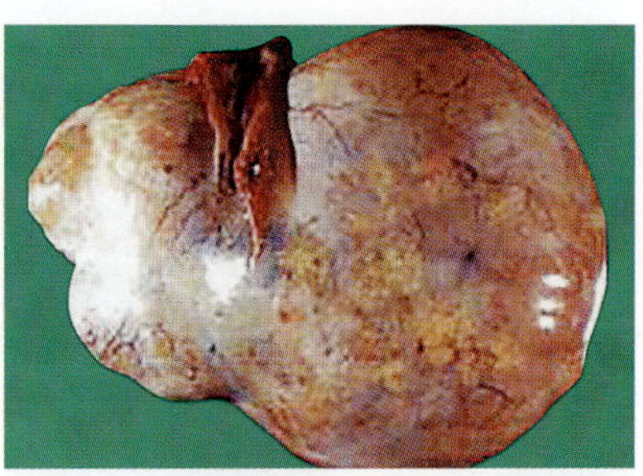 **Fig. 15:** Specimen of an ovarian cystadenocarcinoma.	**Explanation: Figure 15** shows the specimen of ovarian papillary cystadenocarcinoma, in this case obtained at the time of laparotomy. As can be seen in the image, the tumor consists mainly of solid tissue, with papillary projections visible on the surface. Areas of hemorrhage and necrosis can also probably be identified. Multiple blood vessels can also be seen traversing the surface of the ovary. These tumors typically spread by dispersing cancer cells ("seeding") along the peritoneal lining. **Potential questions:** There can be questions related to the characteristic features, presentation, diagnosis, and management of various ovarian neoplasms, including ovarian cancer.

Question	Answer	Comment
Q16. A 50-year-old woman presents with pelvic pain and a palpable mass. Since ultrasound examination was inconclusive, an MRI scan was performed which revealed the findings shown in the image below. What is the most likely diagnosis? 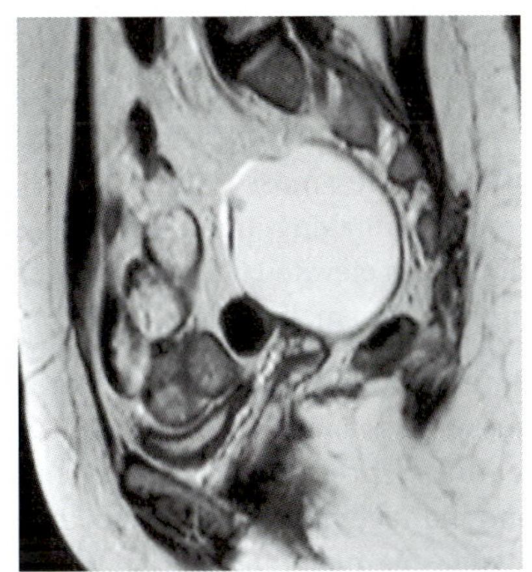 A. Serous cystadenoma B. Mucinous cystadenoma C. Endometrioma D. Fibroma E. Clear cell carcinoma	**Ans: A (Serous cystadenoma)** The adjacent image depicts a T1-weighted MRI scan showing a smooth walled mass, having homogenous consistency with no internal septae or lobulations. Diagnosis of a benign serous cystadenoma was made. **Figure 16** is a specimen showing cut section of an organ, which most likely appears to be ovary, harboring a cystic mass containing clear fluid-like substance. There are no solid areas of hemorrhage or necrosis inside the tumor. Diagnosis of serous cystadenoma was confirmed. 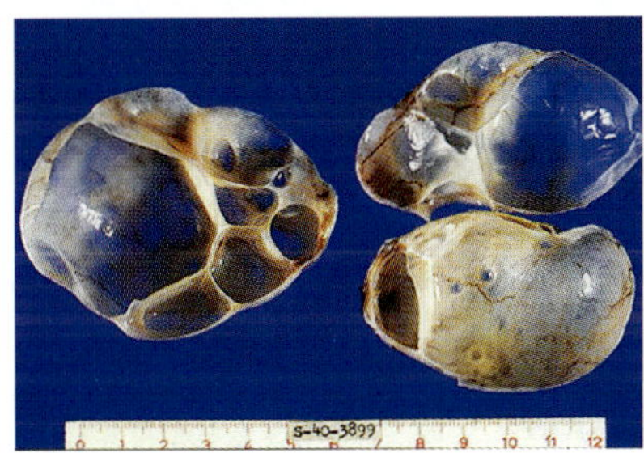 **Fig. 16:** Cut section of ovary showing serous cystadenoma.	**Explanation:** Serous cystadenomas are common benign epithelial ovarian tumors, typically presenting as unilocular or multilocular cystic masses with thin walls and clear serous fluid. They are often asymptomatic but can cause pelvic pain or a palpable mass when they grow larger. Imaging usually shows a well-defined, anechoic mass with posterior acoustic enhancement. Though MRI scans are not routinely used for diagnosing ovarian pathology, they can help in accurate characterization of ovarian tumors and are also particularly helpful for assessing metastatic spread of the cancer to the brain and spinal cord. Treatment often involves surgical removal, especially if the cyst is large or causing symptoms. **Potential questions:** There can be questions related to the characteristic features, presentation, diagnosis, and management of various ovarian neoplasms, including ovarian cancer.

Question	Answer	Comment
Q17. A 55-year-old postmenopausal woman presents with anorexia, bloating, left iliac fossa pain, fatigue, weakness, increased micturition frequency, and significant weight loss over the past month. TVS shows abnormal findings as shown below. Her serum CA-125 levels are elevated. What is the most likely diagnosis based on these clinical and imaging findings? 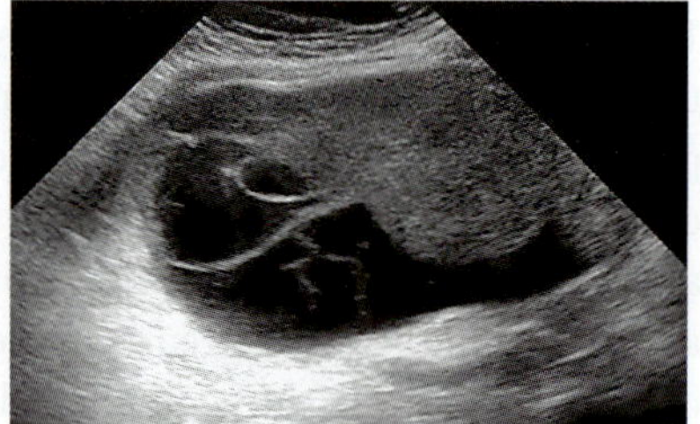 A. Simple ovarian cyst B. Endometrioma C. Ovarian torsion D. Epithelial ovarian cancer E. Functional cyst	**Ans: D (Epithelial ovarian cancer)** TThe TVS shows a multiseptated complex adnexal mass with heterogeneous solid areas. RMI >200 and Doppler findings as seen in **Figure 17** (increased blood flow, pulsatile index <1, resistance index <0.4), indicate presence of malignancy. Biopsy confirmed ovarian cystadenocarcinoma. 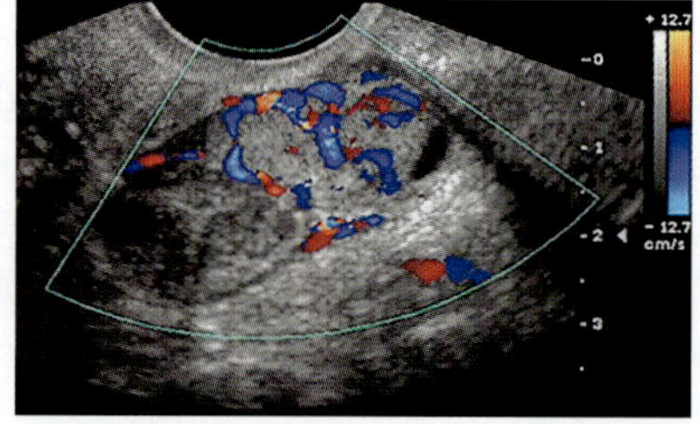 **Fig. 17:** Transvaginal sonography of color Doppler in the same patient.	**Explanation:** Epithelial ovarian cancer is the most common type of ovarian malignancy, particularly in postmenopausal women. The clinical presentation in this case is typical of epithelial ovarian cancer, which often presents late with vague symptoms such as pelvic pain, bloating, and abdominal distension. Due to vague clinical presentation, such lesions are often discovered late at an advanced stage of malignancy. The presence of a complex mass with both solid areas on imaging and elevated RMI along with elevated CA-125 are highly suggestive of malignancy. **Potential questions:** There can be questions related to the characteristic features, presentation, diagnosis, and management of various ovarian neoplasms, including ovarian cancer.

CERVICAL LESIONS

Question	Answer	Comment
Q18. A 45-year-old woman with postcoital bleeding has a polypoid growth protruding from the cervical os as shown in the image. What is the most likely diagnosis? 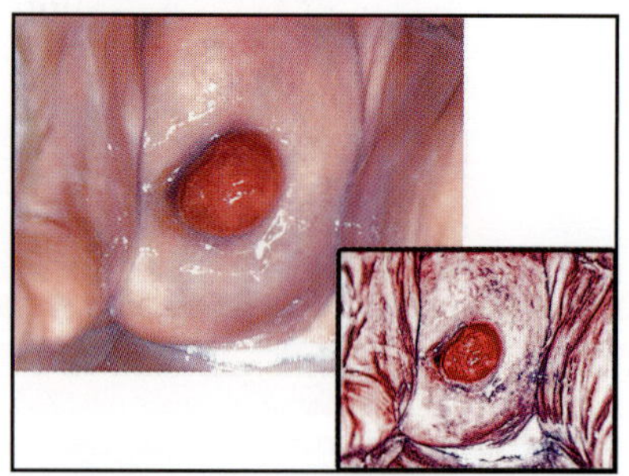 A. Cervical cancer B. Endometrial polyp C. Endocervical polyp D. Cervical fibroid E. Cervical ectropion	**Ans: C (Endocervical polyp)** The adjacent image shows endocervical polyps which are hyperplastic projections of endocervical folds in cervix, resulting in the development of single, red-colored, smooth, elongated masses. These masses, known as endocervical polyps, can be considered as one of the most common benign lesions of the cervix. **Figures 18A to C** shows diagrammatic representation of endocervical polyps. 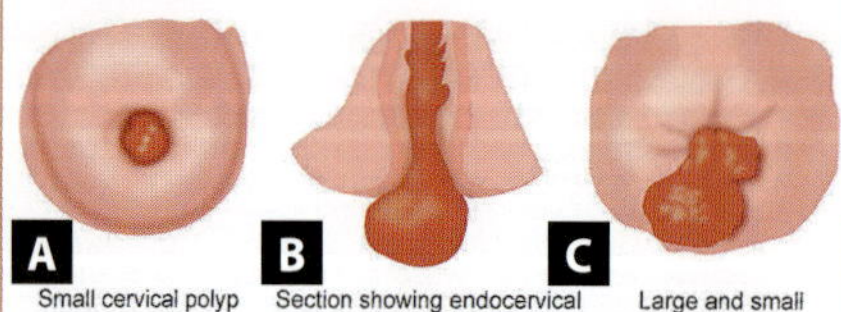 **Figs. 18A to C:** Diagrammatic representation of endocervical polyps.	**Explanation:** Endocervical polyps are polypoid growths protruding through the cervical os, usually asymptomatic but may cause leukorrhea, menorrhagia, or postcoital bleeding. Diagnosis is confirmed histologically after removal. These polyps are rarely malignant but must be routinely biopsied to rule out cervical malignancy. In case of presence of a slender stalk, the polyp can be removed by using ring forceps after twisting it several times about its base in order to strangulate the feeding vessels. **Potential questions:** There may be questions related to different types of cervical lesions (both malignant and nonmalignant).

Question	Answer	Comment
Q19. A 30-year-old woman comes to the clinic with symptoms of vaginal discharge and discomfort. During per speculum examination, the gynecologist notes cervical redness and discharge, suggestive of an inflammatory process as shown in the image below. 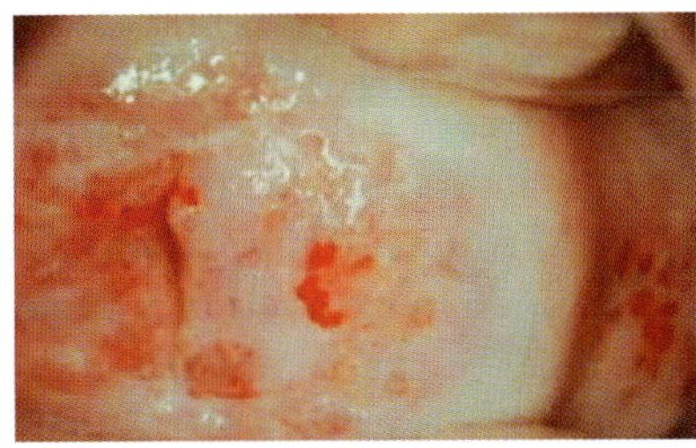 Based on the image, what is the most likely diagnosis? A. Cervical ectropion B. Nabothian cysts C. Cervicitis D. Cervical intraepithelial neoplasia E. Cervical erosion	**Ans: C (Cervicitis)** The adjacent image shows inflammation of the cervix characterized by a purulent endocervical exudate and easily induced endocervical bleeding. This is likely to be caused due to cervicitis, which can be defined as inflammation of cervix **(Fig. 19)**. Cervicitis may frequently cause intermenstrual or postcoital bleeding. Mucopurulent cervicitis may be associated with cervical infection due to organisms such as *Chlamydia trachomatis* and *Neisseria gonorrhoeae*. Cervicitis due to Herpes simplex may result in bleeding. 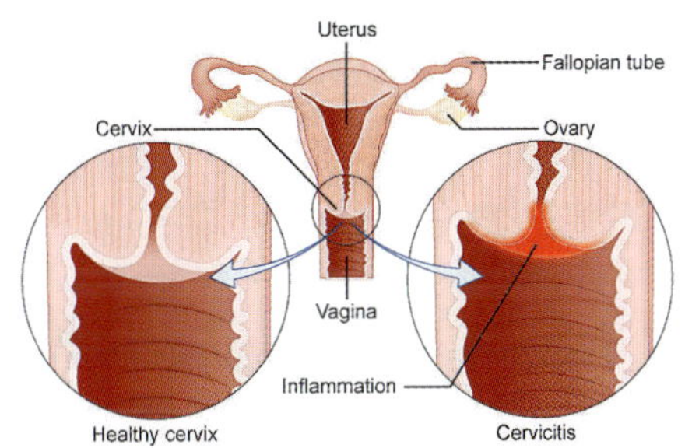 **Fig. 19:** Diagrammatic representation of cervicitis.	**Explanation:** Common causes include sexually transmitted infections, allergic reactions, or chemical irritants. Noninfectious causes may include injury due to some birth control devices like intrauterine contraceptive device, cervical cap or diaphragm. Cervical cancer can be another noninfectious cause of cervicitis. Diagnosis is typically confirmed through nucleic acid amplification testing (NAAT) for specific pathogens. Treatment depends on the cause but often involves administration of antibiotics or antiviral medications. Recommended single-dose treatment for uncomplicated gonococcal infection is either with ceftriaxone 250 mg IM plus azithromycin 1 g or doxycycline 100 mg twice daily for 7 days. Recommended oral treatment for chlamydial infection is azithromycin 1 g or doxycycline 100 mg twice daily for 7 days. **Potential questions:** There may be questions related to different types of cervical lesions (both malignant and nonmalignant).

<table>
<tr><th>Question</th><th>Answer</th><th>Comment</th></tr>
<tr>
<td>

Q20. During a routine pelvic examination, a 25-year-old woman is found to have a reddened, eroded area around the external os of the cervix as shown in the image below. Based on the below image, what is the most likely diagnosis?

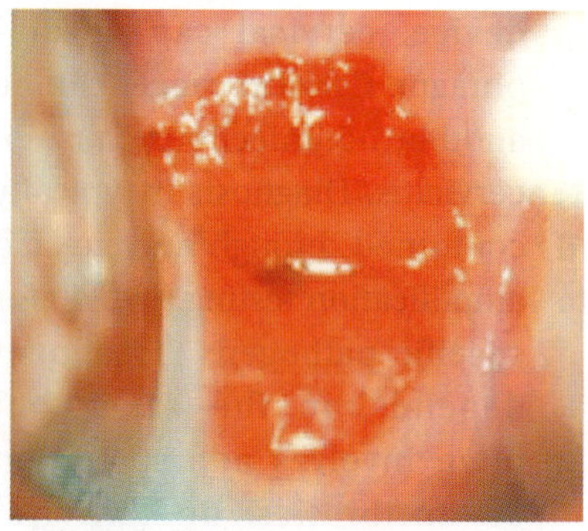

A. Cervical polyp
B. Cervical cancer
C. Cervical erosion
D. Cervicitis
E. CIN

</td>
<td>

Ans: C (Cervical erosion)

The adjacent image shows a reddish area on the cervix, which is indicative of cervical erosion (also known as cervical ectropion/ectopy). This condition occurs when there is migration/eversion of some endocervical tissue onto the vaginal portion of cervix, outward from the endocervical canal **(Fig. 20)**. In prepubertal women, normally the squamocolumnar junction lies at the level of external os. In cases of cervical erosion, the squamocolumnar junction lies external to the os.

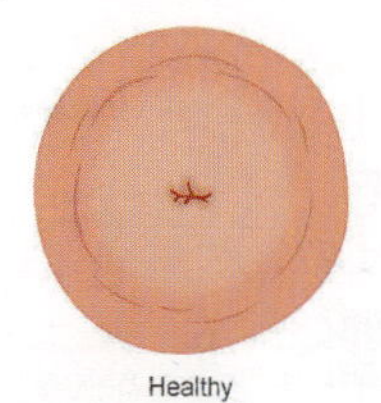

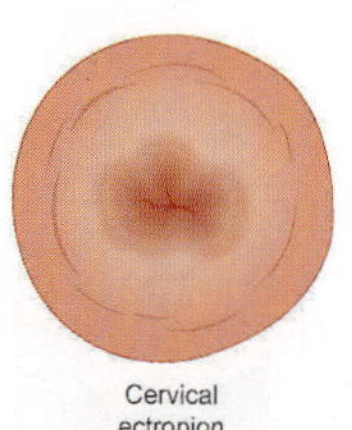

Fig. 20: Diagrammatic representation of cervical ectropion.

</td>
<td>

Explanation: Cervical ectropion is commonly seen in adolescents, pregnant women, and those using estrogen-containing contraceptives. The condition may be associated with excessive but nonpurulent vaginal discharge. Diagnosis is typically made through visual inspection during a speculum examination.

This condition may sometimes be responsible for postcoital bleeding. No treatment is required in asymptomatic cases. In symptomatic cases, hormone therapy may be prescribed. In extremely troublesome cases, it can be ablated under local anesthesia using either cauterization or cryotherapy.

Potential questions: There may be questions related to different types of cervical lesions (both malignant and nonmalignant).

</td>
</tr>
<tr>
<td>

Q21. A 35-year-old woman undergoes a per speculum examination for pelvic pain. On inspection, small, cystic structures are present on the cervix as shown in the image below (depicted by an arrow). The gynecologist discusses the findings with the patient to counsel her about her diagnosis.

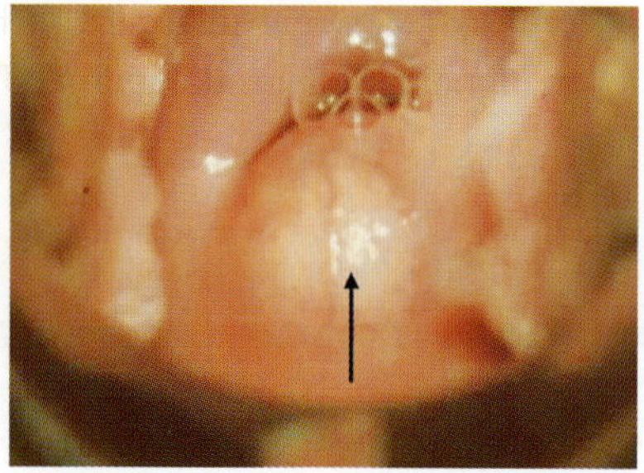

Based on the image, what is the most likely diagnosis?

A. Ectropion
B. Cervical polyp
C. Nabothian cyst
D. Cervical cancer
E. Cervicitis

</td>
<td>

Ans: C (Nabothian cyst)

The adjacent image shows small, well-defined cystic lesion on the cervix, characteristic of Nabothian cyst. These cysts form when the mucus-producing glands of the cervix become covered by squamous epithelium, trapping mucus inside. This might result in the development of smooth, clear, whitish- or yellowish-colored rounded elevations **(Fig. 21)** which may become visible at the time of per speculum examination.

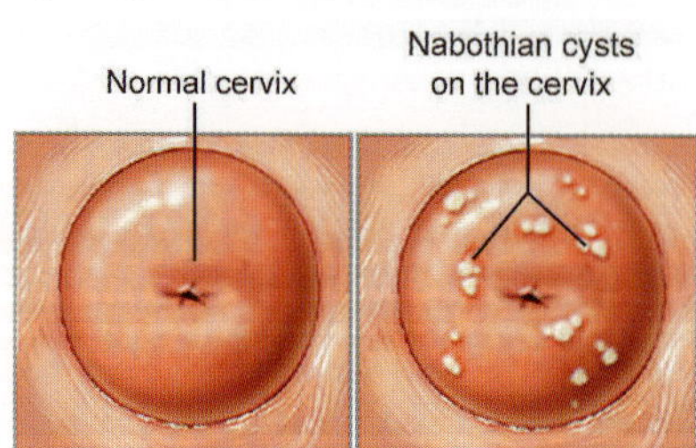

Fig. 21: Diagrammatic representation of Nabothian cysts.

</td>
<td>

Explanation: Nabothian cysts are typically asymptomatic and discovered incidentally during pelvic examinations. They are usually benign and require no treatment unless they are large or symptomatic.

They are mostly harmless but may disappear on their own. If they become large, cause discomfort, or make Pap testing or cervical examination difficult, they can be opened with the help of a biopsy forceps and drained. They can also be removed by electrocautery or cryotherapy. New cysts may sometimes appear even after the treatment.

Potential questions: There may be questions related to different types of cervical lesions (both malignant and nonmalignant).

</td>
</tr>
</table>

Question	Answer	Comment
Q22. A 30-year-old woman undergoes a colposcopy-directed biopsy in view of the presence of abnormal cells on her Pap smear performed during routine screening examination. The histological findings obtained are illustrated in the image below. What should be the next course of action in this case? 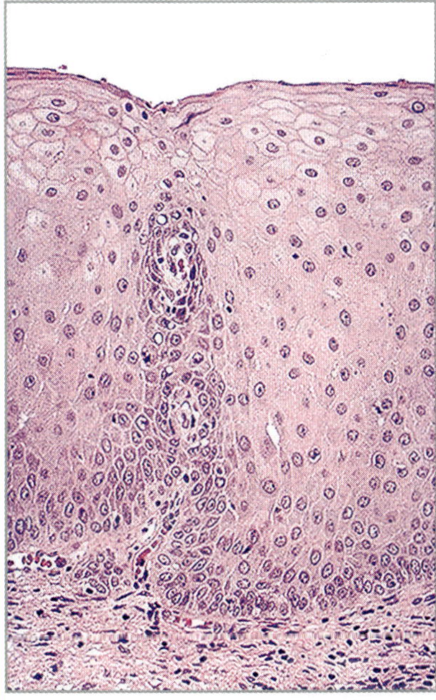 A. Refer her for colposcopy B. Loop electrosurgical excision procedure (LEEP) C. Call for a repeat smear at 6 months D. Human papillomavirus (HPV) testing E. Refer for routine recall	**Ans:** **E (Refer for routine recall)** The adjacent image shows histopathological appearance of normal cervical epithelium. As a result, no treatment or intervention is required in this case and she can be called at 3-yearly intervals for routine recall. Appearance of healthy cervical epithelium on histopathological examination is shown in **Figure 22**. 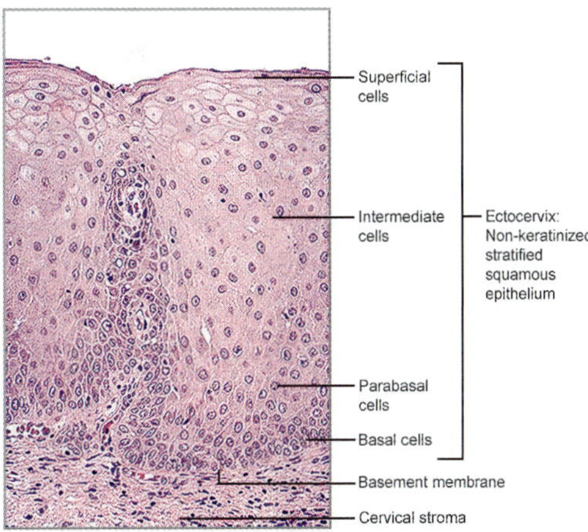 **Fig. 22:** Normal cervical epithelium (HPE).	**Explanation:** Normal ectocervical epithelium is composed of nonkeratinized stratified squamous cells, which are typically identified on Pap smears as large polygonal cells with abundant cytoplasm and small, pyknotic nuclei. The normal stratified squamous epithelium of ectocervix is composed of the following layers: Superficial, intermediate, parabasal, and basal. Cells of healthy cervical epithelium lack features of dysplasia (e.g., increased nuclear size) or viral infection (e.g., perinuclear halos seen in koilocytes). This cytological pattern is common in a normal Pap smear for a healthy cervix. The basement membrane separates the stratified squamous epithelium from cervical stroma. **Potential questions:** There may be questions related to different types of cervical lesions (both malignant and nonmalignant).

PREINVASIVE AND INVASIVE LESIONS OF CERVIX

Question	Answer	Comment
Q23. A 28-year-old woman presents for a routine Pap smear. Her results show atypical squamous cells, and a colposcopy is performed. The biopsy revealed findings as shown in the image below. She is otherwise healthy and has no plans for pregnancy in the immediate future. What is the most appropriate management option for this patient? 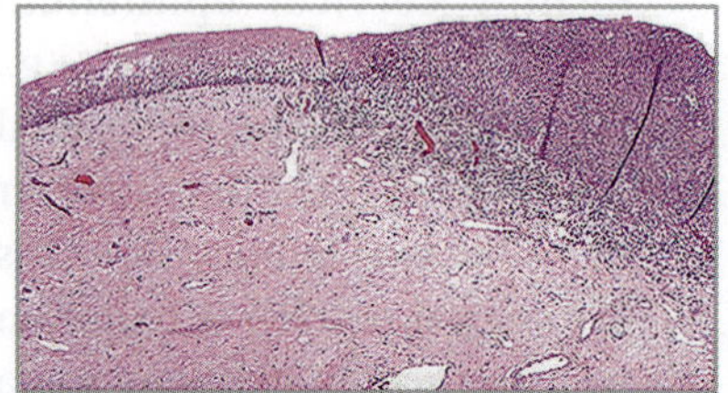 A. Immediate hysterectomy B. Observation with repeat cytology and colposcopy every 6 months C. Human papillomavirus (HPV) vaccination only D. Loop electrosurgical excision procedure (LEEP) E. Chemotherapy	**Ans: D [Loop electrosurgical excision procedure (LEEP)]** The adjacent image shows transformation zone of the normal cervical squamous epithelium on the left-hand side, which gets transformed into dysplastic changes on the right-hand side. Progression of dysplastic changes is shown in **Figure 23**. Biopsy in this case revealed cervical intraepithelial neoplasia grade 2 (CIN II). As per the Bethesda system, CIN II lesions are classified as HSIL (high-grade squamous intraepithelial neoplasia) as these lesions have a high-degree potential to progress to invasive cancer if left untreated. CIN I lesions are treated in adolescents only if the lesion persists beyond 2 years. For CIN II in adult women and CIN III lesions at any age, treatment in the form of loop excision or ablation is recommended. 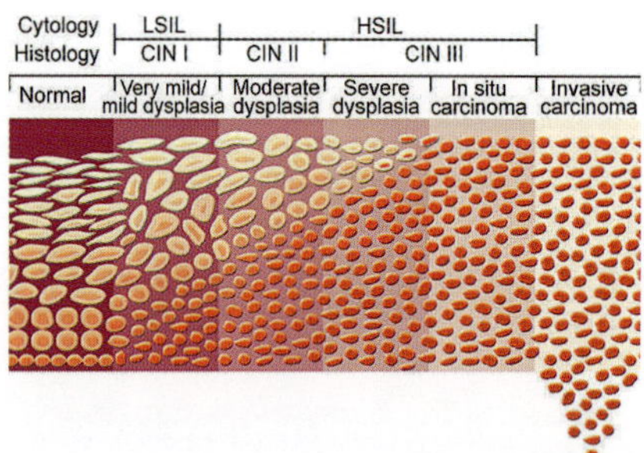 **Fig. 23:** Progression of cervical dysplasia.	**Explanation:** Dysplasia is a process which is associated with an abnormal maturation of cells within a tissue. Treatment of dysplasia at early stages prevents conversion into invasive cancer later. Dysplasias can be graded as follows **(Fig. 23)**: ▪ *Mild dysplasia (CIN-I):* The undifferentiated cells are confined to the lower one-third of the epithelium. ▪ *Moderate dysplasia (CIN-II):* Undifferentiated cells occupy the lower 50–75% of the epithelial thickness. ▪ *Severe dysplasia and carcinoma in situ (CIN-III):* In this grade of dysplasia, the entire thickness of epithelium is replaced by abnormal cells. The basement membrane, however, remains intact and there is no stromal infiltration. **Potential questions:** There may be questions related to different types of cervical lesions (both malignant and nonmalignant).

Question	Answer	Comment
Q24. A 65-year-old woman presents with a history of passing blood-stained dirty discharge per vaginum since the past few months. Per speculum examination revealed a friable growth on cervix. A punch biopsy is taken and sent for histopathological examination. The biopsy results are shown in the image below. What is the most likely diagnosis in this case? 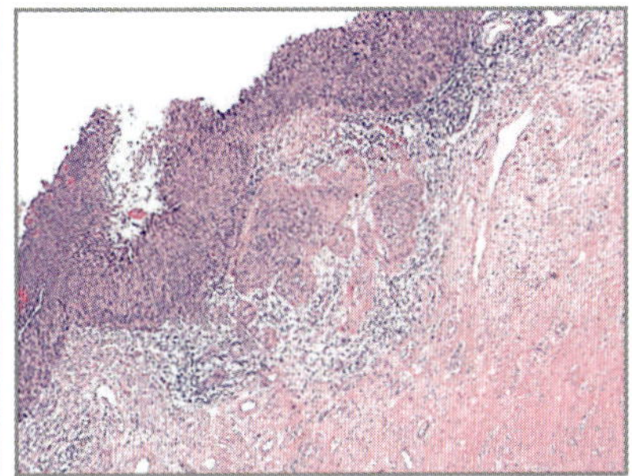 A. Cervicitis B. Cervical ectropion C. Invasive squamous cell carcinoma D. Invasive adenocarcinoma E. Cervical intraepithelial neoplasia	**Ans: C (Invasive squamous cell carcinoma)** Histopathological examination in the adjacent image is suggestive of invasive cervical carcinoma. Small irregular nests of well-differentiated squamous cancer cells have invaded the underlying stroma in the center and left side of the figure (as indicated by arrows in **Fig. 24**). Round eosinophilic structures marked by "KP" can be visualized in this image. These are keratin pearls, created due to the deposition of concentric layers of keratin by the malignant cells. 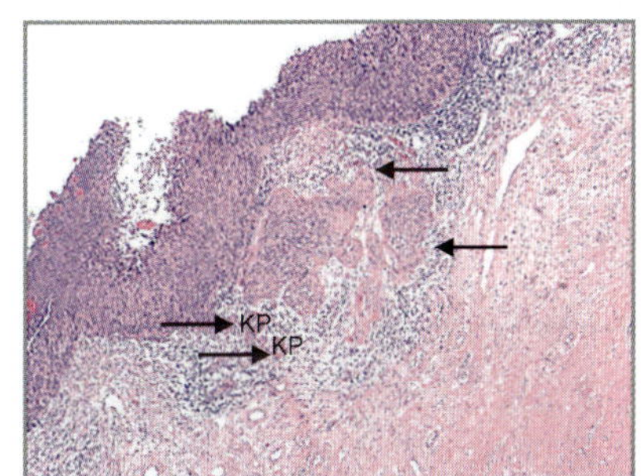 **Fig. 24:** Histopathological image showing the presence of invasive cervical carcinoma (KP: keratin pearls).	**Explanation:** Presence of abnormal results on Pap test or symptoms of cervical cancer may mandate further testing in the form of colposcopy, colposcopic-directed biopsy, punch biopsy and endocervical curettage, which can help in confirming if abnormal cells are dysplastic or cancerous. In case of cervical dysplasia, malignant cells are not able to invade the cervical stroma as the basement membrane remains intact. However, in cases of invasive cervical carcinoma, the basement membrane is breached, and the malignant cells invade the cervical stromal tissue. Squamous cell cancer developing from the cells of ectocervix is the most common type of cervical cancer, followed by adenocarcinoma which develops from the glandular cells of endocervix. **Potential questions:** There may be questions related to different types of cervical lesions (both malignant and nonmalignant).

Question	Answer	Comment
Q25. A 35-year-old woman undergoes a routine cervical cytology screening. The gynecologist explains the procedure to assess for cervical dysplasia or cancer and informs the patient that she shall be using the instruments as shown in the image below. Which of the following devices is used to collect cells from the cervix for the test? 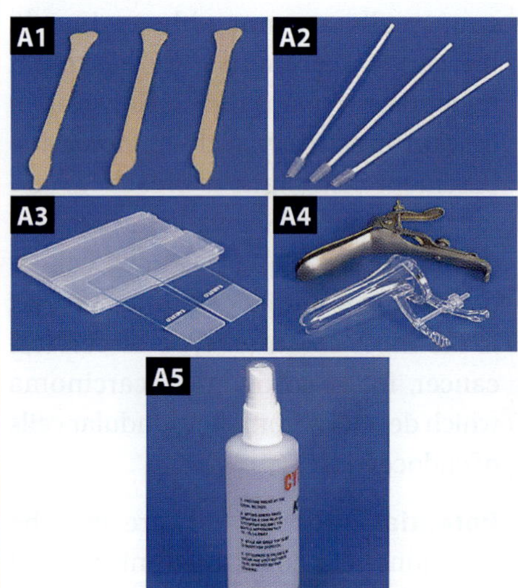 A. Speculum B. Colposcope C. Spatula and brush D. Curette E. Biopsy forceps	**Ans: C (Spatula and brush)** The adjacent images demonstrate the equipment for taking Pap smear, wherein (A1) is Ayre's spatula, (A2) is endocervical brush, (A3) is sides, (A4) is per vaginal speculum, and (A5) is fixative. Liquid-based cytology is a new way of sampling and preparing cervical cells. While the conventional "Pap smear" involves direct preparation of the slide from the cervical scrape obtained, the procedure of "ThinPrep" involves making a suspension of cells from the sample, which is then used to produce a thin layer of cells on the slide **(Figs. 25A and B)**. The advantage of liquid-based Pap smear is that it is associated with fewer drying artifacts and the chances of unsatisfactory smears are reduced. 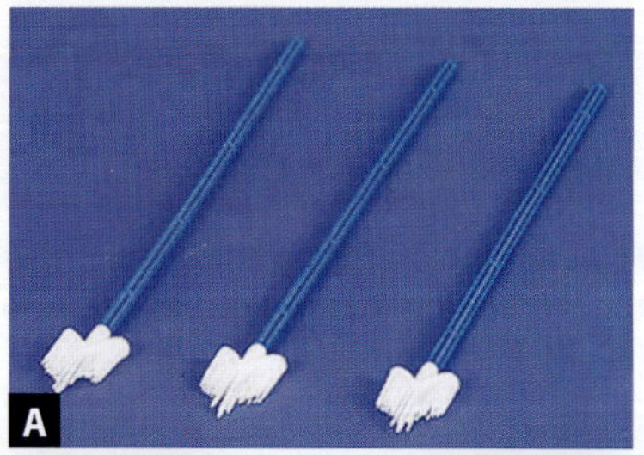 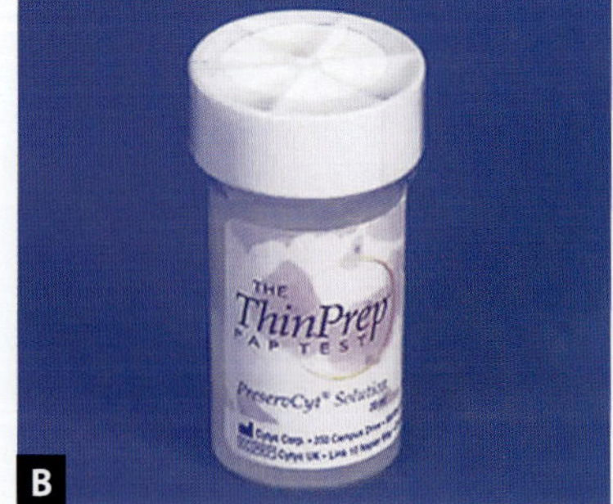 **Figs. 25A and B:** Equipment for liquid-based cytology: (A) Cervex-Brush; (B) ThinPrep vial.	**Explanation:** Since its introduction in the 1940s, cytological screening in the form of Pap smear has become the investigation of choice for detection of precancerous lesions of the cervix. The widespread introduction of the Papanicolaou test for cervical cancer screening has resulted in significantly reducing the incidence and mortality of cervical cancer, especially in the developed countries. Ayre's spatula and endocervical brush are specifically designed to collect cells from the ectocervix and endocervix, respectively, during a Pap smear. This ensures that a complete and representative sample of cervical cells is obtained for cytological examination to detect any abnormal or precancerous changes. Other tools, like the speculum, are necessary for visualizing the cervix, but the actual cell collection is done using the spatula and brush. **Potential questions:** There may be questions related to different types of cervical lesions (both malignant and nonmalignant).

<table>
<tr><th>Question</th><th>Answer</th><th>Comment</th></tr>
<tr><td>Q26. A 32-year-old woman presents for her routine Pap smear. The findings on cytology are shown in the image below. What is the next most appropriate step in the management of this patient?
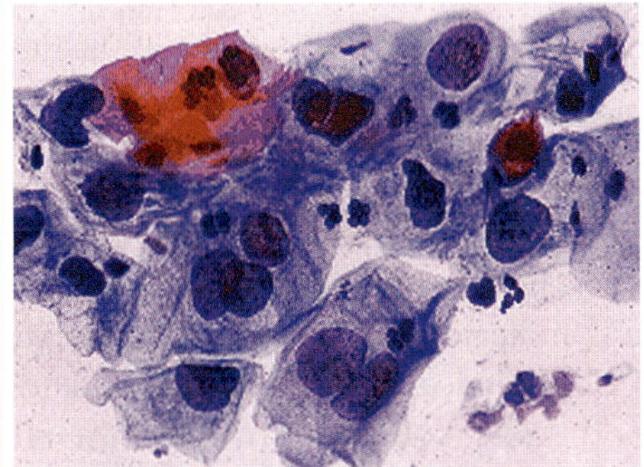
A. Immediate colposcopy
B. Repeat Pap smear in 6 months
C. Human papillomavirus (HPV) DNA testing
D. Endocervical curettage
E. Loop electrosurgical excision procedure (LEEP)</td><td>Ans: C [Human papillomavirus (HPV) DNA testing]
As previously mentioned, the normal ectocervix is composed of nonkeratinized squamous epithelium. Figure 26 shows the histopathological appearance of a normal Pap smear result. In contrast, the adjacent image shows abnormal Pap smear associated with atypical cells having features of atypia and dysplasia suggestive of HSIL.
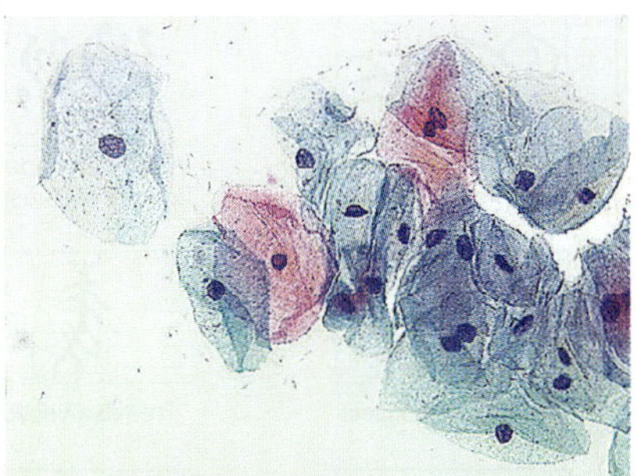
Fig. 26: Histopathological appearance of normal Pap smear result.</td><td>Explanation: Pap smear is an outpatient technique of screening for premalignant cervical changes. This enables early intervention to prevent conversion of premalignant changes into invasive malignant lesions. Changes indicative of HSIL on Pap smear include anisocytosis (abnormality in size), poikilocytosis (abnormality in shape), increased nuclear-cytoplasmic ratio, polymorphism, hyperchromatism of the nuclei, loss of nuclear polarity, presence of mitotic figures, irregular nuclear outline, etc.
Potential questions: There may be questions related to different types of cervical lesions (both malignant and nonmalignant).</td></tr>
</table>

Question	Answer	Comment
Q27. A 35-year-old woman undergoes examination through a specialized instrument as shown in the image below following an abnormal Pap smear. The findings reveal aceto-white epithelium and mosaicism on the cervix. What is the most likely diagnosis? 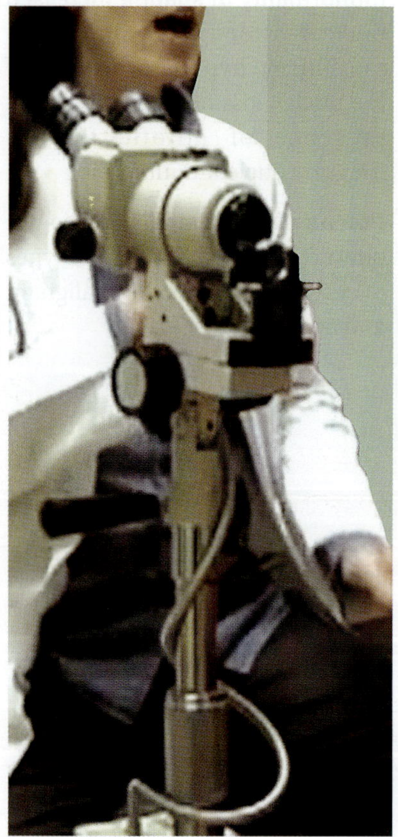 A. Cervicitis B. Normal cervical tissue C. High-grade squamous intraepithelial lesion (HSIL) D. Cervical cancer E. Low-grade squamous intraepithelial lesion	**Ans: C [High-grade squamous intraepithelial lesion (HSIL)]** The instrument depicted in the adjacent image is a colposcope, which is like a small microscope with a light and enables the gynecologist to perform thorough examination of cervix under illumination and magnification before and after application of dilute acetic acid and Lugol's iodine. Appearance of an abnormal vascular pattern on a colposcope is shown in **Figure 27**. 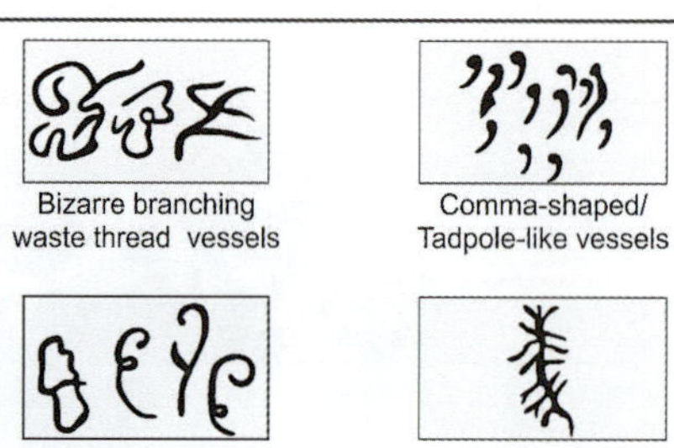 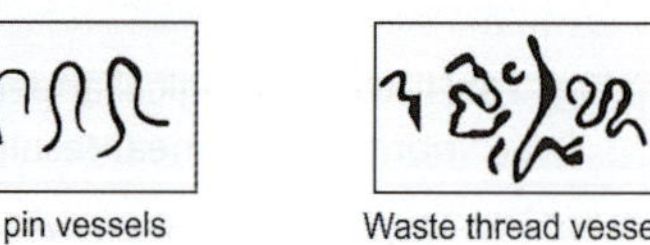 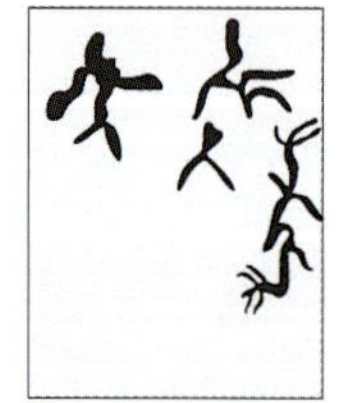 **Fig. 27:** Atypical blood vessel pattern as observed on colposcopic examination exhibiting bizarre variation in caliber, coarse branching pattern, abnormal proliferation, resulting in nonuniform branching pattern, etc.	**Explanation:** If abnormal cells are found in a Pap smear test or liquid-based cytology, the patient may be referred for a colposcopic examination and/or a colposcopic-directed biopsy. While the Pap smear detects abnormal cells, colposcopy helps in locating the abnormal lesions. Aceto-white epithelium and mosaicism observed during colposcopy are characteristic findings of HSIL. These lesions are precancerous and indicate a higher risk for progression to cervical cancer if untreated. Low-grade squamous intraepithelial lesion (LSIL) presents with less distinct colposcopic features. On the other hand, frank cervical malignancy cancer would show more advanced signs such as irregular masses or ulcerations. **Potential questions:** There may be questions related to different types of cervical lesions (both malignant and nonmalignant).

Question	Answer	Comment
Q28. A 29-year-old woman with persistent abnormal Pap smear undergoes a procedure as shown in the image below. Postoperatively, she presents with mild spotting and discharge, but no significant pain. Which of the following would be the most appropriate follow-up management? 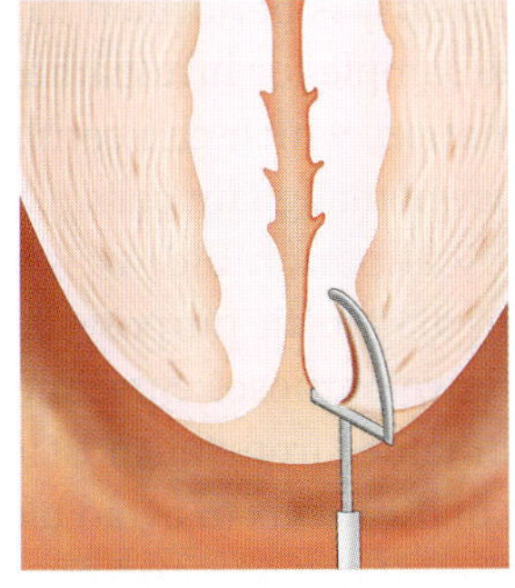 A. Repeat Pap smear in 3 months B. Immediate repeat colposcopy C. HPV test in 6 months D. Pap smear and HPV co-testing in 12 months E. No follow-up required	**Ans: D (Pap smear and HPV co-testing in 12 months)** The adjacent image presents a magnified view showing LEEP, a terminology commonly used in the USA. This procedure is termed "large loop excision of the transformation zone" (LLTZ) in the UK and utilizes a larger loop **(Fig. 28)**. The LEEP equipment comprises a thin wire loop electrode attached to an electrosurgical generator, which generates current to cut away cervical tissue that comes in vicinity of wire loop. 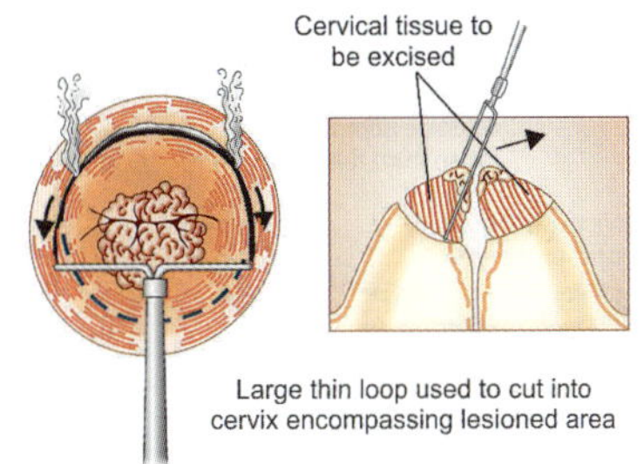 **Fig. 28:** Large loop excision of the transformation zone.	**Explanation:** After a LEEP procedure, the most appropriate follow-up includes co-testing with a Pap smear and HPV test at 12 months to ensure that the abnormal cells have been adequately treated and to monitor for any recurrence of HPV infection or cervical dysplasia. In LEEP, the loop of wire is advanced into the cervix lateral to the lesion until the required depth is reached. The loop is then taken across to the opposite side and a cone of tissue is removed. The excision is usually performed to a depth of 8 mm and extends 4–5 mm beyond the region of the lesion. The area of abnormal cells is removed completely using the loop of wire and electrosurgery. **Potential questions:** There may be questions related to different types of cervical lesions (both malignant and nonmalignant).
Q29. A 48-year-old woman presents with abnormal vaginal bleeding and pelvic pain. A transabdominal sonography shows the following image. What is the most likely diagnosis based on this imaging finding? 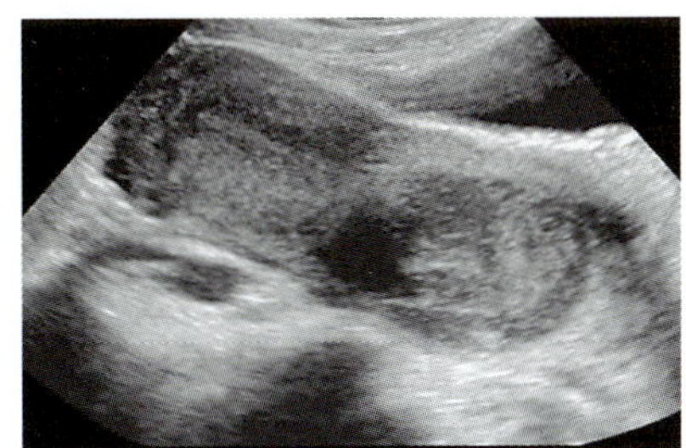 A. Endometrial carcinoma B. Cervical squamous cell carcinoma C. Ovarian germ cell tumor D. Cervical adenocarcinoma E. Benign uterine fibroid	**Ans: B (Cervical squamous cell carcinoma)** The adjacent transabdominal ultrasound image depicts a solid, heterogeneous mass within the cervix, which raises suspicion of cervical malignancy. In the same patient, CT scan **(Fig. 29)** showed large lobulated cervical mass with central hypoattenuation, limited to the cervix (stage I cervical malignancy). 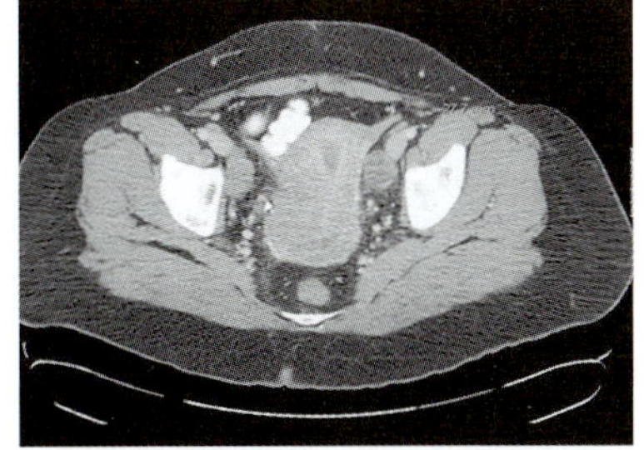 **Fig. 29:** CT scan of the same patient.	**Explanation:** Abnormal vaginal bleeding is the most common manifestation of cervical malignancy and may manifest as irregular vaginal bleeding, postcoital bleeding, bleeding in between periods, etc. The patient's symptoms of abnormal bleeding and the location of the mass on ultrasound further support this diagnosis. Furthermore, the solid heterogeneous appearance of the cervical mass on TAS is highly suggestive of cervical squamous cell carcinoma, which accounts for 80–90% of all cervical cancers. **Potential questions:** There may be questions related to different types of cervical lesions (both malignant and nonmalignant).

Question	Answer	Comment
Q30. A 42-year-old woman presents with postcoital bleeding. On examination, an exophytic/friable growth as shown in the image below is observed on the cervix. What is the next best step of management in this case? 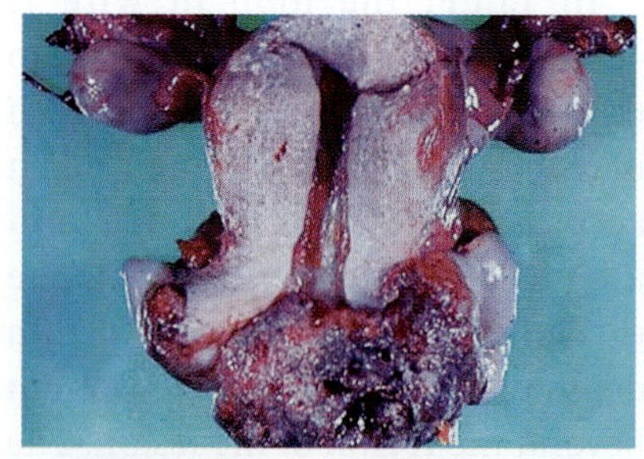 A. Colposcopy B. PET scan C. MRI scan D. Pap smear E. Cervical punch biopsy	**Ans: E (Cervical punch biopsy)** The adjacent image shows a fungating growth on the cervix. Though this is suggestive of malignancy, a biopsy needs to be performed to confirm the diagnosis. Therefore, the next best step of management in this case is to perform cervical biopsy using punch biopsy forceps **(Fig. 30)**. This is usually performed as an outpatient department procedure, in which small pieces of tissue are removed from the affected areas using punch biopsy forceps. 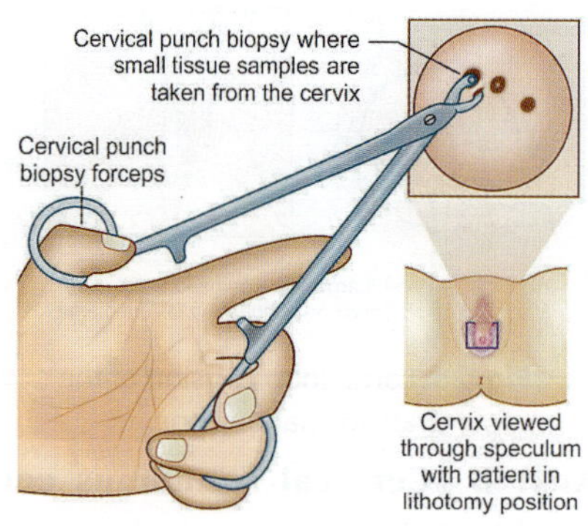 **Fig. 30:** Cervical punch biopsy.	**Explanation:** Presence of a fungating/friable growth on cervix that bleeds on touch and leads to postcoital bleeding is highly suggestive of cervical carcinoma. Cervical carcinoma can present as an exophytic, friable mass that can bleed easily on touch or present as an ulcerative growth. A cervical punch biopsy is performed to obtain a tissue sample for histopathological examination, which can confirm the presence of malignant cells. Cervical punch biopsy is purely used for diagnostic purposes and not for curative purposes. Specimens are firstly obtained from the most inferior aspect of the cervix to avoid bleeding from the biopsy site and obscuring other biopsy sites. Biopsy specimen is then sent for HPE. **Potential questions:** There may be questions related to different types of cervical lesions (both malignant and nonmalignant).

UTERINE CANCER

Question	Answer	Comment
Q31. A 45-year-old woman presents with intermenstrual bleeding since the last 2 weeks. Transvaginal ultrasound revealed an endometrial thickness of 5 mm. She gives a history that her mother died due to endometrial cancer 10 years back. The patient undergoes hysteroscopy, which shows an exophytic growth (marked by an arrow) protruding into the uterine cavity as shown in the image below. Based on the imaging and clinical findings, what is the next best step of management in this case? 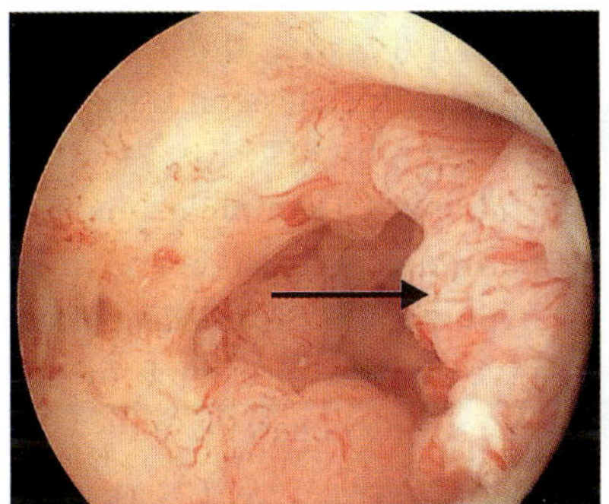 A. Treat for endometrial hyperplasia B. Transcervical resection of endometrium C. Hysteroscopic-directed biopsy D. Treat for endometrial carcinoma E. Endometrial aspiration	**Ans: C (Hysteroscopic directed biopsy)** The arrow in the adjacent image points toward a large exophytic growth arising from the endometrium. The features suggestive of malignancy in this case include: ▪ *Large diffuse growth:* Lesions appears to occupy more than half of the endometrial surface. ▪ *Irregular surface:* The surface of the growth tends to be irregular and has a heterogeneous echotexture ▪ *Abnormal blood vessels:* Abnormal blood vessels are visible over the surface of the lesion. **Figure 31** shows diagrammatic representation of this growth, observed on hysteroscopy. 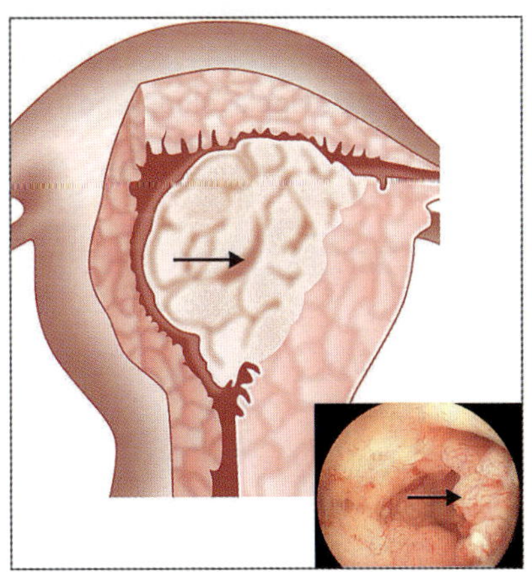 **Fig. 31:** Diagrammatic representation of the exophytic growth arising from the cervix.	**Explanation:** The presence of a large exophytic growth with a heterogeneous echotexture seen during hysteroscopy is highly suspicious of endometrial cancer in the adjacent image. A hysteroscopic-directed biopsy would be required in this case to confirm the diagnosis. Endometrial cancer, characterized by abnormal proliferation of the endometrial epithelium, usually affects menopausal and perimenopausal women, commonly in the age group of 50–65 years. It may commonly present as an exophytic growth or sometimes as an ulcerative lesion. The most important risk factor for endometrial cancer is hyperestrogenism. The most common symptom associated with endometrial cancer is abnormal uterine bleeding. Transvaginal ultrasound is especially indicated in women who are at high risk for endometrial cancer. If the endometrial stripe on ultrasound examination is >4 mm, endometrial sampling/biopsy should be performed. **Potential questions:** There can be questions related to clinical presentation, diagnosis, and management of cases of endometrial hyperplasia as well as malignancy.

Question	Answer	Comment
Q32. A 62-year-old woman presents with postmenopausal bleeding. Transvaginal ultrasound reveals an endometrial thickness of 9 mm. What is the next best step of management? 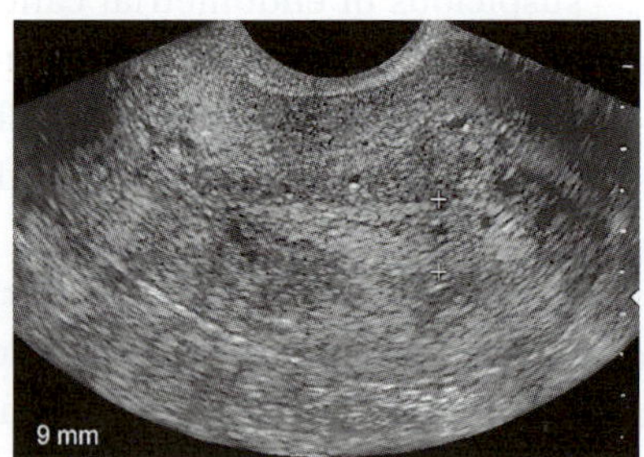 A. Treat for endometrial hyperplasia B. Transcervical resection of endometrium C. Hysteroscopic-directed biopsy. D. Treat for endometrial carcinoma E. Endometrial aspiration/biopsy	**Ans: E (Endometrial aspiration/ biopsy)** The adjacent transvaginal ultrasound image reveals an endometrial thickness of 9 mm. Measurement of endometrial thickness on transvaginal ultrasound has become a routine investigation in patients with abnormal uterine bleeding, especially those belonging to the perimenopausal age groups. Prior to biopsy, Doppler ultrasound was performed in this patient. It revealed endometrial hyperplasia with prominent peripheral vascular signals **(Fig. 32)**. 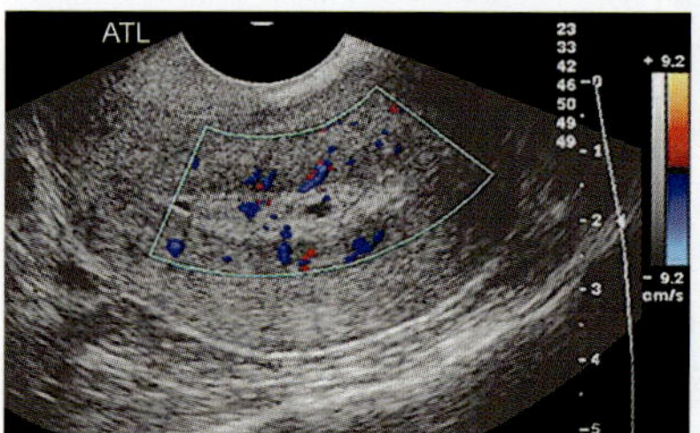 **Fig. 32:** Doppler ultrasound in the same patient.	**Explanation:** Postmenopausal bleeding is a significant clinical symptom that warrants thorough evaluation. An endometrial thickness of >4 mm on transvaginal ultrasound in postmenopausal women with abnormal bleeding is concerning and often prompts further investigation. While endometrial hyperplasia and polyps can also cause increased endometrial thickness, the risk of malignancy, especially in perimenopausal women, necessitates prioritizing the exclusion of endometrial carcinoma. In this case, since the endometrial thickness on transvaginal sonography (TVS) is >4 mm, an endometrial sampling/biopsy was performed to exclude endometrial hyperplasia. Biopsy in this case revealed the presence of endometrial adenocarcinoma. **Potential questions:** There can be questions related to clinical presentation, diagnosis, and management of cases of endometrial hyperplasia as well as malignancy.

Question	Answer	Comment
Q33. A 65-year-old postmenopausal woman presents with postmenopausal bleeding since a month. She also complains of dyspareunia since the last 2 months. The image below shows transvaginal ultrasound performed in this patient. What is the most likely diagnosis? 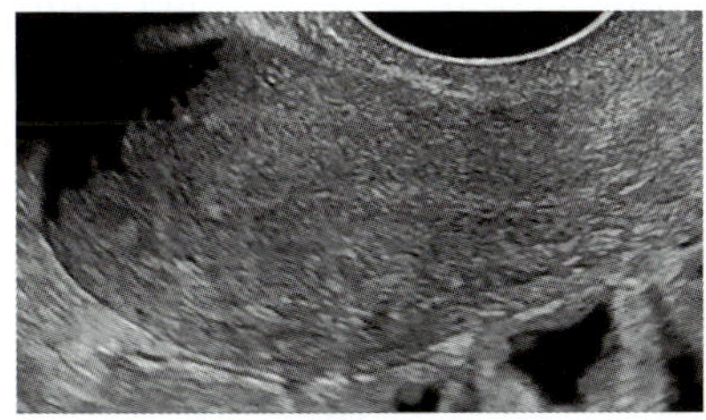 A. Endometrial hyperplasia B. Endometrial carcinoma C. Atrophic endometritis D. Chronic endometritis E. Endometrial polyp	**Ans: C (Atrophic endometritis)** The adjacent transvaginal ultrasound image revealed thin endometrium (thickness = 3 mm) in this patient. Biopsy diagnosed endometrial atrophy. Based on the findings of clinical examination and investigations, a diagnosis of endometrial atrophy was made. On hysteroscopy, atrophic endometrium typically appears as pale or white due to the thinning of the tissue **(Fig. 33)**. There is usually a noticeable reduction in vascularity, although some areas may show hypervascularization. There is also loss of rugae, normally seen in premenopausal women. 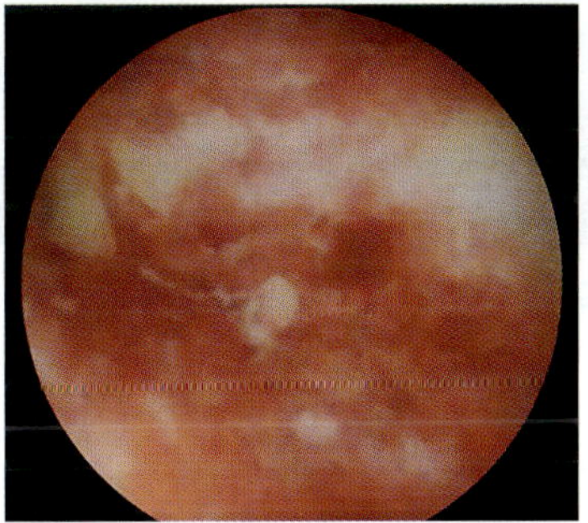 **Fig. 33:** Appearance of atrophic endometrium on hysteroscopy.	**Explanation:** Endometrial atrophy is a benign condition commonly encountered in postmenopausal women. This is related to the deficiency of estrogen, which causes the endometrium, vaginal epithelium, and epithelium of the urinary tract to become thin and atrophic. Atrophic endometritis is characterized by a thin endometrial basalis layer with few narrow tubular glands lined by cuboidal epithelium. Histopathological examination in these cases is essential because there may be hidden areas of hypertrophic endometrium within the areas of atrophic endometrium. Once the diagnosis has been confirmed, treatment usually depends on estrogen replacement. This can be administered systemically or locally (in the form of vaginal topical applications). **Potential questions:** There can be questions related to clinical presentation, diagnosis, and management of cases of endometrial abnormalities (hyperplasia, atrophy, etc.) as well as malignancy.

Question	Answer	Comment
Q34. A 68-year-old postmenopausal woman presents with postmenopausal bleeding. The transvaginal ultrasound image below shows the endometrium. The biopsy has confirmed an endometrial adenocarcinoma stage 1. What is the next most appropriate step in management? 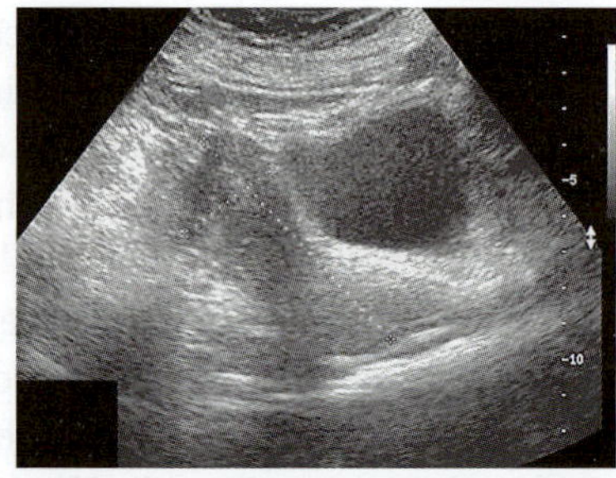 A. Observation and follow-up ultrasound in 6 months B. Hormonal therapy C. Hysteroscopy with biopsy D. Total abdominal hysterectomy with bilateral salpingo-oophorectomy and sentinel lymph node biopsy E. Total abdominal hysterectomy with bilateral salpingo-oophorectomy (TAH + BSO)	**Ans: D (Total abdominal hysterectomy with bilateral salpingo-oophorectomy and sentinel lymph node biopsy)** The adjacent transabdominal ultrasound image shows an enlarged uterine cavity, measuring 77 × 31 mm, with multiple cystic spaces within. Biopsy has confirmed the presence of endometrial cancer. **Figure 34** shows the image on Doppler ultrasound in the same patient. There were prominent peripheral and central vascular signals on ultrasound, which revealed the presence of an advanced stage endometrial adenocarcinoma (Stage 1B). 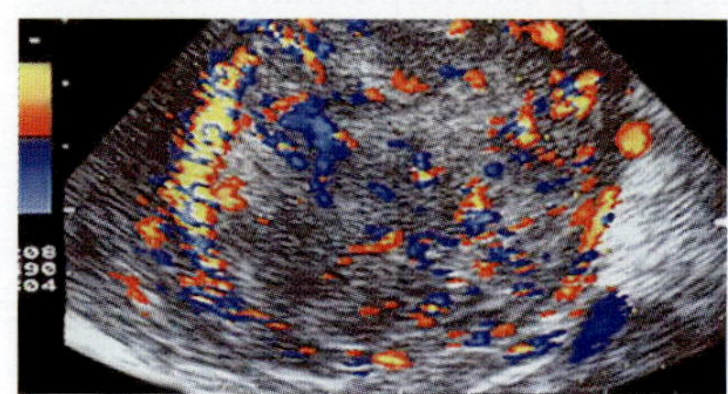 **Fig. 34:** Doppler ultrasound in the same patient.	**Explanation:** The management of endometrial cancer typically involves surgical intervention, especially in postmenopausal women presenting with abnormal uterine bleeding and ultrasound findings suggestive of malignancy. The standard treatment is a total abdominal hysterectomy with bilateral salpingo-oophorectomy with sentinel lymph node biopsy. Bilateral pelvic and paraaortic lymphadenectomy may be required in these cases if sentinel lymph node biopsy is positive. Brachytherapy may be required in cases of low-intermediate risk lesions (G1 and G2, stage 1B). In case of high-intermediate risk lesions (G3, stage 1B), external beam radiotherapy can be administered. **Potential questions:** There can be questions related to clinical presentation, diagnosis, and management of cases of endometrial abnormalities (hyperplasia, atrophy, etc.) as well as malignancy.

Question	Answer	Comment
Q35. A 52-year-old menopausal woman presents with irregular bleeding and offensive vaginal discharge for the past 2–3 months. A transvaginal ultrasound shows the findings depicted in the image below. What is the most likely diagnosis? 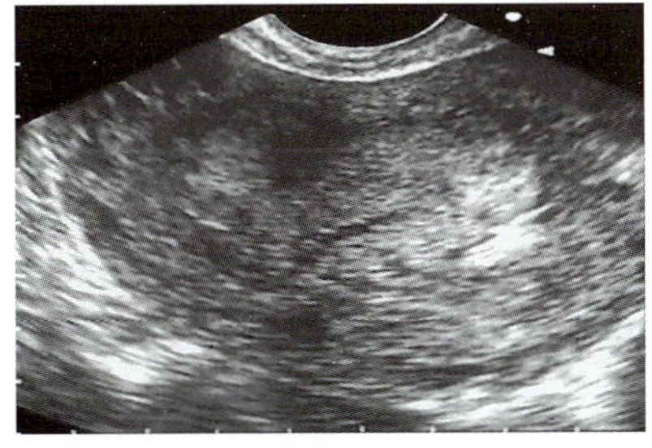 A. Endometrial adenocarcinoma B. Endometrial hyperplasia C. Endometrial polyp D. Atrophic vaginitis E. Squamous cell carcinoma	**Ans: A (Endometrial adenocarcinoma)** The adjacent transvaginal ultrasound image revealed the presence of a heterogeneous mass within the endometrial cavity. This mass was observed to be replacing the normal endometrial stripe. Doppler ultrasound was performed **(Fig. 35)**, which confirmed the suspicion of malignancy. Increased vascular flow was observed on Doppler ultrasound due to increased endometrial angiogenesis in lieu of the underlying malignancy. Hysteroscopic-guided biopsy later confirmed the diagnosis of advanced-stage endometrial cancer. The most common type of endometrial cancer is endometrial adenocarcinoma. 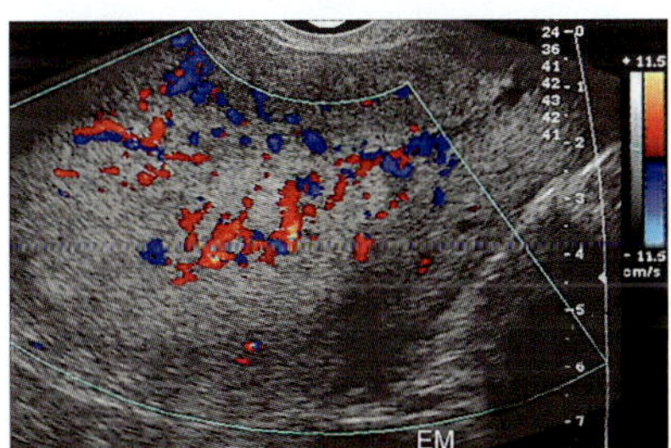 **Fig. 35:** Doppler ultrasound in the same patient.	**Explanation:** Endometrial carcinoma is a common cause of postmenopausal bleeding and can present with symptoms such as irregular bleeding and offensive vaginal discharge. Endometrial cancer is commonly diagnosed using transvaginal ultrasound. The ultrasound finding of a broad-based polypoid mass having heterogeneous echotexture, present within the endometrial cavity, is highly suggestive of malignancy. The mass has also replaced the normal endometrial stripe. Other features that may be seen on ultrasound in these cases include presence of thickened, heterogeneous endometrium with irregular borders, intrauterine fluid collection (suggestive of pyometra or hematometra), presence of calcifications, and disruption of the subendometrial halo, which may suggest myometrial invasion. **Potential questions:** There can be questions related to clinical presentation, diagnosis, and management of cases of endometrial abnormalities (hyperplasia, atrophy, etc.) as well as malignancy.

Question	Answer	Comment
Q36. A 62-year-old woman presents with postmenopausal bleeding and pelvic pain since past 1 week. Doppler ultrasound shows findings as shown in the image below. What is the most appropriate next step in managing this patient? 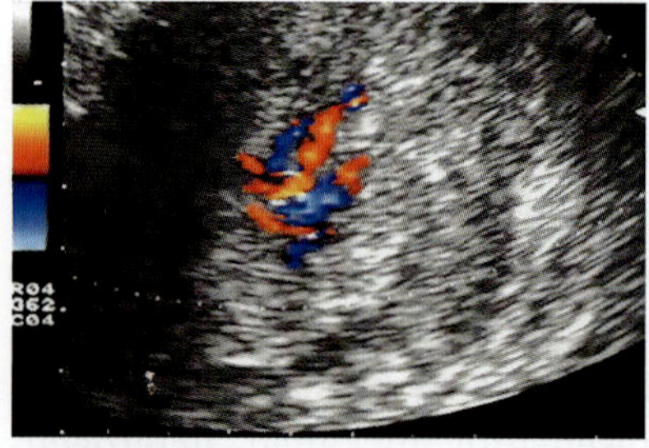 A. Endometrial biopsy B. Repeat Doppler ultrasound in 3 months C. Hormonal therapy D. Total hysterectomy E. Chemotherapy	**Ans: A (Endometrial biopsy)** The adjacent image is a color Doppler ultrasound image revealing thick heterogeneous endometrium with proliferation of blood vessels. A probable diagnosis of advanced-stage endometrial cancer was made. T1-weighted images on MRI examination in the same patient **(Fig. 36)** revealed a large tumor of low signal intensity, expanding within the uterine cavity. There was no spread to distant body organs. 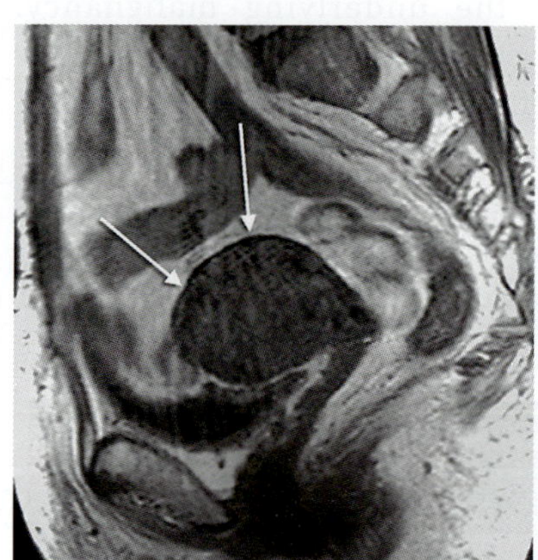 **Fig. 36:** Magnetic resonance imaging scan in the same patient.	**Explanation:** In postmenopausal women with abnormal bleeding and ultrasound findings of thickened endometrium and increased vascularity, endometrial biopsy is the first step to confirm the diagnosis. These findings raise the suspicion of endometrial cancer, and biopsy is necessary to determine the presence of malignancy. Based on biopsy results, further treatment such as TAH + BSO with sentinel lymph node biopsy, with or without lymph node dissection, radiation, or chemotherapy, may be indicated. **Potential questions:** There can be questions related to clinical presentation, diagnosis, and management of cases of endometrial abnormalities (hyperplasia, atrophy, etc.) as well as malignancy.

Question	Answer	Comment
Q37. A 68-year-old postmenopausal woman presents with abdominal pain, abnormal uterine bleeding, offensive discharge, and an enlarging mass per abdomen since past 2 months. The woman had a history of uterine fibroids. A CT scan of the pelvis reveals a heterogeneous uterine mass with areas of necrosis and hemorrhage having irregular margins. A CT-guided biopsy revealed the diagnosis of leiomyosarcoma. What is the most appropriate initial management step for this patient? 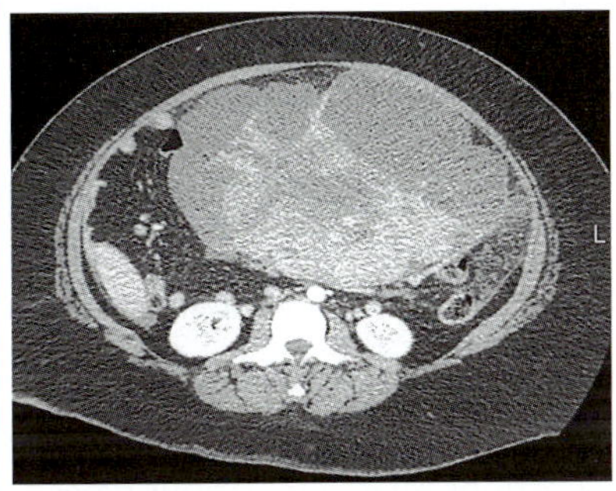 A. Observation with follow-up imaging B. Total abdominal hysterectomy with bilateral salpingo-oophorectomy (TAH-BSO) C. Endometrial biopsy D. Radiotherapy E. Chemotherapy as the first-line treatment	**Ans: B [Total abdominal hysterectomy with bilateral salpingo-oophorectomy (TAH-BSO)]** Leiomyosarcoma is a rare but aggressive malignancy of the uterus, often presenting with rapid growth and symptoms like pelvic pain or bleeding in postmenopausal women. It arises from the smooth muscle fibers of myometrium and can behave in an unpredictable manner. They can remain dormant for long periods of time and then suddenly recur after many years. Computed tomography imaging is useful for evaluating the extent of spread of cancer beyond the uterus into the adjacent structures and organs. CT scan may also be useful in evaluating the patient's response to surgery or presence of any recurrence. Biopsy can be performed using a CT-guided core needle biopsy to confirm the diagnosis. **Figure 37** shows a gross specimen of leiomyosarcoma as obtained upon hysterectomy. 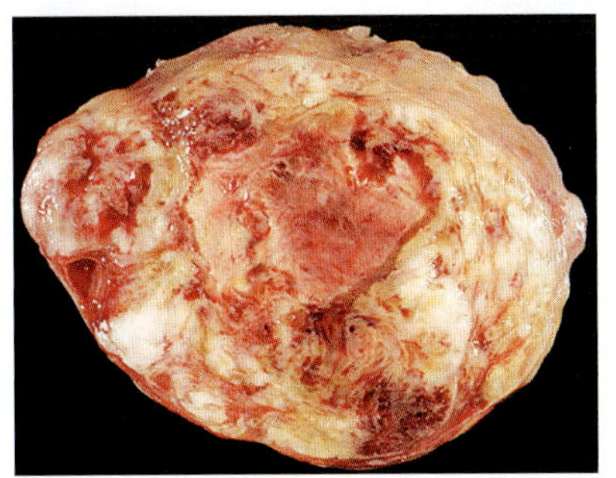 **Fig. 37:** Gross specimen of leiomyosarcoma as obtained upon hysterectomy.	**Explanation:** The rate of conversion of leiomyoma into a leiomyosarcoma is very low, being about 0.5%. Also, the rate of occurrence of uterine leiomyosarcomas is extremely low, with the incidence being about 0.67/1,000 women per year. Since the incidence of sarcomas is so low, it is not clinically justifiable to believe that the growing fibroid in this case indicates malignancy. Since the patient is postmenopausal, any growth in the uterus may be a cause for concern. In this case, efforts were made to first rule out endometrial carcinoma. Biopsy helped in arriving at the correct diagnosis. The definitive management of uterine leiomyosarcoma is surgical, with extrafascial total abdominal hysterectomy with bilateral salpingo-oophorectomy (TAH-BSO) and formal surgical staging being the recommended first-line treatment. While most leiomyosarcomas are usually resistant to radiation and chemotherapy, each case behaves differently and some cases may even respond to radiotherapy or chemotherapy. **Potential questions:** There can be different questions related to the clinical presentation, management, and diagnosis of various benign and malignant lesions arising from uterine muscles.

VULVAR LESIONS

Question	Answer	Comment
Q38. A 55-year-old postmenopausal woman presents with persistent vulvar itching and discomfort. On examination, the gynecologist observes white, thin, and fragile skin in the vulvar area, as shown in the below image. Based on the image, what is the most likely diagnosis in this case? 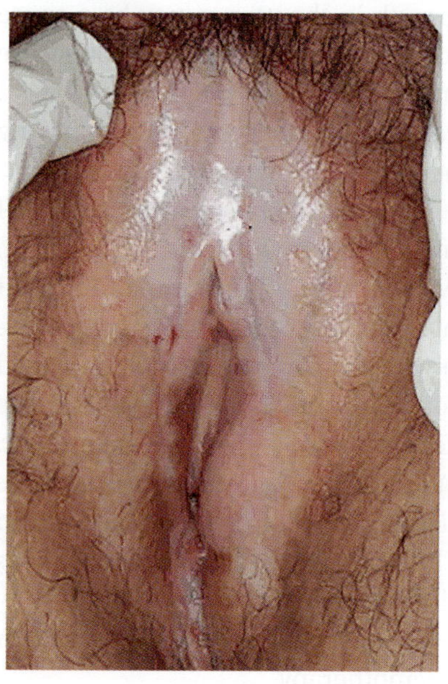 A. Psoriasis B. Lichen planus C. Lichen sclerosis D. Vulvar intraepithelial neoplasia E. Contact dermatitis	**Ans: C (Lichen sclerosis)** The adjacent image shows white, atrophic patches with a crinkled or parchment-like appearance, characteristic of lichen sclerosis. Lichen sclerosis commonly affects postmenopausal women, though it may be frequently also present in premenopausal women. The etiology, largely, remains unknown, though it can be associated with various causes such as infection, hormones, genetic, and autoimmune causes. Though this is a non-neoplastic dermatosis, patients may be at an increased risk of malignancy. Malignant transformation can occur in nearly 4–6% cases. Such women would require surveillance every 6–12 months. 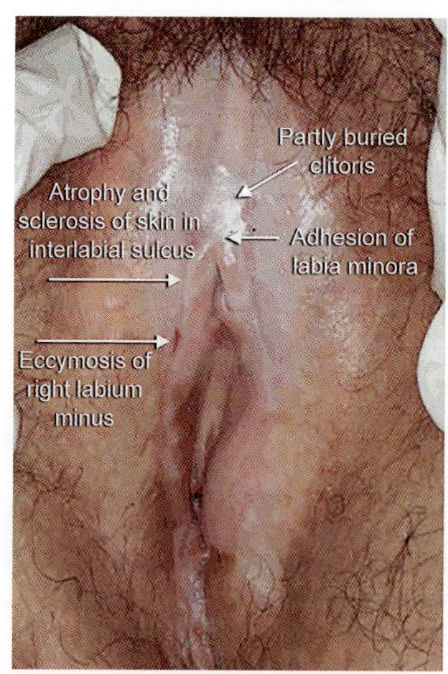 **Fig. 38:** Lesions of lichen sclerosis.	**Explanation:** Most women with lichen sclerosis remain asymptomatic. Symptoms include white, patchy skin that is thinner than normal, itching, and discomfort. Pruritus-induced scratching may result in the development of excoriations and thickening of the vulvar skin. There may be the presence of white atrophic papules, whitish plaques, regression of labia minora, clitoral concealment, and introital stenosis **(Fig. 38)**. Treatment typically involves topical corticosteroids and monitoring for potential malignant transformation. Diagnosis is typically clinical, supported by histopathological findings of thinning epidermis, loss of rete ridges, and a band-like lymphocytic infiltrate in the dermis. **Potential questions:** There can be questions related to various types of vulvar lesions (benign, malignant, and preinvasive)

Question	Answer	Comment
Q39. A 30-year-old woman presents with a painless, unilateral swelling in the posterior aspect of the labia majora. The swelling has been gradually increasing in size over the past few weeks. On examination, the gynecologist identifies a nontender mass near the vaginal opening as shown in the image below. What is the most likely diagnosis? 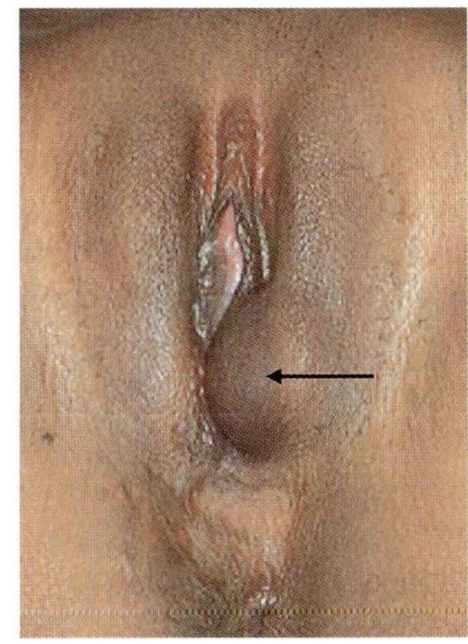 A. Bartholin gland cyst B. Skene's gland cyst C. Gartner duct cyst D. Nabothian cyst E. Vulvar abscess	**Ans: A (Bartholin gland cyst)** Bartholin glands, also known as greater vestibular glands, are located to the left and right of the vaginal introitus, slightly towards the posterior side **(Fig. 39)**. These glands secrete mucus, which helps in lubricating the vagina. These glands are homologous to bulbourethral glands in males. The adjacent image depicts cysts of Bartholin gland (shown by an arrow), which are commonly encountered in routine gynecological practice. They typically measure 1–4 cm in size and are frequently asymptomatic. Larger cysts may result in vaginal pressure symptoms and dyspareunia. A Bartholin gland cyst is usually painless. However, if the cyst becomes infected, it can form an abscess, which is often painful. 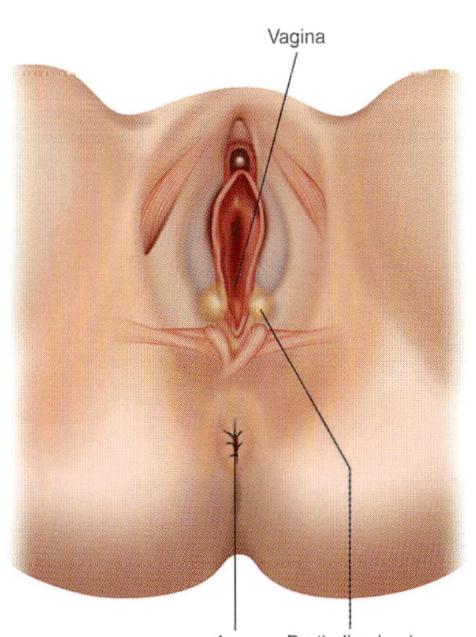 **Fig. 39:** Normal location of Bartholin glands.	**Explanation:** A Bartholin gland cyst occurs when the duct of the Bartholin gland becomes obstructed, leading to the accumulation of mucus and formation of a cyst. The ultrasound image in these cases usually shows a well-defined, fluid-filled cystic structure, which further supports this diagnosis. In contrast, Skene's gland cysts are located near the urethra, Gartner duct cysts are remnants of the mesonephric duct found along the lateral walls of the vagina, Nabothian cysts are found on the cervix, and a vulvar abscess would present with pain and signs of infection. Permanent resolution of the cyst is done either using marsupialization or incision, and drainage with Word's catheter placement. Placement of Word's catheter helps in creating a new epithelialized tract for gland drainage after emptying the cyst cavity through the procedure of incision and drainage. **Potential questions:** There can be questions related to various types of vulvar lesions (benign, malignant, and preinvasive).

<table>
<tr><th>Question</th><th>Answer</th><th>Comment</th></tr>
<tr>
<td>

Q40. A 65-year-old woman presents with a large ulcerative lesion over the right labia majora as shown in the image below. A biopsy confirms squamous cell carcinoma of the vulva. What is the most appropriate initial management for this patient?

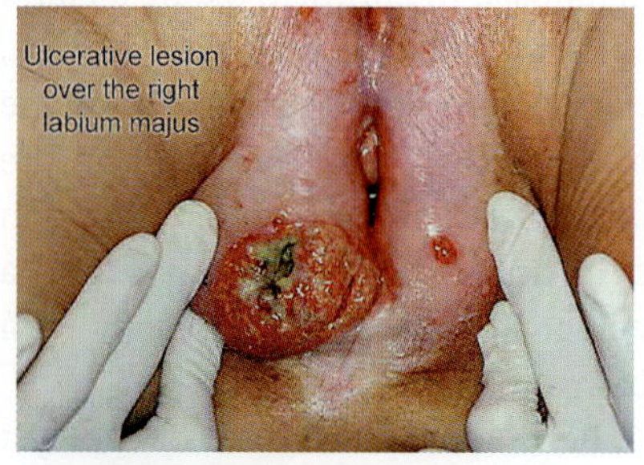

A. Topical imiquimod
B. Radical local excision
C. Radical vulvectomy with inguinal lymphadenectomy
D. Radiation therapy alone
E. Chemotherapy alone

</td>
<td>

Ans: B (Radical local excision)

Vulvar cancer affects the vulva, an area of external female genitalia. Vulva refers to the region of female external genitalia which includes various anatomical structures such as labia majora, mons pubis, labia minora, clitoris, vestibule, and vaginal introitus **(Fig. 40)**.

The lesion in the adjacent image was classified as stage 1 B vulvar cancer (>2 cm in size and stromal invasion of >1 mm^3 confined to vulva with negative lymph nodes).

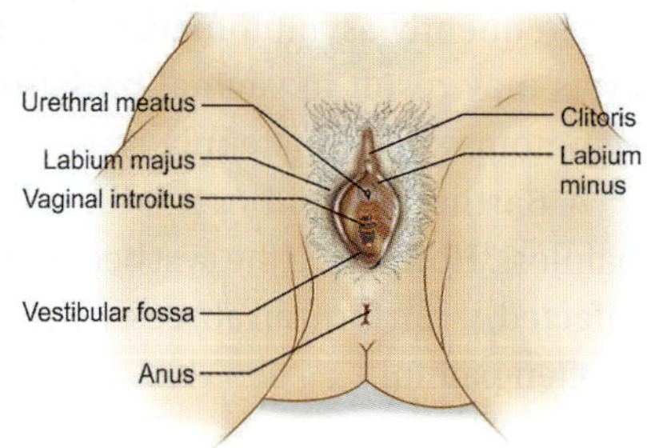

Fig. 40: Normal anatomy of vulva.

</td>
<td>

Explanation: Radical local excision is nowadays preferred over en bloc radical vulvectomy, an approach commonly used in previous times. In recent times, a more conservative approach at the time of surgery is preferred. Stage 1B lesions can be managed with radical partial vulvectomy. Sentinel lymph node biopsy can be performed for this ipsilateral vulvar lesion. If a sentinel lymph node is devoid of malignancy, it implies absence of lymph node metastasis. In case of positive sentinel lymph node, inguinofemoral lymphadenectomy can be done. Topical treatments like imiquimod are generally reserved for preinvasive lesions (vulvar intraepithelial neoplasia). Radiation therapy and chemotherapy alone are not typical first-line treatments but may be used as adjuncts in advanced or recurrent cases.

Potential questions: There can be questions related to various types of vulvar lesions (benign, malignant, and preinvasive).

</td>
</tr>
</table>

CANCER OF THE ADNEXA

Question	Answer	Comment
Q41. A 56-year-old postmenopausal woman presents with complaints of abdominal swelling or bloating since the past 3 months. Transvaginal ultrasound shows an adnexal mass as depicted in the image below. She is found to be a carrier of BRCA1 mutation. Further evaluation with MRI reveals a solid mass involving the fallopian tube. Based on the clinical and imaging findings, what is the next best step in managing her condition? 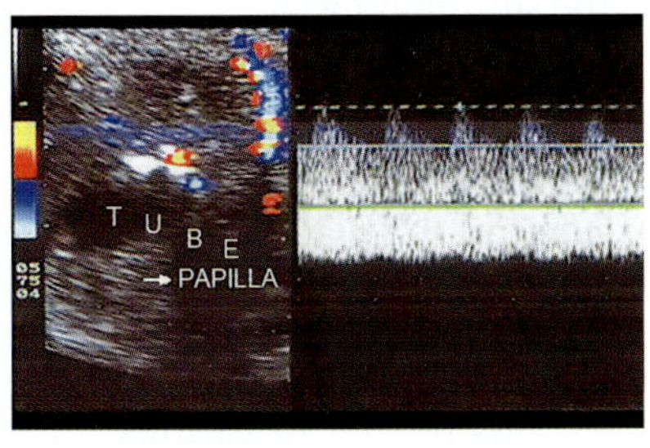 A. Laparoscopic cystectomy with ovarian preservation B. Risk-reducing bilateral salpingo-oophorectomy (RRSO) C. Exploratory laparotomy with staging and cytoreductive surgery D. Neoadjuvant chemotherapy followed by interval debulking surgery E. Surveillance with repeat imaging in 3 months	**Ans: C (Exploratory laparotomy with staging and cytoreductive surgery)** The adjacent ultrasound image shows a sausage-shaped adnexal mass with presence of papillomatous protrusions and solid parts. This is suggestive of carcinoma of fallopian tube. Doppler flow velocimetry shows low-resistance blood flow in the mass, which is indicative of underlying malignancy **(Fig. 41)**. 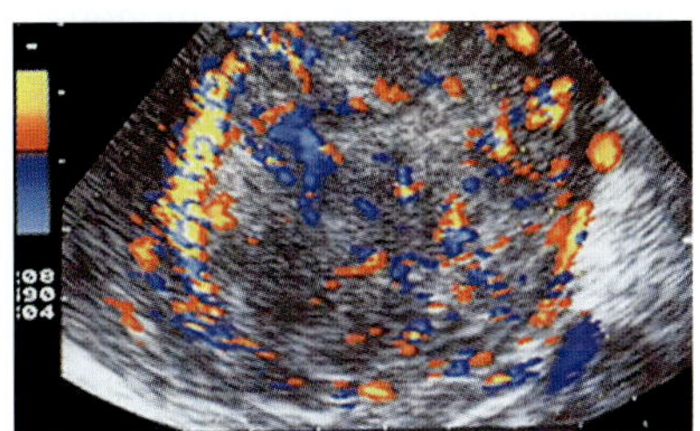 **Fig. 41:** Color Doppler shows increased venous blood flow signals. Fallopian tube cancer, also known as tubal cancer, is very rare and accounts for only 1–2% of all cases of gynecologic cancers. The most common type of Fallopian tube cancer is an adenocarcinoma and typically affects women between the ages of 50 to 60 years. It is bilateral in nearly one-third cases. Women who have inherited the BRCA1 gene (linked with the development of ovarian and breast cancer) are also at an increased risk of developing fallopian tube cancer. This cancer is more common in nulliparous menopausal women. Fallopian tube cancer is a diagnosis of exclusion.	**Explanation:** Exploratory laparotomy with staging and cytoreductive surgery is the gold-standard management for suspected ovarian/fallopian tube carcinoma in a surgically fit patient. This involves TAH with BSO along with omentectomy, peritoneal washings/biopsies with or without pelvic/para-aortic lymph node assessment. The surgery is aimed at maximal cytoreduction, which can be considered as the single most important prognostic factor. In postmenopausal women, cystectomy and ovarian preservation are not appropriate when a solid adnexal mass is seen, especially with BRCA1 mutation, which is associated with a very high malignant potential. This surgery would risk incomplete resection and tumor spillage. Risk-reducing bilateral salpingo-oophorectomy (RRSO) is indicated before malignancy develops, usually at 35–40 years in BRCA1 carriers who have completed childbearing. Neoadjuvant chemotherapy (NACT) followed by interval debulking surgery is reserved for advanced disease not optimally resectable upfront, or poor surgical candidates (frail, comorbidities, etc.) **Potential questions:** There can be questions related to different benign and malignant lesions of the fallopian tube.

BREAST DISEASE

Question	Answer	Comment
Q42. A 32-year-old woman presents with a firm, mobile, painless lump in her breast. In view of a positive family history of breast malignancy, a mammogram was performed, which demonstrated the findings as shown in the image below. What is the most likely diagnosis? 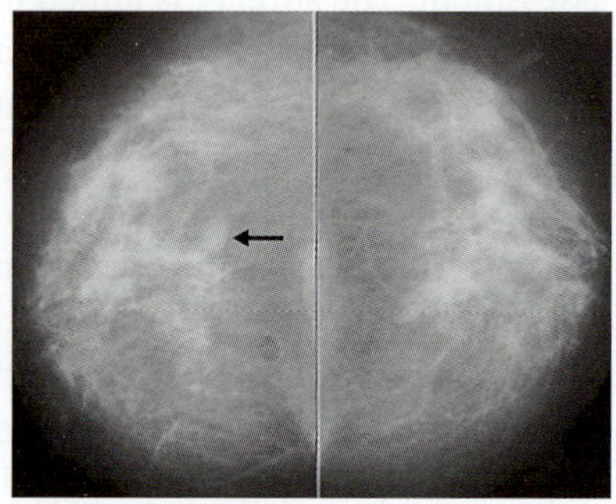 A. Fibroadenoma B. Phyllodes tumor C. Breast cyst D. Invasive ductal carcinoma E. Lipoma	**Ans: A (Fibroadenoma)** The adjacent mammograph showed a homogeneous mass about 1 cm in diameter with well-defined margins in the right breast (indicated by arrow). There were no associated calcifications. These features were suggestive of a benign lesion. The features on clinical examination also pointed toward a non-malignant lesion. Ultrasound examination was performed **(Fig. 42)**, which revealed a hypoechoic, homogeneous round mass with smooth, well-defined walls. An ultrasound-guided biopsy was performed considering the patient's positive family history for malignancy. Biopsy confirmed the diagnosis of a fibroadenoma. 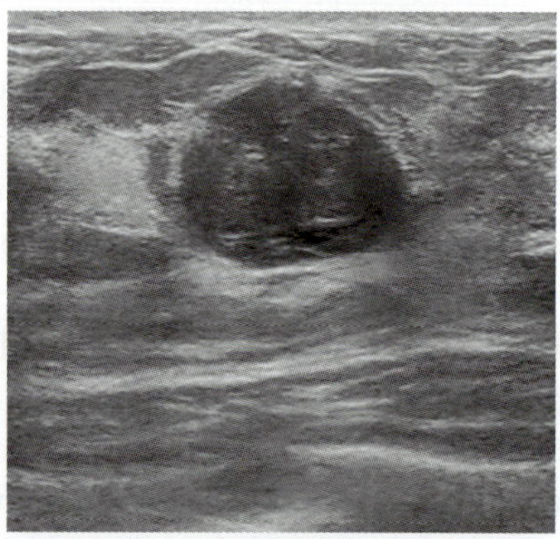 **Fig. 42:** Ultrasound examination of the same patient.	**Explanation:** Fibroadenomas are the most common benign breast tumors, typically encountered in young women. They present as firm, mobile, and painless lumps. On ultrasound, fibroadenomas appear as well-circumscribed, oval, hypoechoic masses with smooth borders, which distinguishes them from other breast lesions. Lipomas are also well-circumscribed breast lesions but are usually isoechoic or hyperechoic compared to the surrounding fat. Sometimes, an ultrasound (with or without a directed biopsy) and/or a core needle biopsy may be required to confirm the diagnosis in cases of breast lumps. **Potential questions:** There can be questions related to various breast lesions (both benign and malignant).

Question	Answer	Comment
Q43. A 45-year-old woman presents with a palpable lump in her right breast. The clinical image at the time of examination is shown below. A mammogram and biopsy confirm invasive ductal carcinoma. What is the most appropriate initial management for this patient? 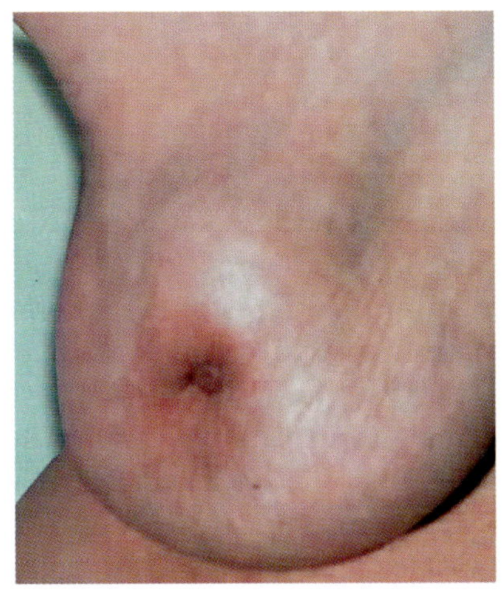 A. Lumpectomy with sentinel lymph node biopsy followed by radiotherapy B. Modified radical mastectomy with axillary clearance C. Surveillance with repeat mammogram in 6 months D. Neoadjuvant chemotherapy followed by breast-conserving surgery E. Primary endocrine therapy with tamoxifen	**Ans: B (Modified radical mastectomy with axillary clearance)** The adjacent image depicts nipple retraction, which can be considered as a sign of underlying pathology, warranting further investigation with imaging and possibly a biopsy. This patient was later diagnosed as stage II invasive ductal carcinoma on mammography **(Fig. 43)**. Mammogram revealed a mass about 3-4 cm in size with fine spikes radiating from the mass. Breast cancer is a malignant growth, arising from the breast tissues (ducts and/or lobules). Although breast cancer primarily occurs in women, it can also affect men. Various types of breast cancers are as follows: Ductal carcinoma in situ (DCIS) (most common type of noninvasive breast cancer), invasive ductal carcinoma (most common invasive lesion), invasive lobular carcinoma, and a few less common ones such as mucinous carcinoma, mixed tumors, medullary carcinoma, inflammatory breast cancer, etc. 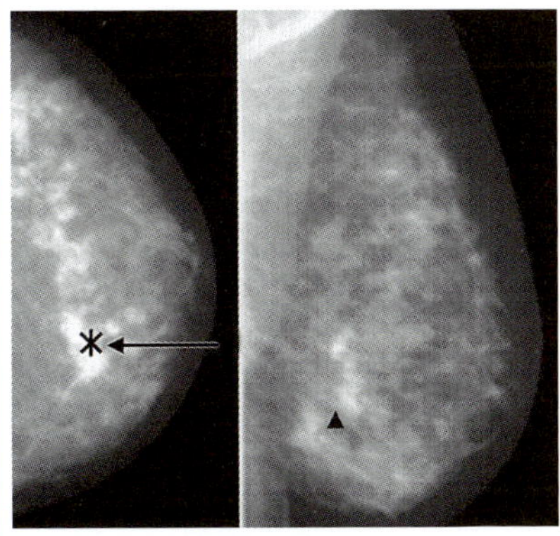 **Fig. 43:** Invasive ductal carcinoma (arrow and the asterisk mark show the location of carcinoma).	**Explanation:** Stage II disease is associated with tumor size greater than 2 cm with/without limited nodal involvement. Since this is an operable disease, so surgery is the initial management. Standard management in this case is modified radical mastectomy (MRM), which removes the entire breast tissue along with axillary lymph node dissection. Lumpectomy with sentinel lymph node biopsy is appropriate for small, peripheral, unifocal tumors without nipple/skin involvement. Therefore, not suitable in this case. Surveillance with repeat mammogram in 6 months is inappropriate for those with confirmed invasive cancer. Neoadjuvant chemotherapy may be considered in locally advanced or inoperable disease. Here, disease appears operable but not suitable for breast conserving surgery. Nipple retraction suggests involvement of the lactiferous ducts/central breast tissue, thereby making breast-conserving surgery less suitable. Endocrine therapy alone is used in elderly/unfit patients with estrogen receptor positive tumors, not in a fit 45-year-old. **Potential questions:** There can be questions related to various breast lesions (both benign and malignant).

CHAPTER 9

Lesions of the Uterus

UTERINE PROLAPSE

Question	Answer	Comment
Q1. A 55-year-old postmenopausal woman presents with a sensation of fullness in the pelvic area and urinary incontinence. On physical examination, a bulge is noted in the anterior vaginal wall. The letter A in the image below shows the condition. What is the most likely diagnosis? 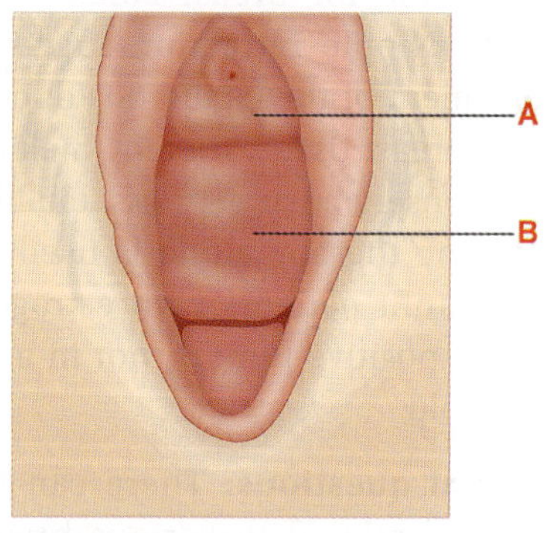 A. Cystocele B. Rectocele C. Urethrocele D. Enterocele E. Vaginal vault prolapse	**Ans: C (Urethrocele)** Letter A in the adjacent image points to a urethrocele, whereas letter B points to a cystocele. Cystocele and urethrocele can be defined as the protrusion of bladder and urethra, respectively, into the anterior vaginal wall, thereby causing its descent **(Fig. 1)**. Cystocele produces a bulge in the upper two-thirds of the anterior vaginal wall, whereas urethrocele produces a bulge in the lower one-third of the anterior vaginal wall. Along with the descent of the vaginal wall, there also occurs prolapse of bladder and/or urethra. 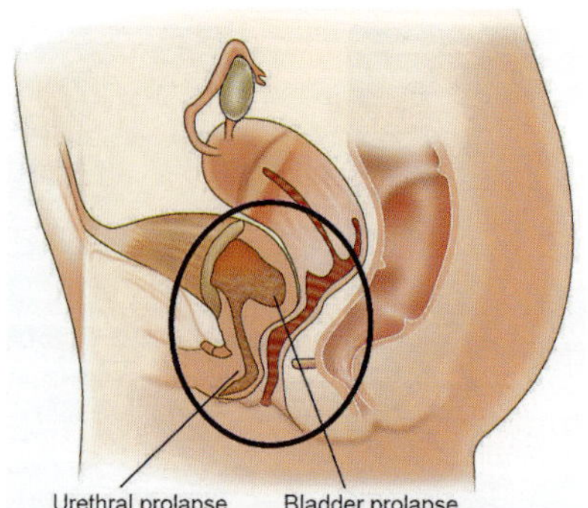 **Fig. 1:** Diagrammatic representation of urethrocele.	**Explanation:** Weakness of the anterior compartment results in cystocele (weakness of upper two-thirds) and urethrocele (weakness of lower one-thirds of the anterior vaginal wall). This condition is often associated with symptoms such as a sensation of fullness or pressure in the pelvic area, difficulty in emptying the bladder, stress urinary incontinence, a visible bulge in the anterior vaginal wall, etc. It is commonly seen in postmenopausal women due to the weakening of pelvic floor muscles and tissues. The tissues around the urethra and bladder can be strengthened with the help of Kegel exercises. **Potential questions:** There can be questions related to clinical presentation, diagnosis, and management of various types of prolapse (urethrocele, cystocele, rectocele, enterocele, vault prolapse, etc.).

Question	Answer	Comment
Q2. A 55-year-old G3P3 woman presents with a 3-month history of vaginal bulging and urinary incontinence. Vaginal examination reveals the finding shown in the image below. What is the most likely diagnosis? 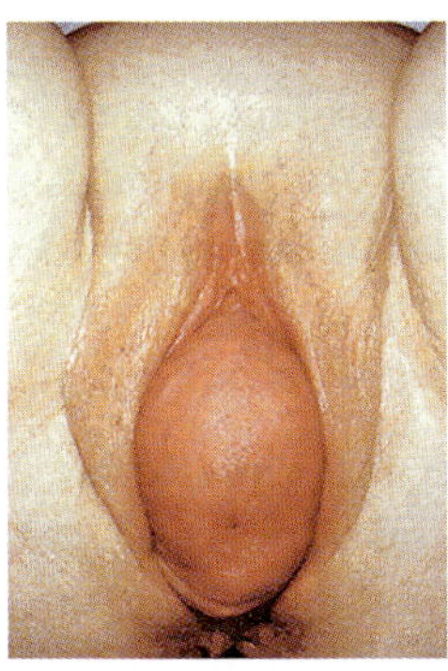 A. Rectocele B. Cystocele (grade 1) C. Cystocele (grade 3) D. Cystocele (grade 2) E. Enterocele	**Ans: C [Cystocele (grade 3)]** The adjacent image depicts a grade 3 cystocele. A cystocele occurs when the bladder descends into the vaginal canal due to weakening of the pelvic floor muscles **(Fig. 2)**. 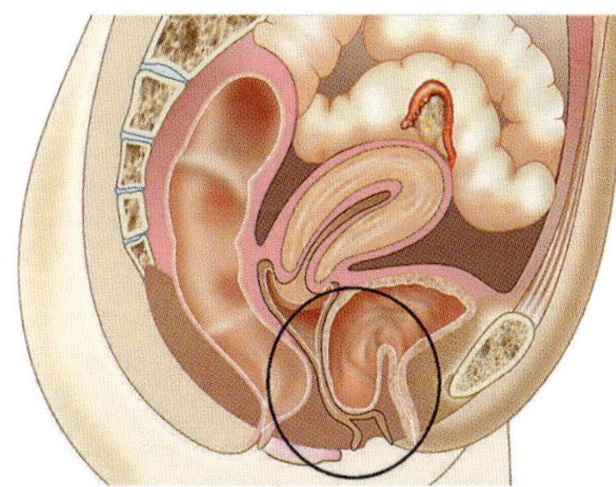 **Fig. 2:** Diagrammatic representation of cystocele.	**Explanation:** Cystocele can be classified as follows: ▪ *Mild (grade I):* The bladder descends halfway up to the vaginal introitus. ▪ *Severe (grade II):* Bladder descends up to the vaginal introitus. ▪ *Advanced (grade III):* Bladder bulges out through the vaginal introitus. **Potential questions:** There can be questions related to clinical presentation, diagnosis, and management of various types of prolapse (urethrocele, cystocele, rectocele, enterocele, vault prolapse, etc.).
Q3. A 54-year-old woman presents with symptoms of pelvic pressure and difficulty with bowel movements. The image below shows the findings of clinical examination. What is the most appropriate management of severe cases with this presentation? 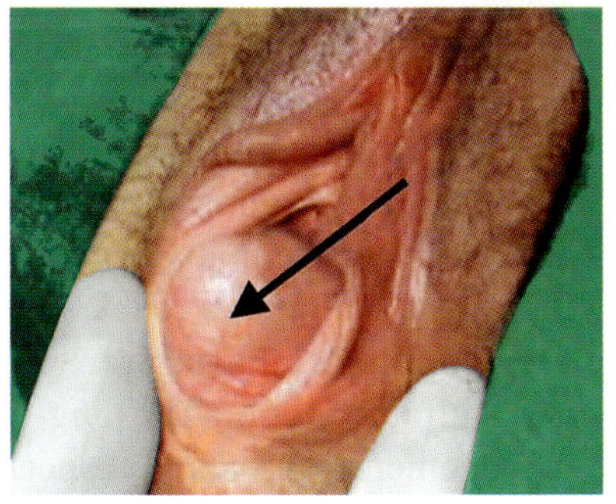 A. Pelvic floor muscle training (PFMT) B. Surgical repair with mesh C. Vaginal estrogen therapy D. Use of a pessary E. Observation and lifestyle modifications	**Ans: B (Surgical repair with mesh)** The adjacent image depicts a significant posterior vaginal wall prolapse or rectocele, which occurs due to the weakness of the lower two-thirds of the posterior vaginal wall. It can be associated with symptoms such as constipation and difficult evacuation with straining. **Figure 3** shows a diagrammatic representation of rectocele. 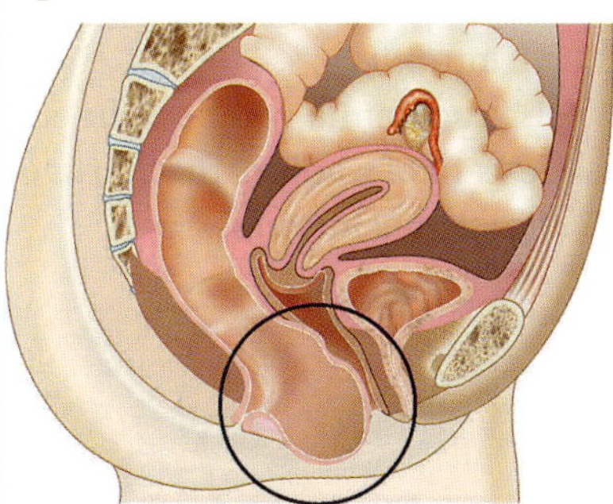 **Fig. 3:** Diagrammatic representation of rectocele.	**Explanation:** The first line of management is conservative. The woman should be advised to avoid constipation by eating a high fiber diet, drinking plenty of fluids (at least 6–8 glasses of water), and avoiding prolonged straining. If this conservative management is not successful, surgical therapy is indicated. For severe cases of rectocele, especially when conservative treatments fail, surgical repair with mesh may be indicated to provide long-term relief and support. **Potential questions:** There can be questions related to clinical presentation, diagnosis, and management of various types of prolapse (urethrocele, cystocele, rectocele, enterocele, vault prolapse, etc.).

<table>
<tr><th>Question</th><th>Answer</th><th>Comment</th></tr>
<tr>
<td>

Q4. A 60-year-old woman presents with a sensation of pelvic pressure and difficulty with bowel movements. On physical examination, a bulge is noted in the upper part of the vagina as shown in the image below. What is the most likely diagnosis?

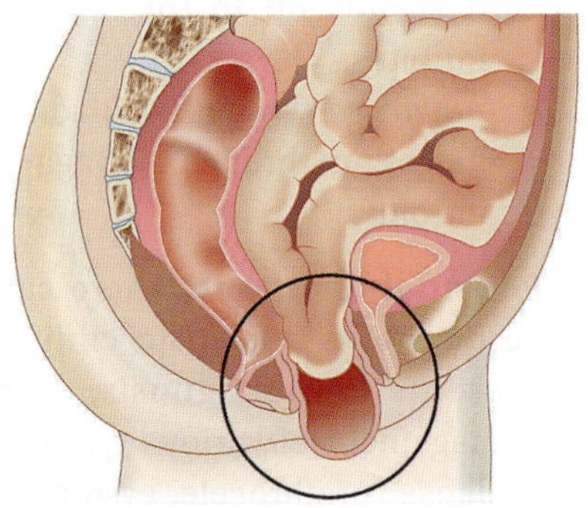

A. Cystocele
B. Rectocele
C. Urethrocele
D. Enterocele
E. Uterine prolapse

</td>
<td>

Ans: D (Enterocele)

Circle in the adjacent image depicts an enterocele. MR image of the same patient is depicted in **Figure 4**.

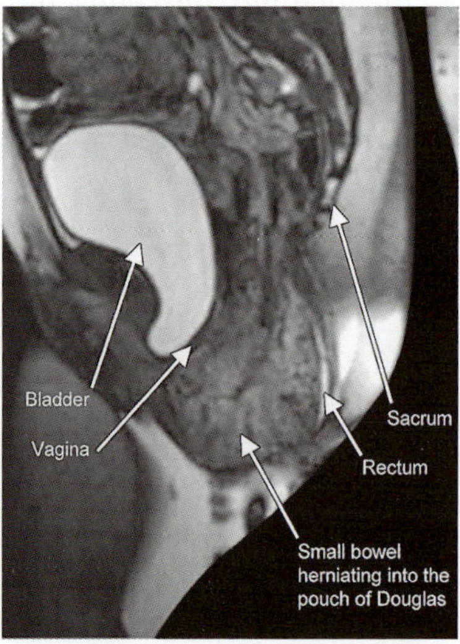

Fig. 4: MR image in the same patient.

</td>
<td>

Explanation: An enterocele, also known as small bowel prolapse, occurs due to the weakness of the posterior compartment (upper one-third of posterior vaginal wall). As a result, the small intestine descends into the lower pelvic cavity and pushes against the upper part of the vagina, creating a bulge.

Surgical treatment is required to replace the prolapsed bowel in its proper place and to strengthen the muscles of pelvic floor.

Potential questions: There can be questions related to clinical presentation, diagnosis, and management of various types of prolapse (urethrocele, cystocele, rectocele, enterocele, vault prolapse, etc.).

</td>
</tr>
<tr>
<td>

Q5. A 64-year-old woman, gravida 4, para 4, reports a feeling of heaviness and protrusion from her vagina. Her findings are depicted in the image below. Which of the following is the most appropriate long-term management option?

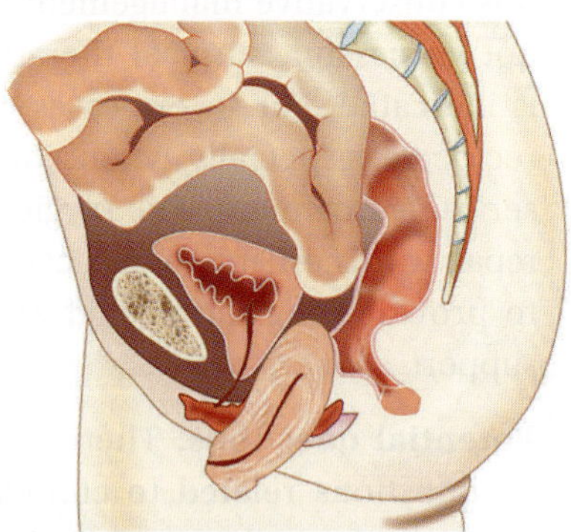

A. Observation and lifestyle modifications
B. Pelvic floor muscle training
C. Use of a vaginal pessary
D. Vaginal hysterectomy
E. Abdominal sacrocolpopexy

</td>
<td>

Ans: D (Vaginal hysterectomy)

The adjacent image depicts complete uterine prolapse. The different stages of uterine descent are described as follows **(Fig. 5)**:

- *First degree:* There is descent of cervix into the vagina.
- *Second degree:* There is descent of cervix up to the vaginal introitus.
- *Third degree:* There is descent of cervix outside the vaginal introitus.

Procidentia can be defined as the descent of whole of the uterus outside the vaginal introitus.

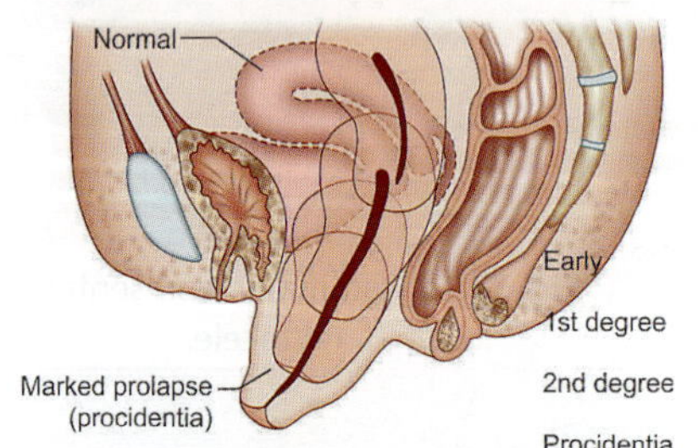

Fig. 5: Stages of uterine prolapse.

</td>
<td>

Explanation: Vaginal hysterectomy is often considered the most appropriate long-term management option for complete uterine prolapse, particularly in elderly patients with significant symptoms who are suitable candidates for surgery. There is no medical treatment available, which can cure prolapse. Though nonsurgical methods (pessary use) and conservative management may provide symptomatic relief, surgery provides the definitive cure. Surgery is a suitable option for long-term management in all patients, especially those with recurrent prolapse or those who prefer a permanent solution and have completed their family.

Potential questions: There can be questions related to clinical presentation, diagnosis, and management of various types of prolapse (urethrocele, cystocele, rectocele, enterocele, vault prolapse, etc.).

</td>
</tr>
</table>

Question	Answer	Comment
Q6. A 55-year-old para 3 woman presents with symptoms of pelvic heaviness and pressure as shown in the image below. Which of the following is the most likely etiology? 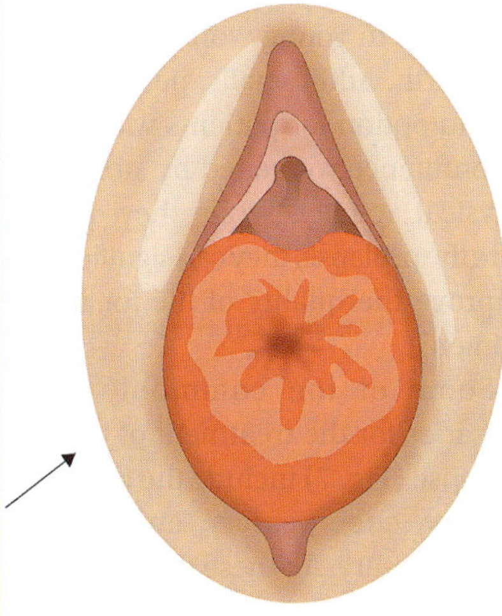 A. Chronic urinary tract infections B. Pelvic inflammatory disease C. Weakening of pelvic floor muscles D. Endometriosis E. Ovarian cysts	**Ans: C (Weakening of pelvic floor muscles)** The adjacent image shows prolapsed uterus visible at the vaginal introitus (as depicted by the arrow). Uterine prolapse usually occurs in postmenopausal and multiparous women, in whom the pelvic floor muscles and the ligaments that support the female genital tract have become slack and atonic. Injury to the pelvic floor muscles during repeated childbirths **(Fig. 6)**, causing excessive stretching of the pelvic floor muscles and ligaments, acts as a major risk factor for causing reduced tone of pelvic floor muscles. 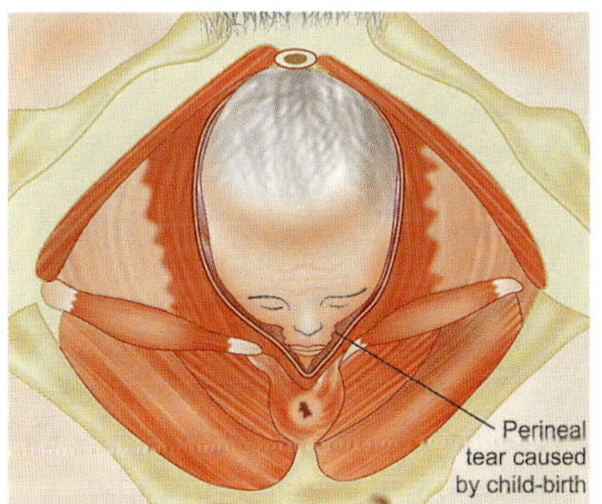 **Fig. 6:** Damage caused by childbirth to the muscles of pelvic floor.	**Explanation:** The pelvic floor muscles and ligaments provide support to the uterus, and when they become weakened or stretched, they can no longer hold the uterus in its proper position, leading to prolapse. Perineal tears occurring at the time of delivery and parturition tend to either divide the decussating fibers of levator ani or cause damage to the perineal body. Both these factors can cause the hiatus urogenitalis to become patulous and result in the development of prolapse. Conditions which result in reduced tone of levator muscles tend to increase the dimensions of hiatus urogenitalis, thereby increasing the tendency of pelvic organs to prolapse. **Potential questions:** There can be questions related to clinical presentation, diagnosis, and management of various types of prolapse (urethrocele, cystocele, rectocele, enterocele, vault prolapse, etc.).

Question	Answer	Comment
Q7. A 88-year-old woman with a history of pelvic organ prolapse is considering nonsurgical management options. The gynecologists shows her some devices as presented in the image below. Which of the following is the most appropriate use of this device for her condition? 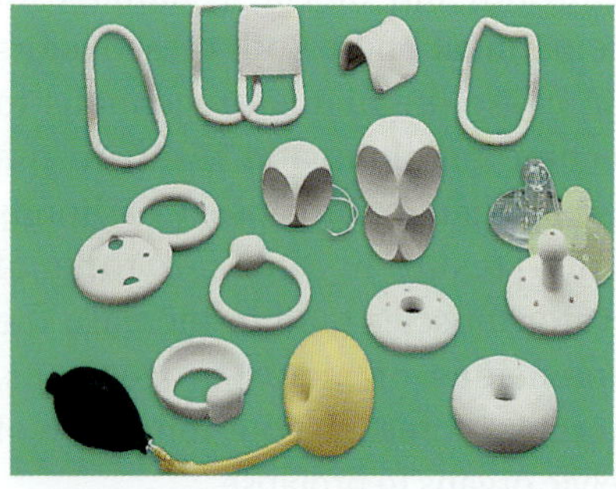 A. To permanently cure the prolapse B. To provide temporary relief until surgery C. To support the vaginal walls and alleviate symptoms D. To prevent urinary tract infections E. To strengthen pelvic floor muscles	**Ans: C (To support the vaginal walls and alleviate symptoms)** The adjacent image shows different types of pessaries which can be used for the treatment of uterine prolapse. Pessaries are a nonsurgical method for supporting the uterine and vaginal structures which can be used for both short-term and long-term management, especially in patients who are not good candidates for surgery or prefer to avoid it. **Figure 7** highlights some of the commonly used pessaries for the treatment of uterine prolapse. 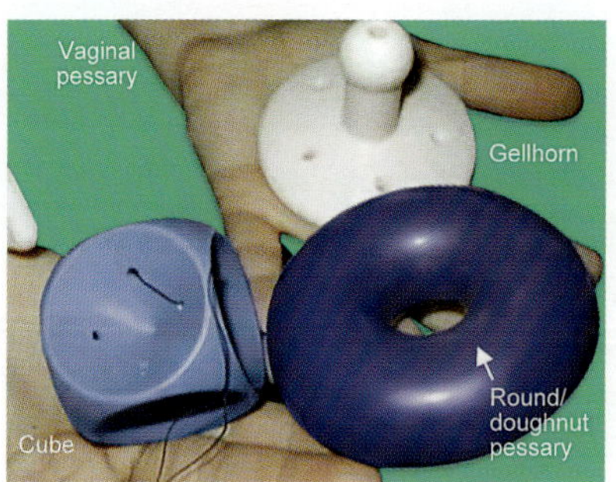 **Fig. 7:** Some commonly used pessaries for the treatment of uterine prolapse.	**Explanation:** Pessaries are usually used for attaining temporary relief in cases with symptomatic prolapse. Pessaries also prove useful in patients who have early-stage prolapse or are too weak for surgery. One of the important indications for using pessary is in young women following childbirth. Additionally, pessaries are a valid option for patients with stress incontinence worsened by strenuous physical activity. While they do not cure the prolapse, they can significantly improve the quality of life for many women. Some of the commonly used pessaries for the treatment of uterine prolapse **(Fig. 7)** include the Gellhorn pessary, cube pessary, and round/donut pessary. All these three types of pessaries can be used in patients with rectoceles and enterocele. **Potential questions:** There can be questions related to various management options for different types of prolapse.

UTERINE RETROVERSION

Question	Answer	Comment
Q8. A 45-year-old woman presents with symptoms of backache and dysmenorrhea. On examination, she is found to have uterine retroversion. The image below shows the pessary prescribed to her. Which of the following is the most appropriate use of this pessary for her condition? 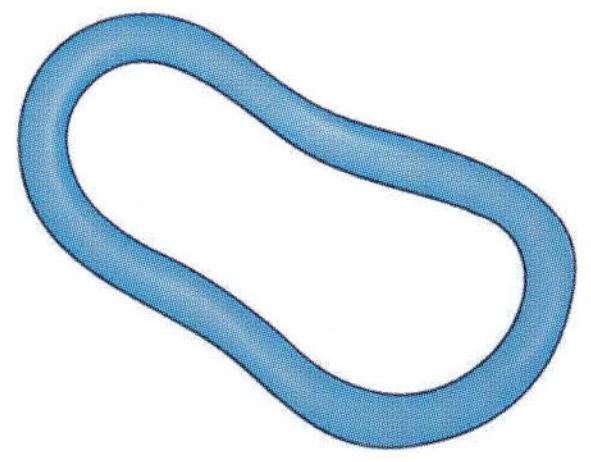 A. To treat stress urinary incontinence B. To support the vaginal walls and alleviate prolapse C. To reposition the uterus and relieve symptoms D. To prevent recurrent urinary tract infections E. To strengthen pelvic floor muscles	**Ans: C (To reposition the uterus and relieve symptoms)** The adjacent image shows a hodge pessary, which is specifically designed to manage uterine retroversion, a condition where the uterus is tilted backward. Diagnosis of retroversion is mainly established on the basis of findings of pelvic examination. Hodge pessary is manually shapeable and fits behind the pubic arch, providing support to the proximal urethra and helps reposition the uterus **(Fig. 8)**. 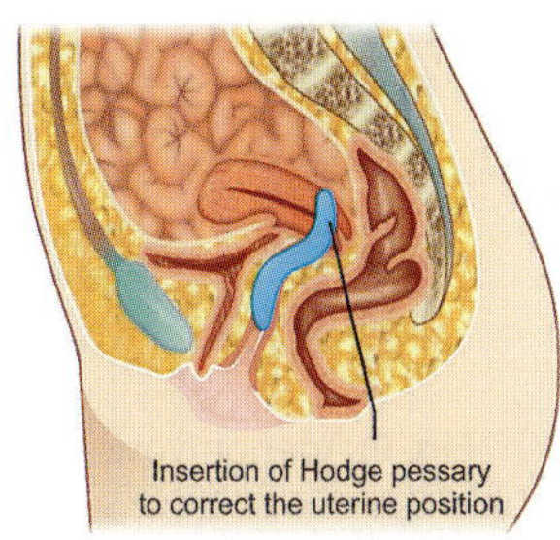 **Fig. 8:** Hodge pessary being used for correction of uterine retroversion.	**Explanation:** Hodge pessary is a nonsurgical option that can be particularly beneficial for women who experience discomfort due to uterine retroversion. This pessary helps reposition the uterus to its normal position, thereby relieving associated symptoms such as backache and dysmenorrhea. It is usually retained in position for 3 months and then removed. Surgical treatment may be required in the cases of fixed retroversion and comprises surgeries such as Modified Gilliam's ventrosuspension, plication of the round ligaments, Baldy-Webster's operation, etc. **Potential questions:** There can be different questions related to clinical presentation, diagnosis, and management of uterine retroversion.

ADENOMYOSIS

<table>
<tr><th>Question</th><th>Answer</th><th>Comment</th></tr>
<tr>
<td>

Q9. A 42-year-old woman presents with chronic pelvic pain and heavy menstrual bleeding. The findings of the transvaginal ultrasound image are shown below. What is the most likely diagnosis?

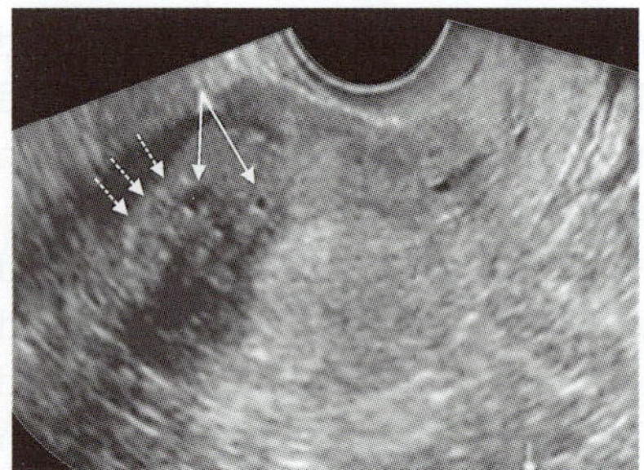

A. Endometrial cancer
B. Uterine fibroids
C. Adenomyosis
D. Endometriosis
E. Ovarian cyst

</td>
<td>

Ans: C (Adenomyosis)

The adjacent ultrasound image demonstrates a diffusely enlarged uterus with heterogeneous myometrial echotexture and small myometrial cysts (depicted by arrows). This is suggestive of adenomyosis **(Fig. 9)**. Other features suggestive of adenomyosis on ultrasound include asymmetrical uterine enlargement, indistinct endometrial–myometrial border, and subendometrial halo thickening.

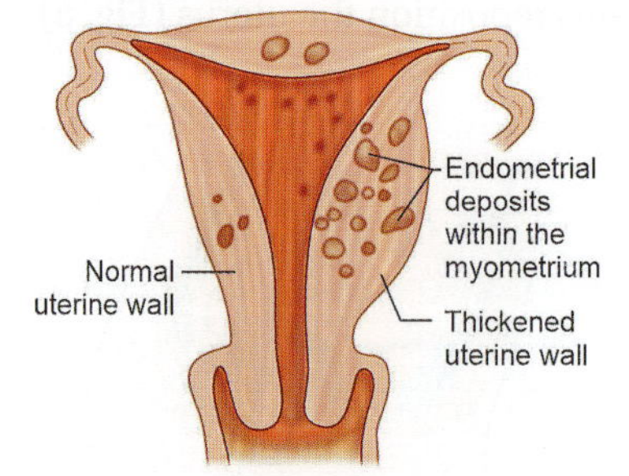

Fig. 9: Adenomyosis.

</td>
<td>

Explanation: Adenomyosis is associated with myometrial hypertrophy, which may be either diffuse or localized (adenomyoma). Patients often present with chronic pelvic pain and heavy menstrual bleeding (unresponsive to hormonal therapy or uterine curettage) and progressively increasing dysmenorrhea. Other symptoms may include, backache, dyspareunia, and subfertility.

Total hysterectomy with or without bilateral salpingo-oophorectomy is the treatment of choice in elderly patients who are past their child-bearing age. Conservative resection may be performed in the younger patients.

Potential questions: There can be questions related to different diagnostic modalities and management of adenomyosis.

</td>
</tr>
<tr>
<td>

Q10. A 38-year-old woman presents with chronic pelvic pain and heavy menstrual bleeding. An MRI is performed, which shows findings as presented in the image below. What is the most likely diagnosis?

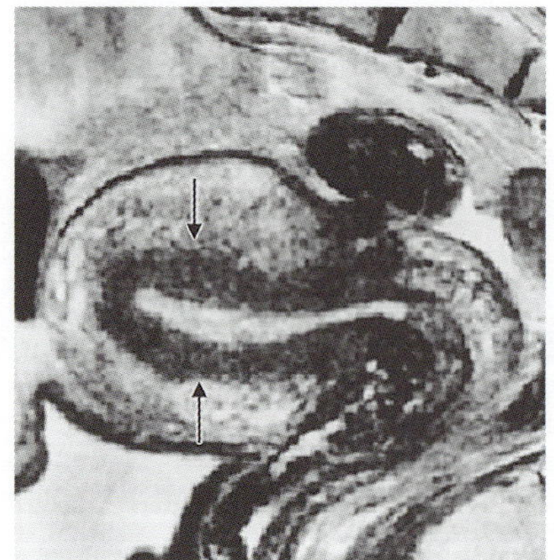

A. Endometrial cancer
B. Uterine fibroids
C. Adenomyosis
D. Endometriosis
E. Ovarian cyst

</td>
<td>

Ans: C (Adenomyosis)

The adjacent image demonstrates a sagittal T2-weighted magnetic resonance (MR) image showing diffuse, even thickening of the junctional zone (as depicted by arrows), which is consistent with the diagnosis of diffuse adenomyosis.

Though MRI is superior to ultrasound for the diagnosis of adenomyosis, the diagnosis of adenomyosis can only be confirmed by pathological examination **(Fig. 10)**.

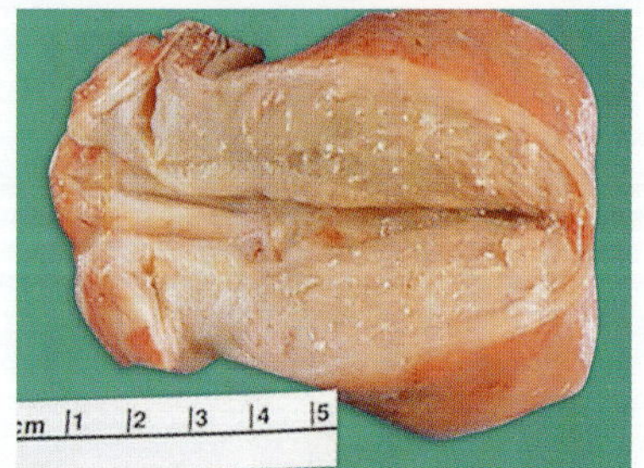

Fig. 10: Cut specimen of uterus showing adenomyosis.

</td>
<td>

Explanation: Adenomyosis is characterized by the presence of ectopic endometrial tissue within the myometrium. On MRI, the most established finding is a thickened junctional zone exceeding 12 mm. High-signal intensity myometrial foci on T2-weighted images are also characteristic. The heterotopic endometrial glands and stroma present in the myometrium appear as bright foci within the myometrium on T2-weighted MR images. Adjacent smooth muscle hyperplasia may present as areas of reduced signal intensity on MRI.

Potential questions: There can be questions related to different diagnostic modalities and management of adenomyosis.

</td>
</tr>
</table>

HYSTERECTOMY

Question	Answer	Comment
Q11. Identify the correct sequence of layers incised during a Pfannenstiel transverse abdominal incision as shown in the image below for an abdominal hysterectomy. 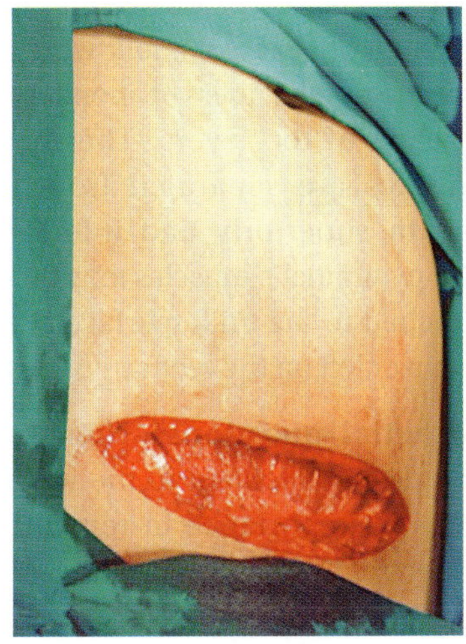 A. Skin, subcutaneous fat, anterior rectus sheath, rectus abdominis muscle, posterior rectus sheath B. Skin, subcutaneous fat, posterior rectus sheath, rectus abdominis muscle, anterior rectus sheath C. Skin, subcutaneous fat, anterior rectus sheath, rectus abdominis muscle, peritoneum D. Skin, subcutaneous fat, rectus abdominis muscle, anterior rectus sheath, peritoneum E. Skin, subcutaneous fat, peritoneum, rectus abdominis muscle, anterior rectus sheath	**Ans: C (Skin, subcutaneous fat, anterior rectus sheath, rectus abdominis muscle, peritoneum)** The adjacent image shows a Pfannenstiel transverse abdominal incision. This involves administration of a transverse incision made just above the pubic symphysis **(Fig. 11)**. This approach minimizes post-operative pain and provides good cosmetic results. Since the transverse incisions may not provide adequate exposure, they are usually reserved for benign uterine pathology, when the uterus is not very large in size. 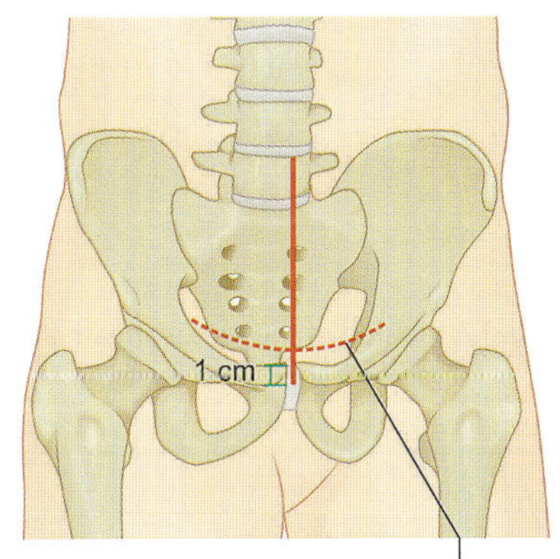 **Fig. 11:** Diagrammatic representation of the Pfannenstiel incision.	**Explanation:** The Pfannenstiel incision, commonly used in gynecological surgeries like abdominal hysterectomy. The sequence of layers incised is as follows: ▪ *Skin*: A transverse incision is made through the skin. ▪ *Subcutaneous fat*: The incision continues through the subcutaneous fat layer. ▪ *Anterior rectus sheath*: This layer is incised next, which is the aponeurosis of the abdominal muscles. ▪ *Rectus abdominis muscle*: The rectus muscles are separated or retracted to expose the underlying structures. ▪ *Peritoneum*: Finally, the peritoneum is incised to enter the abdominal cavity. **Potential questions:** There can be questions related to the various steps of importance in relation to abdominal hysterectomy.

Question	Answer	Comment
Q12. Identify the correct layer of the rectus sheath that is incised first during an abdominal hysterectomy as shown in the image below. This is marked by letter X in this image. 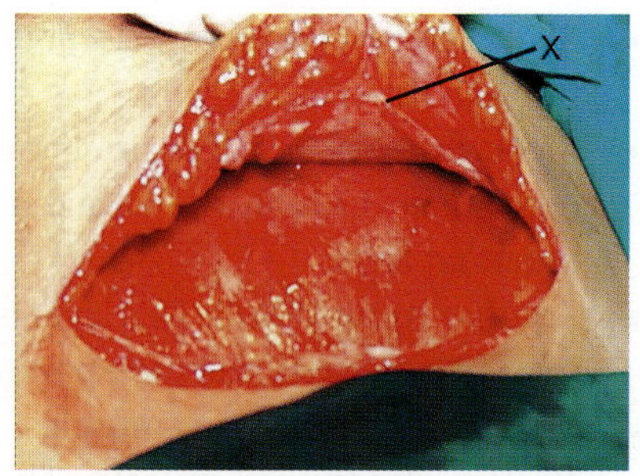 A. External oblique aponeurosis B. Internal oblique aponeurosis C. Transversus abdominis aponeurosis D. Anterior rectus sheath E. Posterior rectus sheath	**Ans: D (Anterior rectus sheath)** The first layer of the rectus sheath encountered is the anterior rectus sheath, which is visible as a glistening white structure (illustrated by letter X in the adjacent image). Anterior rectus sheath is formed by the aponeuroses of the external oblique and the anterior layer of the internal oblique muscles. Incising this layer allows access to the rectus abdominis muscle, which is then retracted to expose the posterior rectus sheath and the underlying peritoneum **(Fig. 12)**. 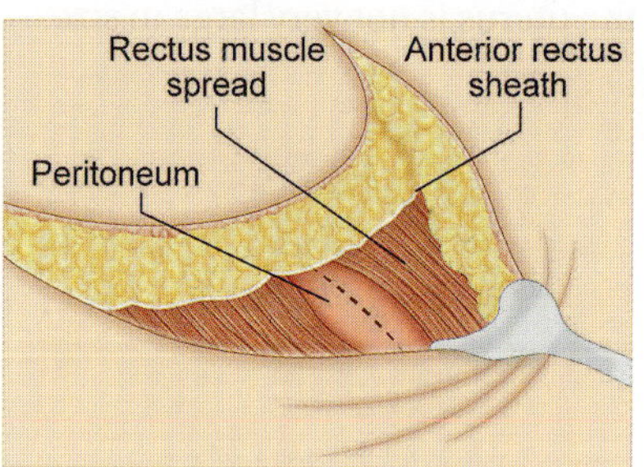 **Fig. 12:** Incision of the rectus sheath at the time of Pfannenstiel incision.	**Explanation:** During an abdominal hysterectomy, the surgeon makes an incision through the skin and subcutaneous tissue to reach the abdominal muscles. As the rectus sheath is encountered, a transverse incision is given with a scalpel in the midline of rectus sheath. It is then extended laterally on both sides with the help of a scissors, following the direction of the fibers of aponeurosis in each of the layers. The rectus muscles are separated from the sheath superiorly and inferiorly. The pyramidalis muscles may be left attached to the undersurface of the fascia or left on the rectus muscles. **Potential questions:** There can be questions related to the various steps of importance in relation to abdominal hysterectomy.

Question	Answer	Comment
Q13. During an abdominal hysterectomy, which structure is being clamped as shown in the image below? 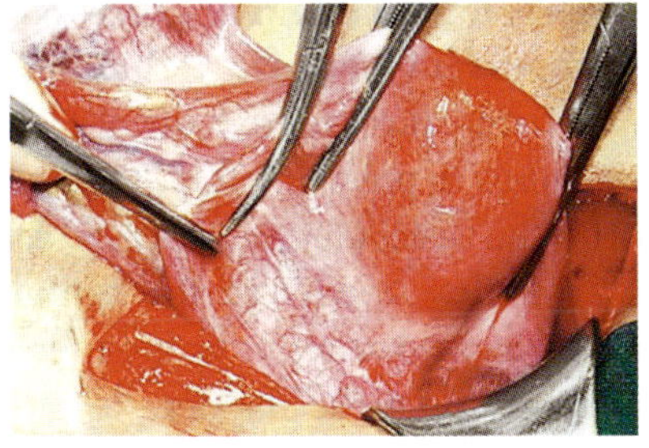 A. Utero-ovarian ligament B. Fallopian tube C. Round ligament D. Broad ligament E. Infundibulopelvic ligament	**Ans: C (Round ligament)** As shown in the adjacent image, the uterus is manually deviated to the left side, thereby stretching the round ligament. Following this, the round ligaments are clamped as shown in the adjacent image. Subsequently, the round ligaments are cut and ligated **(Figs. 13A and B)**. 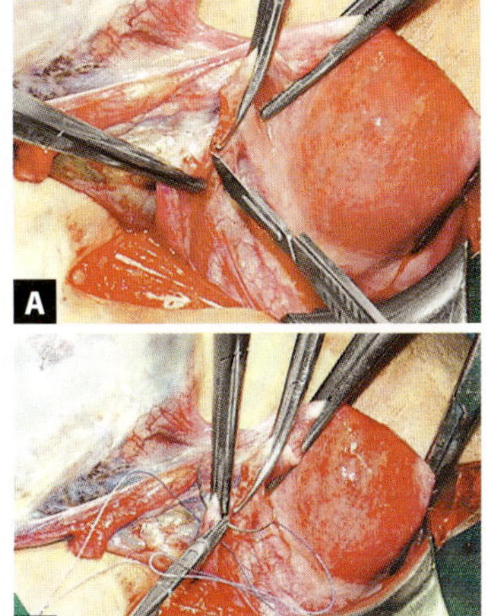 **Figs. 13A and B:** (A) Round ligaments are cut; (B) Round ligaments are ligated.	**Explanation:** In an abdominal hysterectomy, the round ligaments are typically the first structures to be clamped, cut, and ligated. This step is crucial as it helps in mobilizing the uterus and provides better access to other pelvic structures. The round ligaments are located anteriorly and are relatively easy to identify and manage. Clamping, cutting, and ligating the round ligaments first allows the surgeon to proceed with the dissection of other ligaments and structures, such as the utero-ovarian ligament and the fallopian tubes. Once the round ligaments are transected, the anterior leaf of broad ligament is cut out and opened. **Potential questions:** There can be questions related to the various steps of importance in relation to abdominal hysterectomy.
Q14. During an abdominal hysterectomy, which structure is being identified as shown in the image below for subsequently clamping, cutting, and ligating it for controlling the blood supply to the ovaries? 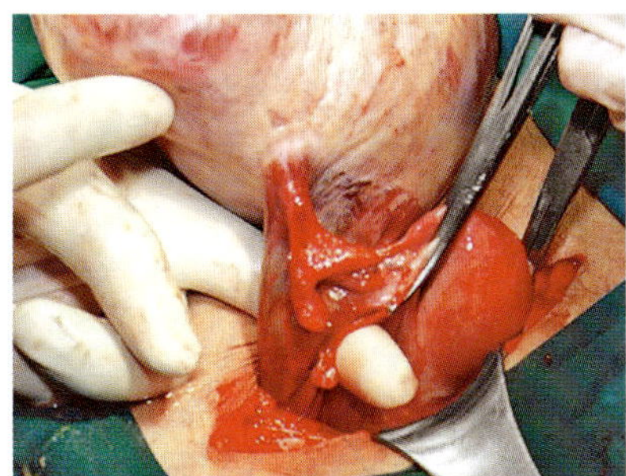 A. Round ligament B. Utero-ovarian ligament C. Uterine artery D. Broad ligament E. Infundibulopelvic ligament	**Ans: E (Infundibulopelvic ligament)** The ligament being identified in the adjacent image is the infundibulopelvic ligament. **Figure 14** illustrates the method of identifying this ligament. 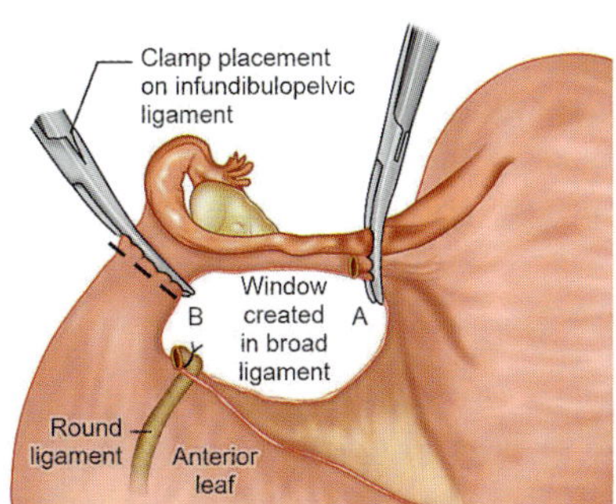 **Fig. 14:** Placement of clamps on the infundibulopelvic ligaments.	**Explanation:** The infundibulopelvic ligament, also known as the suspensory ligament of the ovary, contains the ovarian vessels (artery and vein). During an abdominal hysterectomy, clamping, cutting, and ligating this ligament are essential to control the blood supply to the ovaries, especially if the ovaries are to be removed. This step is important for preventing excessive bleeding and for ensuring safe removal of the ovaries if indicated. The infundibulopelvic ligament is carefully isolated from the ureter before being clamped, cut, and ligated. **Potential questions:** There can be questions related to the various steps of importance in relation to abdominal hysterectomy.

Question	Answer	Comment
Q15. Identify the structure being grasped with the artery forceps in the image below taken during an abdominal hysterectomy. 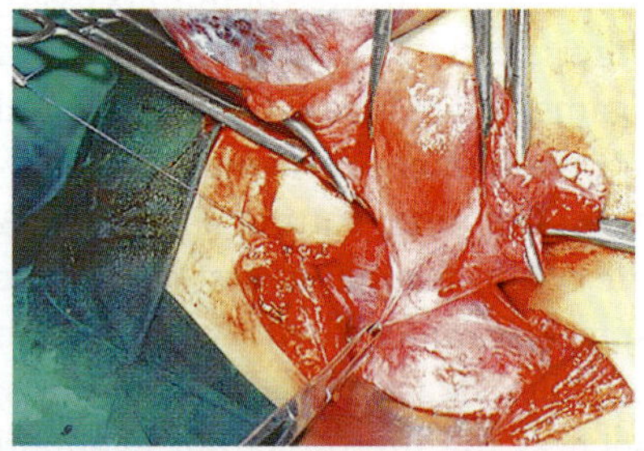 A. The fold between the bladder and the uterus B. The fold between the rectum and the uterus C. The fold between the ovaries and the fallopian tubes D. The fold between the bladder and the rectum E. The fold between the uterus and the abdominal wall	**Ans: A (The fold between the bladder and the uterus)** The adjacent image shows the identification of the vesicouterine fold of peritoneum, which is present between the bladder and the uterus. Following the dissection of the vesicouterine fold of peritoneum **(Fig. 15)**, a curvilinear incision is given over it. After separating the bladder peritoneum from the lower uterine segment, the incision along the vesicouterine fold is then extended over the anterior leaf of broad ligament. 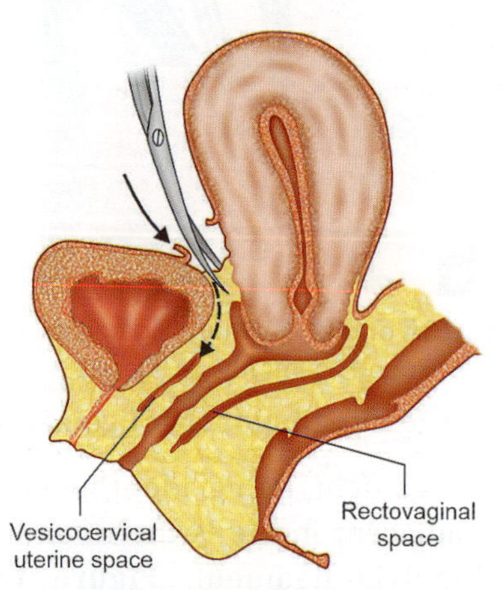 **Fig. 15:** Dissection of the vesicouterine plane to mobilize the bladder.	**Explanation:** The vesicouterine fold of peritoneum is the peritoneal fold extending between the bladder and the uterus. During an abdominal hysterectomy, identifying this fold is important because it helps in mobilizing the bladder away from the uterus to prevent injury. This fold forms the vesicouterine pouch, which is a shallow recess in the female pelvis, located anterior to the uterus and posterior to the bladder. **Potential questions:** There can be questions related to the various steps of importance in relation to abdominal hysterectomy.

Question	Answer	Comment
Q16. During an abdominal hysterectomy, which structure is clamped, cut, and ligated to control the blood supply to the uterus as shown in the image below? 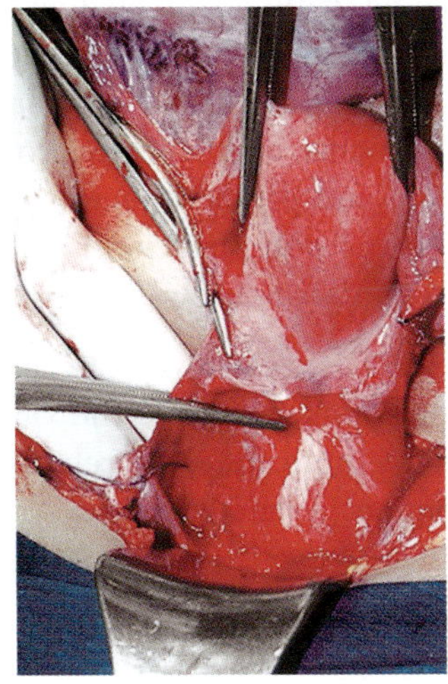 A. Round ligament B. Utero-ovarian ligament C. Uterine artery D. Broad ligament E. Infundibulopelvic ligament	**Ans: C (Uterine artery)** The adjacent image shows the ligation of uterine blood vessels. Before uterine artery ligation, the bladder is sharply dissected off the lower uterine segment and the cervix. The uterus is then retracted cephalad to one side of the pelvis, placing the ligaments in the lower uterine segment on a stretch. Any loose connective tissue overlying the uterine vessels is sharply removed in order to skeletonize the vessels. After the uterine vessels are skeletonized, they are triply clamped and cut **(Figs. 16A and B)**. 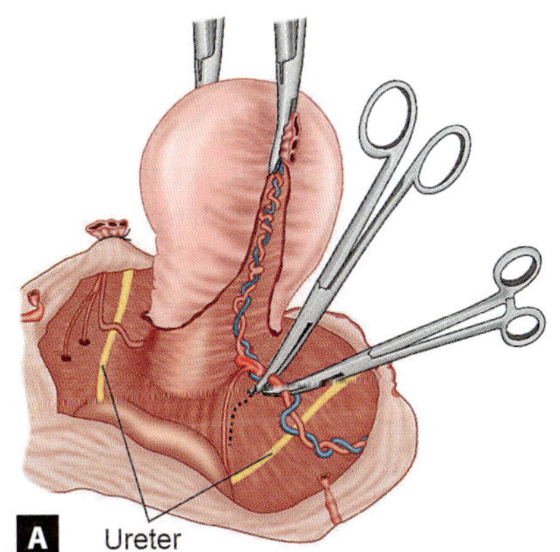 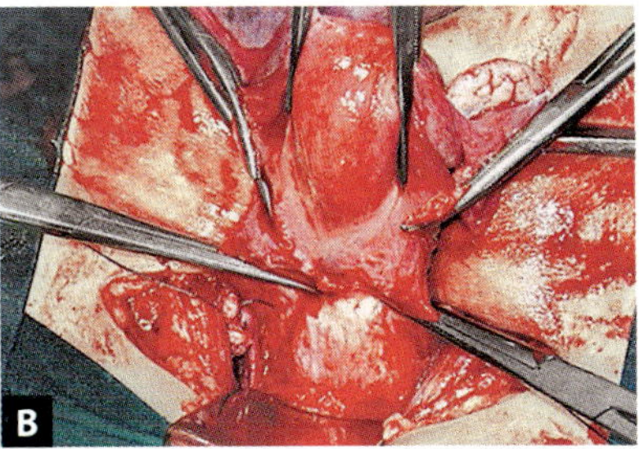 **Figs. 16A and B:** (A) Ligation of uterine vessels; (B) Uterine arteries of both the sides have been clamped.	**Explanation:** Uterine artery is the primary blood supply to the uterus. During an abdominal hysterectomy, clamping, cutting, and ligating the uterine artery is a critical step to control bleeding and safely remove the uterus. Uterine artery arises from internal iliac artery and travels through the broad ligament to reach the uterus. Three cardinal rules must be followed while clamping the uterine vessels in order to avoid clamping the ureters: 1. The lowest clamp must be placed first. 2. The lowest clamp must be placed at the level of internal os. 3. The lowest clamp must be at right angles to the lower uterine segment. The lowest two clamps are replaced by no. 0 delayed absorbable suture ligatures. Following these principles helps in avoiding injury to the ureters. The ureters lie close to the cervix as they travel through the pelvis. By gentle upward uterine traction and downward mobilization of the bladder, the ureters that lie approximately 2 cm lateral to the cervix are further displaced from the uterine vessels. **Potential questions:** There can be questions related to the various steps of importance in relation to abdominal hysterectomy.

Question	Answer	Comment
Q17. During an abdominal hysterectomy, what is the key step when clamping, cutting, and ligating the structure shown in the image below? 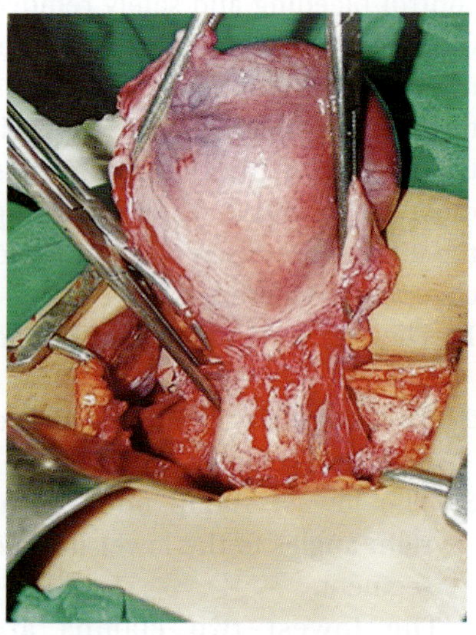 A. Identify and protect the ureter before clamping B. Clamp the ligament close to the uterus to reduce bleeding C. Use a single clamp to secure the ligament before cutting D. Ligate before clamping to prevent slippage E. Avoid electrocautery to prevent thermal damage	**Ans: A (Identify and protect the ureter before clamping.** Mackenrodt's ligaments, also known as cardinal or transverse cervical ligaments, are being identified in the adjacent image. This ligament is found at the base of broad ligament and helps in attaching the cervix and lower uterine segment to the lateral pelvic wall. 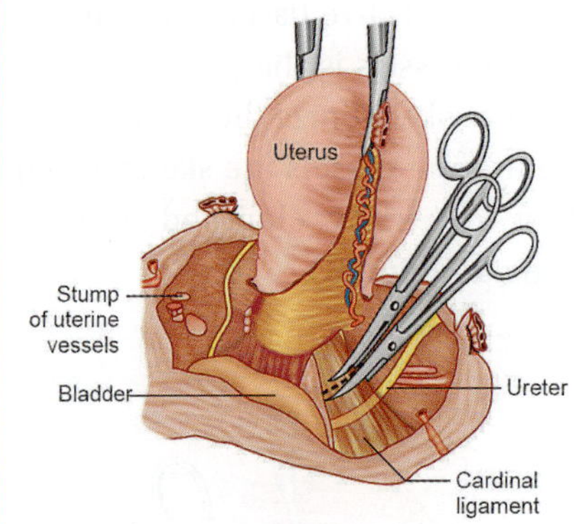 **Fig. 17:** Diagrammatic representation showing clamping and cutting the cardinal ligaments.	**Explanation:** Mackenrodt's ligaments lie in close proximity to the ureters. During an abdominal hysterectomy, it is important to identify and protect the ureters before clamping, cutting, and ligating these ligaments to prevent accidental injury **(Fig. 17)**. The ureters run just beneath the ligaments, and failure to properly identify and protect them can lead to serious complications such as ureteral injury or obstruction. **Potential questions:** There can be questions related to the various steps of importance in relation to abdominal hysterectomy.

Question	Answer	Comment
Q18. During an abdominal hysterectomy, the surgeon is preparing to clamp and cut the structures as shown in the image below. 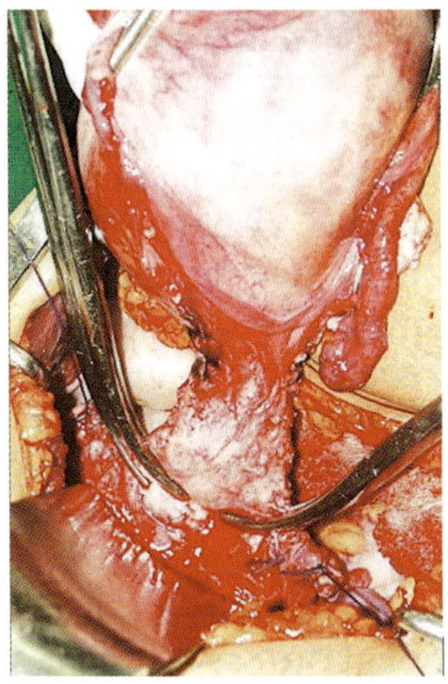 Which structure should be carefully avoided to prevent injury? A. Ureter B. Inferior epigastric artery C. Round ligament D. Ovarian artery E. Uterine artery	**Ans: A (Ureter)** The adjacent image depicts the identification of vaginal angles. **Figures 18A and B** depict the cutting of vaginal angles and separation of cervix from the vaginal vault. 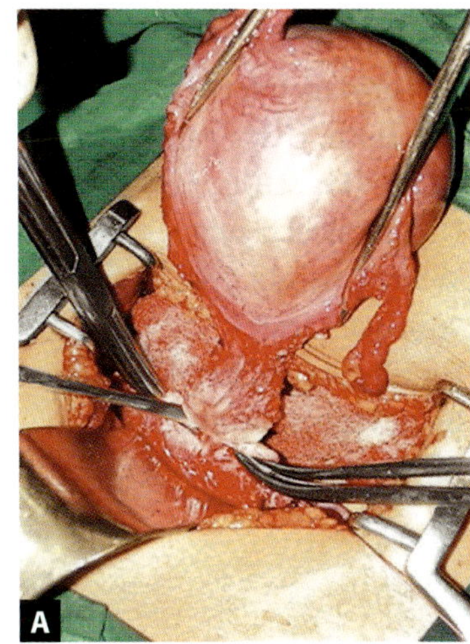 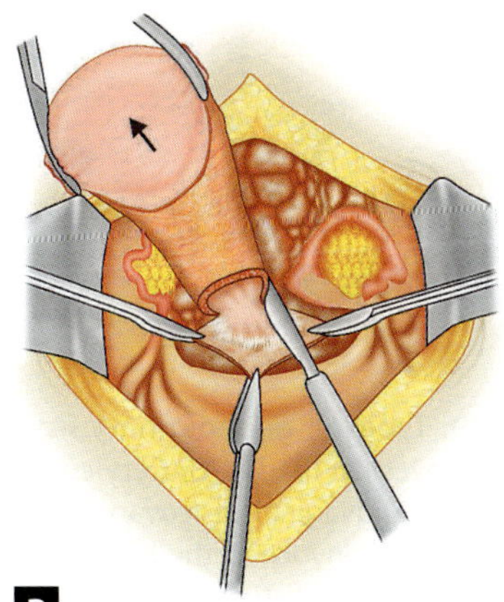 **Figs. 18A and B:** (A) Cutting the vaginal angles; (B) Diagrammatic representation of cutting the cervix from the vaginal vault.	**Explanation:** The ureter runs close to the lateral vaginal fornices and uterine artery, especially at the point where the uterine artery crosses over it. In abdominal hysterectomy, clamping and cutting the vaginal angles require extreme care to avoid damaging the ureter, which can result in significant complications like ureteric obstruction or injury. After the surgeon has determined with certainty that the bladder and rectum have been completely dissected away from the vagina, curved Ochsner's clamps are placed across the vaginal angles. The vagina is entered by a stab wound with a scalpel and is cut across with either a scalpel or scissors. First, the anterior vaginal fornix is opened and the incision is extended circumferentially close to the cervix in order to maintain the length of the vagina. **Potential questions:** There can be questions related to the various steps of importance in relation to abdominal hysterectomy.

GENITOURINARY FISTULAE

Question	Answer	Comment
Q19. A 30-year-old woman, postpartum presents with continuous urinary incontinence. A detailed pelvic examination reveals clear fluid pooling at the apex of her vagina. To counsel the patient about her diagnosis, the gynecologist uses a schematic diagram, as shown below (encircled). Which of the following is a common symptom of this condition? 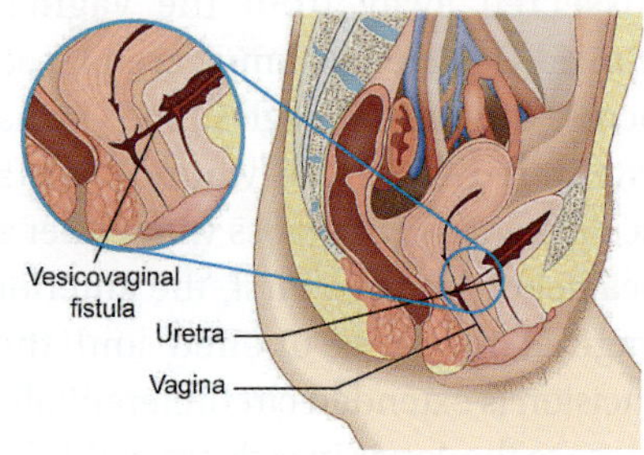 A. Severe pelvic pain B. Continuous urinary leakage from the vagina C. Heavy menstrual bleeding D. Frequent urination without leakage E. Lower back pain	**Ans: B (Continuous urinary leakage from the vagina)** The adjacent image points at genitourinary/urogenital fistula (UGF), which can be defined as abnormal communication tracts (lined with epithelium) between the genital tract and the urinary tract or the alimentary tract or both. UGFs can be classified as follows **(Fig. 19)**: ▪ Uterovesical fistula ▪ Vesical fistula (vesicovaginal or vesicocervical) ▪ Urethrovaginal fistula ▪ Rectovaginal fistula 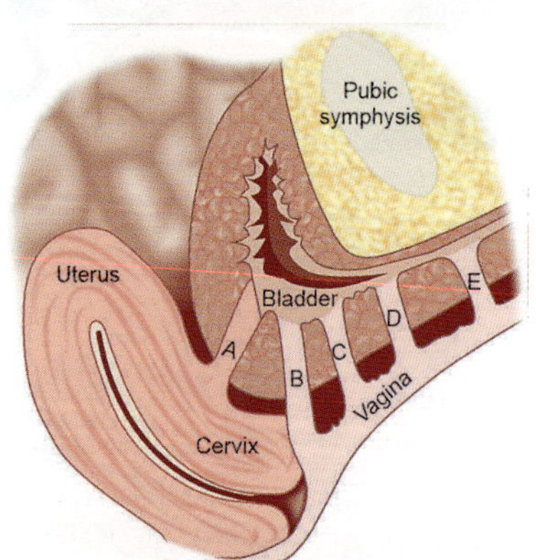 **Fig. 19:** Types of genitourinary fistulas: (A) Uterovesical fistula; (B) Cervicovesical fistula; (C) Midvaginal vesicovaginal fistula (VVF); (D) VVF involving the bladder neck; (E) urethrovaginal fistula.	**Explanation:** The genitourinary fistula often results in continuous urinary leakage from the vagina, as urine bypasses the normal route and leaks out through the fistula. This symptom is a key indicator of the presence of a genitourinary fistula and can significantly impact the patient's quality of life. Other symptoms may include recurrent urinary tract infections, irritation in the vaginal area, or an increase in vaginal discharge. Constant wetness in the genital areas can lead to the excoriation of the vagina, vulva, perineum, and thighs. Presence of recurrent cystitis or pyelonephritis, abnormal urinary stream, and hematuria following surgery may point towards an underlying UGF. **Potential questions:** There can be different questions related to the clinical presentation, diagnosis, and management of UGF.

ABNORMAL MENSTRUAL BLEEDING

Question	Answer	Comment
Q20. A 50-year-old woman, para 3, presents with postmenopausal bleeding. The gynecologist decides to perform an endometrial biopsy (EB) to assess the cause of the bleeding. Prior to performing the biopsy, she shows a cannula-like instrument as depicted in the image below and informs the patient that she shall be using this instrument on her. What is the primary purpose of using this instrument? 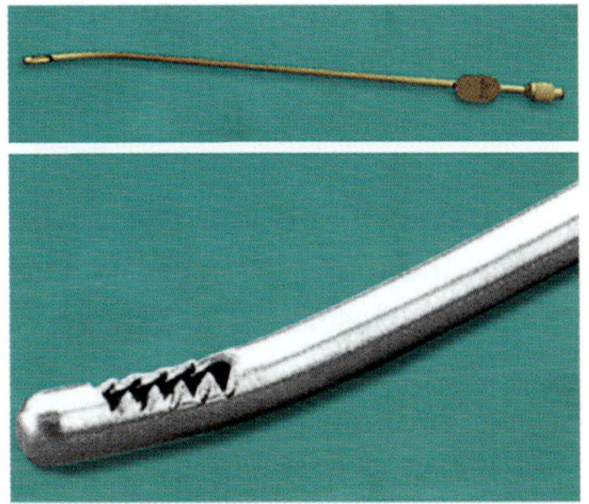 A. To diagnose ovarian cancer B. To collect a sample of endometrial tissue C. To treat uterine fibroids D. To perform a hysteroscopy E. To remove polyps from the cervix	**Ans: B (To collect a sample of endometrial tissue)** The adjacent image shows an EB curette. The EB curette is a narrow metal cannula having serrated edges with side openings on one end and an opening for syringe to be attached at the other end. Application of suction through the syringe helps in aspiration of endometrial curettings, thereby facilitating the procedure of endometrial biopsy **(Fig. 20)**. This tissue obtained is sent for the histopathological examination of the endometrium. 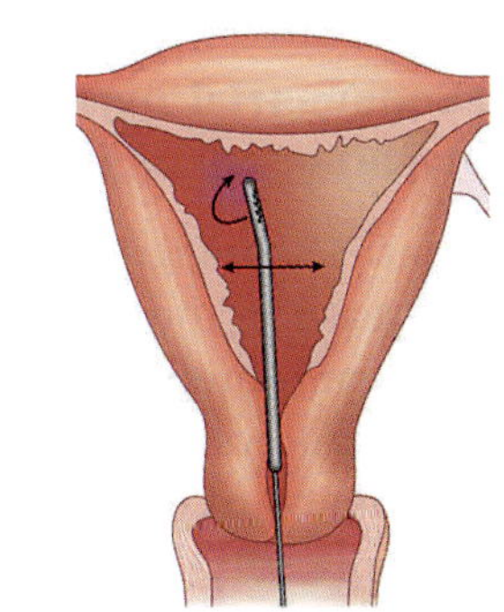 **Fig. 20:** Transverse section of endometrial cavity showing the endometrial biopsy curette.	**Explanation:** A curette is a surgical instrument used for endometrial biopsy, i.e., to scrape and collect tissue from the uterine endometrium. This procedure is often performed to diagnose conditions such as endometrial hyperplasia, endometrial cancer, and other abnormalities of the uterine endometrium. This method is particularly useful when a more substantial tissue sample is needed compared to less invasive techniques like endometrial aspiration using pipelle device. In case the endometrial thickness is >4 mm on transvaginal ultrasound examination in a postmenopausal patient with abnormal uterine bleeding (AUB), endometrial studies (endometrial aspiration, biopsy, etc.) should be done in order to exclude endometrial hyperplasia or even potential malignancy. **Potential questions:** There can be different questions related to the etiology, diagnosis and management of various cases of AUB.

Question	Answer	Comment
Q21. Which of the following is a common indication for performing an endometrial biopsy using the device shown in the image below? 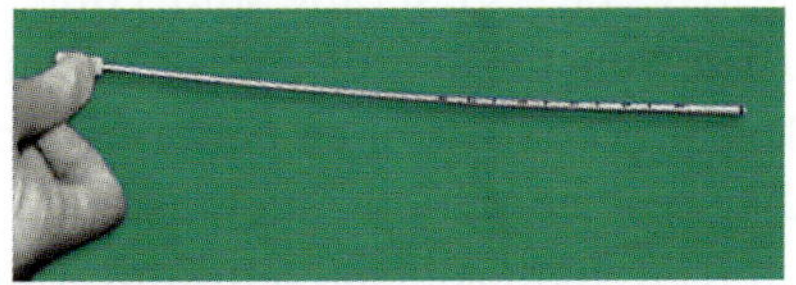 A. Evaluation of endometrial cancer B. Investigation of abnormal uterine bleeding C. Evaluation of suspected endometrial hyperplasia D. Evaluation of the size of uterine fibroids E. Infertility evaluation for endometrial receptivity	**Ans: B (Investigation of abnormal uterine bleeding)** The adjacent image shows a pipelle device, used for endometrial aspiration/biopsy to investigate the cause of AUB, such as heavy, prolonged, or irregular menstrual periods, as well as postmenopausal bleeding. This is a minimally invasive procedure that provides valuable diagnostic information **(Fig. 21)**. 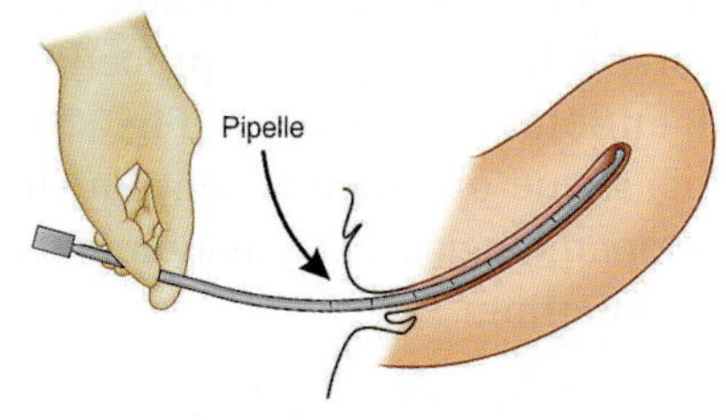 **Fig. 21:** Endometrial aspiration.	**Explanation:** The procedure of endometrial aspiration/biopsy helps in diagnosing conditions such as endometrial hyperplasia, endometrial cancer, and other endometrial abnormalities. Since no dilatation of the internal os is required prior to the insertion of a pipelle device, the procedure can be performed as an outpatient procedure without any requirement of anesthesia. Following the procedure, the endometrial sample obtained is sent for histopathological examination. **Potential questions:** There can be different questions related to the etiology, diagnosis, and management of various cases of AUB.
Q22. A 52-year-old woman presents with abnormal uterine bleeding. An endometrial biopsy is performed, and the HPE reveals findings as shown in the image below. What is the most likely diagnosis? 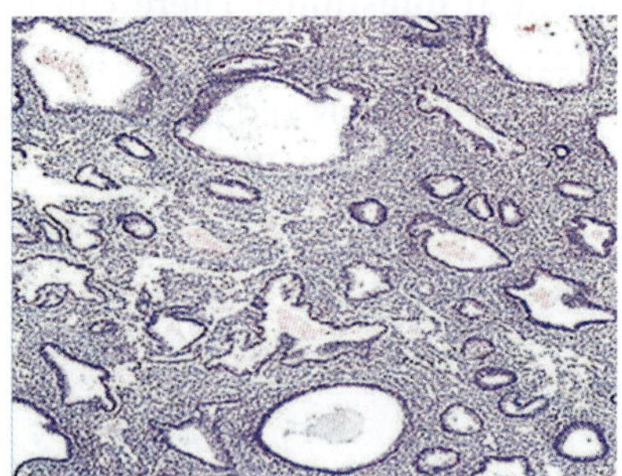 A. Endometrial carcinoma B. Endometrial polyp C. Complex endometrial hyperplasia D. Endometrial hyperplasia without atypia E. Endometrial hyperplasia with atypia	**Ans: D (Endometrial hyperplasia without atypia)** The adjacent HPE image demonstrates an increase in the number of glands and endometrial stroma. Some glands are cystically dilated. There is presence of an increased gland-to-stroma ratio with glands that are irregular in size and shape **(Fig. 22)**. However, the epithelium does not show any atypical features. This is suggestive of simple endometrial hyperplasia or endometrial hyperplasia without atypia. 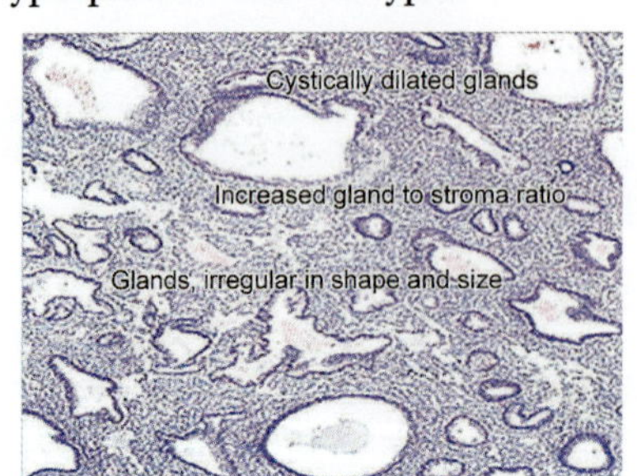 **Fig. 22:** Histopathological appearance of simple endometrial hyperplasia.	**Explanation:** Endometrial hyperplasia without atypia is characterized by features described in **Figure 25**. However, the epithelial cells lining these glands do not show atypical features. This distinguishes it from endometrial carcinoma, which would show cytological atypia and invasive growth. Most individuals with simple hyperplasia without any atypia can be managed with hormonal therapy using medroxyprogesterone (Provera), 10 mg daily every 5 days for 3 months or with close follow-up. Progestin may be administered orally, intramuscularly, in the form of an intrauterine device (IUD), or as a vaginal cream. A follow-up endometrial biopsy after 3–12 months can be done. **Potential questions:** There can be different questions related to different types of endometrial hyperplasias.

Question	Answer	Comment
Q23. A 55-year-old woman presents with postmenopausal bleeding. An endometrial biopsy is performed, and the HPE reveals findings as shown in the image below. What is the most likely diagnosis? 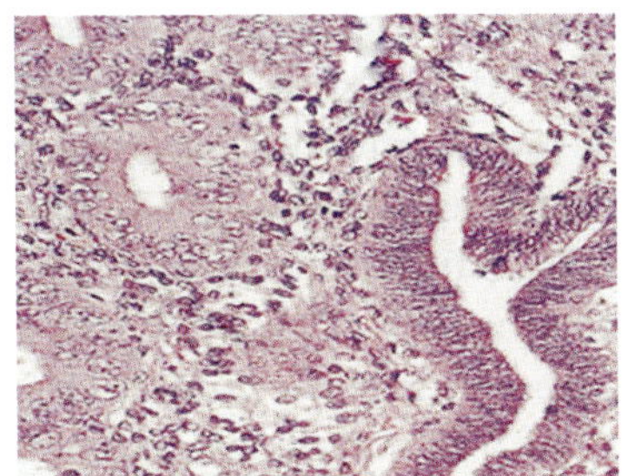 A. Endometrial carcinoma B. Endometrial polyp C. Simple endometrial hyperplasia D. Endometrial hyperplasia with atypia E. Complex endometrial hyperplasia	**Ans:** **D (Endometrial hyperplasia with atypia)** The adjacent HPE image shows features of endometrial hyperplasia as well as cytological atypia **(Fig. 23)**. This is a premalignant lesion that may progress to cancer in 30–45% of women. Additionally, atypical endometrial hyperplasia may be associated with a co-existing endometrial cancer in approximately 20% of patients. 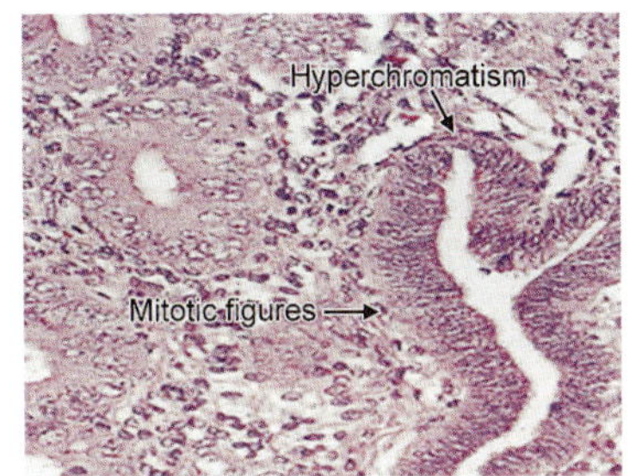 **Fig. 23:** Histopathological appearance of complex endometrial hyperplasia with atypia.	**Explanation:** Endometrial hyperplasia with atypia, also known as atypical endometrial hyperplasia, is characterized by features of hyperplasia such as an increased gland-to-stroma ratio with glands that are irregular in size and shape. The presence of cytological features of atypia, such as nuclear enlargement/hyperchromatism, stratification, and loss of polarity, mitotic figures, etc., distinguishes it from nonatypical hyperplasia. Though most physicians treat complex hyperplasia with or without atypia with hormonal therapy, hysterectomy may be considered for complex or high-grade cases of hyperplasia with atypia. **Potential questions:** There can be different questions related to different types of endometrial hyperplasias.
Q24. A 58-year-old postmenopausal woman presents with a history of prolonged and abnormal uterine bleeding. After initial investigations, an endometrial biopsy is performed. The histopathological imaging of the biopsied tissue shows the findings as depicted in the image below. What is the most likely diagnosis? 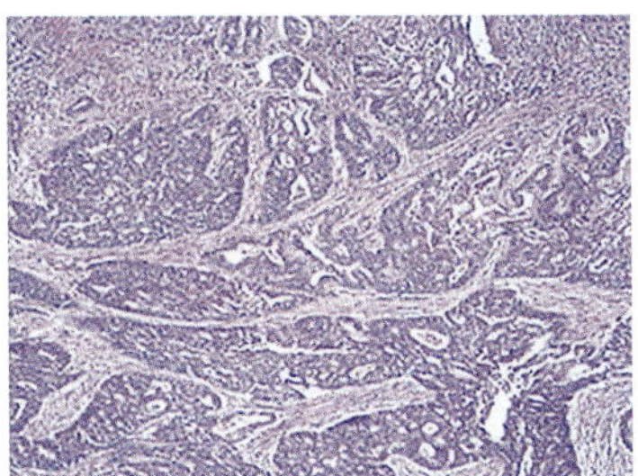 A. Endometrial hyperplasia B. Endometrial polyp C. Endometrial carcinoma D. Adenomyosis E. Uterine sarcoma	**Ans:** **C (Endometrial carcinoma)** The adjacent image shows replacement of normal uterine endometrium with frank invasive cancer showing invasion of the basement membrane. This is suggestive of frank endometrial cancer. **Figure 24** is the hysterectomy specimen in the same patient showing an enlarged uterus with a fungating growth, which is localized in the upper part of the uterine cavity close to the fundus. 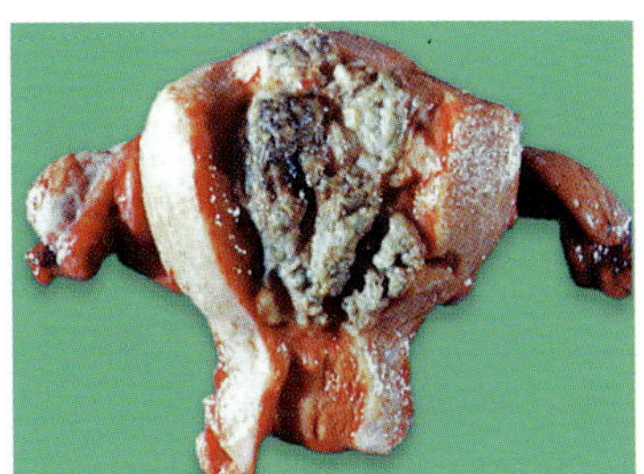 **Fig. 24:** Hysterectomy specimen of endometrial cancer.	**Explanation:** Endometrial carcinoma is characterized histopathologically by the presence of atypical glandular cells with increased mitotic activity with the invasion of basement membrane. There may be invasion into the myometrium based on the stage of cancer. These features distinguish it from endometrial hyperplasia, which lacks basement membrane/myometrial invasion. Laparotomy with total abdominal hysterectomy and bilateral salpingoo-ophorectomy along with staging laparotomy is required in these cases in order to determine the stage of uterine cancer. Treatment is then directed based on the stage of cancer. **Potential questions:** There can be different questions related to different types of endometrial hyperplasias.

Question	Answer	Comment
Q25. A 40-year-old woman presents with abnormal uterine bleeding. TVS is performed, which reveals the findings as shown in the image below. Based on clinical suspicion, SIS was subsequently performed, which revealed presence of a focal lesion. 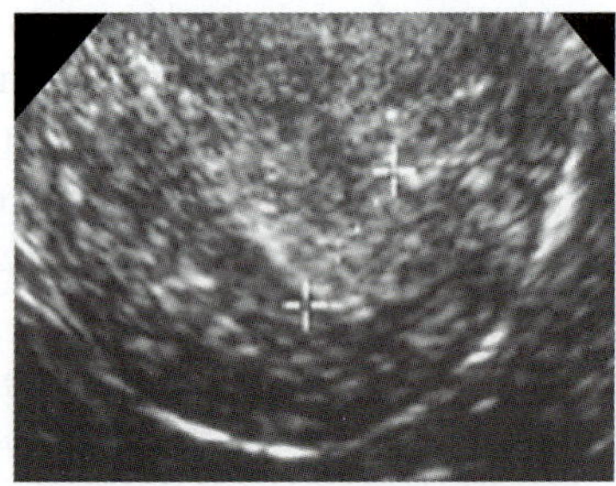 What is the most likely diagnosis? A. Submucosal fibroid B. Endometrial polyp C. Endometrial hyperplasia D. Endometrial cancer E. Uterine septum	**Ans: B (Endometrial polyp)** The adjacent TVS image shows presence of thickened endometrium (>4 mm). In a premenopausal patient, endometrial thickness >4 mm is not of much significance. Based on the clinical suspicion of endometrial polyp, SIS was performed, which revealed the presence of an endometrial polyp **(Fig. 25)**. 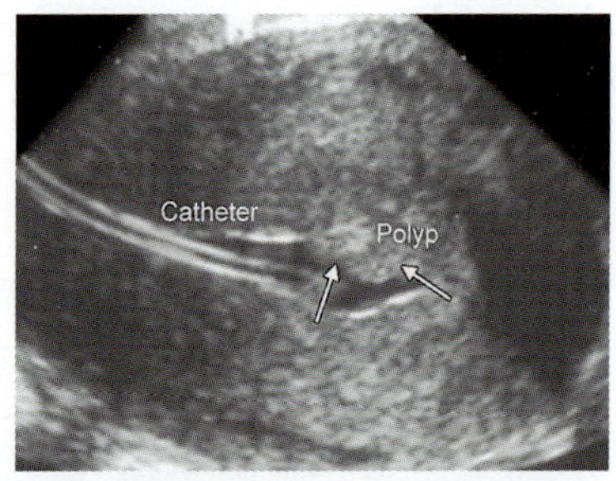 **Fig. 25:** In the same patient, SIS revealed the presence of an endometrial polyp.	**Explanation:** Endometrial polyps are benign growths that protrude into the endometrial cavity. They are often identified on transvaginal ultrasound as solitary, homogeneous, and echogenic lesions. Sometimes, they may just result in an increased endometrial thickness on transvaginal ultrasound and may require SIS for polyp localization. SIS is able to clearly delineate the masses or defects inside the uterine cavity. It helps in differentiating between focal lesions (polyps and submucosal myomas) and global endometrial thickening. Hysteroscopic resection and guided biopsy have been considered as the most effective treatment for the management of endometrial polyps. **Potential questions:** There can be different questions related to the diagnosis and management of cases with AUB.

MENOPAUSE

Question	Answer	Comment
Q26. In the image below, identify the hormone labeled A, responsible for hot flashes, night sweats, and vaginal dryness. 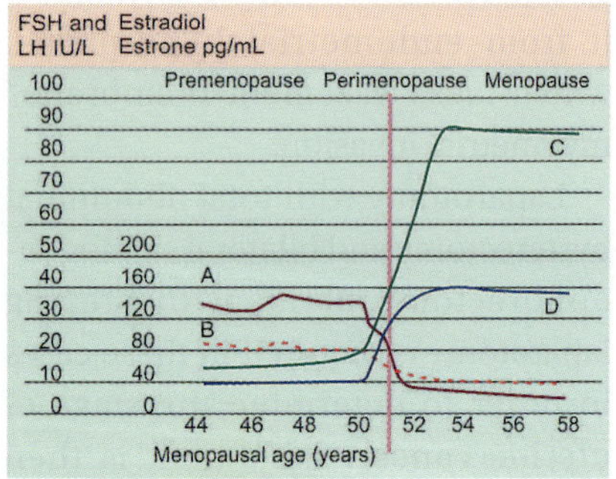 A. Progesterone B. Estrogen C. Follicle-stimulating hormone (FSH) D. Luteinizing hormone (LH) E. Testosterone	**Ans: B (Estrogen)** The hormone labeled A is estrogen. A significant drop in estrogen during menopause causes symptoms like hot flashes, night sweats, and vaginal dryness. **Figure 26** shows hormone level changes during menopause. 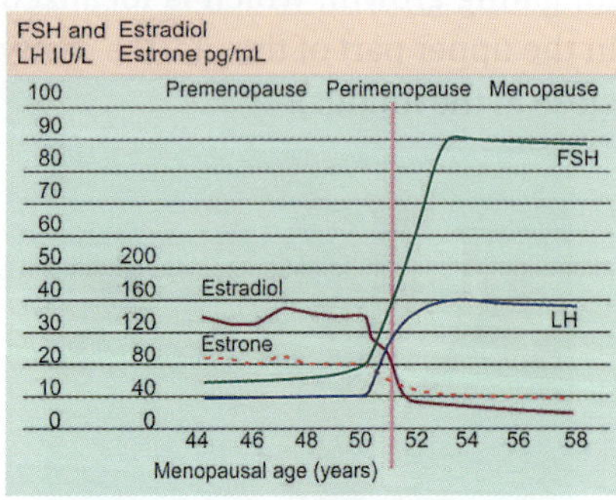 **Fig. 26:** Changes in the level of various hormones at the time of menopause.	**Explanation:** Menopause occurs due to decline in the ovarian activity. There is failure of ovulation, formation of corpus luteum, and of secretion of progesterone by the ovaries. Estrogenic activity is reduced and there occurs endometrial atrophy, resulting in amenorrhea. Initially, there is a rebound increase in the secretion of FSH and LH by the anterior pituitary. However, with further advancing years, the gonadotropic activity of pituitary glands also ceases and a fall in FSH levels eventually occurs. **Potential questions:** There can be questions pertaining to changes in levels of various other hormones during menopause.

Question	Answer	Comment
Q27. A 65-year-old woman presents with sudden onset of back pain after lifting a heavy object. An X-ray of the spine shows an abnormality depicted in the image below. What is the most likely underlying condition? 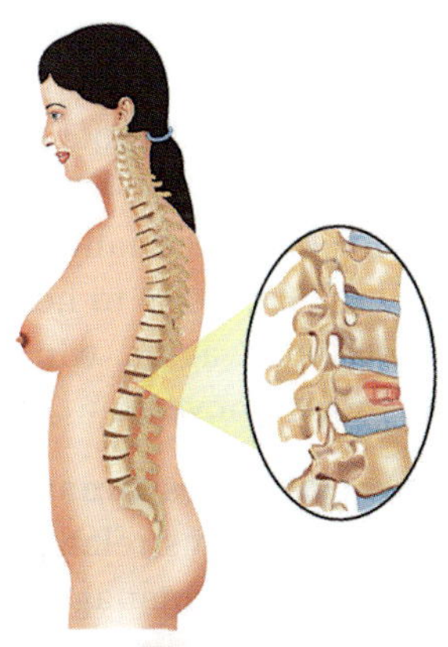 A. Osteoarthritis B. Osteopetrosis C. Osteoporosis D. Osteomalacia E. Spondylolisthesis	**Ans: C (Osteoporosis)** The adjacent image shows the presence of vertebral compression fracture. The sudden onset of back pain following minimal trauma, such as lifting a heavy object, points towards the diagnosis of vertebral compression fracture. Since the woman is menopausal, this is likely to be due to osteoporosis. Changes in bone marrow density with age and gender are illustrated in **Figure 27**. Peak bone density in women normally occurs at about 25 years of age, following which the bone loss starts to occur. After the age of 35 years, men and women normally lose 0.3–0.5% of their bone density per year as a part of normal aging process. 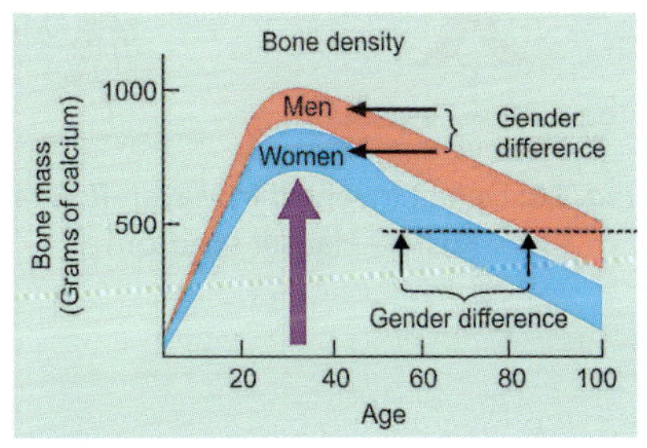 **Fig. 27:** Changes in bone marrow density with age and gender.	**Explanation:** Osteoporosis is a condition characterized by decreased bone density and increased bone fragility, leading to a higher risk of fractures. This condition is particularly common in postmenopausal women because menopause results in falling estrogen levels, which may result in the development of primary osteoporosis. As the regulatory effect of estrogen on bone resorption is lost, the resorption process is accelerated and not adequately balanced by compensatory bone formation. Diagnosis is typically confirmed through bone mineral density (BMD) testing using dual-energy X-ray absorptiometry (DEXA). Management includes lifestyle modifications, calcium and vitamin D supplementation, and pharmacological treatments such as bisphosphonates to strengthen bones and reduce fracture risk. **Potential questions:** There can be questions pertaining to clinical presentation, diagnosis, management, and complications of menopause.

MÜLLERIAN ABNORMALITIES

Question	Answer	Comment
Q28. A 20-year-old woman with Mayer-Rokitansky-Küster-Hauser (MRKH) syndrome presents for treatment. She is advised to use a set of smooth, cylindrical plastic tubes of varying sizes as shown in the image below. 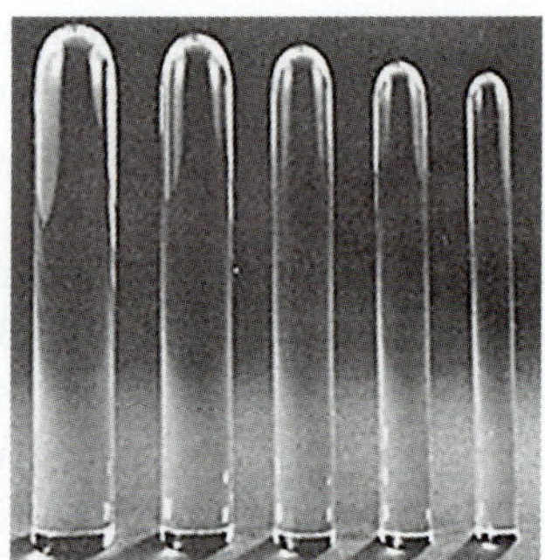 What is the primary purpose of using this device in MRKH syndrome? A. To treat urinary incontinence B. To prevent vaginal stenosis C. To create a functional vaginal canal D. To diagnose vaginal stenosis E. To manage infertility	**Ans: C (To create a functional vaginal canal)** The adjacent image shows vaginal dilators with progressively increasing size. In MRKH syndrome, the vagina is either absent or underdeveloped **(Fig. 28)**. Vaginal dilators are used to gradually stretch the vaginal tissue and create a functional vaginal canal. This process helps patients achieve a vaginal length that allows for comfortable sexual intercourse, thereby improving their quality of life. 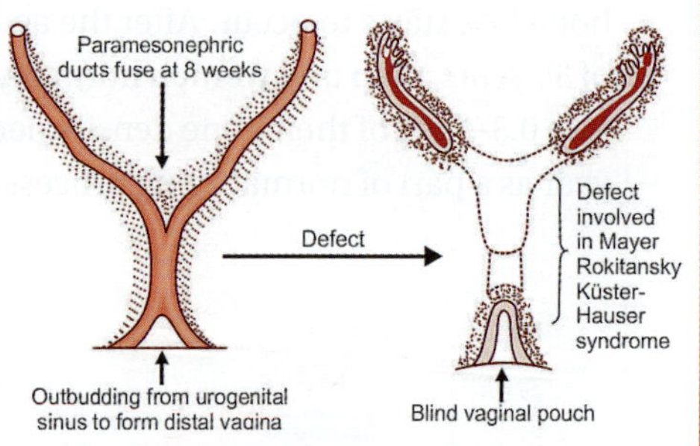 **Fig. 28:** Defect involved in Mayer–Rokitansky–Küster– Hauser syndrome.	**Explanation:** Surgery is the most effective treatment for vaginal agenesis, but nonsurgical options like dilator use are also effective. Dilators can be used with Frank's method (active dilatation) or Ingram's method (passive dilatation). In Frank's method, the woman applies manual pressure with a dilator for 15–20 minutes, twice a day, gradually increasing the dilator size to help form a functional vagina, which may take months or years. **Potential questions:** There can be questions related to the diagnosis and management of various uterine malformations such as Mullerian agenesis, bicornuate uterus, unicornuate uterus, septate uterus, etc.

Question	Answer	Comment
Q29. The following hysterosalpingography (HSG) image shows a uterine anomaly. What is the most likely diagnosis? 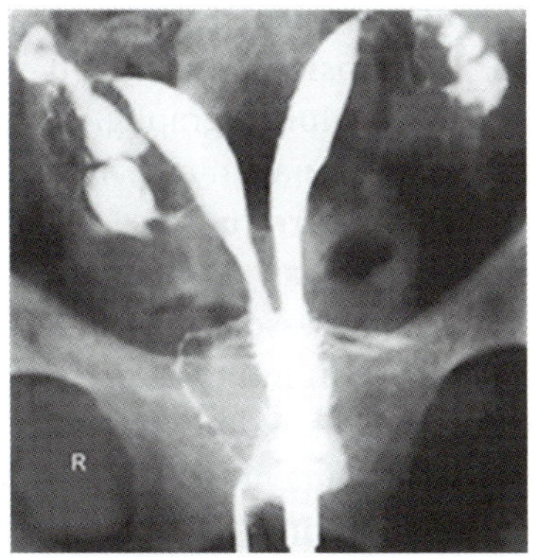 A. Bicornuate uterus B. Uterine septum C. Arcuate uterus D. Unicornuate uterus E. Didelphys uterus	**Ans: B (Uterine septum)** The adjacent HSG image shows the presence of uterine septum which was later confirmed on hysteroscopy **(Fig. 29)**. HSG shows the presence of an elongated fibrous structure arising from the uterine fundus, which is observed to be dividing the uterine cavity. This is noticed as a linear filling defect on HSG extending from the fundus towards the cervix, creating two separate endometrial cavities. This defect is usually seen in the midline and can vary in length and thickness. 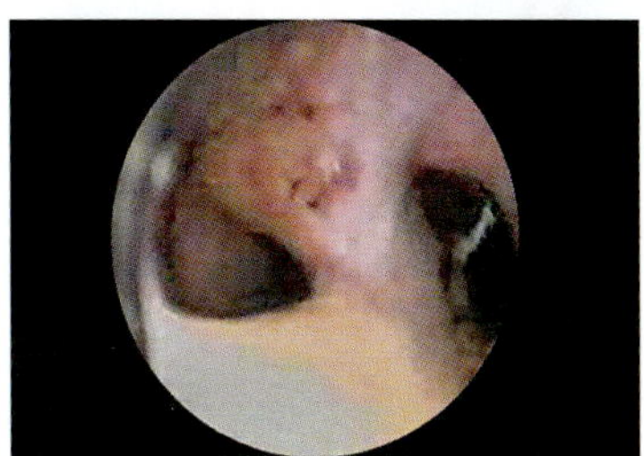 **Fig. 29:** Uterine septum as observed on hysteroscopic examination.	**Explanation:** A uterine septum is a congenital anomaly where a fibrous or muscular septum divides the uterine cavity. Differentiating a uterine septum from other anomalies like a bicornuate uterus is important, as the latter involves an external indentation of the uterine fundus, which is not visible on HSG alone. Further imaging with 3D ultrasound or MRI may be required for definitive diagnosis. The uterine septum can be treated by removing it surgically, either through metroplasty (reconstructive uterine surgery) or through hysteroscopic resection. **Potential questions:** There can be questions related to the diagnosis and management of various uterine malformations such as Müllerian agenesis, bicornuate uterus, unicornuate uterus, septate uterus, etc.
Q30. The three-dimensional ultrasound image shown below depicts a uterine anomaly. What is the most likely diagnosis? 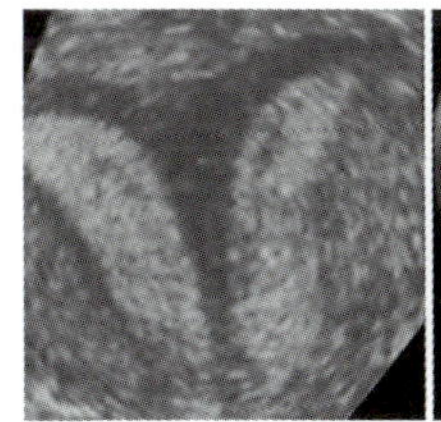 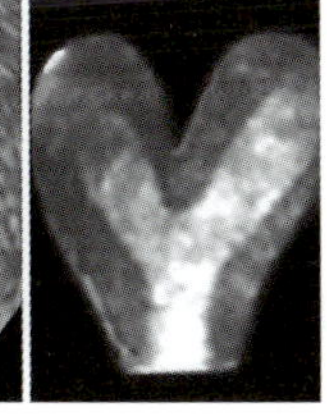 A. Septate uterus B. Bicornuate uterus C. Arcuate uterus D. Unicornuate uterus E. Didelphys uterus	**Ans: B (Bicornuate uterus)** On three-dimensional ultrasound, the central myometrial tissue extends up to internal cervical os and there are two endometrial cavities. The outer fundal contour was not round but instead showed an indentation (>1 cm), which confirmed the diagnosis of bicornuate uterus **(Fig. 30)**. 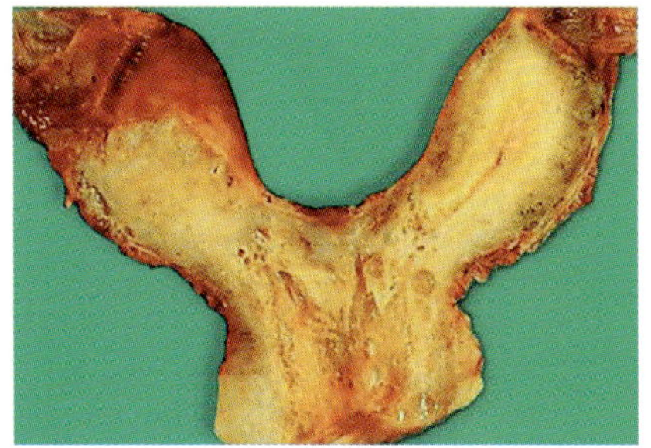 **Fig. 30:** Specimen showing cut section of a bicornuate uterus with a single cervix.	**Explanation:** A bicornuate uterus is a congenital uterine anomaly resulting from the incomplete fusion of the Müllerian ducts, leading to a heart-shaped uterus with two distinct cavities. On hysterosalpingography, it is characterized by a deep fundal cleft and widely divergent uterine horns. The angle between the horns is typically more than 105°, which helps differentiate it from a septate uterus, where the angle is less than 75°. Other investigations, which help in confirming the diagnosis of bicornuate uterus, include laparoscopic (invasive) and MRI (noninvasive) examination. **Potential questions:** There can be questions related to the diagnosis and management of various uterine malformations such as Mullerian agenesis, bicornuate uterus, unicornuate uterus, septate uterus, etc.

Question	Answer	Comment
Q31. During a routine fertility assessment, a 29-year-old woman undergoes pelvic imaging. The gynecologist evaluates the unusual uterine shape observed in the scan and discusses its implications for her fertility and pregnancy, by drawing a diagram of the anatomical anomaly as shown below. What is the most likely diagnosis? 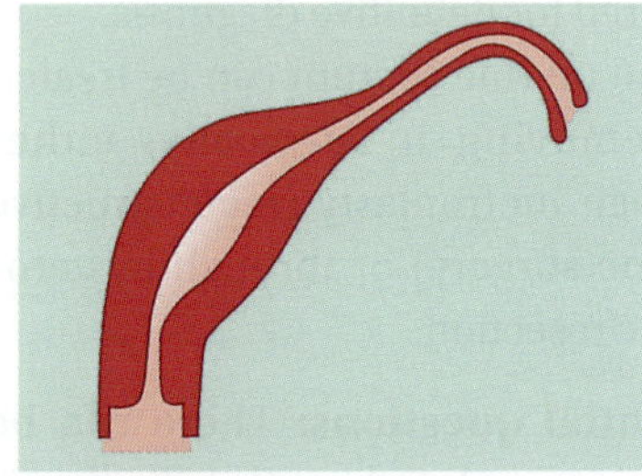 A. Bicornuate uterus B. Septate uterus C. Uterus didelphys D. Unicornuate uterus E. Arcuate uterus	**Ans: D (Unicornuate uterus)** A unicornuate uterus, as shown in the image, is a congenital anomaly where only one Müllerian duct develops, resulting in a banana-shaped uterine cavity. This condition typically includes a single fallopian tube, cervix, and vagina. It may also involve a rudimentary horn, with or without a uterine cavity and functional endometrium, sometimes communicating with the main uterine cavity **(Figs. 31A to D)**. 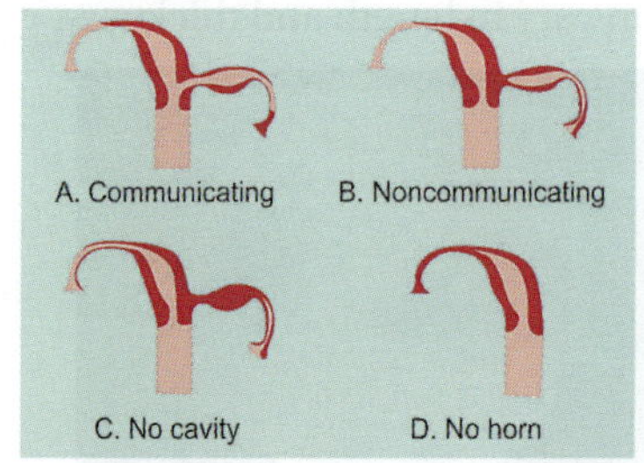 **Figs. 31A to D:** Buttram and Gibbons's classification of unicornuate uterus.	**Explanation:** Women with unicornuate uterus may face recurrent pregnancy loss, pelvic pain, and pregnancy complications due to reduced uterine volume and abnormal shape. Diagnosis is confirmed via MRI, hysterosalpingography, or 3D ultrasound. Management involves addressing reproductive issues, monitoring renal abnormalities, and excising accessory horns during laparoscopic hemihysterectomy. Symptomatic hematometra with a functioning rudimentary horn can be treated with endometrial ablation via the hysteroscopic route. **Potential questions:** There can be questions related to the diagnosis and management of various uterine malformations such as Mullerian agenesis, bicornuate uterus, unicornuate uterus, septate uterus, etc.
Q32. A 28-year-old woman presents with recurrent miscarriages and dysmenorrhea. An MRI of the pelvis in this case is shown in the image below. What is the most likely diagnosis? 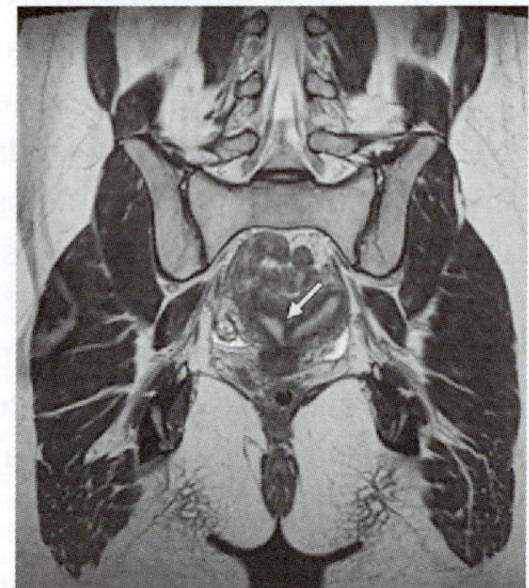 A. Bicornuate uterus B. Septate uterus C. Uterus didelphys D. Unicornuate uterus E. Arcuate uterus	**Ans: C (Uterus didelphys)** The MRI image shows a didelphus uterus with two divergent uterine horns (depicted by the arrow), a large fundal cleft, and two separate cervices. It features two hemiuteri, each connected to one fallopian tube **(Fig. 32)**, and may have one or two vaginas with a complete or partial longitudinal vaginal septum. 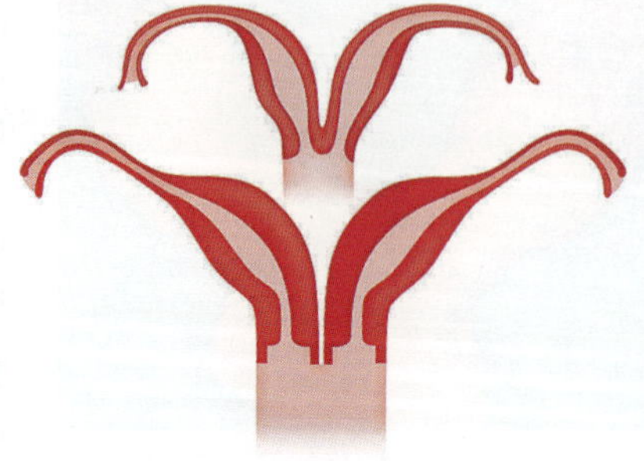 **Fig. 32:** Didelphus uterus.	**Explanation:** Uterus didelphys is a Müllerian duct anomaly caused by incomplete fusion of the uterine ducts between weeks 12–16 of gestation. It leads to duplication of the uterine horns and cervices. Common issues include recurrent miscarriages, preterm birth, cervical incompetence, and dysmenorrhea. A key symptom is tampon use being ineffective during menstruation, and patients may also have a history of second-trimester spontaneous abortions. **Potential questions:** There can be questions related to the diagnosis and management of various uterine malformations such as Müllerian agenesis, bicornuate uterus, unicornuate uterus, septate uterus, etc.

Question	Answer	Comment
Q33. A 19-year-old woman reports difficulty using tampons and experiencing discomfort during intercourse. She also mentions having two separate menstrual flows. On physical examination, the gynecologist discovers an anatomical anomaly, as shown below. What is the most likely diagnosis? 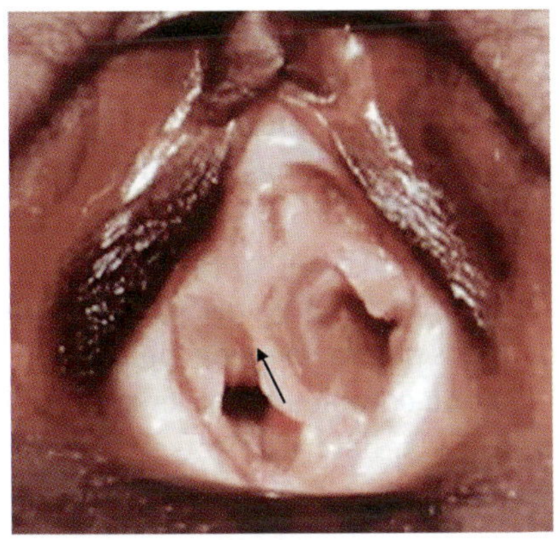 A. Transverse vaginal septum B. Longitudinal vaginal septum C. Vaginal atresia D. Imperforate hymen E. Vaginal agenesis	**Ans: B (Longitudinal vaginal septum)** The longitudinal vaginal septum results due to incomplete fusion of the lower parts of the Müllerian ducts. Presence of a longitudinal vaginal septum results in a double vagina **(Fig. 33)**. Sometimes, the defect in fusion may extend towards the upper parts of the Müllerian ducts, resulting in a double cervix and/or uterus didelphys. 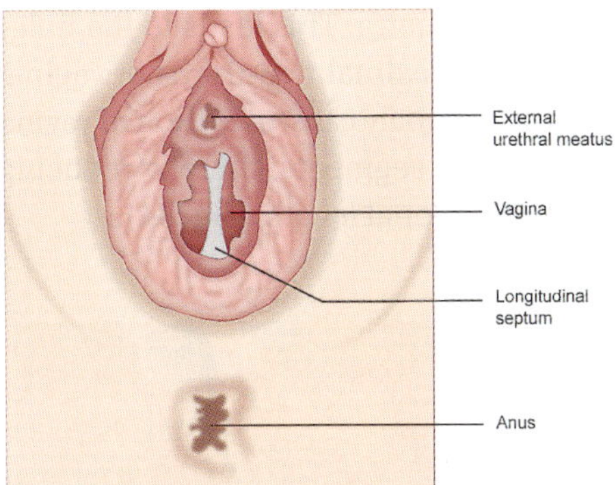 **Fig. 33:** Longitudinal vaginal septum.	**Explanation:** A longitudinal vaginal septum is a congenital anomaly resulting from incomplete fusion of the Müllerian ducts. It presents as a vertical partition within the vaginal canal, which can be partial or complete. On MRI, it appears as a linear structure dividing the vaginal lumen into two separate channels. This condition can be asymptomatic or associated with symptoms such as dyspareunia, difficulty with tampon use, or obstructed labor. The diagnosis of a vaginal septum is usually made on clinical examination. If the longitudinal vaginal septum causes dyspareunia or some other symptom, it can be surgically excised. **Potential questions:** There can be questions related to the diagnosis and management of various uterine malformations such as Müllerian agenesis, bicornuate uterus, unicornuate uterus, septate uterus, etc.

AMENORRHEA

<table>
<tr><th>Question</th><th>Answer</th><th>Comment</th></tr>
<tr>
<td>Q34. A 16-year-old girl presents with primary amenorrhea and cyclic pelvic pain. She has normal breast development and pubic and axillary hair. On examination, her external genitalia appear normal, but no vaginal opening can be visualized. The MRI image below shows the vaginal anomaly in this case. What is the most likely diagnosis?

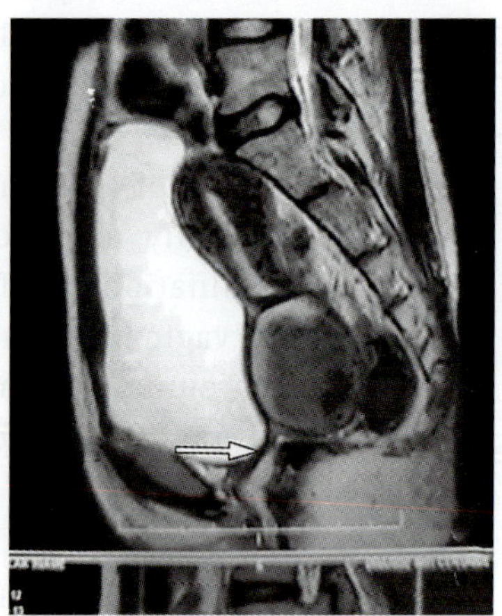

A. Imperforate hymen
B. Transverse vaginal septum
C. Vaginal atresia
D. Mayer-Rokitansky-Küster-Hauser (MRKH) syndrome
E. Vaginal agenesis</td>
<td>Ans: B (Transverse vaginal septum)

The adjacent MRI image demonstrates the absence of the lower one-third of vagina (as shown by the arrow), a condition termed transverse vaginal septum or vaginal atresia. As a result, there could be accumulation of menstrual debris resulting in development of hematocolpos or hematometra. This leads to the bulging of proximal two-thirds of vagina. This anomaly causes division of vagina into two segments, thereby reducing its functional length (Fig. 34).

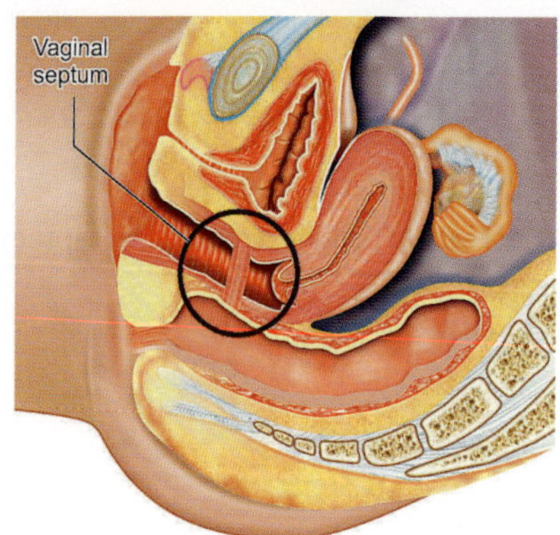

Fig. 34: Transverse vaginal septum (encircled).</td>
<td>Explanation: A transverse vaginal septum is a congenital anomaly resulting from incomplete fusion or canalization of the vaginal plate and the caudal end of the Müllerian ducts. This septum can cause obstruction, leading to symptoms such as primary amenorrhea, cyclic pelvic pain, and hematocolpos. Incomplete vaginal septum may sometimes result in dyspareunia, menstrual abnormalities, difficulty with intercourse, reproductive issues, obstructed labor, etc.

In case of an incomplete vaginal septum, complete surgical excision of the septum may be performed. Ideally, a complete transverse vaginal septum must be incised before menarche to allow for the discharge of menstrual secretions.

Potential questions: There can be questions related to various causes of primary amenorrhea such as imperforate hymen, transverse vaginal septum, MRKH syndrome, androgen insensitivity syndrome, Turner syndrome, etc.</td>
</tr>
</table>

<table>
<tr><th>Question</th><th>Answer</th><th>Comment</th></tr>
<tr>
<td>

Q35. A 14-year-old girl with absent menstruation presents with recurrent lower abdominal pain and a palpable mass in the lower abdomen. She reports normal development of pubic and axillary hair. On per speculum examination, the gynecologist discovers an anatomical anomaly as shown in the image below. What is the most likely diagnosis?

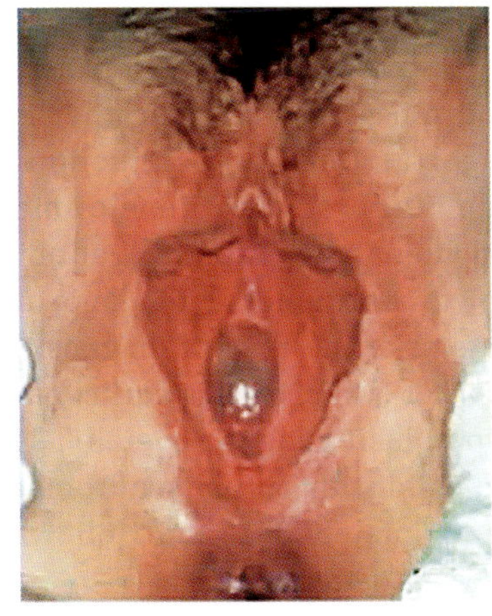

A. Hydrocolpos
B. Hematocolpos
C. Vaginal cyst
D. Endometrioma
E. Ovarian torsion

</td>
<td>

Ans: B (Hematocolpos)

The adjacent image depicts an anomaly due to imperforate hymen, which occurs as a result of abnormal or incomplete embryologic development. Since a bluish discoloration is visible behind the translucent membrane, hematocolpos (accumulation of blood in the vaginal canal) is also present **(Figs. 35A and B)**. This condition commonly causes amenorrhea, usually associated with cyclical abdominal pain, which tends to worsen over time.

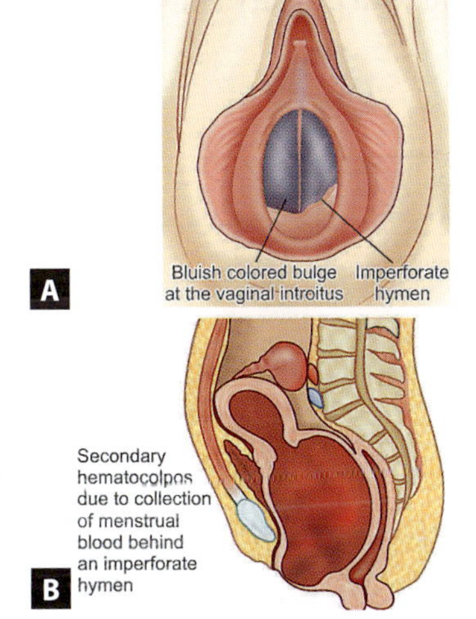

Figs. 35A and B: (A) Imperforate hymen; (B) Accumulation of blood in the uterine cavity as a result of imperforate hymen.

</td>
<td>

Explanation: Hematocolpos is a condition characterized by the accumulation of menstrual blood in the vagina due to an anatomical obstruction, most commonly an imperforate hymen. Patients typically present with primary amenorrhea, cyclic pelvic pain, and a palpable lower abdominal mass. Differentiating hematocolpos from hydrocolpos is essential, as the latter involves the accumulation of nonbloody fluid, often due to congenital anomalies or infections.

In case an adolescent girl presents with hematometra (accumulation of blood in the uterine cavity) or hematocolpos, surgical correction (hymenotomy) should be performed as an emergency but with an appropriate preoperative evaluation. The objective of the hymenotomy procedure is to open the hymenal membrane in such a way as to form a normally patent vaginal orifice, without scarring. During hymenotomy, the hymenal orifice is enlarged by giving either a circular or a cruciate incision along the diagonal diameters of hymen.

Potential questions: There can be questions related to various causes of primary amenorrhea such as imperforate hymen, transverse vaginal septum, MRKH syndrome, androgen insensitivity syndrome, Turner syndrome, etc.

</td>
</tr>
</table>

Question	Answer	Comment
Q36. A 18-year-old girl presents with short stature, webbed neck, and primary amenorrhea. An ultrasound of the pelvis shows streak ovaries. A karyotype analysis was done which revealed the findings as shown in the image below. What is the most likely diagnosis? 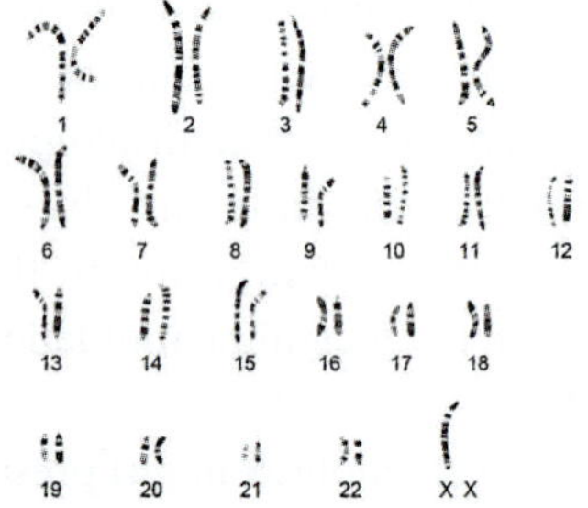 A. Klinefelter syndrome B. Turner syndrome C. Androgen insensitivity syndrome D. Polycystic ovary syndrome E. Congenital adrenal hyperplasia	**Ans: B (Turner syndrome)** The adjacent image of karyotype analysis shows absence of one X chromosome (45, X karyotype). This is associated with a chromosomal defect known as Turner syndrome and is characterized by clinical features such as short stature, webbed neck, shield chest, increased carrying angle at the elbow, and hypergonadotropic hypoestrogenic amenorrhea **(Fig. 36)**. Due to the presence of streak gonads, which lack ovarian follicles, no gonadal sex hormones are produced at the time of puberty and the patients present with primary amenorrhea. 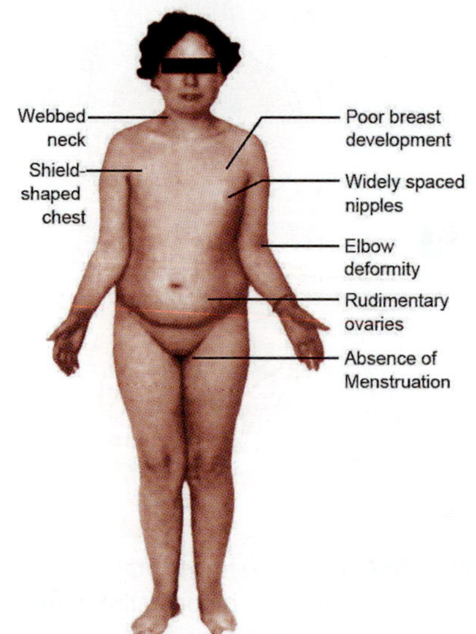 **Fig. 36:** Physical appearance of a girl diagnosed to be suffering from Turner syndrome.	**Explanation:** Other common findings in these cases can include lymphedema, low-set ears, and a broad chest with widely spaced nipples. Diagnosis is confirmed through karyotype analysis. Management involves hormone replacement therapy and monitoring for associated conditions such as cardiovascular anomalies and osteoporosis. The main aims of treatment in the case of a patient with Turner's syndrome are increasing the final height attained and induction of secondary sexual development and menarche. Administration of growth hormone at the age of 4 years or at the time of diagnosis of disorder (whichever is earlier) may help in increasing the overall height of a child with Turner syndrome by approximately 8–10 cm (following 3–7 years of treatment). Estrogen replacement therapy is often started at the time of expected puberty (12 or 13 years) to help trigger the development of secondary sexual characteristics. **Potential questions:** There can be questions related to various causes of primary amenorrhea such as imperforate hymen, transverse vaginal septum, Mayer-Rokitansky-Küster-Hauser (MRKH) syndrome, androgen insensitivity syndrome, Turner syndrome, etc.

CHAPTER 10

Abnormalities in Conception

DIAGNOSIS OF INFERTILITY

Question	Answer	Comment
Q1. A 28-year-old woman, trying to conceive, presents to the clinic for an evaluation of her ovulatory cycle. The gynecologist examines her cervical mucus under a microscope, looking for a specific pattern, as shown in the image below. What does the presence of this pattern of cervical mucus indicate in the context of infertility treatment? 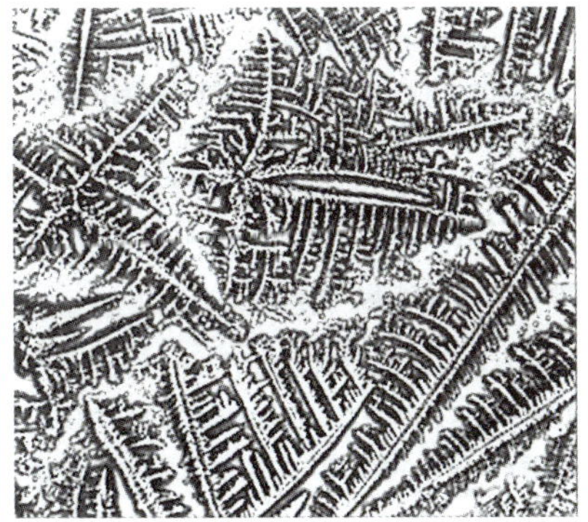 A. Low estrogen levels B. High progesterone levels C. Ovulation D. Menstrual bleeding E. Anovulation	**Ans: C (Ovulation)** The adjacent image shows a fern-like pattern of the cervical mucous when it is allowed to dry on a slide under the microscope. This pattern indicates that the woman is in her fertile period and ovulation is about to occur. During this phase, the cervical mucous also shows the Spinnbarkeit phenomenon. 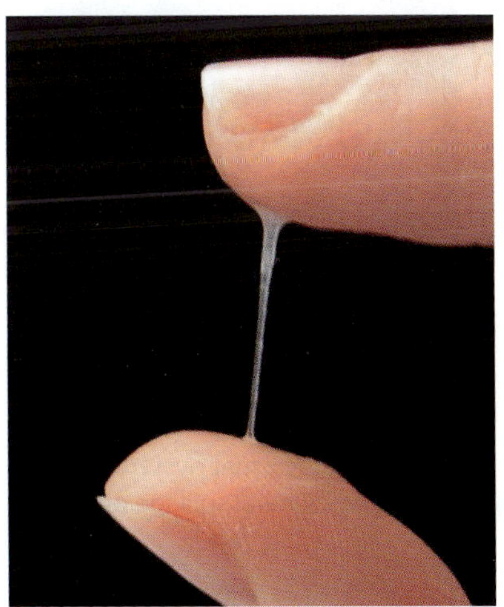 **Fig. 1:** Estrogen-dominant cervical mucus: Spinnbarkeit test.	**Explanation:** Nearly 24–48 hours prior to ovulation, the cervical mucus becomes thin, watery, alkaline, profuse, stretchable, acellular, and elastic in appearance. It has a high content of sodium chloride in it due to which it forms a characteristic fern-like pattern when dried on a glass slide. It has great elasticity and can withstand stretching up to 10 cm. This is also known as the Spinnbarkeit test or the thread test **(Fig. 1)**, an evidence of estrogenic activity. Following ovulation, under the effect of progesterone, the cervical mucus changes its character and becomes opaque and viscid, which is hostile to the sperms. The fern pattern also cannot be demonstrated during this phase. **Potential questions:** There can be various questions related to the characteristics of cervical mucus during different phases of menstrual cycle.

Question	Answer	Comment
Q2. A 32-year-old woman presents to the gynecology clinic with a history of primary infertility since the past 2 years. She has regular menstrual cycles and no significant past medical history. Her partner's semen analysis is normal. She undergoes hysterosalpingography (HSG) as part of her infertility workup. The findings are shown in the image below. What does the HSG indicate? 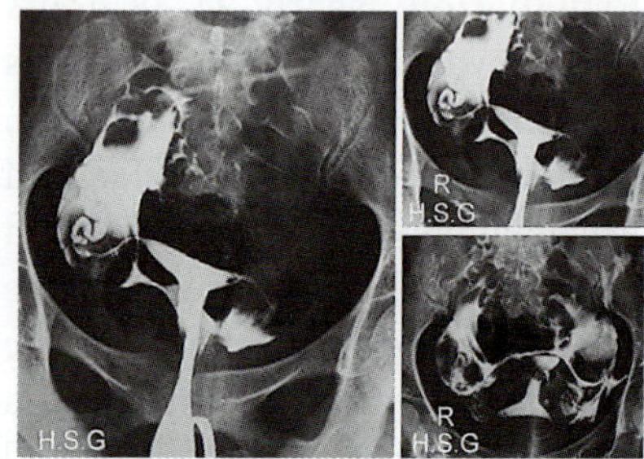 A. Blocked fallopian tubes B. Uterine fibroids C. Normal patency of fallopian tubes D. Endometrial polyps E. Uterine septum	**Ans: C (Normal patency of fallopian tubes)** The adjacent image shows a normal HSG showing bilateral spillage of dye into the peritoneum. The HSG is the most frequently used diagnostic tool for evaluation of endometrial cavity as well as tubal pathology. A normal HSG depicts a smooth triangular uterine outline with opacification of both fallopian tubes, showing spillage of dye into the peritoneal cavity on both sides **(Figs. 2A and B)**. 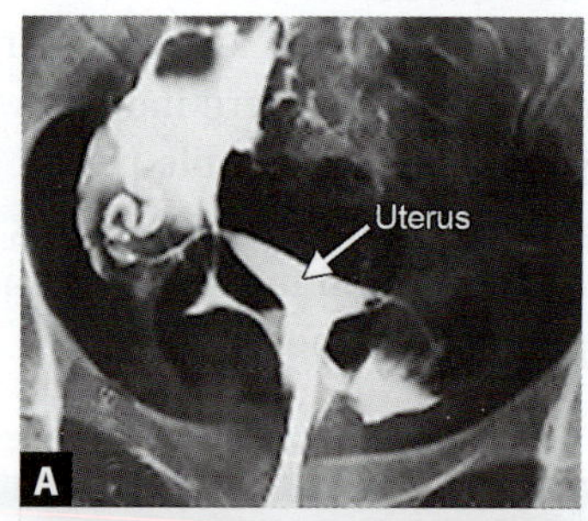 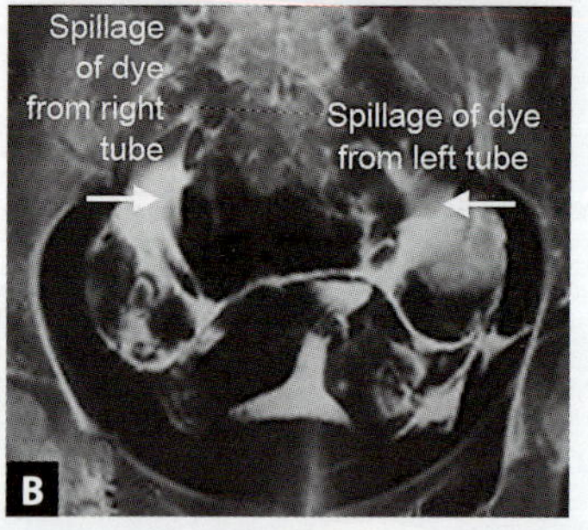 **Figs. 2A and B:** Normal hysterosalpingogram showing bilateral spillage of dye.	**Explanation:** Finding of patent tubes on HSG is an important finding in the evaluation of infertility. It suggests that the fallopian tubes are not obstructed, allowing for the possibility of natural conception. Besides the tubal patency, HSG also helps in providing accurate information about the endocervical canal, endometrial cavity, cornual ostium, and status of the fimbriae. HSG can accurately define the shape and size of the uterine cavity. Normal uterine cavity is symmetrical and triangular. It is widest at the level of cornual orifices near the fundus. HSG can help in diagnosing uterine developmental anomalies, (e.g., unicornuate uterus, septate uterus, bicornuate uterus, and uterus didelphys), submucous myomas, intrauterine adhesions and endometrial polyps. During hysterosalpingography, a diluted, water-soluble, hyperosmolar iodinated contrast agent is injected into the uterine cavity via Foley's catheter. Following this, X-ray images are taken to visualize the flow of the dye through the fallopian tubes. **Potential questions:** There can be questions related to the interpretation of various anomalies encountered on HSG.

Question	Answer	Comment
Q3. A 32-year-old woman with a history of pelvic inflammatory disease presents with infertility. The pelvic ultrasound done by the gynecologist reveals findings, marked by the letter X as shown in the image below. What is the most common cause of this abnormality seen on the ultrasound? 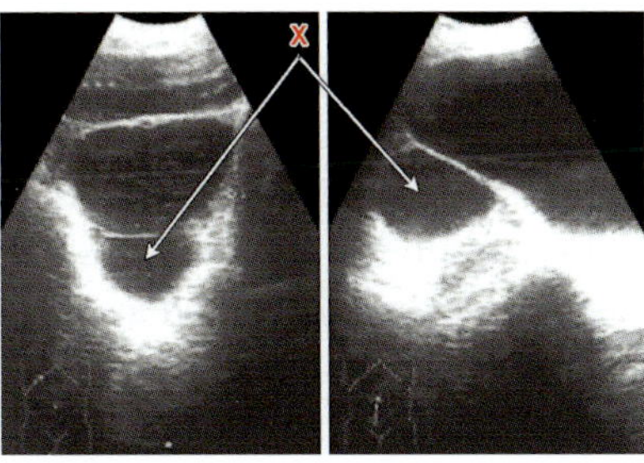 A. Endometriosis B. Pelvic inflammatory disease (PID) C. Bilateral hydrosalpinx D. Ovarian cysts E. Ectopic pregnancy	**Ans: C (Bilateral hydrosalpinx)** The adjacent TAS reveals the presence of bilateral, cystic tubal masses with multiple internal echoes suggestive of hydrosalpinx. **Figure 3** shows the findings of hysterosalpingography (HSG) in the same patient, demonstrating the presence of tubular convoluted structures on both sides of the uterus, representing bilateral hydrosalpinges. No intraperitoneal spillage of contrast was seen. 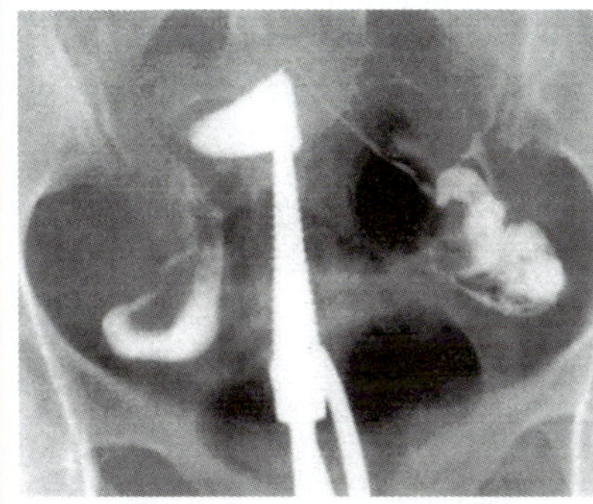 **Fig. 3:** HSG in the same patient showing the presence of mass bilaterally.	**Explanation:** Hydrosalpinx is a condition where a fallopian tube is blocked and filled with serous or clear fluid, often leading to infertility. The most common cause of hydrosalpinx is pelvic inflammatory disease (PID), which is usually a result of an ascending infection by sexually transmitted bacteria such as *Chlamydia trachomatis* or *Neisseria gonorrhoeae*. These infections cause inflammation and scarring of the fallopian tubes, leading to blockage and fluid accumulation. This condition can impair fertility by preventing the egg from traveling through the fallopian tube and by affecting the uterine environment. **Potential questions:** There can be questions related to interpretation of various tubal/ovarian pathologies on USG/HSG reports.
Q4. What is the most likely cause of the abnormality observed in a HSG image shown below? 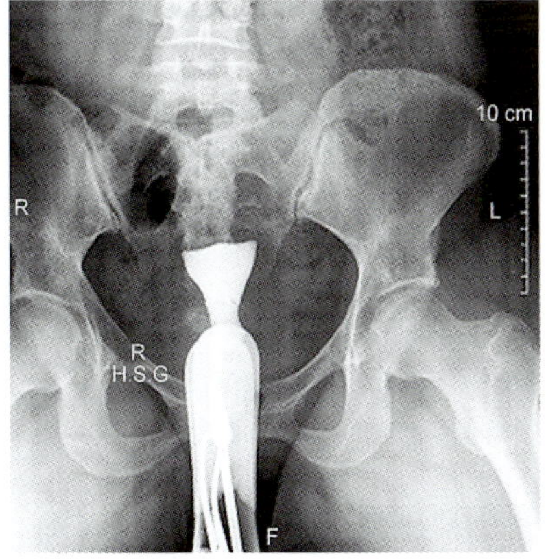 A. Endometriosis B. Pelvic inflammatory disease (PID) C. Congenital anomalies D. Tubal ligation E. Uterine fibroids	**Ans: B [Pelvic inflammatory disease (PID)]** HSG in the adjacent image shows a triangular-shaped uterine cavity. There is no movement of dye beyond the tubal cornu on both sides, demonstrating bilateral cornual blockage **(Fig. 4)**. 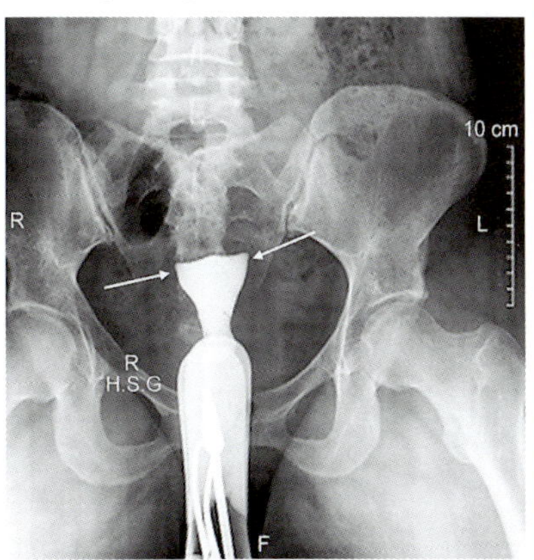 **Fig. 4:** HSG showing bilateral cornual block (as indicated by arrows).	**Explanation:** Bilateral cornual block on a HSG typically indicates that there is an obstruction at the junction where the fallopian tubes meet the uterus. The most common cause of this type of blockage is pelvic inflammatory disease. PID is an infection of the female reproductive organs, often caused by sexually transmitted bacteria such as *Chlamydia trachomatis* or *Neisseria gonorrhoeae*. The infection can lead to inflammation and scarring of the fallopian tubes, resulting in blockages at the cornual ends. This condition can significantly impact fertility by preventing the passage of eggs from the ovaries to the uterus. **Potential questions:** There can be questions related to interpretation of various tubal/ovarian pathologies on USG/HSG reports.

Question	Answer	Comment
Q5. What observation is indicated by the below image showing the findings of laparoscopic chromopertubation performed in a woman with 3 years' history of secondary infertility? 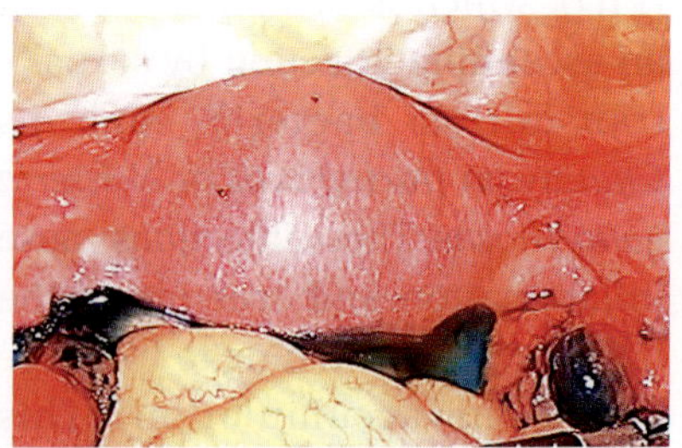 A. Left tube blocked B. Right tube blocked C. Left-side hydrosalpinx D. Right-side hydrosalpinx E. Bilateral patent tubes	**Ans: E (Bilateral patent tubes)** **Figure 5** demonstrates laparoscopic chromopertubation, which is nowadays being regarded as the gold standard for the assessment of fallopian tubes, especially in women with infertility suspected to be due to tubal pathology. This test has now become part of the routine assessment for infertility. The adjacent image shows bilateral spillage of dye into the peritoneal cavity, thereby indicating the patency of tubes. 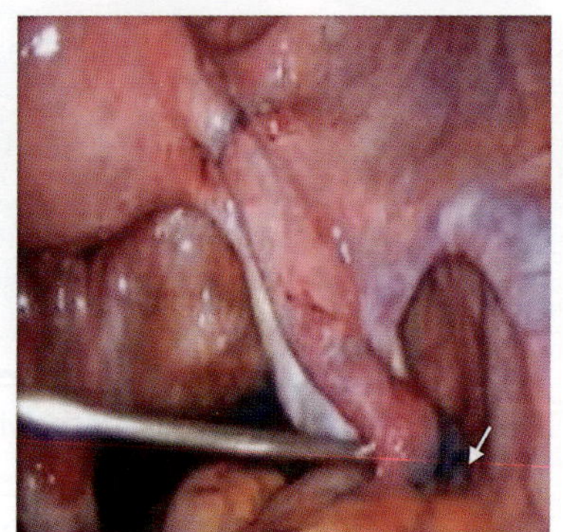 **Fig. 5:** Magnified view showing the spillage of dye from the left tube (indicated by the arrow).	**Explanation:** Laparoscopic chromopertubation is a diagnostic procedure used to evaluate the patency of the fallopian tubes. Laparoscopic examination also allows visualization of fallopian tubes, ovary and pelvis. During the procedure, a dye (usually methylene blue or indigo carmine) is injected into the uterine cavity through a plastic or metal cannula placed in the cervical canal under laparoscopic guidance. If both the fallopian tubes are patent, they first become slightly distended as they fill with the dye. As the injection of dye is continued, it spills out through the tubal ostia into the peritoneal cavity, which is observed laparoscopically. In the beginning, the spillage may be in the form of bubbles. **Potential questions:** There can be questions related to the findings of various diagnostic modalities (HSG and laparoscopic chromopertubation for the diagnosis of tubal factor infertility).

<table>
<tr><th>Question</th><th>Answer</th><th>Comment</th></tr>
<tr><td>

Q6. A 28-year-old woman with a 2-year history of primary infertility and intermittent pelvic pain, previously treated for PID, underwent an ultrasound revealing the findings shown below. What appears to be the most likely diagnosis in this case?

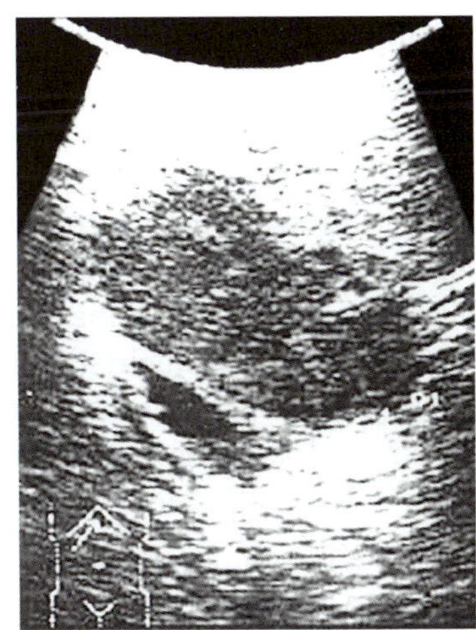

A. Ovarian cyst
B. Ectopic pregnancy
C. Hydrosalpinx
D. Endometrioma
E. Uterine fibroid

</td><td>

Ans: C (Hydrosalpinx)

The adjacent ultrasound image shows an anechoic elongated, retort-shaped/sausage-shaped mass with mixed echogenicity arising from the left adnexa. This is suggestive of a tubo-ovarian mass, most likely a hydrosalpinx. Laparoscopic examination **(Fig. 6)** helps in confirming the diagnosis of a left-sided hydrosalpinx.

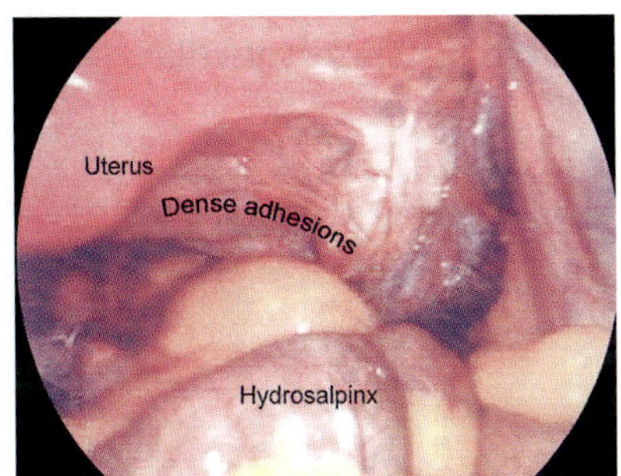

Fig. 6: Laparoscopic appearance of hydrosalpinx arising from the left tube.

</td><td>

Explanation: Hydrosalpinx is formed due to distal occlusion of the fallopian tubes (commonly due to PID). As the blocked fallopian tube gets distended with fluid, it develops into a retort-shaped structure called hydrosalpinx. Women with bilateral hydrosalpinx may be infertile. In these cases, either tubal surgery in the form of neosalpingostomy or in vitro fertilization (IVF) may be required to achieve pregnancy.

Potential questions: There can be questions related to interpretation of various tubal/ovarian pathologies on USG/HSG reports.

</td></tr>
</table>

Question	Answer	Comment
Q7. During a hysteroscopic examination, the tubal ostia are visualized as shown in the image below. What is the typical appearance of the tubal ostia in a normal hysteroscopic assessment? 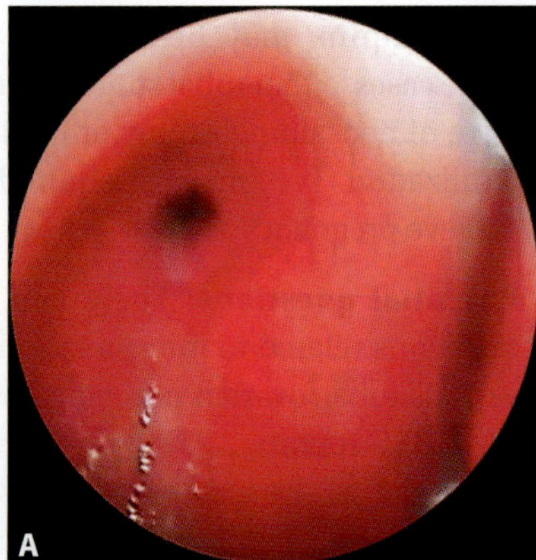 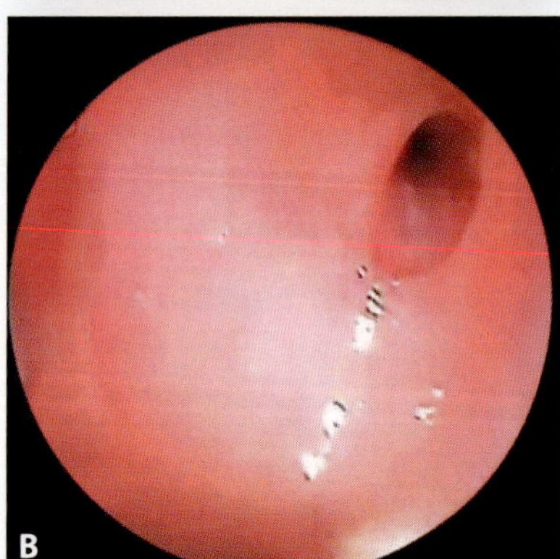 A. Two small, oval openings located at the 2 and 10 o'clock positions B. Two small, round openings located at the 2 and 10 o'clock positions C. Two small, round openings located at the 1 and 11 o'clock positions D. Two small, oval openings located at the 3 and 9 o'clock positions E. Two elongated slits located at the 4 and 8 o'clock positions	**Ans: B (Two small, round openings located at the 2 and 10 o'clock positions)** The adjacent images show (A) right and (B) left tubal ostia as visualized on hysteroscopic examination. Tubal ostia refer to the opening where the fallopian tube enters the uterine cavity **(Fig. 7)**. Evaluation of both the tubal ostia is important because the presence of membrane or any other blockage over the tubal ostia (especially if bilateral) may be responsible for infertility. 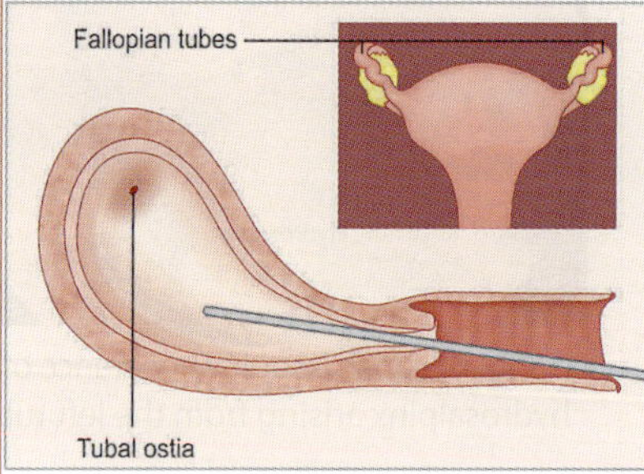 **Fig. 7:** Diagrammatic representation of the anatomy of tubal ostia.	**Explanation:** In a normal hysteroscopic assessment, the tubal ostia appear as two small, round openings situated at the 2 and 10 o'clock positions on the uterine cavity wall. These openings represent the entry points of the fallopian tubes into the uterus. Visualizing these structures is important for confirming the correct positioning of the hysteroscope and for assessing the patency and anatomical integrity of the fallopian tubes. Diagnostic hysteroscopy is a commonly performed procedure, which can help evaluate the endocervical canal, endometrial cavity, and tubal ostia. In case of suspected endometrial pathology, endometrial biopsy can be performed. **Potential questions:** There can be different questions related to the normal anatomical appearance of various pelvic organs during diagnostic hysteroscopy and laparoscopy.

Question	Answer	Comment
Q8. During laparoscopic examination, an ovary with a developing follicle is visualized as shown in the image below. What is the typical appearance of this follicle in the ovary? 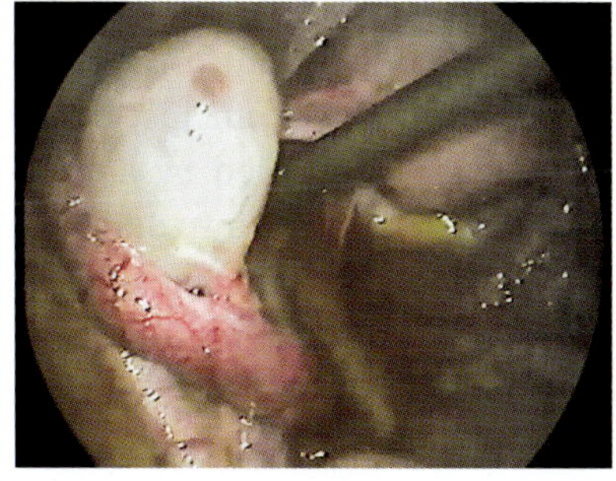 A. A small, solid mass with no fluid-filled cavity B. A large, fluid-filled cyst with irregular borders C. A small, fluid-filled structure with a clear antrum D. A solid mass with multiple small fluid-filled cavities E. A large, solid mass with a central necrotic area	**Ans: C (A small, fluid-filled structure with a clear antrum)** Laparoscopic examination can help visualize the ovary. The adjacent image shows the presence of a single dominant (preovulatory) follicle protruding from the surface of ovary, just a few hours prior to ovulation. The preovulatory follicle has an ovum surrounded by cumulus oophorus, composed of granulosa cells. This is surrounded by a large antrum composed of follicular fluid **(Fig. 8)**. 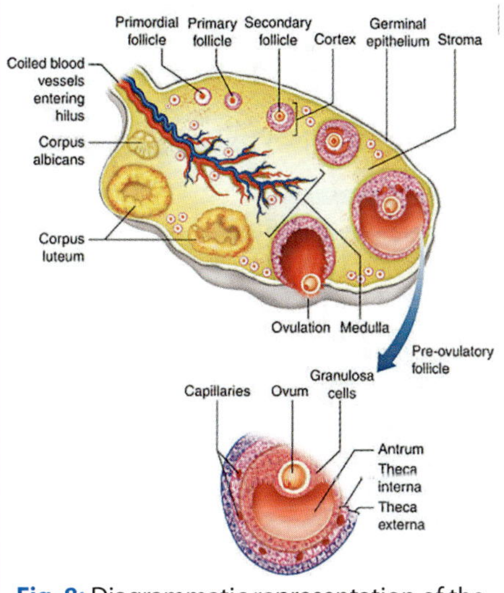 **Fig. 8:** Diagrammatic representation of the preovulatory follicle.	**Explanation:** In a laparoscopic view, a developing follicle in the ovary typically appears as a small, fluid-filled structure with a clear antrum. This antrum is a fluid-filled cavity that forms during the secondary follicle stage of development. The presence of the antrum is a distinguishing feature of a developing follicle, indicating that the follicle is progressing toward the preovulatory stage. The granulosa cells surrounding the antrum play a crucial role in the production of estrogen, which is essential for the maturation of the oocyte. **Potential questions:** There can be different questions related to the normal anatomical appearance of various pelvic organs during diagnostic hysteroscopy and laparoscopy.

Question	Answer	Comment
Q9. What does the basal body temperature (BBT) chart below indicate about the timing of ovulation? 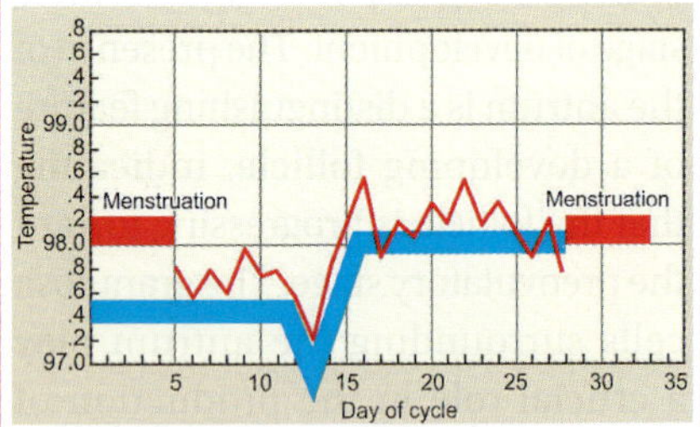 A. Ovulation occurred on day 5 B. Ovulation occurred on day 10 C. Ovulation occurred on day 14 D. Ovulation occurred on day 18 E. Ovulation did not occur	**Ans: C (Ovulation occurred on day 14)** Basal body temperature charts can be used for predicting ovulation. In the adjacent BBT chart, just prior to day 14, there occurs a slight dip in temperature followed by a significant rise. This rise is sustained in the subsequent days, confirming that ovulation has indeed occurred. This biphasic pattern is evident in ovulatory women **(Fig. 9)**. 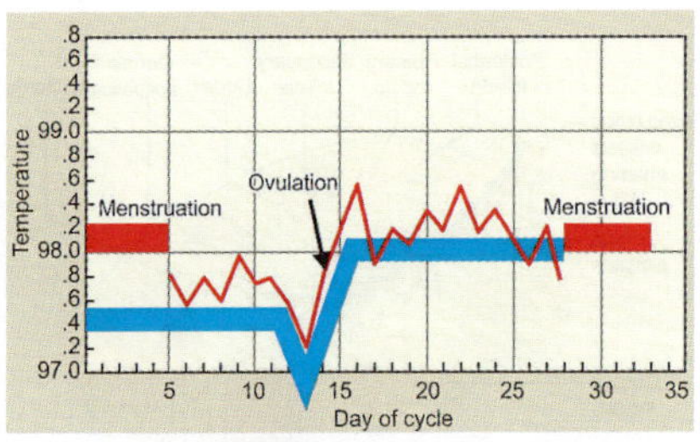 **Fig. 9:** Basal body temperature method for predicting ovulation.	**Explanation:** The BBT method involves tracking the body's temperature at rest each morning before any activity. A typical BBT chart shows a biphasic pattern: ▪ *Follicular phase:* BBT remains relatively low, usually between 97.0 to 97.5°F. ▪ *Ovulation:* A slight dip in temperature may occur just before ovulation, followed by a significant rise of about 0.5–1.0°F due to the thermogenic effect of increased progesterone levels. ▪ *Luteal phase:* BBT stays elevated until the onset of menstruation. ▪ *Menses:* The temperature again falls to baseline just before or after the onset of menses. **Potential questions:** There could be questions related to different tests for ovulation, tubal patency, cervical factor, etc.

<table>
<tr><th>Question</th><th>Answer</th><th>Comment</th></tr>
<tr>
<td>

Q10. Which of the following is a common sign related to the event marked by X in the below image?

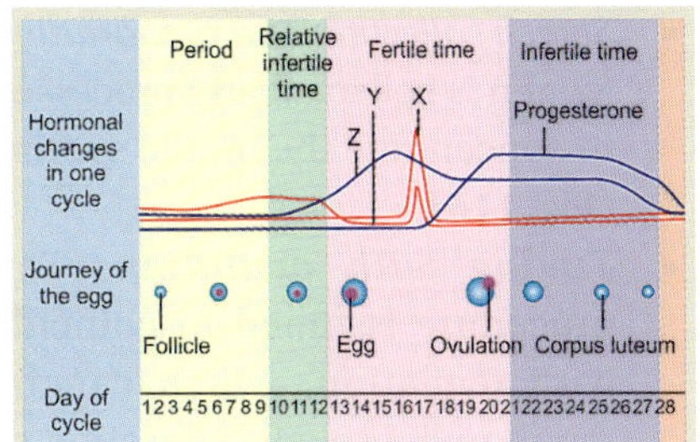

A. Decreased basal body temperature
B. Increased cervical mucus
C. Decreased libido
D. Heavy menstrual bleeding
E. Breast tenderness

</td>
<td>

Ans: B (Increased cervical mucus)

The events preceding ovulation are as follows: Peak in estrogen production (>200 pg/mL for more than 24 hours), peak of follicle-stimulating hormone (FSH), and surge of luteinizing hormone (LH). Ovulation occurs about 10–12 hours after LH surge and 24–36 hours after the peak of estradiol levels have been attained.

The event related to the letter X in the adjacent image is LH surge, which is the most reliable indicator of impending ovulation.

Hormonal changes suggestive of ovulation in a 28-day cycle are depicted in **Figure 10**.

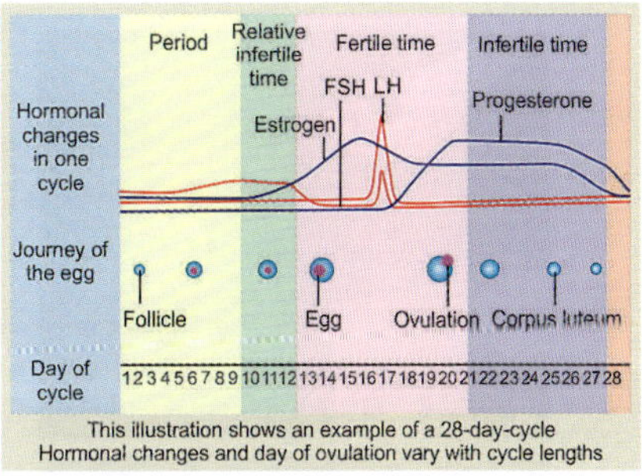

Fig. 10: Hormonal changes suggestive of ovulation in a 28-day cycle.

</td>
<td>

Explanation: During ovulation, the body produces more cervical mucus, which becomes clear, stretchy, and slippery, resembling egg whites. This change in cervical mucus helps sperm travel through the cervix into the uterus to fertilize the egg. Monitoring cervical mucus is a common method used to predict ovulation and identify the most fertile days in the menstrual cycle.

A surge of LH takes place just prior to ovulation. LH initiates luteinization and progesterone production in the granulosa layer. A preovulatory rise in progesterone facilitates the positive feedback action of estrogen which may be required to induce the midcycle FSH peak.

Potential questions: There could be different questions related to various hormonal changes and their effects occurring at the time of ovulation.

</td>
</tr>
</table>

ASSISTED REPRODUCTIVE TECHNIQUES FOR THE TREATMENT OF INFERTILITY

Question	Answer	Comment
Q11. What is the primary purpose of the procedure shown in the image below? 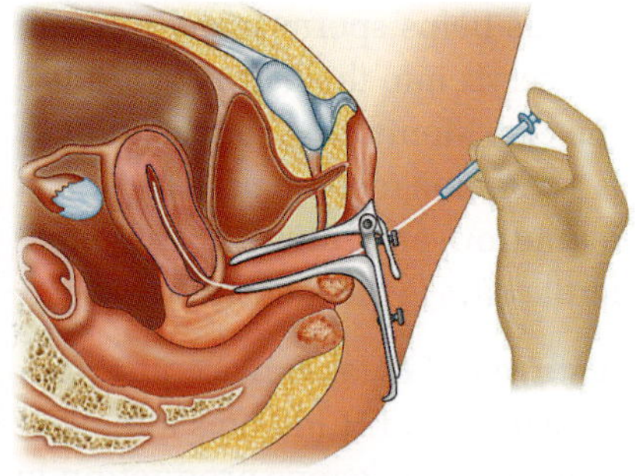 A. To diagnose uterine abnormalities B. To treat endometriosis C. To enhance sperm motility D. To facilitate fertilization by placing sperm directly into the uterus E. To monitor ovarian follicle development	**Ans: D (To facilitate fertilization by placing sperm directly into the uterus)** The adjacent image depicts the procedure of artificial insemination, a fertility treatment procedure, which is performed by depositing the sperms either at the level of internal cervical os (cervical insemination) or inside the endometrial cavity [intrauterine insemination (IUI)] **(Figs. 11A to C)**. The primary purpose of IUI is to increase the number of sperms that reach the fallopian tubes, thereby enhancing the chances of fertilization. This procedure is often used for couples with unexplained infertility, mild male factor infertility, or cervical mucus problems. 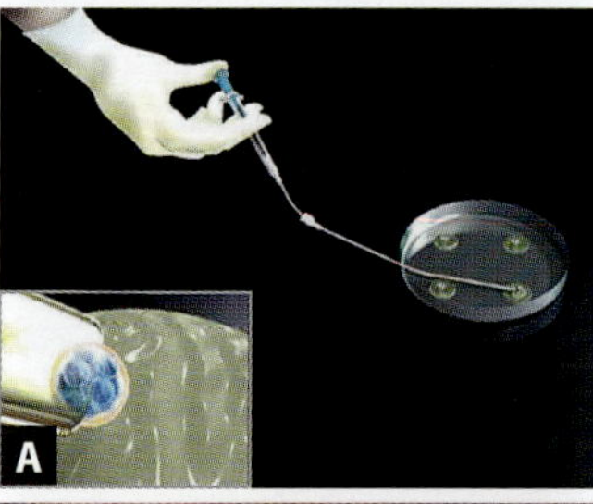 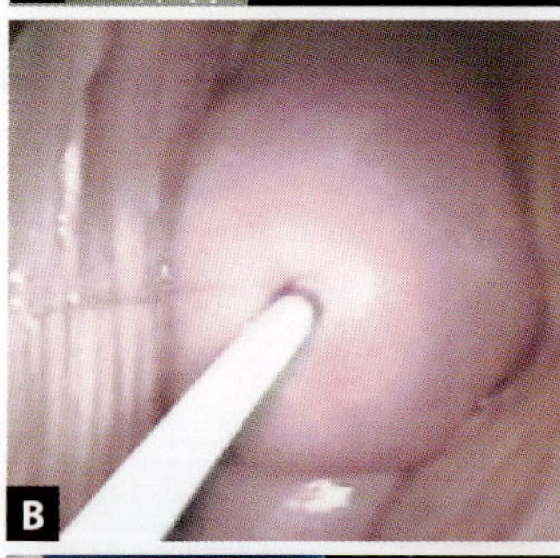 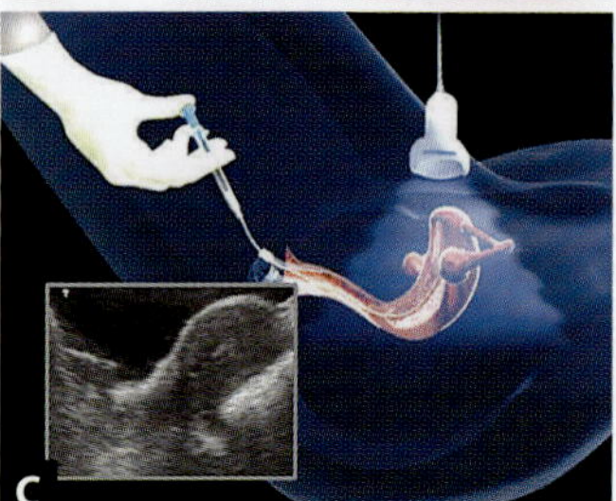 **Figs. 11A to C:** Procedure of intrauterine insemination.	**Explanation:** As shown in **Figure 11**, the procedure of IUI comprises the following steps: ▪ *Semen collection and preparation:* Semen is collected and processed to concentrate the motile sperms **(Fig. 11A)**. ▪ *Timing with ovulation:* The procedure is timed to coincide with ovulation, which can be monitored through ultrasound or ovulation predictor kits. ▪ *Introduction of IUI catheter through the cervix:* Using a "no touch" technique, IUI catheter is introduced through the cervix up to the uterine fundus under ultrasound guidance **(Figs. 11B and C)**. ▪ An amount of 0.3–05 mL of processed semen is then slowly injected through the catheter. **Potential questions:** There can be different questions related to different procedure used for assisted reproductive technology (ART), their indications, steps, and complications.

Question	Answer	Comment
Q12. A 29-year-old woman with polycystic ovarian syndrome (PCOS) and a 4-year history of primary infertility presents for assisted reproductive technology. Her baseline ultrasound shows an antral follicle count of 22, and her AMH is 7.5 ng/mL. She is commenced on daily recombinant FSH injections along with GnRH antagonist to prevent premature LH surge. Serial transvaginal scans are performed to monitor follicular growth, and serum estradiol levels are checked to guide further management. Identify the step of the in vitro fertilization (IVF) process shown in the image below. 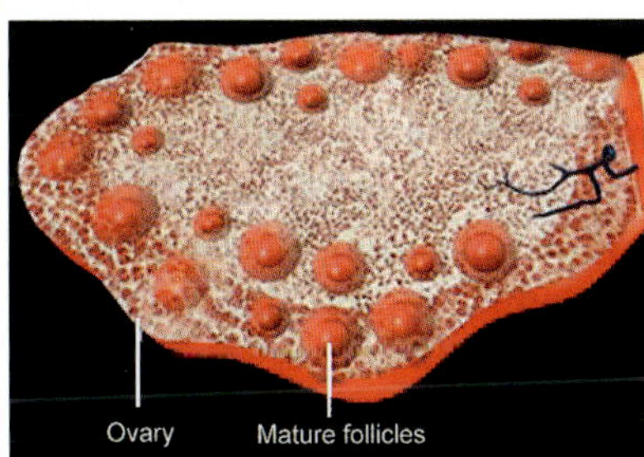 A. Follicular stimulation B. Egg retrieval C. Oocyte insemination with multiple sperms D. Embryo transfer E. Follicular aspiration	**Ans: A (Follicular stimulation)** The adjacent image shows the ovary with multiple follicles simultaneously maturing, one of the first steps of in vitro fertilization (IVF). Due to multifollicular development, more than one oocyte can be harvested. IVF is an ART procedure, involving the following **(Fig. 12)**: Follicular stimulation, retrieving a preovulatory oocyte from the ovary, fertilizing it with sperm in the laboratory, and subsequently transferring the embryo within the endometrial cavity. 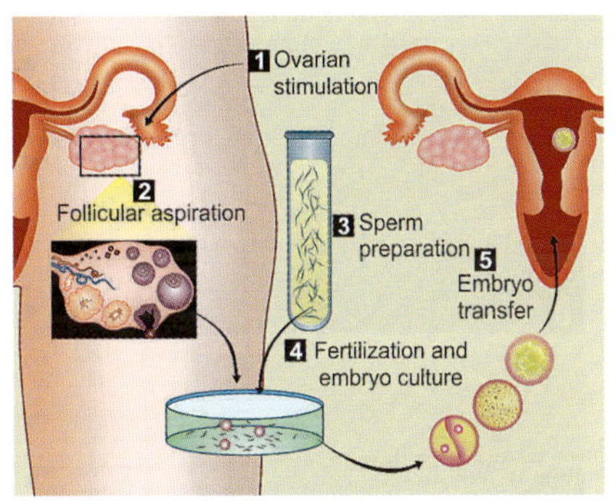 **Fig. 12:** Diagrammatic representation of the procedure of in vitro fertilization (IVF).	**Explanation:** The IVF process typically involves the following steps: 1. *Follicular stimulation:* Gonadotropins are usually administered to stimulate the ovaries to produce multiple eggs. 2. *Egg retrieval:* Once the eggs are mature, they are retrieved from the ovaries using a needle under ultrasound guidance. 3. *Semen preparation:* This step involves washing and processing the semen sample to separate motile sperm from seminal fluid, debris, and non-motile sperm, ensuring a high-quality sample for fertilization. 4. *Fertilization:* The retrieved eggs are then fertilized with sperms in a laboratory to form embryos. 5. *Embryo transfer:* The best-quality embryos are selected and transferred into the uterus for implantation. **Potential questions:** There can be different questions related to various steps of the IVF procedure.

<table>
<tr><th>Question</th><th>Answer</th><th>Comment</th></tr>
<tr>
<td>

Q13. What is the primary purpose of the procedure shown in the image below?

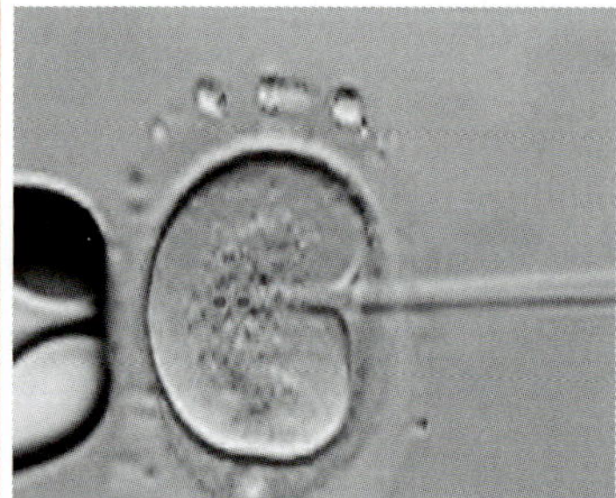

A. To diagnose genetic disorders in embryos
B. To enhance sperm motility
C. To facilitate fertilization by injecting a single sperm directly into an egg
D. To monitor ovarian follicle development
E. To treat endometriosis

</td>
<td>

Ans: C (To facilitate fertilization by injecting a single sperm directly into an egg)

The adjacent image illustrates the procedure of intracytoplasmic sperm injection (ICSI). ICSI is a specialized form of IVF used primarily for male infertility. The steps of ICSI are illustrated in **Figures 13A to E**.

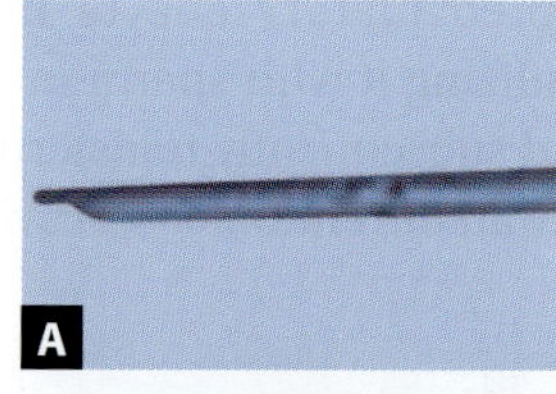

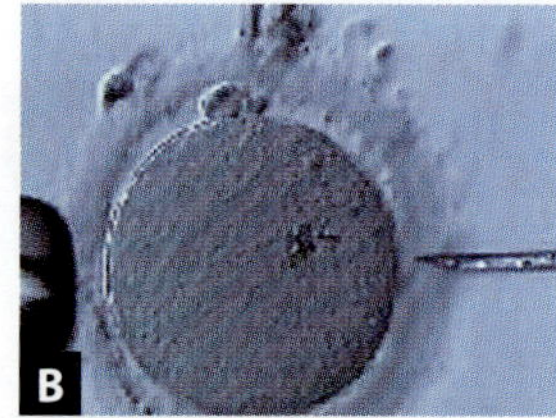

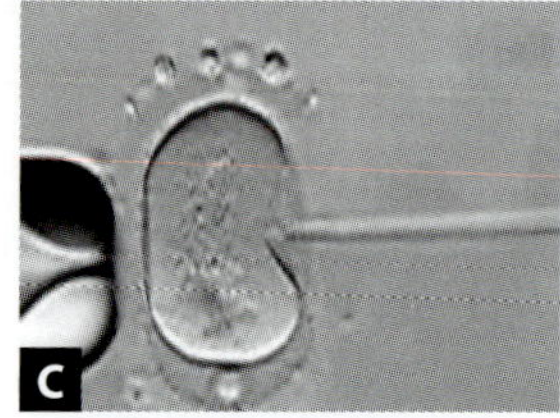

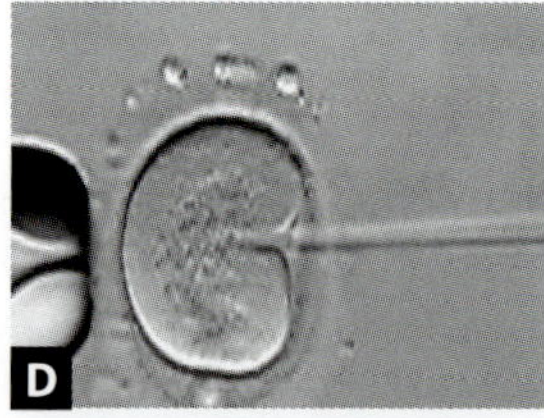

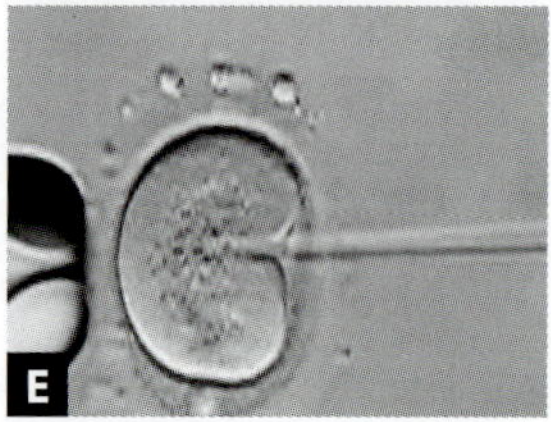

Figs. 13A to E: (A) Microneedle is loaded with a sperm; (B) The microneedle approaches the oocyte; (C) The microneedle pierces the oocyte membrane; (D) The microneedle is advanced deeper inside the cytoplasm; (E) The spermatozoon is released inside the oocyte.

</td>
<td>

Explanation: ICSI significantly increases the chances of fertilization by ensuring that the sperm reaches the egg, which is crucial for couples facing male infertility issues. Indications for ICSI include the following:

- Severe male infertility (low sperm count, poor motility, abnormal morphology).
- Failure of fertilization in a previous IVF cycle.
- Absence of sperm in the ejaculate (azoospermia), with sperm retrieved via testicular biopsy or aspiration.
- Obstructive or non-obstructive azoospermia.
- Inability to achieve fertilization with conventional IVF.
- Male factor infertility due to prior vasectomy, ejaculation issues, or retrograde ejaculation.
- Use of frozen sperm with poor motility or quality.

The procedure involves following steps:

- *Sperm selection:* The sperms can be obtained through masturbation, epididymal aspiration, testicular biopsy or needle puncture of the testes. A single sperm is selected based on its morphology and motility. The sperm is paralyzed by stroking the distal portion of its tail.
- *Injection:* The oocyte is stripped from the cumulus using a solution of hyaluronidase. To inject the sperm, first the oocyte is stabilized with a micropipette, then the sperm is loaded, tail first, into a microneedle.
- *Fertilization:* The microinjected oocyte is kept in the incubator.

Potential questions: There can be different questions related to the indications, steps, and complications of ICSI.

</td>
</tr>
</table>

Question	Answer	Comment
Q14. What is the most likely diagnosis for the ultrasound image shown below? 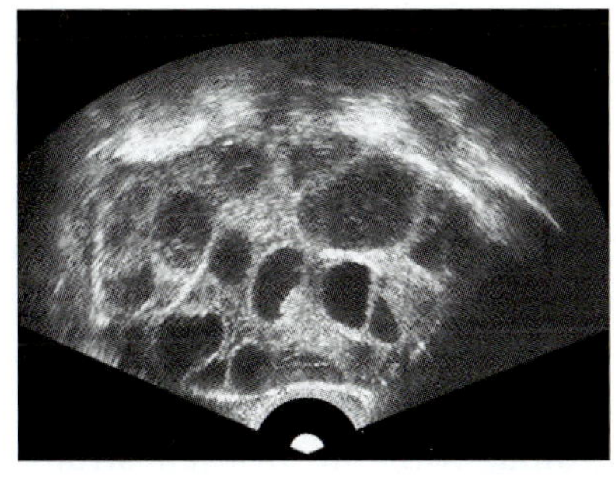 A. Polycystic ovary syndrome (PCOS) B. Ovarian torsion C. Ovarian hyperstimulation syndrome (OHSS) D. Endometriosis E. Ovarian cystadenoma	**Ans: C [Ovarian hyperstimulation syndrome (OHSS)]** The adjacent transvaginal ultrasound image shows a "wheel-spoke appearance" suggestive of ovarian hyperstimulation syndrome (OHSS). OHSS is the most common iatrogenic complication occurring due to ovarian stimulation during assisted reproductive technology (ART) and other infertility treatments. Various risk factors for OHSS include raised levels of luteinizing hormone (cases of polycystic ovarian disease), administration of human chorionic gonadotropin, administration of high doses of stimulation-causing drugs, and the size and number of ovarian follicles. The pathophysiology of OHSS is shown in **Figure 14**. 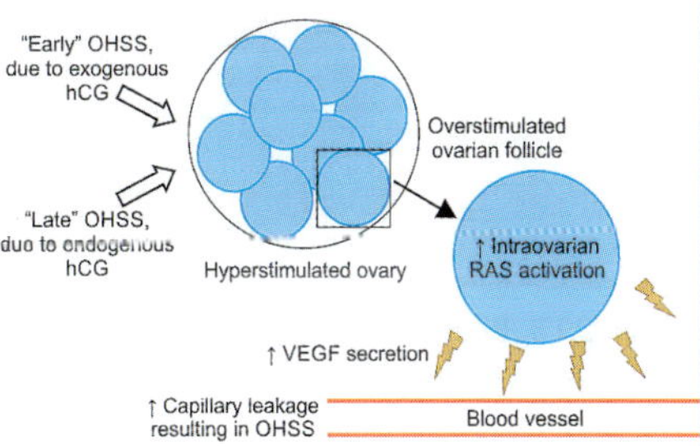 **Fig. 14:** Pathophysiology of OHSS (OHSS; ovarian hyperstimulation syndrome; RAS: renin–angiotensin system; VEGF: vascular endothelial growth factor)	**Explanation:** The condition is diagnosed based on clinical presentation and ultrasound findings. Ultrasound shows bilateral symmetric enlargement of ovaries (often > 12 cm in size). There may be the presence of multiple cysts, having varying sizes. This is often termed the "wheel-spoke appearance". Associated ascites and pleural effusion with or without pericardial effusion (which is due to capillary leak) may also be present. According to Galen's classification, OHSS has been classified into three classes: Mild, moderate, and severe. Symptoms of OHSS include abdominal pain, bloating, nausea, and in severe cases, significant fluid shifts resulting in ascites and pleural effusion. **Potential questions:** There can be questions related to various complications associated with ART.

POLYCYSTIC OVARIAN DISEASE

<table>
<tr><th>Question</th><th>Answer</th><th>Comment</th></tr>
<tr>
<td>Q15. A 24-year-old woman with irregular menstrual cycles, acne, and hirsutism is evaluated for a possible hormonal disorder. The gynecologist considers a range of diagnostic tests, including hormonal profiles and an ultrasound, whose findings are shown below. Identify the most likely diagnosis in this case.
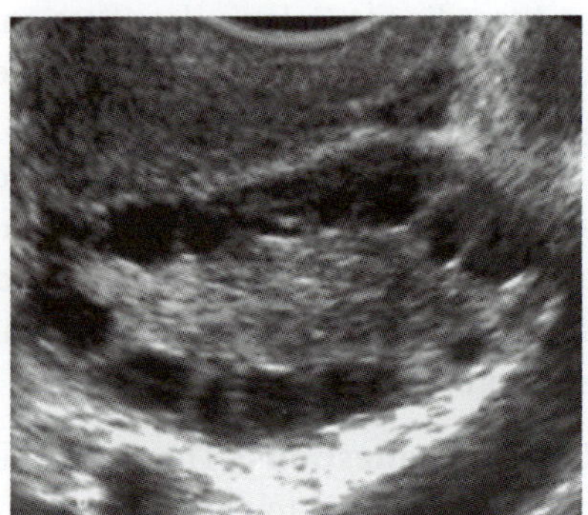
A. Endometriosis
B. Ovarian cystadenoma
C. Polycystic ovary disease (PCOD)
D. Ovarian torsion
E. Follicular cyst</td>
<td>Ans: C [Polycystic ovary disease (PCOD)]
The adjacent ultrasound image demonstrates multiple small follicles arranged peripherally, giving it an appearance of string of pearls or a pearl necklace appearance. This is suggestive of polycystic ovarian morphology.
When observed on laparoscopic examination, the polycystic ovaries appear large (nearly 1.5–3 times larger than the normal ovaries), round in shape, and are surrounded by a thick, white capsule (Fig. 15).
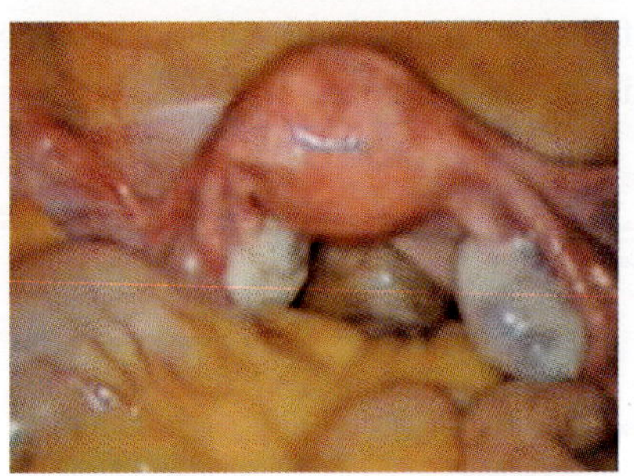
Fig. 15: Bilateral polycystic ovaries as observed on laparoscopic examination.</td>
<td>Explanation: Polycystic ovary disease (PCOD) is characterized by the presence of multiple small follicles (usually more than 20) arranged peripherally around the ovary, giving it a "string of pearls" appearance on ultrasound. This occurs due to the hormonal imbalance that leads to anovulation and the accumulation of immature follicles. The ovaries are often enlarged and have a dense stroma, with the ovarian stromal volume being ≥10 mL. This ultrasound finding, along with clinical features such as irregular menstrual cycles, hirsutism, and obesity, supports the diagnosis of PCOD.
Potential questions: There can be different questions related to the etiology, clinical presentation, diagnosis, and management of the cases of PCOD.</td>
</tr>
</table>

<table>
<tr><th>Question</th><th>Answer</th><th>Comment</th></tr>
<tr>
<td>Q16. A 27-year-old woman with polycystic ovary syndrome (PCOS) and infertility is counseled about surgical treatment options. The first step of this laparoscopic procedure is shown in the image below. Identify the procedure shown in the image.
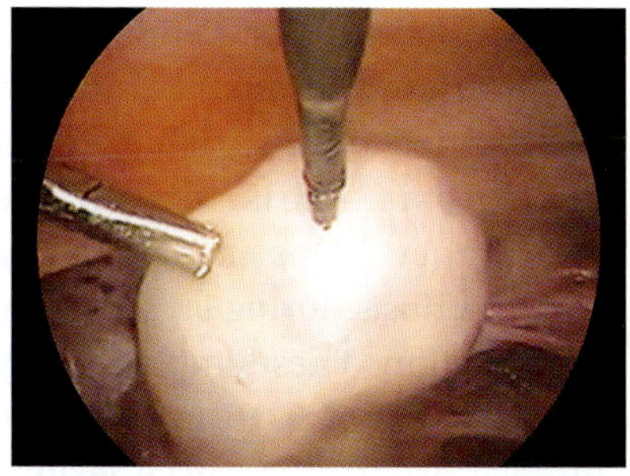
A. Laparoscopic cystectomy
B. Laparoscopic ovarian drilling (LOD)
C. Laparoscopic salpingectomy
D. Laparoscopic cyst aspiration
E. Laparoscopic oophorectomy</td>
<td>Ans: B [Laparoscopic ovarian drilling (LOD)]
The adjacent image demonstrates a laparoscopic procedure in which the ovaries are lifted out of the ovarian fossa and placed over the cervicouterine junction. This forms the first step of the procedure of laparoscopic ovarian drilling (LOD). The number of holes to be made during LOD is usually decided based on the ovarian size and volume, and preoperative ultrasound appearance of the ovaries. Figures 16A and B typically show the laparoscopic needle making small punctures in the ovary.
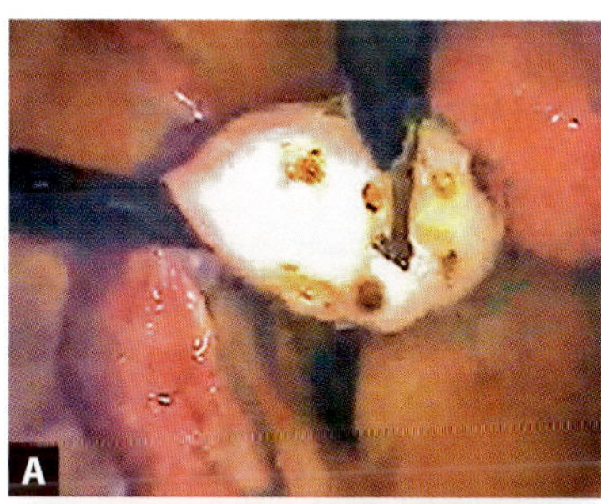
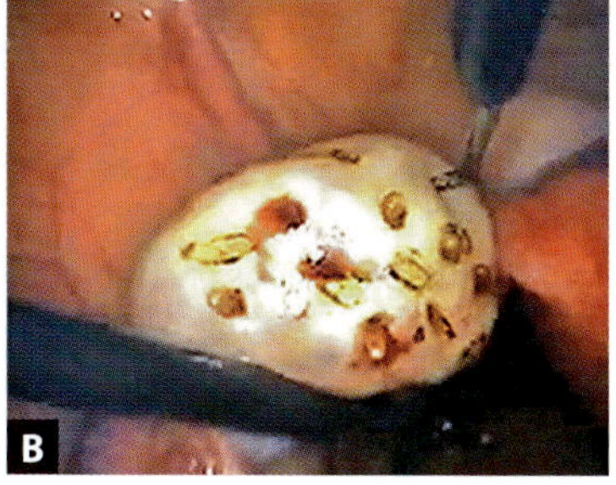
Figs. 16A and B: (A) Laparoscopic ovarian drilling using electrocauterization; (B) Appearance of the ovary following the procedure.</td>
<td>Explanation: The procedure of LOD involves using a laparoscope to create multiple punctures in the ovarian capsule with a diathermy needle. This helps to reduce the androgen-producing stroma and restore regular ovulation. LOD is used for treating women with clomiphene citrate-resistant PCOS or in cases where other treatments for inducing ovulation have failed.
LOD is performed utilizing pure cutting current equivalent to 40 watts. The number of holes varying from 4 to 20 are usually made in each ovary. In moderately enlarged ovaries, 10–12 holes are made. However, if the ovaries are extremely voluminous, i.e., 50–60 mm in size, the number of cautery points can be increased further. The holes which are to be made are usually 3 mm wide and 3–4 mm deep.
Potential questions: There can be different questions related to the etiology, clinical presentation, diagnosis, and management of the cases of PCOS.</td>
</tr>
</table>

ENDOMETRIOSIS

Question	Answer	Comment
Q17. A 32-year-old woman presents with complaints of chronic pelvic pain for the past 8 months, worsening during menstruation. No significant finding was observed on physical examination or ultrasound. Diagnostic laparoscopy was done which revealed findings as shown in the image below. Identify the condition based on the below laparoscopic image. 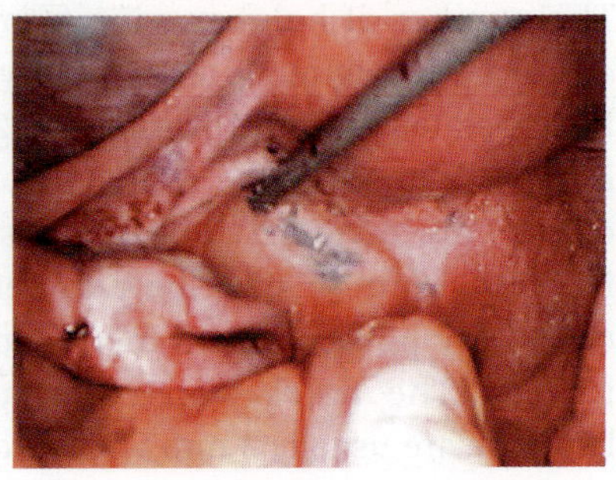 A. Ovarian cystadenoma B. Pelvic inflammatory disease (PID) C. Endometriosis D. Tubo-ovarian abscess E. Uterine fibroids	**Ans:** C (Endometriosis) The adjacent laparoscopic image shows black, dark-brown, or bluish puckered lesions on the peritoneum. This is suggestive of endometriosis. These lesions are also known as "powder burn" or "gunshot" lesions and are typical of endometriosis. Endometriotic lesions are typically located over the pelvic organs and pelvic peritoneum and may acquire variable colors such as red, white, reddish-pink, yellow, yellowish-brown, black, or blackish-blue. Endometrial lesions may appear as smooth blebs on the peritoneal surface, as holes or defects in the peritoneum, or as flat stellate lesions surrounded by scar tissue **(Fig. 17)**. 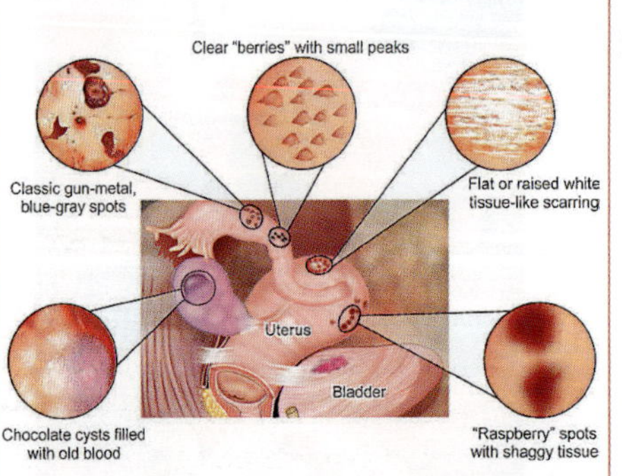 **Fig. 17:** Different lesions of endometriosis.	**Explanation:** Endometriosis is characterized by presence of endometrial-like tissue outside the uterus, which induces a chronic inflammatory reaction. The "powder burn" lesions of endometriosis are nodules or small cysts containing old hemorrhage/accumulated menstrual blood surrounded by a variable extent of fibrosis. This distinctive appearance helps in diagnosing endometriosis during laparoscopic examination. These implants may attain a size of 5–10 mm. As the disease progresses, these lesions may increase in size and number, and there may be development of extensive adhesions. **Potential questions:** There can be questions related to distinctive lesions of endometriosis, their diagnosis, and management.

Question	Answer	Comment
Q18. A 35-year-old woman who presented with long-standing history of infertility, dyspareunia, and dysmenorrhea underwent a diagnostic laparoscopy. This revealed the findings as shown in the image below. What is the best management of choice in this case? 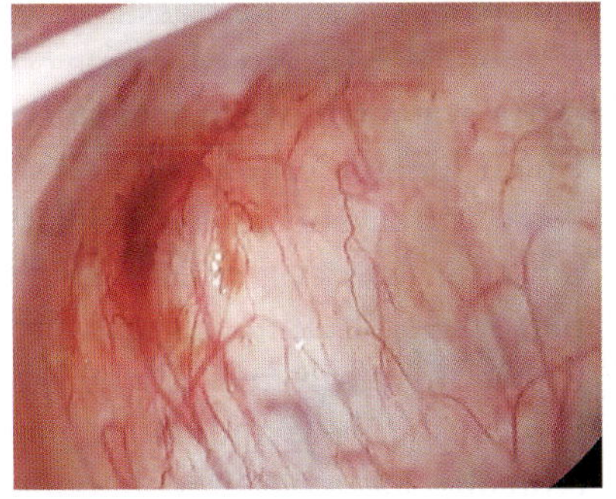 A. Emergency laparotomy B. Laser excision of the lesions C. Prescription of gonadotropin-releasing hormone (GnRH) agonists D. Prescription of (nonsteroidal anti-inflammatory drugs) NSAIDs E. Laparoscopic ablation of the uterine nerve	**Ans: B (Laser excision of the lesions)** The adjacent image shows reddish-brown plaque-like lesions of endometriosis. Since the patient in this case desires fertility, surgery would form the treatment of choice. Specific endoscopic procedures, which can be performed, include ablation of endometriotic implants **(Fig. 18)**, adhesiolysis, ovarian cystectomy, oophorectomy, and salpingectomy. 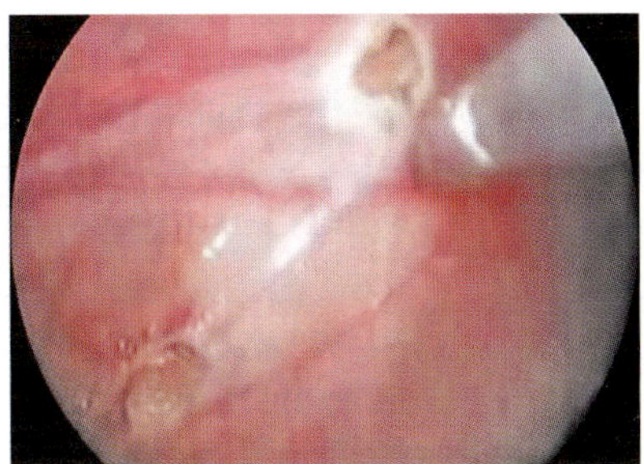 **Fig. 18:** Laser ablation of the endometriotic lesions.	**Explanation:** Endometriosis is characterized by the presence of endometrial-like tissue outside the uterus, which can cause chronic pelvic pain, dysmenorrhea, and infertility. Endometriotic lesions may be either superficial or may deeply invade the peritoneum or pelvic organs. Laparoscopic surgery is nowadays considered for most of the cases of endometriosis. Surgery in case of patients presenting with infertility may involve the following: ▪ Removal or destruction of endometrial implants ▪ Removal or destruction of ovarian endometriomas ▪ Removal, lysis, or destruction of adhesions **Potential questions:** There can be questions related to distinctive lesions of endometriosis, their diagnosis, and management.
Q19. A 28-year-old woman presents with chronic pelvic pain and infertility. The picture obtained at the time of diagnostic laparoscopy is shown below. Which of the following is the most likely diagnosis? 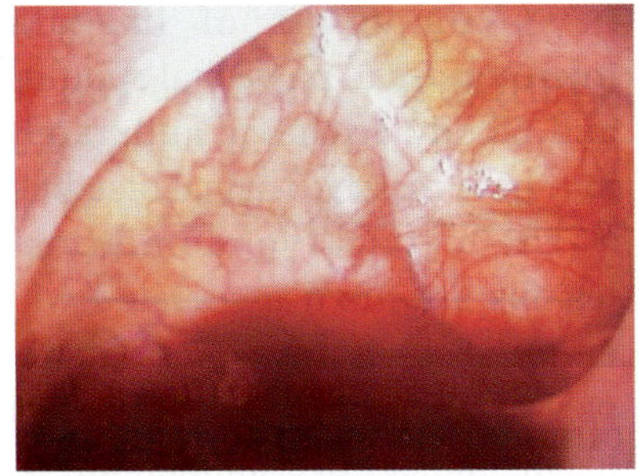 A. Ectopic pregnancy B. Pelvic inflammatory disease (PID) C. Endometriosis D. Ovarian torsion E. Ruptured ovarian cyst	**Ans: C (Endometriosis)** The adjacent laparoscopic image depicts the presence of blood in cul-de-sac. Laparoscopy can help detect the presence of blood or endometriotic deposits **(Fig. 19)** in the cul-de-sac. 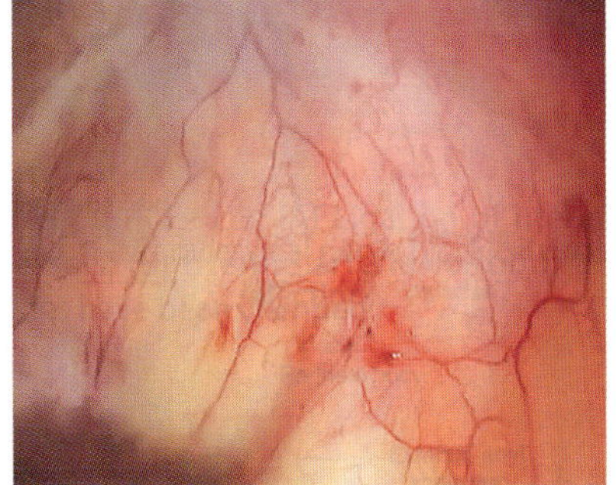 **Fig. 19:** Presence of endometriotic deposits in the pouch of Douglas (POD).	**Explanation:** Endometriosis is characterized by the presence of endometrial-like tissue outside the uterus, which can cause chronic inflammation and bleeding. During menstruation, this ectopic endometrial tissue can bleed, leading to the accumulation of blood in the pelvic cavity, including the pouch of Douglas. The presence of free blood or endometriotic deposits in the pouch of Douglas, observed during laparoscopy, is a common finding in endometriosis. **Potential questions:** There can be questions related to distinctive lesions of endometriosis, their diagnosis, and management.

Question	Answer	Comment
Q20. A 32-year-old woman presents with chronic pelvic pain and dysmenorrhea. A laparoscopic examination revealed the findings as shown in the image below. What is the most likely diagnosis? 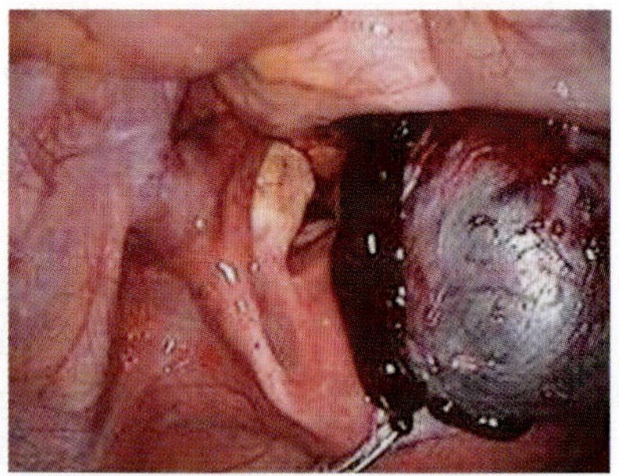 A. Functional cyst B. Physiologic cyst C. Ovarian endometrioma D. Ovarian teratoma E. Germ cell tumor	**Ans: C (Ovarian endometrioma)** The adjacent laparoscopic image shows brown-colored cyst-like growth filled with a tarry, thick, chocolate-colored content, adherent to the pelvic side uterine wall. The clinical features in this case strongly suggests an endometrioma. **Figure 20** shows diagrammatic representation of a chocolate cyst. 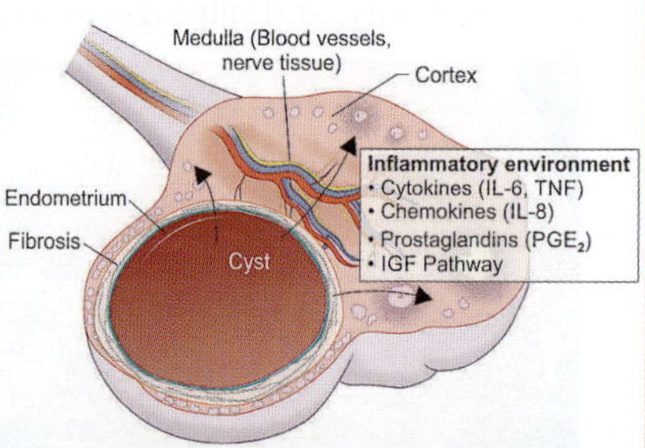 **Fig. 20:** Diagrammatic representation of a chocolate cyst. (IL-6: interleukin-6; TNF: tumor necrosis factor; IL-8: interleukin-8; PGE2: prostaglandin E2; IGF: insulin-like growth factor)	**Explanation:** The presence of chronic pelvic pain and dysmenorrhea, along with the laparoscopic findings, strongly suggests endometriosis. In the ovary, endometrial cysts may get enlarged to several centimeters resulting in the development of endometriomas or chocolate cysts. The classic lesion of endometriosis is a chocolate cyst of the ovary that contains old blood which has undergone hemolysis. Once intracystic pressure inside the chocolate cyst rises, the cyst perforates, spilling its contents within the peritoneal cavity. This can cause severe abdominal pain typically associated with endometriosis exacerbations. **Potential questions:** There can be questions related to distinctive lesions of endometriosis, their diagnosis, and management.
Q21. A 33-year-old woman presents to the clinic complaining of dyspareunia and vaginal spotting for 3–4 months. Bimanual examination is uncomfortable for her. Per speculum examination reveals the findings as shown in the image below. What is the diagnosis? 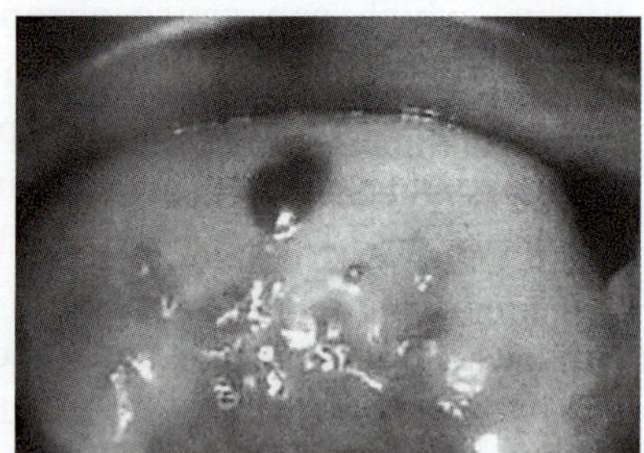 A. Actinomycosis B. Cervical endometriosis C. Nabothian cyst D. Cervical ectopic E. Chronic cervicitis	**Ans: B (Cervical endometriosis)** The adjacent image shows the presence of small, bluish-black, or fresh red nodules that have a diameter of <1.5 cm. The most likely diagnosis appears to be cervical endometriotic lesions. **Figure 21** depicts a magnified view of cervix showing the endometriotic lesions over cervix. 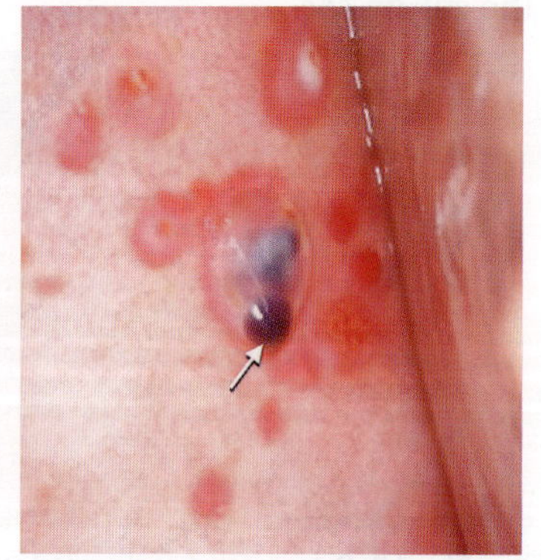 **Fig. 21:** Magnified view of cervix showing the endometriotic lesion (depicted by an arrow).	**Explanation:** The cervix is a rare location for endometriosis. Cervical endometriosis is characterized by the presence of endometrial-like tissue on the cervix. This condition can cause symptoms such as postcoital bleeding, chronic pelvic pain, and dysmenorrhea. According to literature reports, most patients are asymptomatic; however, some have complaints of irregular intermenstrual, postcoital spotting, and bloody discharge and, rarely, may have massive vaginal bleeding. The cervical endometriosis lesions are often associated with endometriosis elsewhere in the pelvis and can be confirmed through histopathological examination. **Potential questions:** There can be questions related to distinctive lesions of endometriosis, their diagnosis, and management.

GENITAL INFECTIONS

Question	Answer	Comment
Q22. A 35-year-old woman presents with chronic pelvic pain, menstrual irregularities, and infertility. The hysterosalpingography reveals findings shown in the image below. What is the most likely diagnosis? 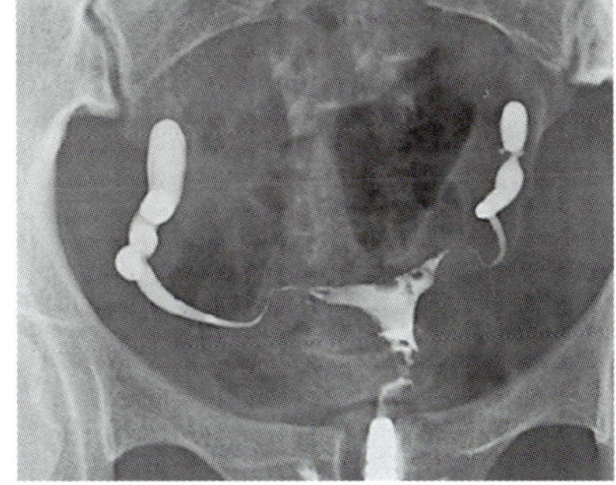 A. Endometriosis B. Pelvic inflammatory disease C. Ovarian cancer D. Genital tuberculosis E. Uterine fibroids	**Ans:** D (Genital tuberculosis) The adjacent hysterosalpingography (HSG) image shows lead pipe-like appearance of fallopian tubes and bilateral tubal obstruction along with bilateral hydrosalpinx. This has been depicted with the help of arrows in **Figure 22**. Diagnosis of genital tuberculosis was made. Tubercular infection of the genital tract first affects the fallopian tubes resulting in pelvic inflammatory disease. Later, it spreads downward causing uterine synechiae and Asherman's syndrome. Cervical and vulvar lesions are rare. 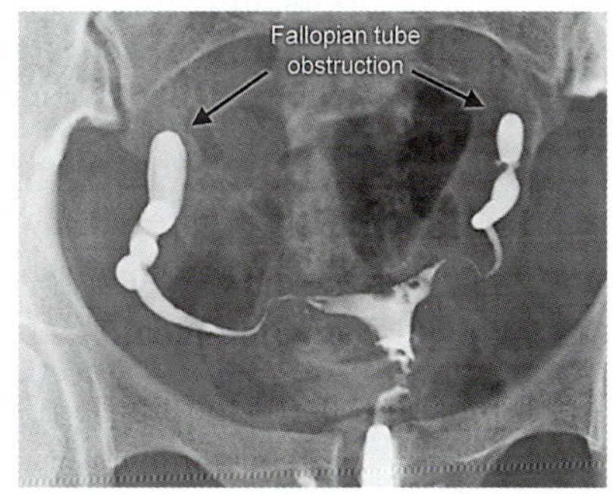 **Fig. 22:** Hysterosalpingogram findings in a patient with genital tuberculosis.	**Explanation:** Genital tuberculosis often presents with chronic pelvic pain, menstrual irregularities, and infertility. Diagnosis is confirmed through microbiological tests, histopathology, or molecular methods. Various findings suggestive of tubercular salpingitis, if HSG is done in an asymptomatic woman, include the following: ▪ Lead pipe appearance of the tubes ▪ Beading and variations in the filling density ▪ Tobacco pouch appearance ▪ Calcification of tube and jagged fluffiness of the tubal outline ▪ Cornual block ▪ Distorted uterine contour ▪ Vascular or lymphatic intravasation of the dye **Potential questions:** There can be questions pertaining to different findings encountered on HSG in cases of infertility due to tubal factors.

CHAPTER 11

Contraception

LONG-ACTING REVERSIBLE CONTRACEPTION (LARC) METHODS

Question	Answer	Comment
Q1. Identify the correct procedure for inserting the contraceptive device as shown in the image. 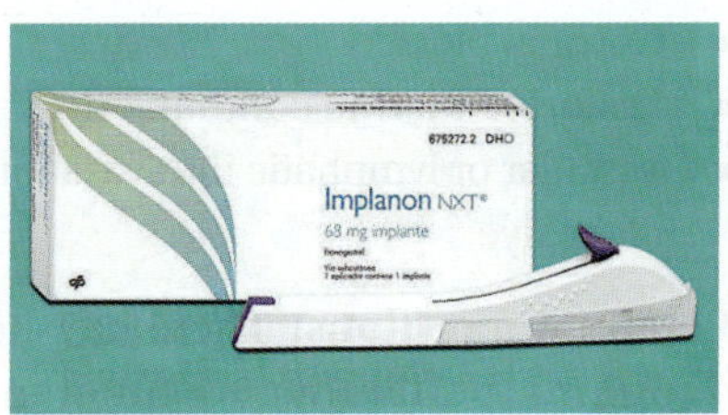 A. Clean the insertion site, make a small incision, insert the implant, apply a bandage B. Make a small incision, insert the implant, clean the insertion site, apply a bandage C. Clean the insertion site, insert the implant, make a small incision, apply a bandage D. Clean the insertion site, insert the implant using an applicator, apply a bandage E. Insert the implant, clean the insertion site, make a small incision, apply a bandage	**Ans: D (Clean the insertion site, insert the implant using an applicator, apply a bandage)** The adjacent image shows Implanon (or Nexplanon) subdermal implant along with its applicator. Subdermal implant is a long acting-reversible contraception (LARC), containing 68 mg of the synthetic progestin etonogestrel. It provides contraception for up to 3 years. Implanon is inserted subdermally in the inner side of the woman's upper, nondominant arm **(Fig. 1)**. The specific site is: ▪ 3–5 cm posterior to the sulcus (groove) between the biceps and triceps muscles ▪ 8–10 cm proximal to the medial epicondyle of the humerus 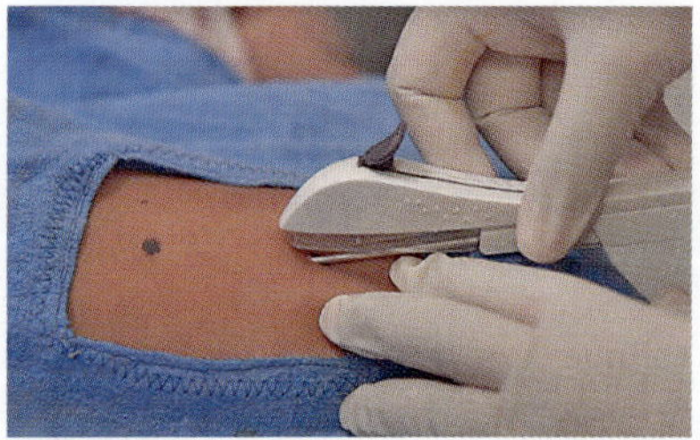 **Fig. 1:** Insertion of implanon subdermal implant using an applicator.	**Explanation:** The correct procedure for inserting the implanon contraceptive implant involves the following steps: 1. *Clean the insertion site:* The skin where the implant will be inserted is cleaned with an antiseptic solution to prevent infection. 2. *Insert the implant using an applicator:* The implanon implant is preloaded in a sterile applicator. The healthcare provider uses this applicator to insert the implant just under the skin of the upper arm. 3. *Apply a bandage:* After the implant is inserted, a small bandage is applied to the insertion site to protect it and help it heal. This method ensures that the implant is placed correctly and minimizes the risk of infection **Potential questions:** There can be questions related to the composition, method of insertion, advantages, and complications associated with the use of subdermal implants.

Question	Answer	Comment
Q2. Identify the primary mechanism of action of the device shown in the image below. 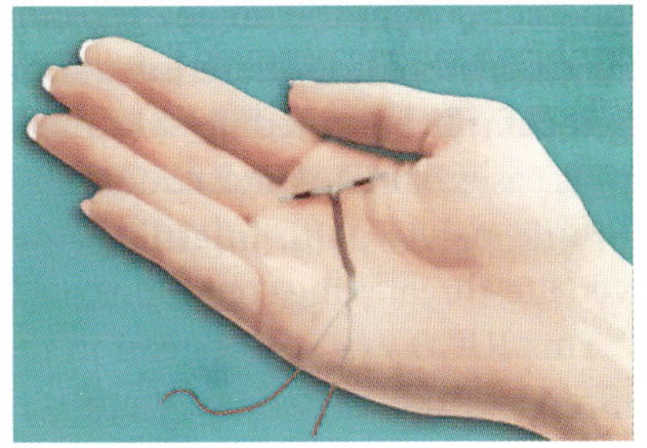 A. Inhibition of ovulation B. Thickening of cervical mucus C. Prevention of sperm from reaching the egg D. Suppression of endometrial growth E. Release of hormones to prevent pregnancy	**Ans: C (Prevention of sperm from reaching the egg)** The adjacent image shows copper-T 380A, which is a third-generation intrauterine copper device, being marketed as ParaGard in the US. Copper wire is wound on its arms and stem and amounts to a total of 380 mm^2 of copper. There are two nylon strings attached at one of its end **(Fig. 2)**. It has been approved for 10 years of continuous use. 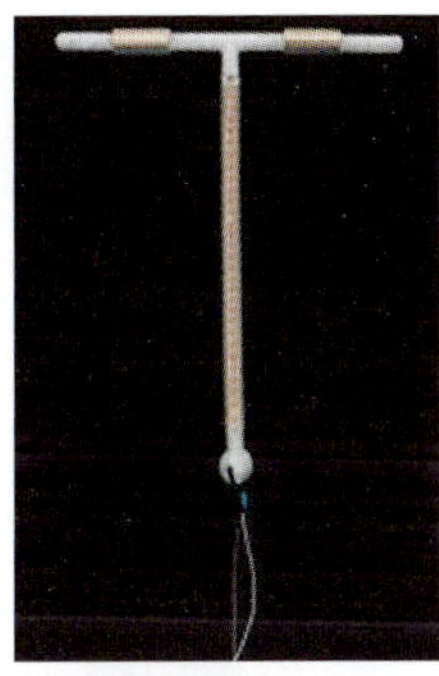 **Fig. 2:** Magnified view of Copper-T 380A.	**Explanation:** The Cu-T 380A intrauterine device (IUD) primarily works by releasing copper ions into the uterine cavity, which creates an inflammatory reaction that is toxic to sperm and eggs. This reaction prevents sperm from fertilizing the egg. Unlike hormonal IUDs, the Cu-T 380A does not inhibit ovulation or release hormones. Instead, its effectiveness is due to the spermicidal effect of copper, which disrupts sperm motility and viability, thereby preventing fertilization. Common side effects associated with its use include menstrual irregularities, cramping, and increased risk of intrauterine infection. **Potential questions:** There can be questions related to mode of action, method of insertion, and complications of various intrauterine devices.
Q3. What is the typical duration of effectiveness for the intrauterine device shown in the below image? 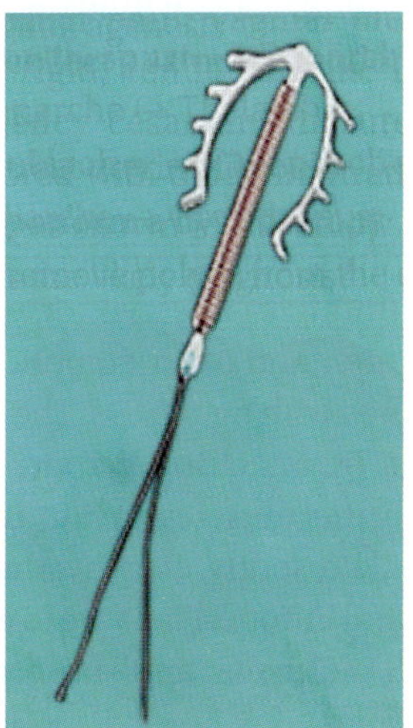 A. 1 year B. 3 years C. 5 years D. 7 years E. 10 years	**Ans: C (5 years)** The adjacent image shows Multiload 375 IUD. Multiload is a third-generation IUD, used for long acting-reversible contraception. It has a stem and two small flexible side-arms. A copper wire is wound around the stem. A nylon thread with two ends is attached to the bottom end of the stem. **Figure 3** demonstrates. Multiload 375 IUD, inserted inside the uterus. 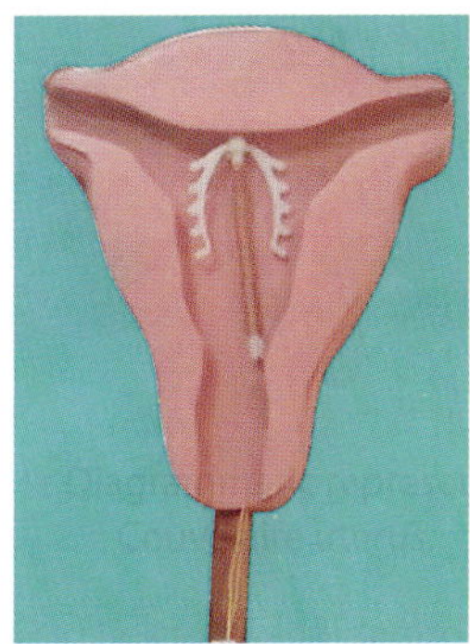 **Fig. 3:** Multiload 375 IUD, inserted inside the uterus.	**Explanation:** Two types of Multiload devices which are commonly available are: ▪ Multiload Cu-250 (having a surface area of 250 mm^2), whose action lasts for a period of 3 years ▪ Multiload Cu-375 has a copper wire with a surface area of 375 mm^2 and its action lasts for a period of 5 years. Multiload Cu-375 comes in two sizes, standard and short length, which are used based on the uterine size. It releases copper ions into the uterine cavity, which creates an environment that is toxic to sperm, thereby preventing fertilization **Potential questions:** There can be questions related to mode of action, method of insertion, and complications of various intrauterine devices.

Question	Answer	Comment
Q4. What complication is most commonly associated with the use of the device shown below? 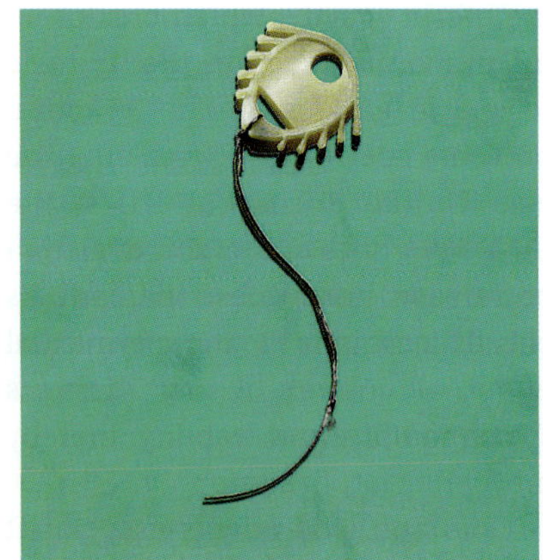 A. Ectopic pregnancy B. Pelvic inflammatory disease (PID) C. Uterine perforation D. Menorrhagia E. Endometrial cancer	**Ans: B [Pelvic inflammatory disease (PID)]** The adjacent image shows Dalkon Shield, an IUD in shape of a triangle with five fin-like structures on each of the lower sides. The tail made up of monofilament had wicking properties. The fins acted as a predisposing factor for the IUD to get embedded inside the uterine walls **(Fig. 4)**. The Dalkon Shield was associated with a high incidence of PID. 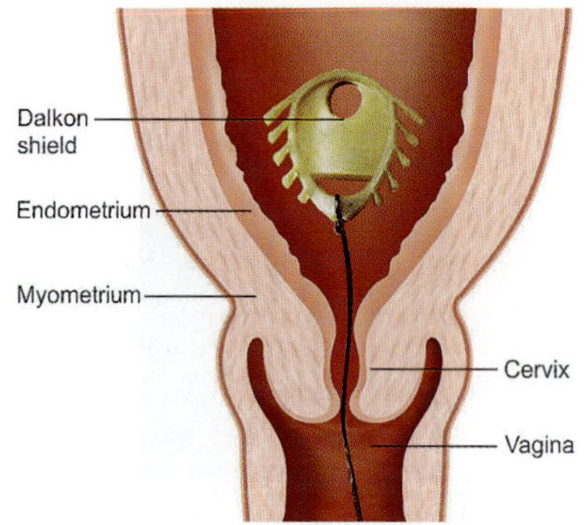 **Fig. 4:** Dalkon Shield intrauterine device.	**Explanation:** The design of the Dalkon Shield, particularly its multi-filament string, facilitated the ascent of bacteria from the vagina into the uterus, leading to severe infections. This complication resulted in numerous cases of PID, which could cause chronic pelvic pain, infertility, and even life-threatening conditions. This IUCD was introduced in the US during the 1970s and went into dispute due to numerous problems related to its safety. It was eventually withdrawn from the market by 1974. The company manufacturing Dalkon Shield had to pay 485 million dollars in settlements and legal costs, following which the company declared bankruptcy in 1986. **Potential questions:** There can be questions related to mode of action, method of insertion, and complications of various IUDs.
Q5. What is a notable advantage of the device shown in the image below in comparison to traditional T-shaped intrauterine device (IUDs)? 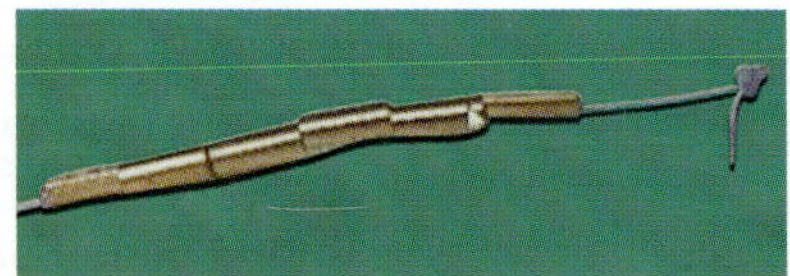 A. Lower risk of uterine perforation B. Higher copper content C. Frameless design D. Longer duration of effectiveness E. Easier insertion process	**Ans: C (Frameless design)** The adjacent image depicts an IUD known as Flexiguard 330/GyneFix. It is an innovative contraceptive device which is implanted in the wall of uterus **(Fig. 5)**. It comprises four to six mini copper tubes, threaded on a length of nylon. Knots at the two ends keep the device in place. This is an anchored, frameless, and flexible IUCD. Its action lasts for 5 years. 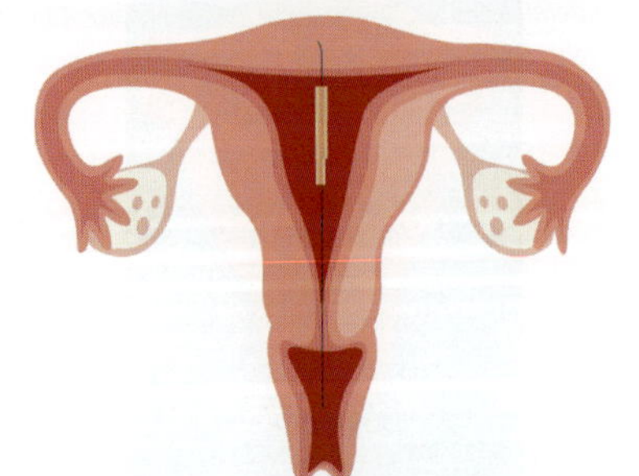 **Fig. 5:** Intrauterine insertion of GyneFix.	**Explanation:** The GyneFix IUD is unique due to its frameless design, which distinguishes it from traditional T-shaped IUDs. This design allows the GyneFix to be more flexible and adaptable to the shape of the uterus, reducing the risk of expulsion and discomfort. The frameless nature also minimizes the risk of uterine perforation and other complications associated with rigid IUDs. The device is fitted by attaching the anchoring knot to the muscles in the uterine fundus. Presently, it is available in China and Europe. Plans are to market it to USA, Canada, and subsequently worldwide. **Potential questions:** There can be questions related to mode of action, method of insertion, and complications of various IUDs.

<table>
<tr><th>Question</th><th>Answer</th><th>Comment</th></tr>
<tr>
<td>
Q6. What is a primary therapeutic benefit of the IUD shown in the image below?
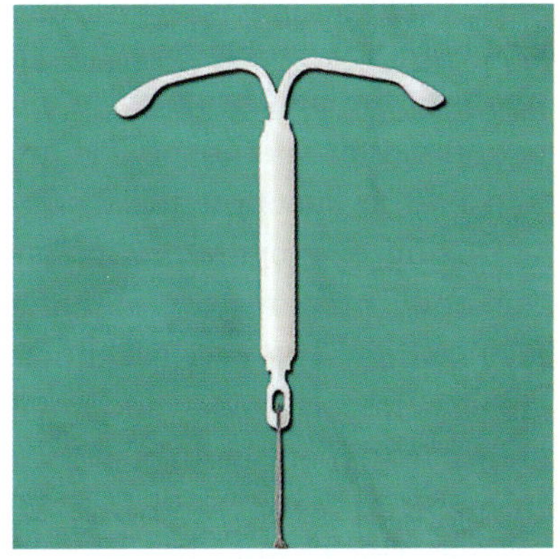
A. Treatment of endometriosis
B. Management of heavy menstrual bleeding
C. Management of uterine fibroids
D. Prevention of ectopic pregnancy
E. Treatment of ovarian cysts
</td>
<td>
Ans: B (Management of heavy menstrual bleeding)

The adjacent image shows a Mirena device. It is a type of progestogen-containing IUCD. It is available in the form of a T-shaped polyethylene structure **(Fig. 6)**. The stem is encased by a cylinder, which contains polydimethylsiloxane and levonorgestrel. At the end of the vertical stem are two threads. The effects of Mirena last for about 5 years.
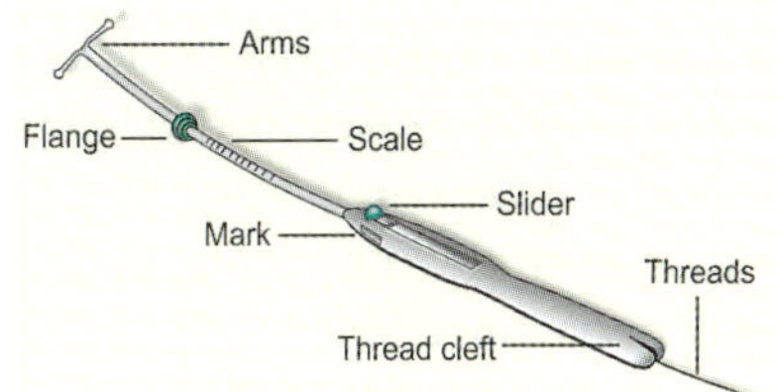

Fig. 6: Parts of levonorgestrel-intrauterine system device.
</td>
<td>
Explanation: The LNG IUS not only is an effective contraceptive but also provides significant therapeutic benefits, particularly in reducing heavy menstrual bleeding. It contains 52 mg of levonorgestrel, which is released at the rate of 20 µg/day. This helps to make the endometrial lining thin, thereby reducing menstrual blood flow and cramping. This makes it a valuable option for women suffering from heavy menstrual bleeding (HMB) and painful periods. Mirena is also indicated for the treatment of menorrhagia/HMB in women who want to use IUCD as their method of contraception.

Potential questions: There can be questions related to modes of action, methods of insertion, and complications of various IUDs.
</td>
</tr>
<tr>
<td>
Q7. A 32-year-old woman presents with severe lower abdominal pain and abnormal bleeding. She has a history of Cu-T 380A IUD insertion 6 months ago. She has been unable to feel thread of Cu-T device since past few days. A pelvic ultrasound reveals the findings as shown below. What should be the next best step of management in this case?
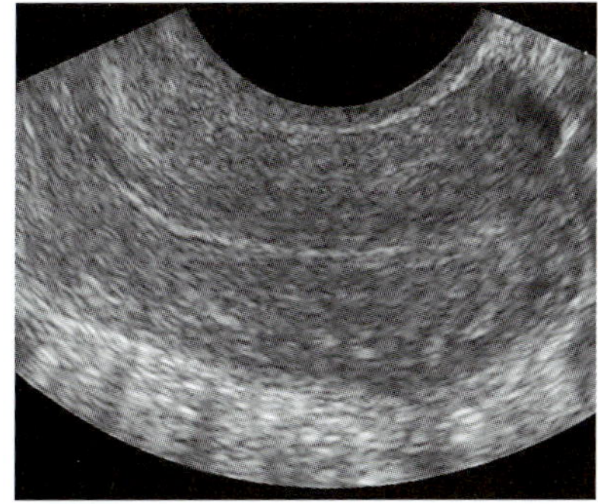
A. Emergency laparotomy
B. X-ray abdomen
C. MRI imaging
D. Reinsertion of the Cu-device
E. Removal of the Cu-device
</td>
<td>
Ans: B (X-ray abdomen)

The adjacent ultrasound image shows an empty uterine cavity with no echogenic shadow of the copper device, suggesting its absence. If IUCD strings are missing, ultrasound is the first step to locate it. If not seen in the uterus or pelvis, an abdominal X-ray is performed. As shown in **Figure 7**, X-ray confirms uterine perforation, with the device present outside the uterine cavity.
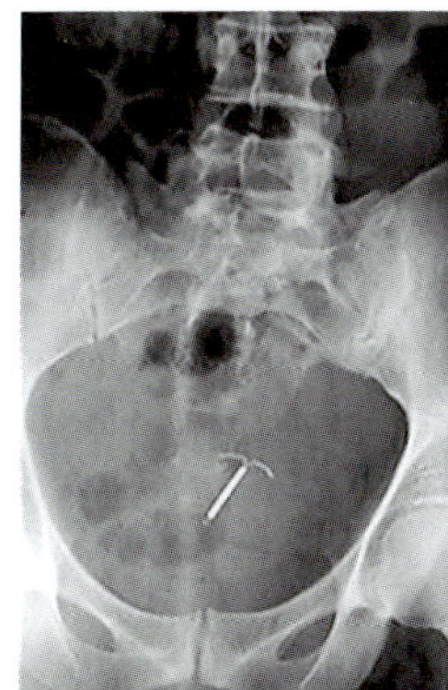
Fig. 7: X-ray showing intrauterine device inside the abdominal cavity.
</td>
<td>
Explanation: The missing threads indicate that the IUD may have migrated through the uterine wall, necessitating further imaging studies like ultrasound or X-ray to locate the device.

Uterine perforation is a rare but serious complication of IUD insertion, occurring in less than 1 in 1,000 insertions. It can happen during the insertion process or later due to uterine contractions. Symptoms may include severe pelvic pain, abnormal bleeding, and missing IUD threads. Immediate medical attention is required to manage the condition and prevent further complications.

Potential questions: There can be questions related to mode of action, method of insertion, and complications of various IUDs.
</td>
</tr>
</table>

NATURAL FAMILY PLANNING METHODS

Question	Answer	Comment
Q8. A 28-year-old woman presents to the clinic seeking advice on natural family planning methods. She has regular menstrual cycles and prefers to avoid hormonal contraceptives. She is interested in using the cervical mucus method to identify her fertile window. During her visit, she provides a sample of her cervical mucus, which is examined under a microscope. The image observed under the microscope is shown below. This pattern is indicative of which phase in the menstrual cycle? 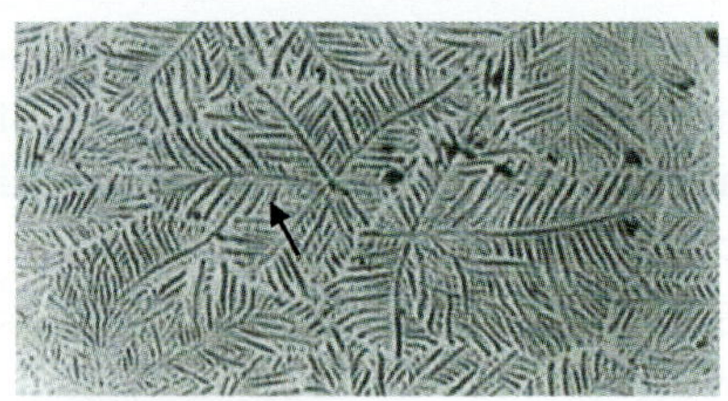 A. Menstrual phase B. Follicular phase C. Ovulatory phase D. Luteal phase E. Postmenstrual phase	**Ans: C (Ovulatory phase)** The adjacent image shows a ferning pattern of cervical mucus. Under the effect of estrogens, cervical mucus becomes thin, watery, clear, and profuse. It has a high content of sodium chloride in it due to which it forms a characteristic pattern of ferning when dried on a glass slide. It has great elasticity and can withstand stretching up to 10 cm. This is also known as the Spinnbarkeit or the thread test, which provides evidence of estrogenic activity. On the other hand, under the effect of progesterone, the mucus becomes thick, tenacious, and highly viscous. It loses its property of Spinnbarkeit and easily fractures when put under tension. This property is known as tack. **Figure 8** demonstrates the appearance of progesterone-dominant mucus under the microscope. 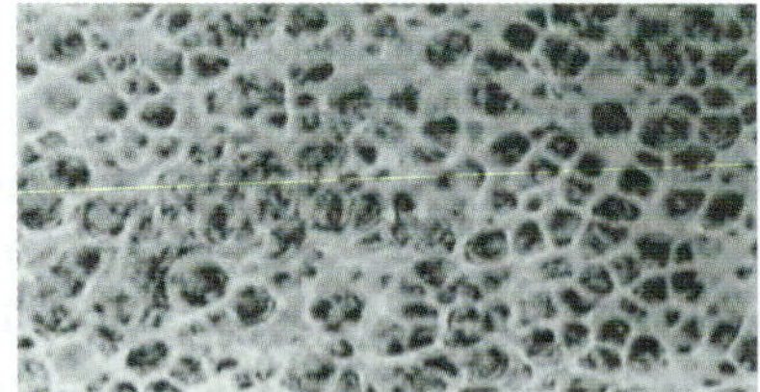 **Fig. 8:** Progesterone-dominant cervical mucus.	**Explanation:** The ferning pattern of cervical mucus is a characteristic sign observed during the ovulatory phase of the menstrual cycle and is optimal for sperm survival and transport, facilitating fertilization. During the ovulatory phase, the body prepares for potential fertilization. The cervical mucus changes in consistency and appearance to support sperm movement through the cervix and into the uterus. The ferning pattern is a reliable indicator of this fertile period, helping women using natural family planning methods to identify the best time for conception or to avoid intercourse if they wish to prevent pregnancy. Cervical mucus method is one of the natural fertility awareness methods. This method is safe and there are no side effects. However, this method is associated with a high failure rate of approximately 20–25 pregnancies per 100 women-years of use. The high failure rate associated with this method commonly results due to irregular ovulation or irregular menstrual cycles. **Potential questions:** There can be questions related to the characteristics of cervical mucus during various phases of the menstrual cycle.

Question	Answer	Comment
Q9. A 30-year-old woman is using the device shown below for family planning. She starts her period on the red bead and moves the ring one bead each day. On which days should she avoid unprotected intercourse to prevent pregnancy? 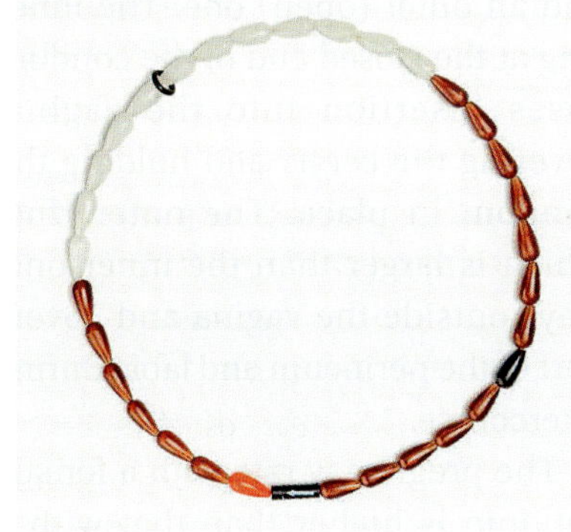 A. Days 1–7 B. Days 8–19 C. Days 20–26 D. Days 1–5 E. Days 15–28	**Ans: B (Days 8–19)** The adjacent image shows CycleBeads. This is a natural family planning method, which is designed for women with cycles between 26 to 32 days. The fertile period in these women lasts from 8th to 19th day, which can be identified by the presence of white beads. Brown beads mark the "safe days" or the period during which the woman is likely to be least fertile **(Fig. 9)**. During this time, the couple can have unprotected intercourse. A rubber band is moved head to head every day to track the cycle. 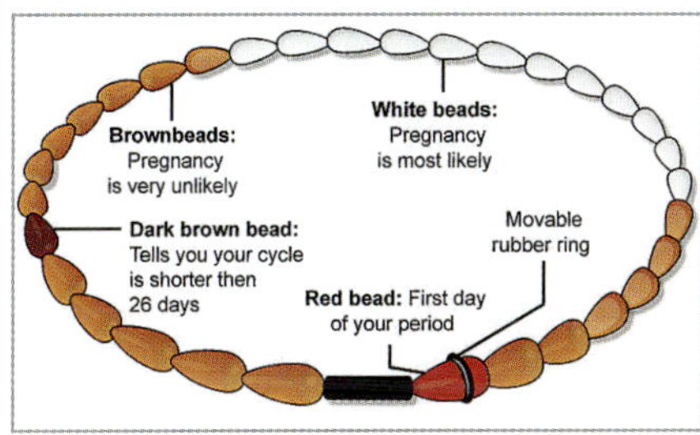 **Fig. 9:** CycleBeads.	**Explanation:** CycleBeads is a visual tool used to track the menstrual cycle and identify fertile days based on the Standard Days Method. This method helps in preventing unwanted pregnancies, using the "Standard Days" method. The users are instructed to avoid unprotected sexual intercourse by using a condom or abstaining during days 8–19 of the cycle (identified by the white beads). **Potential questions:** There can be different questions pertaining to various natural methods for family planning.
Q10. The graph below shows a woman's basal body temperature chart over a menstrual cycle. Based on the temperature shift observed, which phase of the menstrual cycle is indicated by the rise in basal body temperature (BBT)? 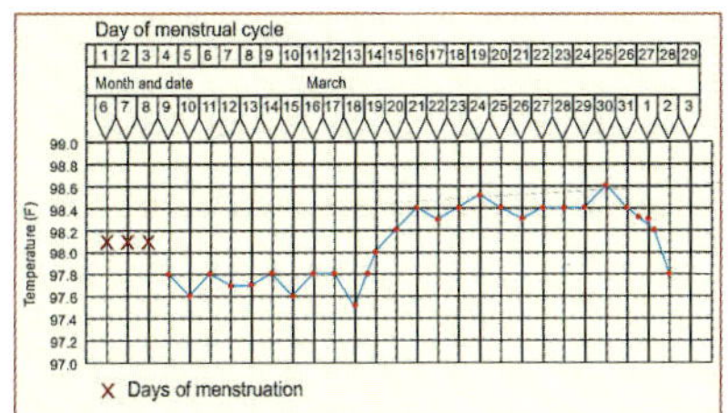 A. Menstrual phase B. Follicular phase C. Ovulatory phase D. Luteal phase E. Premenstrual phase	**Ans: D (Luteal phase)** The BBT method involves tracking a woman's body temperature at rest each morning before any physical activity **(Fig. 10)**. A slight increase in BBT, typically by about 0.5–1°F, occurs after ovulation due to hormone progesterone. This temperature rise indicates the transition from the follicular phase to the luteal phase. If pregnancy does not occur, progesterone levels drop, leading to a decrease in BBT and start of the menstrual phase. 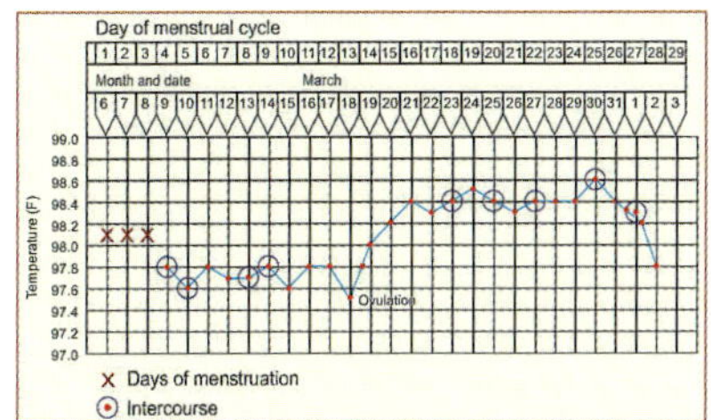 **Fig. 10:** Basal body temperature method.	**Explanation:** This method is based on the fact that BBT increases by 0.3–0.6°C following ovulation under the thermogenic effect of hormone progesterone. Therefore, the couple must be instructed that the safest way to use BBT for avoiding pregnancy is to avoid intercourse or use a barrier method during at least the first half of the menstrual cycle until 3 days after there has been a rise in BBT. **Potential questions:** There can be different questions pertaining to various natural methods for family planning.

BARRIER METHODS

Question	Answer	Comment
Q11. A 28-year-old woman is using a method for contraception as shown in the image below for the first time. She wants to ensure that she is using it correctly. Which of the following statements about the use of this method is true? 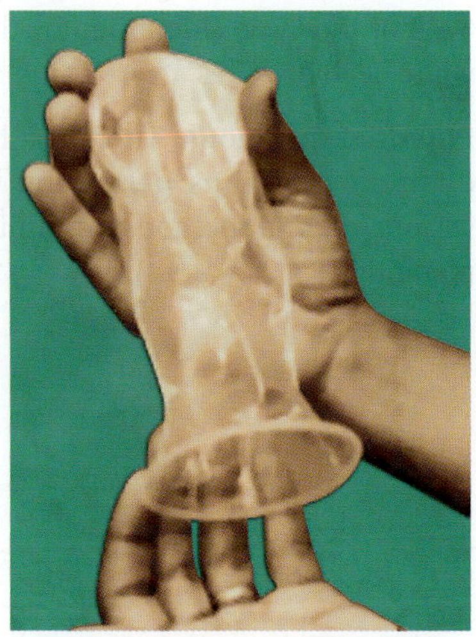 A. The inner ring should be removed before insertion B. The condom should be twisted before insertion C. The outer ring should remain outside the vagina D. The condom should be inserted only halfway E. The condom can be reused after washing	**Ans: C (The outer ring should remain outside the vagina)** The adjacent image shows a female condom. When using a female condom, the inner ring is inserted into the vagina to hold the condom in place, while the outer ring remains outside the vagina, covering the external genitalia **(Fig. 11)**. This ensures that the condom stays in place during intercourse and provides effective protection against pregnancy and sexually transmitted infections (STIs). 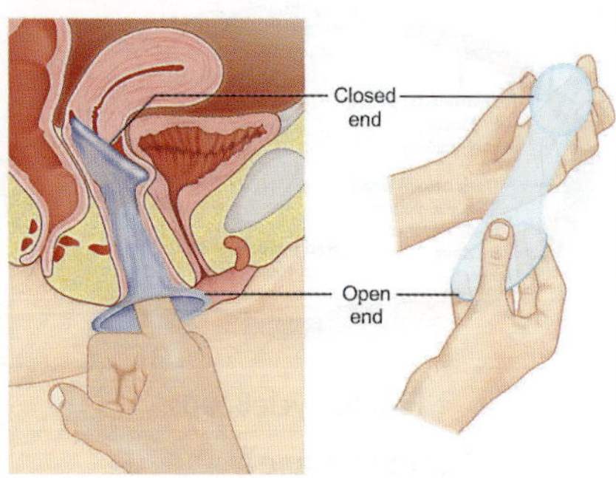 **Fig. 11:** Method of insertion of the female condom.	**Explanation:** The female condom comprises a strong, soft, transparent polyurethane sheath, which is approximately 15 cm in length and 7 cm in diameter. It has two flexible rings, the inner (closed ring) ring and an outer (open) one. The inner ring at the closed end of the condom eases insertion into the vagina, covering the cervix and holding the condom in place. The outer ring, which is larger than the inner one, stays outside the vagina and covers part of the perineum and labia during intercourse. The pregnancy rate with a female condom is higher than that with a male condom. Female condoms may be expensive or limited in their availability and may be difficult to insert. **Potential questions:** There can be different questions pertaining to various barrier methods for family planning (both male and female).

Question	Answer	Comment
Q12. A 32-year-old woman is considering using a device as shown in the image below for contraception. She wants to know the correct way to use it. Which of the following steps is correct for using this device? 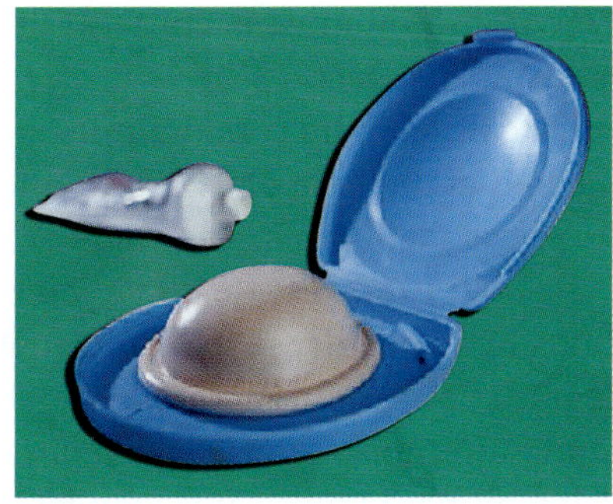 A. Insert the diaphragm without any additional products B. Insert the diaphragm immediately after intercourse C. Use the diaphragm with spermicide D. Remove the diaphragm immediately after intercourse E. Use the diaphragm only during menstruation	**Ans: C (Use the diaphragm with spermicide)** The adjacent image shows cervical diaphragm which is a shallow rubber dome with firm flexible rim. It covers the cervix to prevent sperm from entering the uterus. Though it is available in many sizes ranging from 50 to 105 mm, the most used size in clinical practice is 75 mm. Different types of cervical diaphragms are available **(Figs. 12A to D)**. These include latex arcing spring, coil spring, flat spring, and silicone wide seal rim. 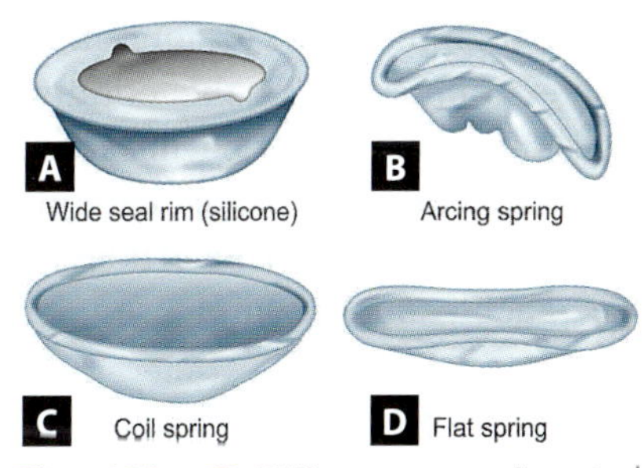 **Figs. 12A to D:** Different types of cervical diaphragms.	**Explanation:** Cervical diaphragm is an immediately effective and reversible method of contraception, which can be inserted up to 6 hours before intercourse. However, it must not be left inside the vagina for more than 24 hours. For maximum effectiveness, cervical diaphragm should be used with spermicide, which kills or immobilizes sperm. The latex arcing spring diaphragm has a firm rim, which makes its insertion in the posterior fornix easier. This can be used in women with a narrow vaginal canal or who prefer a lighter and more comfortable option. The rim of a coil spring diaphragm is soft and flexible, which does not form an arc when folded. This is usually used in women with moderate tone of vaginal muscles. The flat spring diaphragm is similar to coil spring but has a thinner and more delicate rim. It may be used in women with good tone of vaginal muscles. The silicone wide seal rim type cervical diaphragm is used in woman with normal tone of vaginal muscles. **Potential questions:** There can be different questions pertaining to various barrier methods for family planning (both male and female).

Question	Answer	Comment
Q13. A 25-year-old man visits the clinic for advice on contraceptive methods. He is particularly interested in using a male method of contraception as illustrated in the images below. Which of the following statements about this method of male contraception is correct? 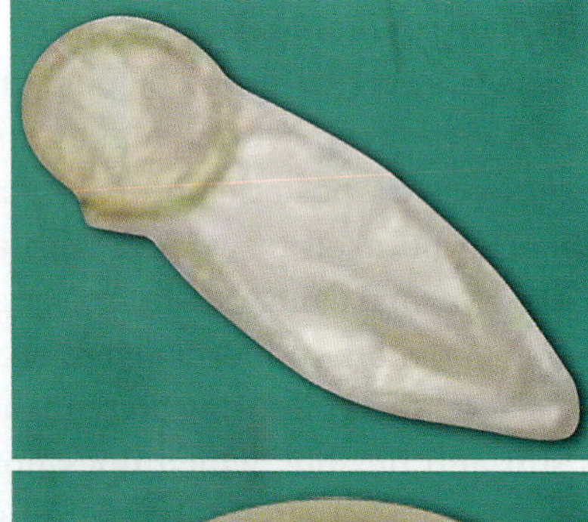 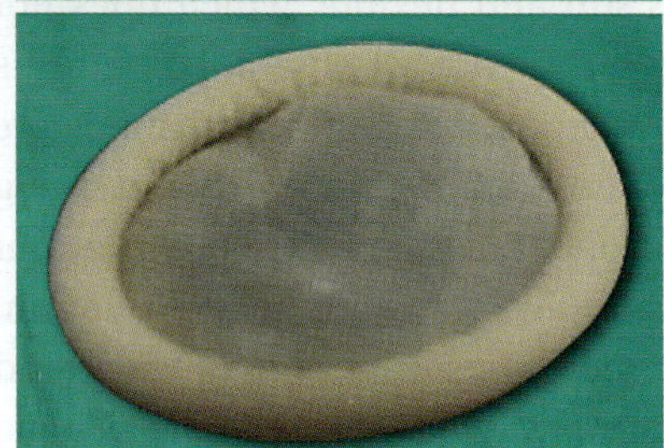 A. Male condoms are made from nitrile and can be reused B. Male condoms provide protection against pregnancy but not sexually transmitted infections (STIs) C. Male condoms should be stored in a cool, dry place to maintain their effectiveness D. Male condoms can be used with oil-based lubricants for better comfort E. Male condoms are less effective than female condoms in preventing STIs	**Ans: C (Male condoms should be stored in a cool, dry place to maintain their effectiveness)** A male condom is a thin sheath made of latex, polyurethane, or polyisoprene and is designed for single use only. Latex is the most used material. They may be available in different sizes. The main advantage of using condoms is that they provide protection against various STDs. Condoms also help prevent premalignant cervical changes, probably by blocking the transmission of human papilloma virus. The procedure for application of male condom is depicted in **Figures 13A to D**. The man puts the condom on his erected penis, while the condom holds the semen. After having sexual intercourse, the man must carefully take off the condom so that it does not leak. Each condom can be used only once. 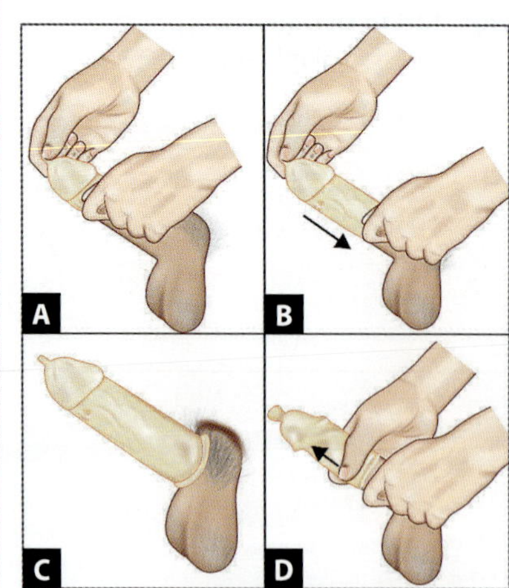 **Figs. 13A to D:** Application of male condom.	**Explanation:** Various precautions, which must be observed to ensure maximal effectiveness of condoms are as follows: ▪ It must be used with every act of coitus. ▪ It must be applied before penis has any contact with the vagina. ▪ Withdrawal must occur with the penis still erect. ▪ The base of the condom must be held at the time of withdrawal to prevent it from slipping out. It is important to store condoms in a cool, dry place to prevent degradation of the material, which can compromise their effectiveness. Using oil-based lubricants with latex condoms is not recommended as these can cause the latex to break down, increasing the risk of breakage. Condoms are an effective form of contraception and when used by motivated couples, failure rates as low as 3–4 per 100 couple-years of exposure have been obtained. However, perfect use rarely occurs and in practical life, high failure rates (10–14 per 100 couple-years of use) may be achieved. **Potential questions:** There can be different questions pertaining to various barrier methods for family planning (both male and female).

NON HORMONAL CONTRACEPTION

Question	Answer	Comment
Q14. A 30-year-old woman is prescribed nonhormonal contraceptive tablets as shown in the image below She is curious about their usage and effectiveness. Which of the following statements about this contraceptive pill is correct? 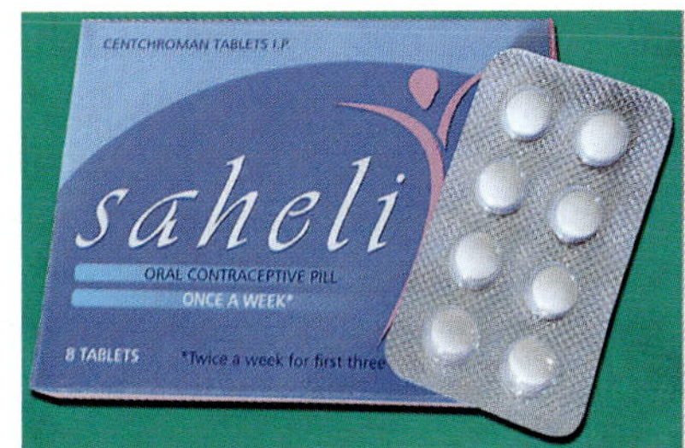 A. Centchroman needs to be taken daily for effective contraception B. Centchroman is a steroidal contraceptive pill C. Centchroman is safe for use in breastfeeding women D. Centchroman is effective immediately after the first dose E. Centchroman causes significant weight gain as a side effect	**Ans: C (Centchroman is safe for use in breastfeeding women)** The adjacent image depicts Centchroman tablets primarily used for contraception in India. These were developed by the Central Drug Research Institute (CDRI) in Lucknow and introduced into the Indian national family planning program. Centchroman is available in some markets in India under the brand name of Saheli® tablets which is used as a contraceptive. This can be purchased over the counter. Centchroman has also been introduced in the Indian public health system under the brand name Chhaya® **(Fig. 14)**. This is available free of cost in the Indian public health system. 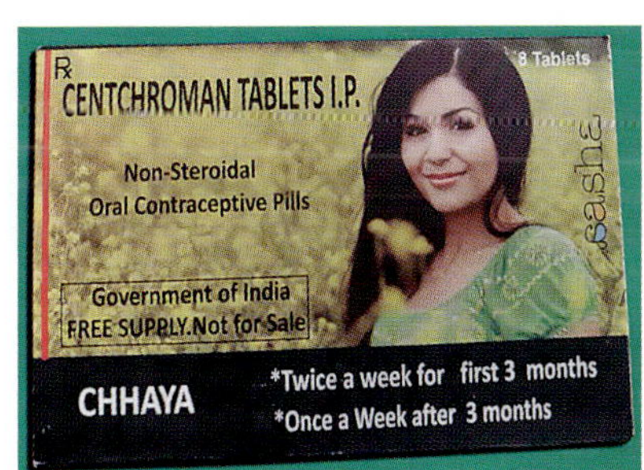 **Fig. 14:** Centchroman available as Chhaya®.	**Explanation:** Centchroman (also known as Ormeloxifene) is a nonsteroidal oral contraceptive pill that acts as a selective estrogen receptor modulator. Centchroman tablets are taken twice a week for the first 3 months and then once a week thereafter. They are safe for use in both breastfeeding and nonbreastfeeding women, making it a versatile option for postpartum contraception. Unlike steroidal/hormonal contraceptives, these do not cause significant weight gain and have a different mechanism of action. They are not effective immediately after the first dose and require consistent use as per the prescribed schedule to ensure effectiveness. **Potential questions:** There can be questions related to various hormonal and nonhormonal oral contraceptive pills, their mechanism of action, complications, etc.

COMBINED HORMONAL CONTRACEPTION

Question	Answer	Comment
Q15. A 30-year-old woman comes to your clinic seeking advice on contraception. She is interested in using the method of contraception as shown in the image below. Which of the following statements about this method is correct? 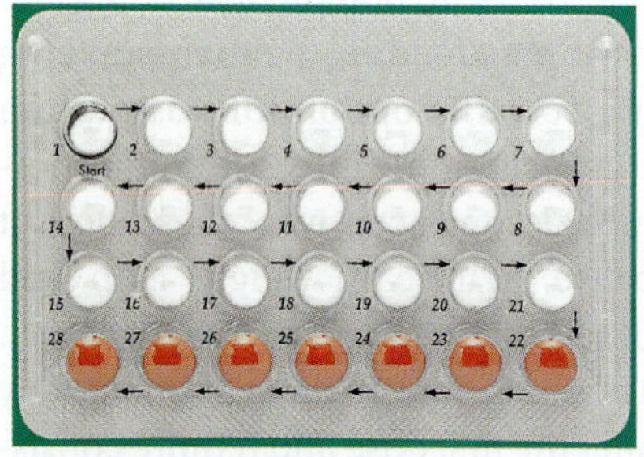 A. These tablets need to be taken only during the menstrual period B. These tablets provide protection against sexually transmitted infections (STIs) C. These tablets can be taken at any time of the day without affecting their efficacy D. These tablets help reduce the risk of ovarian and endometrial cancer E. These tablets are effective immediately after the first dose	**Ans: D (These tablets help reduce the risk of ovarian and endometrial cancer)** The adjacent image depicts a blister packet of combined oral contraceptive pills (COCPs), containing 21 active (hormonal tablets) and 7 inactive pills (nonhormonal pills). Active and inactive pills often use different colors to help users distinguish between them. Pills are arranged in a blister pack, usually in rows, with each pill in its own compartment. **Figure 15** shows the method of using these oral contraceptive pills in case one or more pill is missed. Missed 2 or more of these 7? • Take 1 immediately. • Take others in the row, one each day and then start a new pack. • Use condoms for 7 days. Missed 2 or more of these 14? • Take 1 as soon as remembered. • Take all the others as usual. • Use condoms for 7 day. 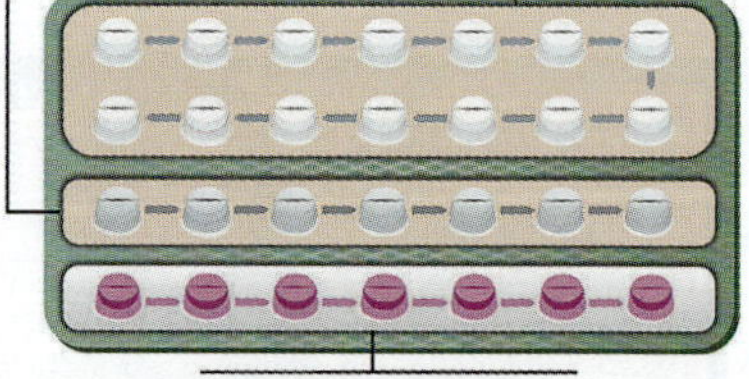 Missed any of these 7? • Throw the missed pills away. • Take all the others as usual. **Fig. 15:** Method of using oral contraceptive pills.	**Explanation:** COCPs contain both estrogen and progestin and can be considered as a highly effective method of reversible contraception. Active or the hormonal pills (white) are to be consumed for 21 days starting from the first day of menstrual periods. This should be followed by 7 inactive or the nonhormonal pills (red) which do not contain the hormone. They are taken daily, ideally at the same time each day, to maintain consistent hormone levels and ensure maximum efficacy. One of the significant benefits of COCPs is their ability to reduce the risk of ovarian and endometrial cancer, and probably even the colorectal cancer. However, they do not provide protection against STIs, and their effectiveness can be compromised if not taken consistently. COCPs typically require 7 days of consistent use before they become fully effective. **Potential questions:** There can be questions related to various hormonal and nonhormonal oral contraceptive pills, their mechanism of action, complications, etc.

Question	Answer	Comment
Q16. A 27-year-old woman is considering using a contraceptive device as shown in the image below for contraception. She asks you about its usage and benefits. Which of the following statements about the vaginal ring is correct? 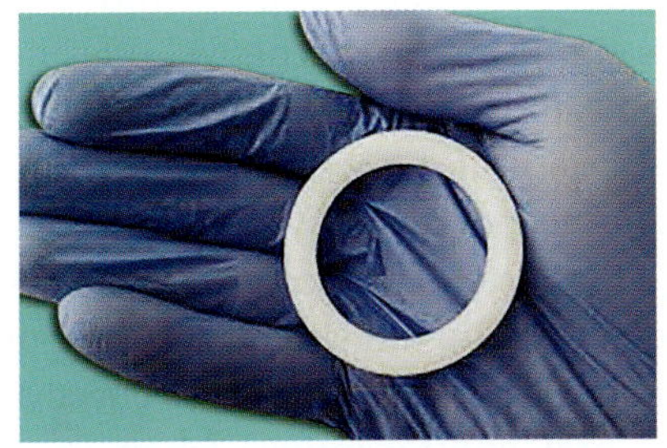 A. Daily replacement is required B. Provides protection against sexually transmitted infections (STIs) C. Monthly insertion with a break for 1 week D. Continuous use is required E. Less-effective hormonal method	**Ans: C (Monthly insertion with a break for 1 week)** The adjacent image shows a vaginal ring which is a type of combined hormonal, reversible method of contraception. The ring works by preventing ovulation, thickening the cervical mucus and thinning the endometrial lining. Placement of the vaginal ring is shown in **Figure 16**. The vaginal ring is inserted once a month and remains in place for 3 weeks, followed by a ring-free week. 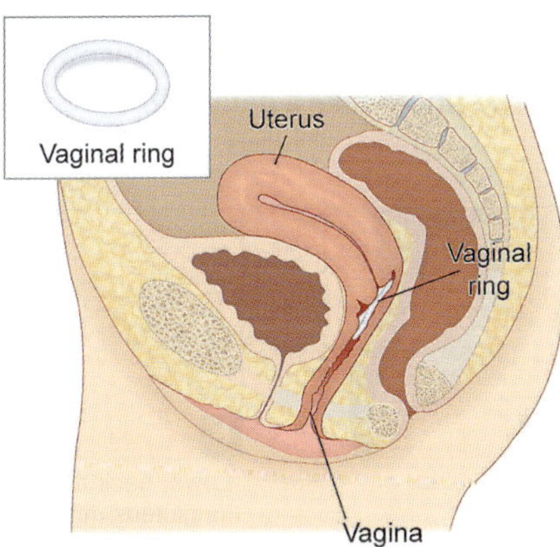 **Fig. 16:** Placement of the vaginal ring.	**Explanation:** The vaginal ring is a flexible, plastic ring that is inserted inside the vagina where it releases a combination of estrogen and progestin hormones to prevent pregnancy. NuvaRing®, a combined hormonal contraceptive vaginal ring manufactured by Merck®, releases 120 µg of etonogestrel and 15 µg of ethinyl estradiol daily. The vaginal ring is inserted once a month on the first day of the menstrual cycles. Once inserted inside the vagina, it is left in place for 3 weeks, followed by a 1-week break during which the users will have their menstrual period. This method is convenient as it does not require daily attention and is as effective as other hormonal contraceptive methods when used correctly. However, it does not provide protection against STIs. **Potential questions:** There can be questions related to various formulations of combined hormonal contraception methods such as pill, transdermal patches, vaginal ring etc. There can be questions related to the method of use, their mechanism of action, complications, etc.

<table>
<tr><th>Question</th><th>Answer</th><th>Comment</th></tr>
<tr><td>

Q17. A 28-year-old woman visits your clinic seeking a reliable contraceptive method that does not require daily administration. You suggest a method as shown in the image below. Which of the following statements about this device is correct?

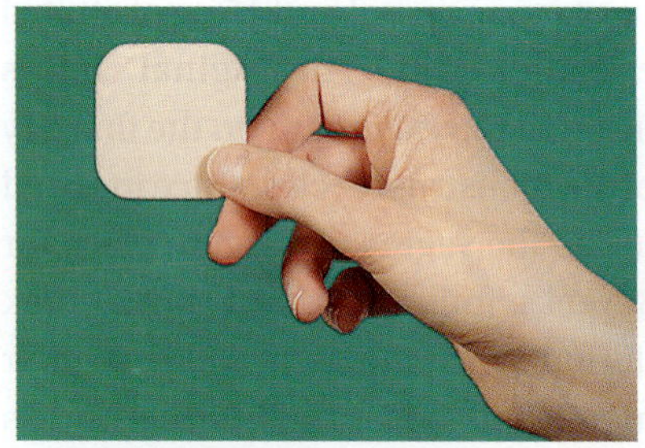

A. It needs to be changed daily
B. It is applied once a week for 3 weeks, followed by a device-free week
C. It is less effective than oral contraceptives
D. It must be applied to the same skin area repeatedly
E. It provides protection against sexually transmitted infections (STIs)

</td><td>

Ans: B (It is applied once a week for 3 weeks, followed by a device-free week)

The adjacent image shows contraceptive patch, a form of combined hormonal contraception. The transdermal patch releases hormones estrogen and progestin to prevent pregnancy. Various body parts where this patch can be applied are shown in **Figures 17A to D**.

It is applied to the skin once a week for 3 consecutive weeks, followed by a patch-free week during which the user has their menstrual period. This method is convenient for those who prefer not to take a daily pill.

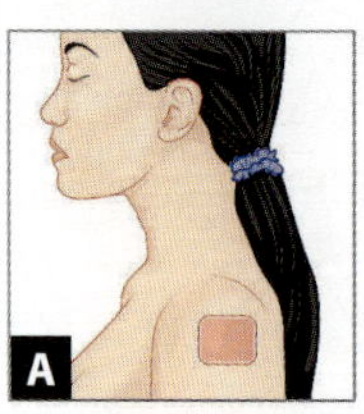

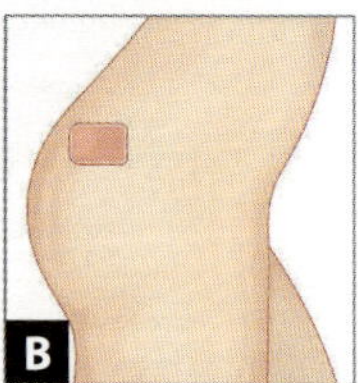

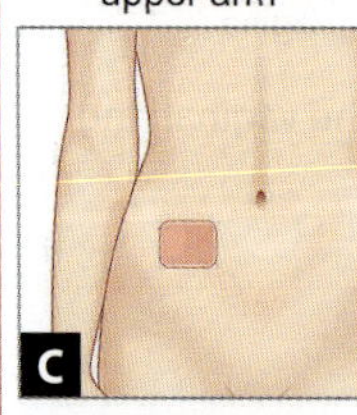

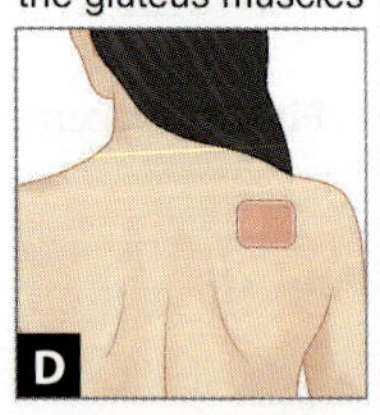

Figs. 17A to D: Placement of the contraceptive patch over the various body parts.

</td><td>

Explanation: Evra® Patch is the first transdermal patch contraceptive releasing 20 µg of estradiol and 150 µg of norelgestromin every 24 hours. Evra® was officially discontinued in the United States in 2017, with its phase-out occurring at different times in other regions. In many markets, Xulane® was introduced as the primary alternative, offering the same active ingredients (ethinyl estradiol and norelgestromin) and contraceptive efficacy.

Its efficacy, cycle control, and side-effect profile are similar to those of other COCPs. The patch is as effective as oral contraceptives when used correctly. It should be applied to a different skin area each week to avoid irritation. However, it does not provide protection against sexually STIs.

Potential questions: There can be questions related to various formulations of combined hormonal contraception such as pill, transdermal patches, vaginal ring etc. There can be questions related to the method of use, their mechanism of action, complications, etc.

</td></tr>
</table>

PERMANENT METHODS OF CONTRACEPTION

Laparoscopic Sterilization

Question	Answer	Comment
Q18. A 32-year-old woman undergoes tubal ligation using a device shown in the image below. Six months later, she presents with lower abdominal pain and a positive pregnancy test. Which of the following is the most likely explanation for her condition? 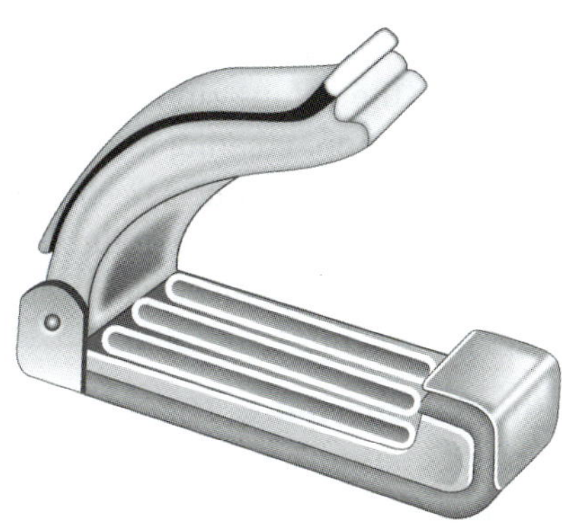 A. Incorrect placement of Filshie's clips B. Migration of Filshie's clips causing tubal recanalization C. Ectopic pregnancy unrelated to sterilization D. Filshie's clips removed in a later surgery E. Pregnancy existed at the time of sterilization	**Ans: B (Migration of Filshie's clips causing tubal recanalization)** The adjacent image shows Filshie's clips. Filshie's clips are silicone-lined titanium clips used for tubal ligation, which occlude the fallopian tubes by inducing avascular necrosis. The technique of tubal ligation using Filshie's clip **(Fig. 18)** is widely used in Canada, United Kingdom, and Australia and was first approved for use in the United States in 1997. 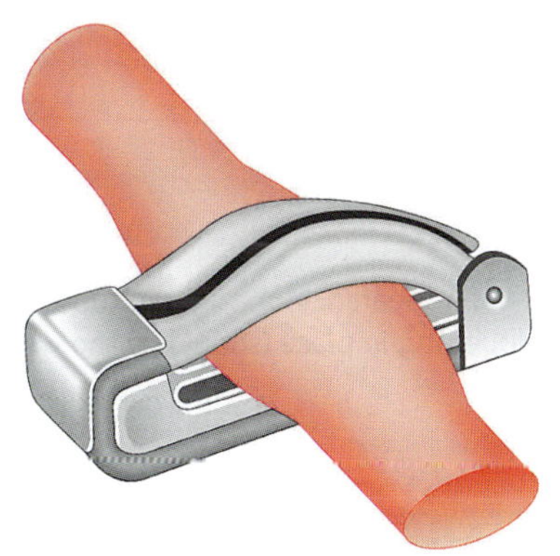 **Fig. 18:** Tubal ligation using Filshie's clip.	**Explanation:** The technique of tubal ligation using Filshie's clips involves application of a 12.7-mm long clip of titanium with a silicone rubber lining. The clip is applied laparoscopically with an applicator at right angles to the isthmus approximately 2–2.5 cm from the uterotubal junction. However, there is a rare possibility of the clips migrating from their original position, which can lead to tubal recanalization and subsequent pregnancy. This migration can cause the fallopian tubes to reopen, allowing for the possibility of fertilization and pregnancy. Proper placement and follow-up are crucial to ensure the effectiveness of the procedure. **Potential questions:** There can be different questions related to various permanent methods of sterilization, both male and female.

Question	Answer	Comment
Q19. A 35-year-old woman undergoes laparoscopic sterilization using the device shown in the image below. What is the primary mechanism by which this device achieves sterilization during a laparoscopic tubal ligation? 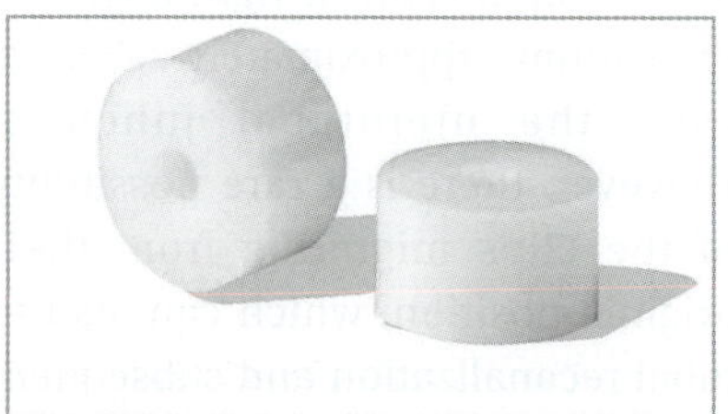 A. Electrocoagulation of the fallopian tubes B. Mechanical occlusion of the fallopian tubes C. Chemical sclerosing of the fallopian tubes D. Thermal ablation of the fallopian tubes E. Removal of a segment of the fallopian tubes	**Ans: B (Mechanical occlusion of the fallopian tubes)** The adjacent image shows Falope rings. These are small silastic (silicone rubber) bands used for tubal ligation during the process of female sterilization. **Figure 19** shows the appearance of ligated fallopian tube with a Falope ring in place. 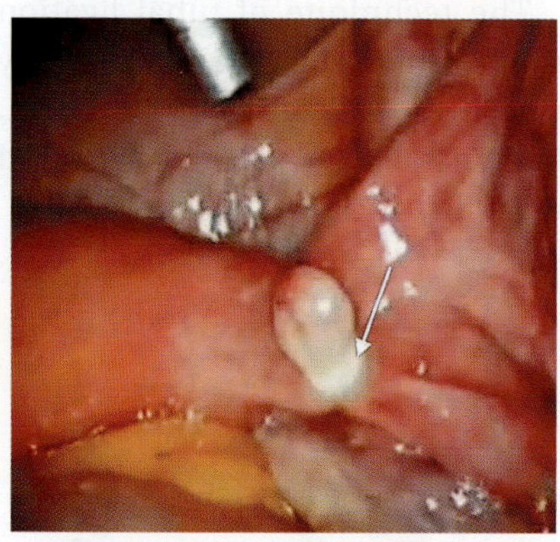 **Fig. 19:** Appearance of a ligated tube with a Falope ring in place (shown by the white arrow).	**Explanation:** Laparoscopic tubal ligation is most commonly used as an interval procedure for female sterilization. This procedure can be carried out using various techniques, such as electrodessication of tubes using electrosurgery or mechanical blockage of tubes using Falope rings or Filshie's clips. Falope rings achieve sterilization by mechanically occluding the fallopian tubes. During this procedure, a loop of the fallopian tube is drawn into the applicator, and the Falope ring is placed around the loop, creating a knuckle **(Fig. 19)**. This mechanical occlusion prevents the egg from traveling through the fallopian tube to meet the sperm, thereby preventing fertilization. **Potential questions:** There can be different questions related to various permanent methods of sterilization, (both male and female): The procedure, efficacy, and complications.

Question	Answer	Comment
Q20. A 35-year-old woman is considering permanent contraception and asks about the device shown in the image below. 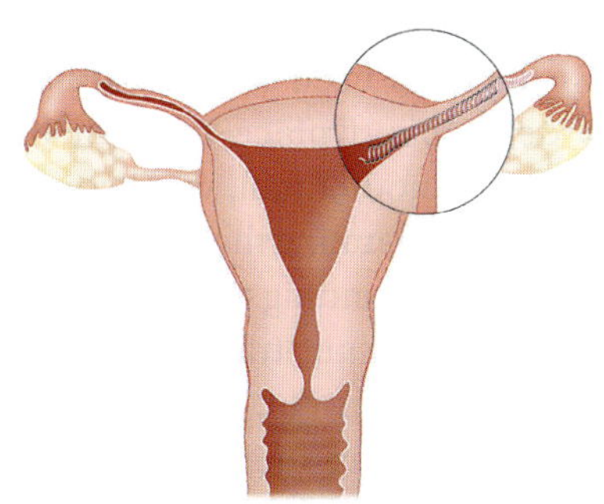 Which of the following statements about this device is correct? A. Hormonal contraceptive method B. Requires laparotomy for insertion C. Placement of flexible metal coil in fallopian tubes D. Provides immediate contraception E. Easily removable without surgery	**Ans: C (Placement of flexible metal coil in fallopian tubes)** The adjacent image depicts the Essure system, which is a nonhormonal, permanent contraceptive device that consists of small, flexible metal coils inserted into the fallopian tubes through the vagina and cervix, using a hysteroscope, without the need for an incision. **Figures 20A to C** depict the procedure of Essure hysteroscopic sterilization. 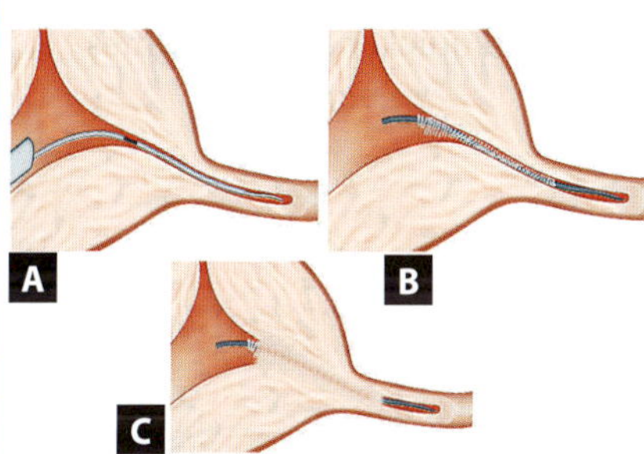 **Figs. 20A to C:** Essure hysteroscopic sterilization: A) Hysteroscopic cannulation of tubal lumen; (B) Microinsert device inserted inside the tubal ostium; (C) Fibrosis develops over the "Essure" Microinsert device over a period of time, resulting in tubal occlusion.	**Explanation:** Once the coils of the Essure system are in place, scar tissue forms around them, which blocks the fallopian tubes and prevents sperm from reaching the egg. It typically takes about 3 months for the scar tissue to form and for the device to become fully effective, so additional contraception is needed during this period. The device is designed to be permanent and is not easily removed. This method was designed as a less invasive alternative to tubal ligation. However, due to reports of complications such as chronic pain and device migration, the manufacturer, Bayer, discontinued its sale in 2018. **Potential questions:** There can be different questions related to various permanent methods of sterilization (both male and female): Procedure, efficacy, and complications.

Question	Answer	Comment
Q21. A 35-year-old male, father of two, in a stable relationship, is seeking permanent contraception. The surgeon performs the procedure using the instrument shown in the image below. Identify the primary advantage of the technique performed using this equipment in comparison to the traditional technique 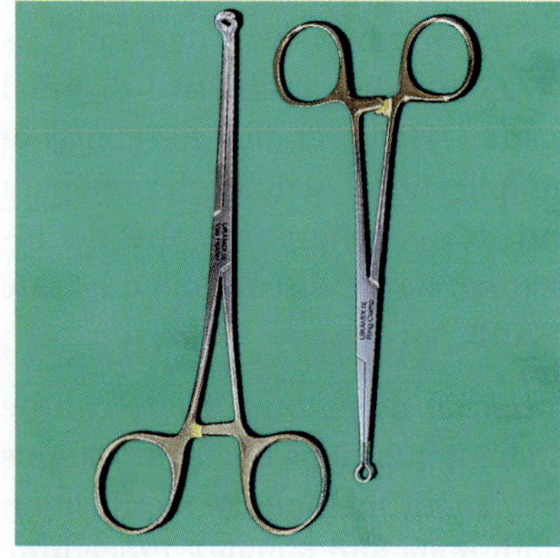 A. Reduced risk of postoperative hematomas B. Provides reversible contraception without additional procedures C. Eliminates the need for semen analysis post-procedure D. Increases the rate of spontaneous recanalization E. Enhances fertility in cases of obstructive azoospermia	**Ans: A (Reduced risk of postoperative hematomas)** The adjacent image shows vas ring clamp, a tool used for holding and stabilizing the vas deferens during the procedure of no-scalpel vasectomy (NSV). Being a noninvasive procedure, NSV technique is associated with several advantages over the traditional incisional method, the primary benefit being reduced risk of postoperative hematomas. It is also associated with fewer complications, including reduced pain, fewer infections, and quicker recovery times. 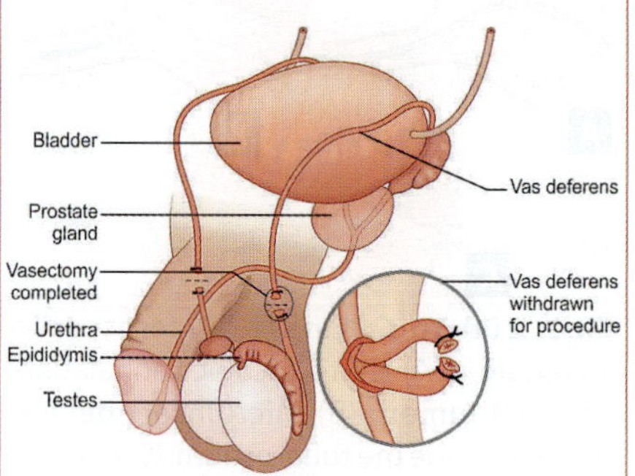 **Fig. 21:** Procedure of vasectomy.	**Explanation:** No-scalpel vasectomy is a minimally invasive procedure for male sterilization, which does not require incisions unlike traditional vasectomy. Instead, a small puncture is made in the scrotum. The vas ring clamp is used for holding the vas deferens in place through the puncture. Another tool, vas dissector is used for separating the vas deferens from the surrounding tissues without causing significant trauma. The vas deferens is then cut, and the ends are sealed using methods such as cauterization, tying, or clipping **(Fig. 21)**. Since the puncture is very small, no stitches are required and the wound heals on its own. Even with NSV, semen analysis is still required. The risk of recanalization is not increased. This is permanent, not reversible procedure and does not treat the causes of infertility. **Potential questions:** There can be different questions related to various permanent methods of sterilization, (both male and female): Procedure, efficacy, and complications.

CHAPTER 12

Infections of the Genital Tract

VAGINAL DISCHARGE

Question	Answer	Comment
Q1. A 35-year-old woman presents with complaints of vaginal itching, burning, and a thick, white discharge. She mentions that her symptoms worsen after taking antibiotics. The findings on per speculum examination are shown in the image below. Based on the clinical image and scenario, what is the most likely diagnosis? 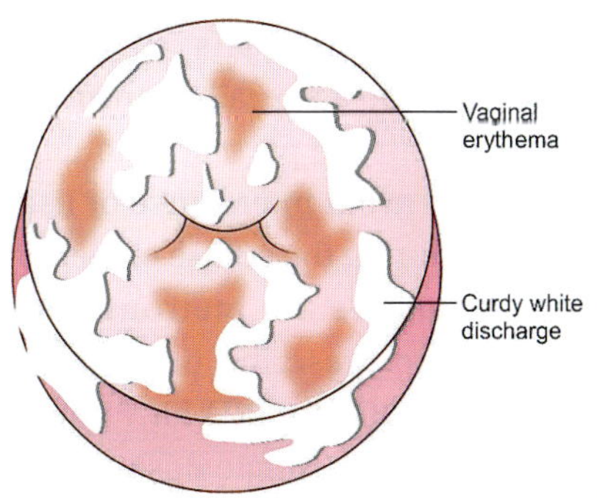 A. Bacterial vaginosis B. Trichomoniasis C. Candidal vaginitis D. Atrophic vaginitis E. Herpes simplex virus infection	**Ans: C (Candidal vaginitis)** The adjacent image shows presence of thick, white curdy discharge and vaginal erythema. These findings and the clinical features point the diagnosis of vulvovaginal candidiasis (VVC). Women with VVC frequently complain of pruritus, vaginal irritation, dysuria, vulvar and vaginal erythema, and occasionally scaling and fissures of vulvar tissue. Diagnosis is confirmed by microscopic examination of the wet mount and potassium hydroxide (KOH) preparations, showing budding yeast cells and pseudohyphae **(Fig. 1)**. 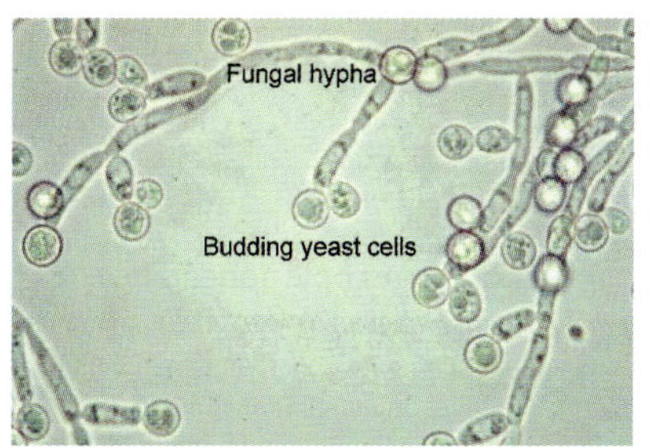 **Fig. 1:** Appearance of wet-mount preparation of *Candida albicans.*	**Explanation:** The infecting agent of candidal vaginitis, or vulvovaginal Candidiasis in most of the cases, is the yeast *Candida albicans.* This infection is characterized by symptoms such as intense itching, burning, and a thick, white, curd-like discharge. Pruritus vulva is a cardinal feature of this condition. This condition is often triggered or exacerbated by antibiotic use, which can disrupt the normal vaginal flora and allow *Candida* species to overgrow. Treatment usually involves antifungal medications, either topical or oral. Imidazoles and triazoles are presently the most extensively used antifungal drugs for treatment of VVC. Imidazole antifungal preparations, which can be used in the form of creams and pessaries for treatment of VVC, include butoconazole, clotrimazole, and miconazole. Triazole preparations include systemically acting agents such as fluconazole. **Potential questions:** There can be questions related to diagnosis and management of common vulvovaginitis encountered in women: Candidiasis, trichomoniasis, and bacterial vaginosis.

Question	Answer	Comment

Question

Q2. A 30-year-old woman presents with complaints of frothy, yellow-green vaginal discharge, vaginal itching, and a foul odor. She also reports pain during intercourse and urination. The appearance of cervix on per speculum examination is shown in the image below. Based on the clinical image and scenario, what is the most likely diagnosis?

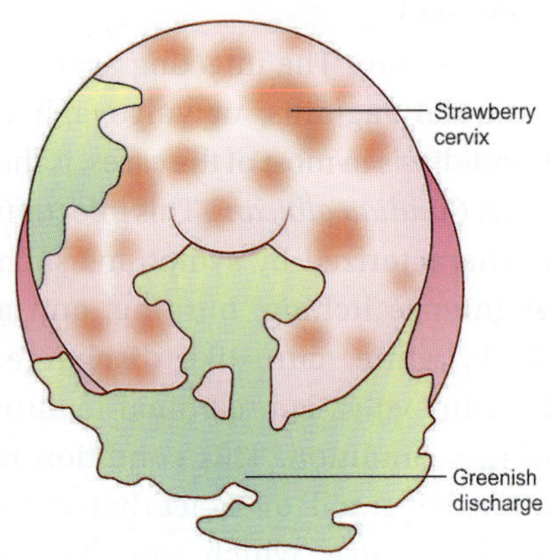

A. Bacterial vaginosis
B. Trichomoniasis
C. Candidal vaginitis
D. Atrophic vaginitis
E. Herpes simplex virus infection

Answer

Ans: B (Trichomoniasis)

The adjacent image shows presence of a greenish yellowish discharge along with strawberry cervix. This is characteristic of vaginal trichomoniasis. The typical discharge associated with this infection is profuse, purulent, thin, creamy or slightly green in color, irritating and frothy associated with pruritis and dysuria. The "strawberry cervix" appearance, which refers to punctate hemorrhages on the cervix, is a classic finding in trichomoniasis.

Microscopic examination of wet mounts showing motile trichomonads are **(Fig. 2)** is diagnostic of trichomonas infection.

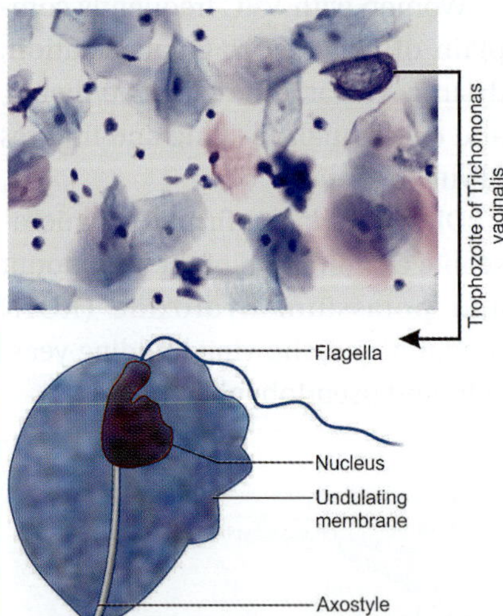

Fig. 2: Microscopic appearance of *Trichomonas vaginalis.*

Comment

Explanation: Trichomoniasis is a sexually transmitted infection caused by the motile protozoan parasite *Trichomonas vaginalis*. Besides the typical clinical presentation, the diagnosis is typically confirmed by microscopic examination of the vaginal discharge, which reveals motile trichomonads.

Additionally, tests using DNA probes, polymerase chain reaction tests, nucleic acid amplification test (NAAT), latex agglutination test, etc., which are associated with high rates of sensitivity and specificity, may also be performed.

Metronidazole in the dose of 200 mg TDS or 375 mg BID must be prescribed to both the partners for a period of 7 days. The Centers for Disease Control and Prevention (CDC), however, recommends a single dose of 2 g of metronidazole. Since trichomoniasis is largely believed to be a sexually transmitted disease, both the partners should be advised to avoid intercourse or use a condom during the course of therapy. An alternative to metronidazole could be to prescribe tinidazole in the dose of 300 mg BID for 7 days or secnidazole in a single dose of 1,000 mg daily for 2 days.

Potential questions: There can be questions related to diagnosis and management of common vulvovaginitis encountered in women: Candidiasis, trichomoniasis, and bacterial vaginosis.

Question	Answer	Comment
Q3. A 30-year-old woman presents with a complaint of abnormal vaginal discharge. The discharge is thin and grayish-white and has a fishy odor. The findings on per speculum examination are shown in the image below. What is the most likely diagnosis? 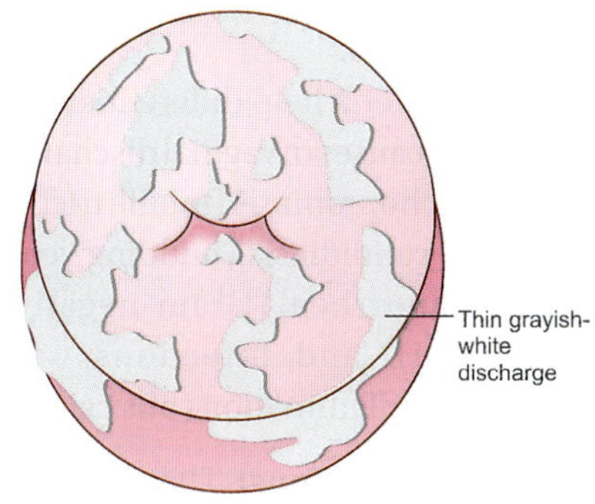 A. Trichomoniasis B. Candidiasis C. Bacterial vaginosis D. Gonorrhea E. Chlamydia	**Ans: C (Bacterial vaginosis)** The adjacent image shows presence of grayish-white vaginal discharge adherent to the vaginal walls. The clinical examination is otherwise normal. The discharge has a fishy odor, and the pH of discharge is more than 4.5. These are the characteristic features of bacterial vaginosis (BV). Another characteristic feature in these cases is the presence of positive whiff test **(Fig. 3)**. Initially also known as bacterial vaginitis, bacterial vaginosis is primarily caused due to the alteration of normal vaginal flora, rather than due to any specific infection. 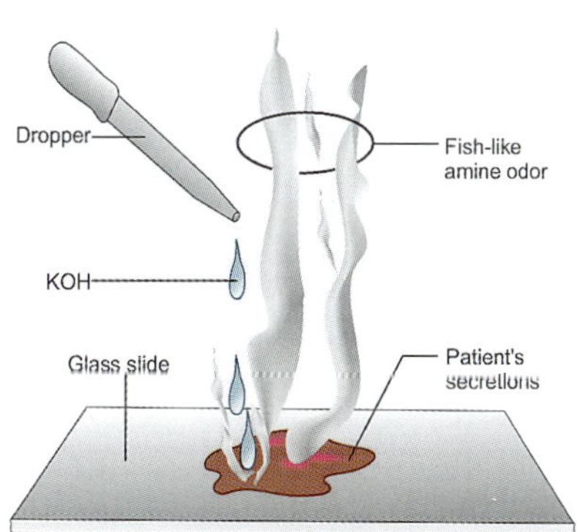 **Fig. 3:** Whiff test.	**Explanation:** Bacterial vaginosis is typically associated with a reduction in the number of the normal hydrogen peroxide-producing *Lactobacilli* in the vagina (which is toxic to other aerobic and anaerobic bacteria). The resultant change in pH allows proliferation of organisms that are normally suppressed such as *Hemophilus vaginalis, Gardnerella mobiluncus, Mycoplasma hominis, Gardnerella vaginalis, Peptostreptococcus* species, etc. This is responsible for causing bacterial vaginosis. The whiff test or the amine test **(Fig. 3)** is diagnostic of bacterial vaginosis and is performed using 10% KOH solution. The test is said to be positive if a fishy odor is produced when the discharge of a woman with bacterial vaginosis is mixed with 10% KOH solution. The fishy odor is produced due to production of amino metabolites from various organisms. Presence of clue cells in the wet mount is another characteristic feature of this disease. **Potential questions:** There can be questions related to diagnosis and management of common vulvovaginitis encountered in women: Candidiasis, trichomoniasis, and bacterial vaginosis.

Question	Answer	Comment
Q4. A 28-year-old woman presents with a complaint of abnormal vaginal discharge. The discharge is thin and white and has a fishy odor. A wet mount preparation of the vaginal discharge is shown in the image below. What is the most likely finding on this wet mount? 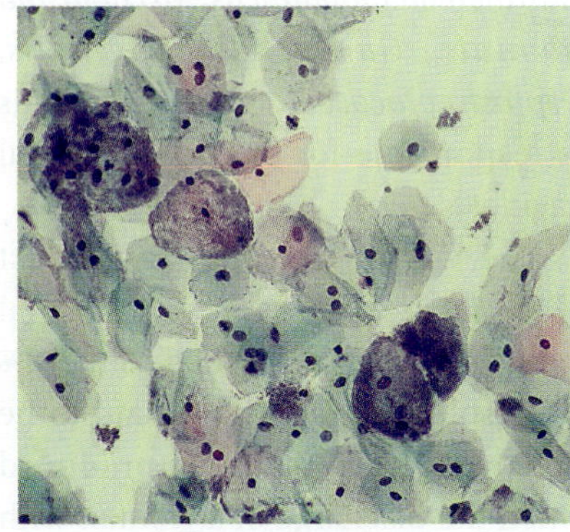 A. Motile trichomonads B. Budding yeast cells C. Clue cells D. Gram-negative diplococci E. Pus cells	**Ans: C (Clue cells)** The clinical features in the adjacent case are suggestive of bacterial vaginosis. A typical sign of bacterial vaginosis on microscopic examination is the presence of an unusual vaginal cell known as "clue cell" **(Fig. 4)**. Clue cells are vaginal epithelial cells covered with bacteria, giving them a stippled or a granular appearance. This finding is a hallmark of bacterial vaginosis. 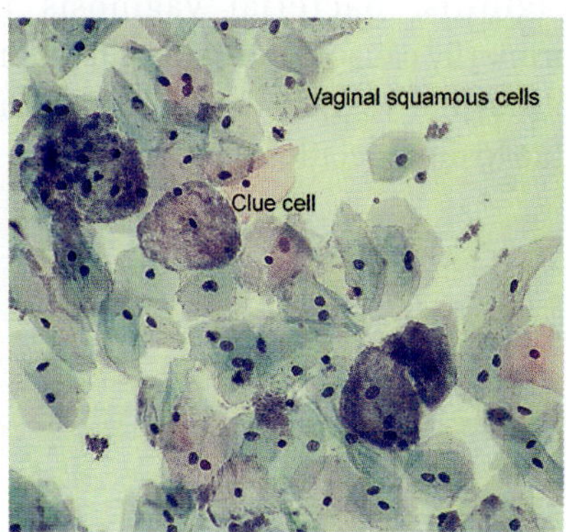 **Fig. 4:** Clue cells.	**Explanation:** Diagnosis of bacterial vaginosis can be established through Amsel's criteria, which require at least three of the following four signs: (1) homogeneous grayish-white vaginal discharge, (2) Positive Whiff test, where the addition of 10% potassium hydroxide produces a fishy odor, (3) Presence of clue cells on a saline wet mount, and (4) Vaginal pH greater than 4.5. These criteria help differentiate BV from other causes of vaginal discharge, such as trichomoniasis (motile trichomonads), candidiasis (budding yeast cells), gonorrhea (Gram-negative diplococci), and infections with significant inflammation (pus cells). **Potential questions:** There can be questions related to diagnosis and management of common vulvovaginitis encountered in women: Candidiasis, trichomoniasis, and bacterial vaginosis.

SEXUALLY TRANSMITTED DISEASES

Question	Answer	Comment
Q5. A 28-year-old woman presents with painful vesicular lesions on her vulva as shown in the image below. She reports a tingling sensation before the lesions appeared. What is the most likely diagnosis? 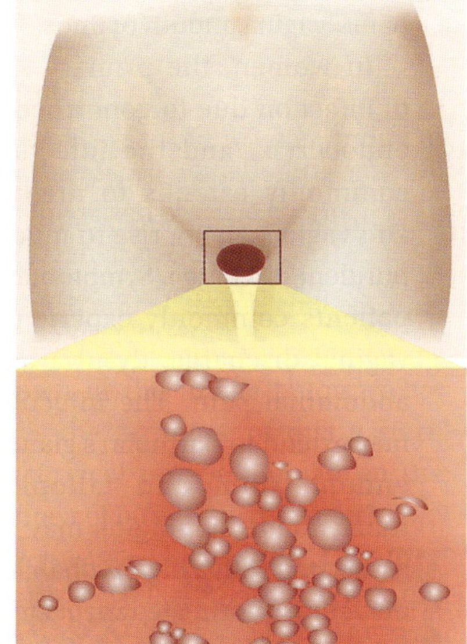 A. Syphilis B. Genital herpes C. Bacterial vaginosis D. Candidiasis E. Trichomoniasis	**Ans: B (Genital herpes)** The adjacent image shows the presence of small, vesicular reddish-white fluid-filled blisters on an erythematous base. This characteristic presentation is suggestive of genital herpes. These lesions may be painful or itchy and are often preceded by a prodrome of tingling, itching, or burning sensations. **Figure 5** shows the magnified view of these lesions. These vesicles can rupture, leading to shallow ulcers that eventually crust over and heal. The initial outbreak is usually the most severe and may be accompanied by systemic symptoms such as fever, malaise, and lymphadenopathy. 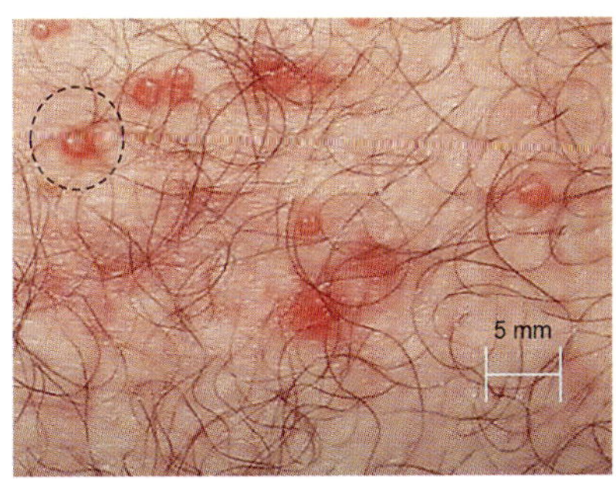 **Fig. 5:** Magnified view showing herpetic lesions in women.	**Explanation:** Genital herpes is caused by the herpes simplex virus (HSV), typically HSV-2. This virus is transmitted through sexual contact. The virus enters through mucous membrane of the genital tract via microscopic tears. From there the virus travels to the nerve roots near the spinal cord and settles down permanently. The primary infection may be associated with constitutional symptoms like fever, malaise, vulval paresthesia, itching or tingling sensation on the vulva and vagina followed by redness of the skin. Finally, the formation of blisters and vesicles begins, which eventually develop into shallow and painful ulcers within a period of 2–6 weeks. In women, these lesions may appear on the vulva, vagina, cervix, perianal area, or inner thigh and are frequently accompanied by itching and a mucoid vaginal discharge. When the blisters break, they are usually very painful to touch. **Potential questions:** There can be questions related to the clinical presentation, diagnosis, and management of lesions related to various sexually transmitted diseases.

Question	Answer	Comment
Q6. A 30-year-old woman presents with vaginal pruritus and mucopurulent discharge as shown in the image below. On pelvic examination, the cervical os is erythematous and bleeds easily upon contact. Based on the image provided, what is the most likely diagnosis? 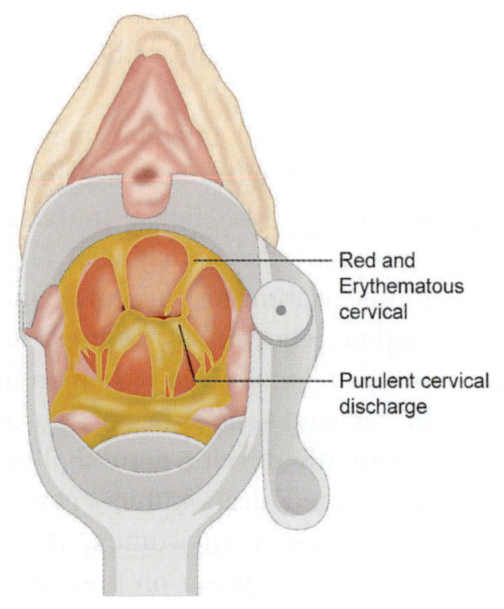 A. Bacterial vaginosis B. Trichomoniasis C. Gonorrhea D. Chlamydia E. Genital herpes	**Ans: C (Gonorrhea)** The adjacent image shows mucopurulent cervical discharge, which is a hallmark of cervicitis. The cervix may appear erythematous and friable, bleeding easily upon contact. This is likely to be suggestive of gonorrhea. This infection can also cause vaginal pruritus and intermenstrual bleeding. Early diagnosis and treatment are crucial to prevent complications such as pelvic inflammatory disease, infertility, and chronic pelvic pain. Various lesions of gonorrhea in women are illustrated in **Figure 6**. 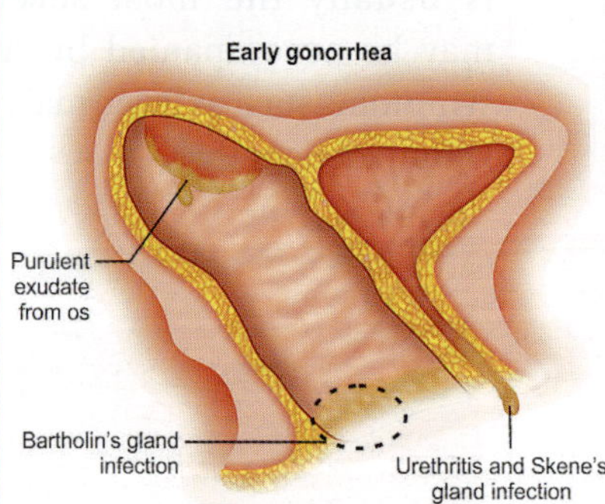 **Fig. 6:** Lesions due to early gonorrhea infection.	**Explanation:** Gonorrhea is a sexually transmitted disease, which is caused by the bacterium *Neisseria gonorrhoeae.* The disease is characterized by adhesion of the gonococci to the surface of urethra or other mucosal surfaces. Gonorrhea is spread through contact with the penis, vagina, mouth or anus. In women, the primary site of infection due to gonorrhea is endocervix, and the infection commonly extends to urethra and vagina, giving rise to mucopurulent discharge. Symptomatic patients commonly experience vaginal discharge, dysuria and abdominal pain. The infection may extend to Bartholin's glands, endometrium and fallopian tubes. Acute salpingitis may be associated with a high probability of sterility, if not treated adequately. **Potential questions:** There can be questions related to the clinical presentation, diagnosis, and management of lesions related to various sexually transmitted diseases.

Question	Answer	Comment
Q7. A 28-year-old woman presents with a painless ulcer on her labia that has been present for 3 weeks. She reports having unprotected sexual intercourse with a new partner about a month ago. The physical examination reveals a firm, round, and nontender ulcer as shown in the image below. What is the most likely diagnosis? 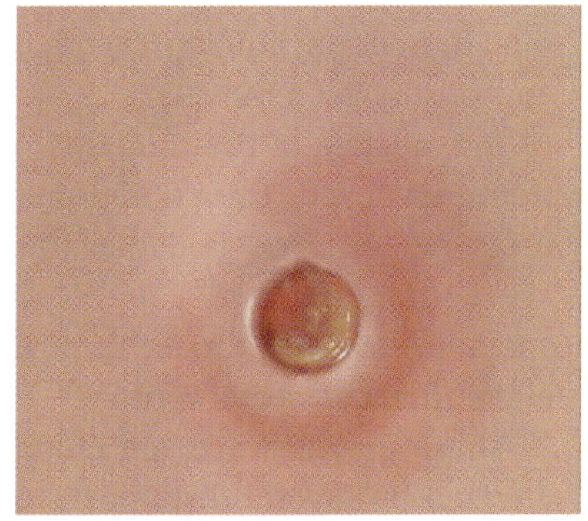 A. Genital herpes B. Chancroid C. Hard chancre of syphilis D. Genital warts E. Molluscum contagiosum	**Ans: C (Hard chancre of syphilis)** The presence of a painless ulcer and the patient's history of unprotected sexual intercourse strongly suggest primary syphilis. The adjacent image shows a hard chancre, the primary lesion of syphilis. The hard chancre typically appears as a firm, round, relatively avascular, circumscribed, indurated, painless, and superficially ulcerated lesion at the site of infection, usually on the genitals, within 3 weeks of exposure. In women, it can be found on the labia, cervix, or vaginal walls. The ulcer is nontender and has a clean base, which helps differentiate it from other STIs like chancroid (which is painful) and genital herpes (which presents with multiple painful vesicles). 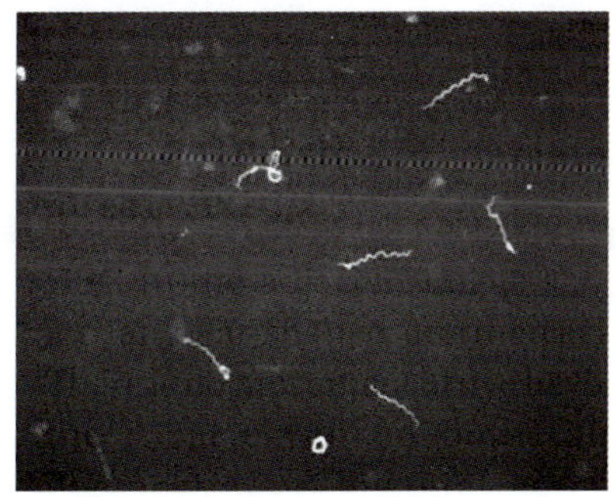 **Fig. 7:** Appearance of treponema pallidum under dark ground microscopy.	**Explanation:** Syphilis is a sexually transmitted disease caused by the bacterium *Treponema pallidum* **(Fig. 7)**. It is typically characterized by three stages: Primary, secondary, and tertiary. Primary lesions appear approximately 10–90 days after the initial exposure. Primary lesion of syphilis, also known as a hard chancre, often appears at the point of contact, usually the external genitalia. The "hard chancre" of syphilis usually persists for about 4–6 weeks and heals spontaneously. Syphilis is usually diagnosed based on the results of serological tests such as Kahn test, venereal disease research laboratory (VDRL) test, rapid plasma reagin test, etc. A single dose of benzathine penicillin G (2.4 million units) intramuscularly is sufficient for the treatment of primary, secondary or latent syphilis of less than 1 year duration. An alternative to penicillin is oral doxycycline 100 mg BID. **Potential questions:** There can be questions related to the clinical presentation, diagnosis and management of lesions related to various sexually transmitted diseases.

<table>
<tr><th>Question</th><th>Answer</th><th>Comment</th></tr>
<tr>
<td>Q8. A 26-year-old woman presents with multiple flesh-colored, verrucous papules on her vulva as shown in the image below. She reports that the lesions have been increasing in number over the past few weeks and are sometimes painful during intercourse. What is the most likely diagnosis?
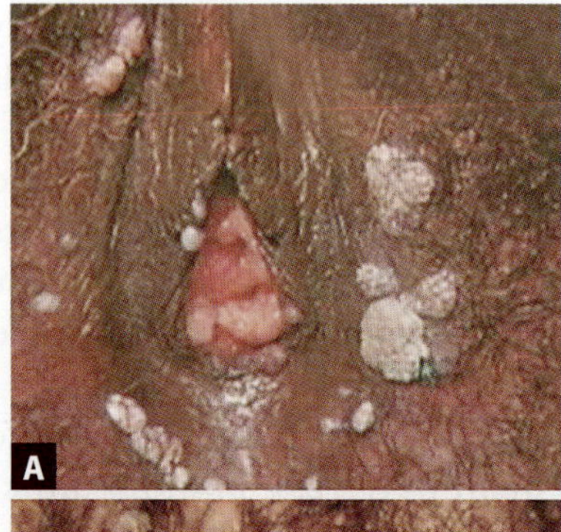
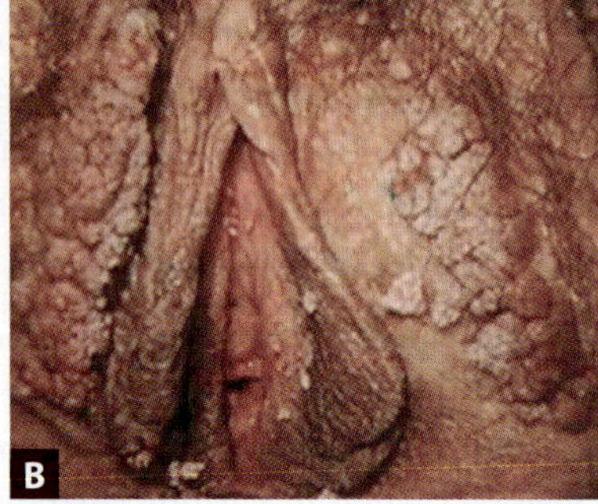
A. Genital herpes
B. Chancroid
C. Condyloma acuminatum
D. Genital warts
E. Molluscum contagiosum</td>
<td>Ans: C (Condyloma acuminatum)
The adjacent image shows soft, flesh-colored, verrucous papules on the external genitalia, perianal skin, perineum, or groin suggestive of condyloma acuminatum. Being a sexually transmitted disease, it commonly develops at the sites of sexual contact or trauma such as urogenital and anogenital regions. The lesions appear as broad-based pink masses, whose surface is covered with short, blunted projections, resulting in a raspberry or mulberry-like appearance. Condylomas can be multiple and clustered, with the average size of the lesions being about 1–1.5 cm.
Figure 8 shows the histological appearance of condyloma acuminatum
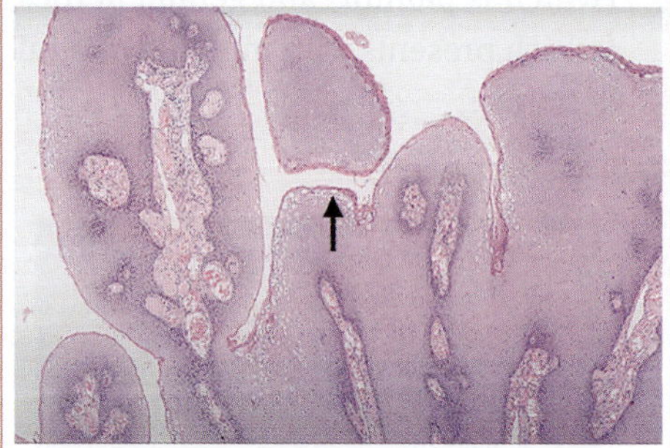
Fig. 8: Histological appearance of condyloma acuminatum (arrow indicating the koilocytes).</td>
<td>Explanation: Condyloma acuminatum, also known as anogenital warts, is caused by the human papillomavirus (HPV), primarily types 6 and 11. These lesions can be painful and itchy or cause discomfort during sexual intercourse. The diagnosis is usually clinical, based on the characteristic appearance of the lesions. Treatment options include topical agents like imiquimod or podophyllotoxin, cryotherapy, or surgical removal.
Irrespective of the modality of treatment used, the condylomas must be removed because they are contagious and capable of spreading to other surface through either direct or sexual contact.
These genital warts are characterized by several distinct histopathological features (Fig. 8) such as epidermal acanthosis (thickening of the epidermis), papillomatosis, koilocytes (vacuolated keratinocytes with shrunken nuclei), hyperkeratosis, and parakeratosis.
Potential questions: There can be questions related to the clinical presentation, diagnosis, and management of lesions related to various sexually transmitted diseases.</td>
</tr>
</table>

PELVIC INFLAMMATORY DISEASE

Question	Answer	Comment
Q9. A 25-year-old woman presents with acute right upper quadrant abdominal pain, fever, and a history of PID. A contrast-enhanced CT scan shows perihepatic enhancement. The gynecologist considers a rare complication involving the liver and plans for appropriate diagnostic laparoscopy which reveals the image shown below. What is the most likely diagnosis? 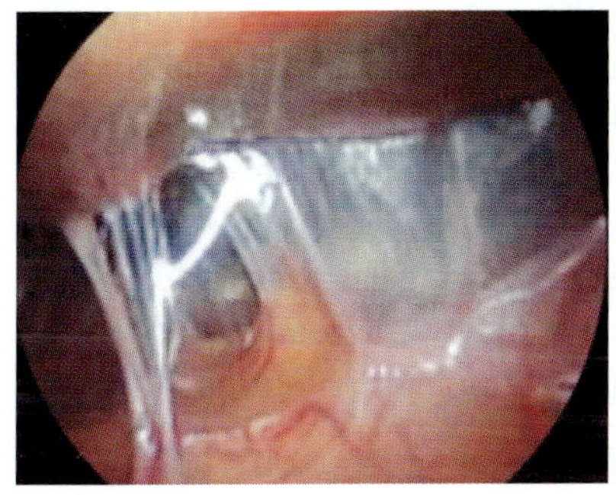 A. Cholecystitis B. Hepatitis C. Fitz-Hugh-Curtis syndrome D. Pulmonary embolism E. Appendicitis	**Ans: C (Fitz-Hugh-Curtis syndrome)** The adjacent image shows the presence of typical violin-string adhesions between the liver and parietal peritoneum on laparoscopic examination. This finding as well as the clinical presentation and the history of PID suggests the diagnosis of Fitz-Hugh-Curtis syndrome. This syndrome is characterized by the presence of acute-onset right quadrant pain in the abdomen. This may increase upon breathing, coughing, sneezing, etc. Symptoms of pelvic infection such as nausea, vomiting, chills, fever, headache, etc., may also be present. The diagnosis is usually confirmed on laparoscopy which shows the typical violin string adhesions **(Fig. 9)**. 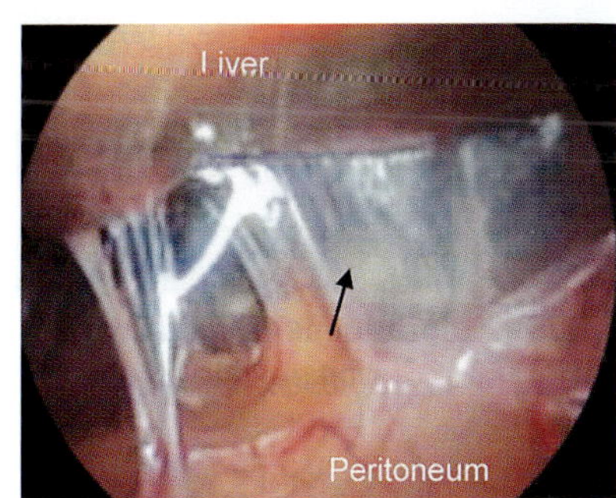 **Fig. 9:** Fitz-Hugh-Curtis syndrome (shown by the arrow).	**Explanation:** Fitz-Hugh-Curtis syndrome is characterized by perihepatic inflammation. It is usually caused by pelvic inflammatory disease, often due to *Chlamydia trachomatis* or *Neisseria gonorrhoeae* infection. This infection may rarely result in peritoneal spread from pelvis to liver causing perihepatic inflammation. This leads to the development of characteristic violin string adhesions between the liver and the abdominal wall. The CT scan typically shows perihepatic enhancement, which helps identify perihepatic inflammation. Laparoscopy remains the gold standard investigation of choice for confirming the diagnosis. Management of this syndrome primarily comprises the treatment of underlying gonococcal/chlamydial infection. The violin string adhesions may require laparoscopic excision. **Potential questions:** There can be different questions related to the diagnosis, management, and potential complications associated with PID.

Question	Answer	Comment
Q10. A 32-year-old woman presents with lower abdominal pain, fever, and vaginal discharge. A pelvic ultrasound reveals findings as shown in the image below. What is the most likely diagnosis? 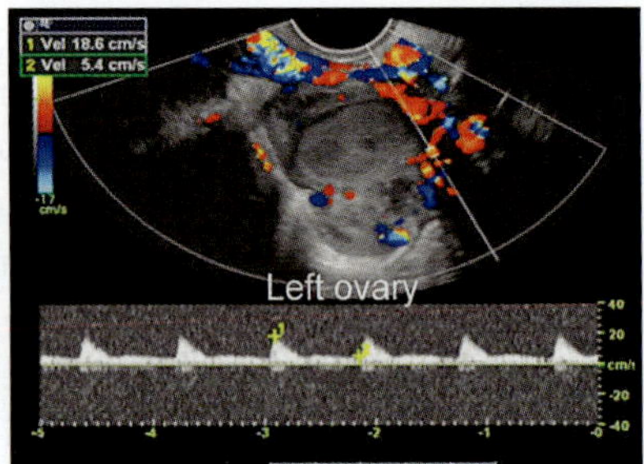 A. Ovarian cyst B. Ectopic pregnancy C. Tubo-ovarian abscess D. Endometrioma E. Uterine fibroid	**Ans: C (Tubo-ovarian abscess)** The adjacent transvaginal sonography shows a complex cystic-solid adnexal mass with thick irregular walls and septations. On color flow Doppler, there is prominent vascular perfusion with low-moderate vascular impedance. A diagnosis of tubo-ovarian abscess (TOA) was established based on clinical presentation and the ultrasound findings. **Figure 10** demonstrates the laparoscopic appearance of a TOA. Laparoscopy not only helps in the diagnosis of a TOA, but can also be useful for therapeutic purposes. 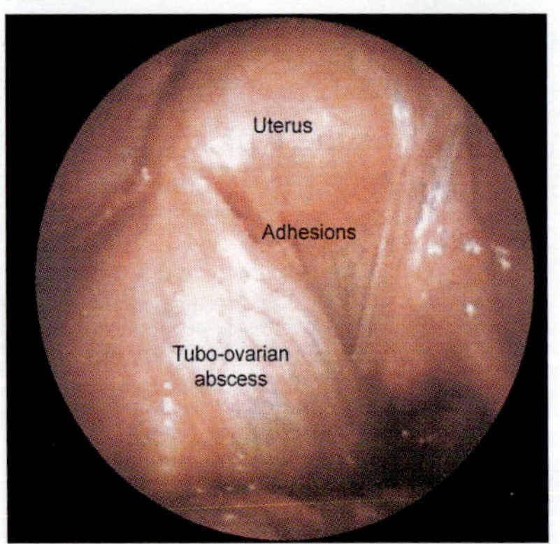 **Fig. 10:** Laparoscopic appearance of a tubo-ovarian abscess.	**Explanation:** Tubo-ovarian abscess can be defined as the collection of pus involving the tubes and the ovary. It is a serious complication of PID and is characterized by an inflammatory mass involving the fallopian tube, ovary, and sometimes adjacent pelvic organs. It typically presents with lower abdominal pain, fever, and vaginal discharge. This condition requires prompt medical or surgical intervention to prevent severe complications such as rupture and sepsis. For evaluation of cases of tubo-ovarian abscess, transvaginal rather than transabdominal approach is preferable. Surgery is rarely required in cases of PID. However, it may be required in the following cases of TOA: Drainage of a pelvic abscess, presence of a pyoperitoneum, ruptured TOA, etc. **Potential questions:** There can be different questions related to the diagnosis, management, and potential complications associated with PID.

Question	Answer	Comment
Q11. A 32-year-old woman presents with a history of infertility and intermittent pelvic pain. A transvaginal ultrasound is performed, revealing findings shown in the image below. What is the most likely diagnosis? 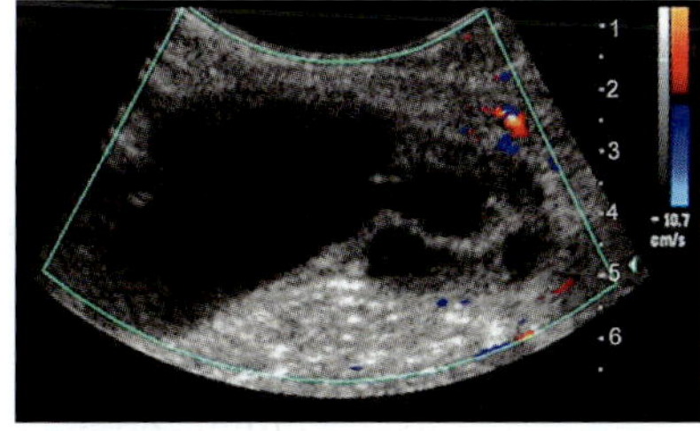 A. Ovarian cyst B. Ectopic pregnancy C. Hydrosalpinx D. Endometrioma E. Pelvic inflammatory disease (PID)	**Ans: C (Hydrosalpinx)** The adjacent transvaginal ultrasound image shows presence of a retort-shaped, fluid-filled, elongated, tubular structure in the adnexal region, distinct from the ovary. This mass appears to be arising from the fallopian tubes and is suggestive of hydrosalpinx. Presence of peripheral vascularization and poor vascularization of septa on Doppler sonography is also highly indicative of a hydrosalpinx. The presence of thin-walled, longitudinal folds/septa, which may produce a "cogwheel" appearance, and the "waist sign" are pathognomonic features of hydrosalpinx. **Figure 11** shows diagrammatic representation of hydrosalpinx. 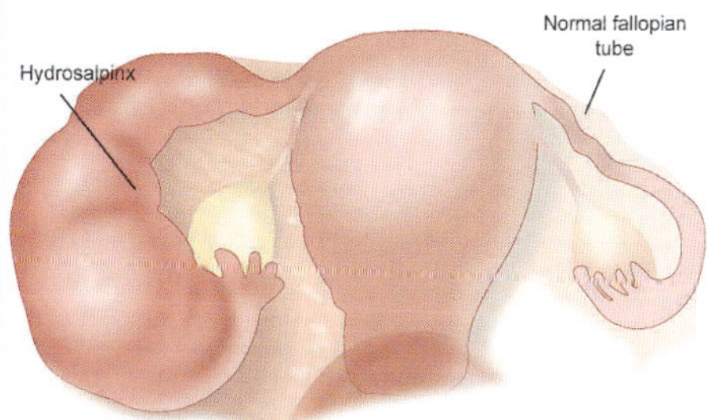 **Fig. 11:** Diagrammatic representation of a hydrosalpinx.	**Explanation:** Hydrosalpinx refers to a fluid-filled dilatation of the fallopian tube, often resulting from an obstruction at the distal end of the tube. Formation of peritoneal adhesions secondary to PID can compromise the motility of fallopian tubes. Furthermore, obstruction of the distal end of the fallopian tubes due to adhesions results in accumulation of the normally secreted tubal fluid, creating distension of the tube. This subsequently causes damage to the epithelial cilia and may result in development of hydrosalpinx. The major clinical significance of a hydrosalpinx is its adverse effect on fertility, thereby resulting in a reduced pregnancy rate. A hydrosalpinx, although sterile, can be re-infected later leading to formation of a pyosalpinx. **Potential questions:** There can be different questions related to the diagnosis, management, and potential complications associated with PID.

SECTION 3

Obstetrics and Gynecology

CHAPTER 13

Imaging in Obstetrics and Gynecology

NORMAL ANATOMY ON ULTRASOUND

Question	Answer	Comment
Q1. A 32-year-old woman presents for a routine gynecological checkup. She has a regular 28-day menstrual cycle and is currently on day 12 of her cycle. A transvaginal ultrasound is performed, which shows findings depicted in the image below. Based on the transvaginal ultrasound image, what do the findings indicate? 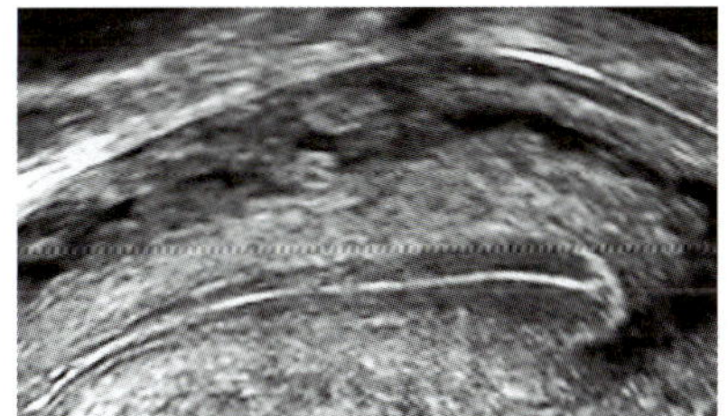 A. Thin, bright endometrium with a single-layered appearance B. Thick, echogenic endometrium with homogeneous texture C. Trilaminar endometrium D. Endometrium measuring < 4 mm E. Endometrium > 4 mm	**Ans: C (Trilaminar endometrium)** The adjacent transvaginal sonography (TVS) image of the uterus depicts the proliferative phase, showing the presence of a well-defined "three-line sign". This trilaminar appearance is a normal finding, typically observed in women of reproductive age group around the time of ovulation. During this phase, the ovary may show the presence of a dominant follicle **(Fig. 1)** with several other follicles in different stages of development. 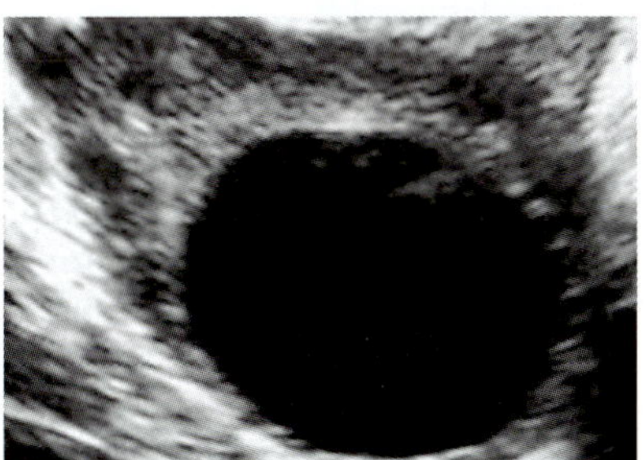 **Fig. 1:** Ovary showing the presence of a dominant follicle.	**Explanation:** In the proliferative phase on TVS, the endometrium appears as a trilaminar pattern, meaning it has three distinct layers: An inner echogenic layer, a central hypoechoic layer, and an outer echogenic layer. The central hyperechoic reflection represents the endometrial cavity and the additional hyperechoic reflections represent the thin developing layer of the endometrium on either side. The outer lines represent the interface between endometrium and myometrium. There is a hypoechogenic functional layer. The general hypoechogenic character of the functional layer of the proliferative endometrium is related to the simple configuration of the glands and blood vessels. There is minimal or absent posterior acoustic enhancement during this phase. **Potential questions:** There can be questions related to normal anatomical findings of the internal reproductive organs in both premenopausal women during various phases of menstrual cycle and postmenopausal women.

Question	Answer	Comment
Q2. Based on the below transvaginal ultrasound image showing the endometrium during the luteal phase of the menstrual cycle, what is the most likely normal finding? 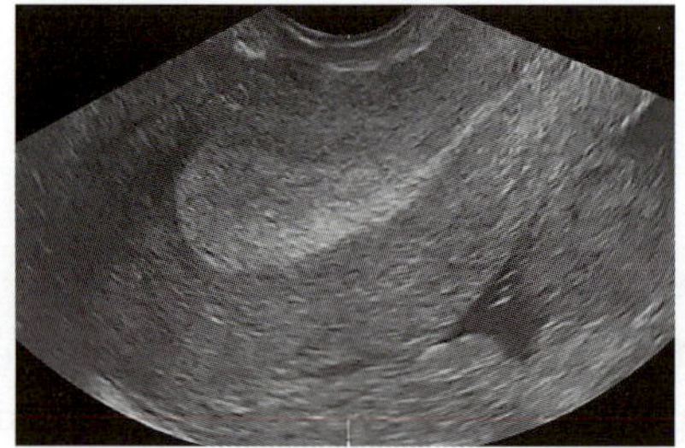 A. Thin endometrium with a trilaminar appearance B. Thick, echogenic endometrium with homogeneous texture C. Endometrium measuring < 4 mm with no corpus luteum D. Trilaminar endometrium with a dominant follicle in one ovary E. Endometrium with cystic degeneration and irregular thickness	**Ans: B (Thick, echogenic endometrium with homogeneous texture)** The adjacent transvaginal sonography image depicts the endometrium in luteal phase showing uniformly hyperechogenic endometrium. In the immediate pre and postovulatory period (2 days postovulation), an additional inner hyperechogenicity of variable thickness, which corresponds to a relatively high fluid content of these inner functional layers, can be seen with TVS **(Fig. 2A)**. **Figures 2B and C** show corpus luteum, which appears during this phase. It presents as an echogenic structure within the ovary with prominent peripheral vascularization. 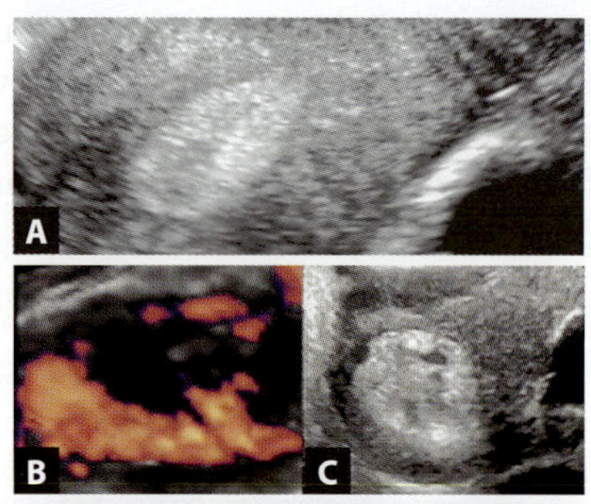 **Figs. 2A to C:** (A) Transvaginal sonography in the luteal phase showing uniformly hyperechogenic endometrium; (B and C) Two small pictures in the bottom half show corpus luteum, which appears as an echogenic structure within the ovary with prominent peripheral vascularization.	**Explanation:** During the luteal phase of the menstrual cycle (which typically occurs after ovulation, from days 15 to 28), the endometrium becomes more thickened and echogenic due to progesterone secretion by the corpus luteum. This phase prepares the endometrium for potential implantation, resulting in a homogeneous, bright appearance on TVS. The total double-layer thickness in the luteal phase ranges from 4 to 12 mm with an average of 7.5 mm. During this phase, there is presence of posterior acoustic enhancement and "three-line sign" is absent. The presence of a corpus luteum in one of the ovaries during this phase is also a normal finding, as it forms after ovulation to maintain hormonal support until the next cycle or pregnancy. **Potential questions:** There can be questions related to normal anatomical findings of the internal reproductive organs in both premenopausal women during various phases of menstrual cycle and postmenopausal women.

EARLY PREGNANCY SCANS

Question	Answer	Comment
Q3. The transvaginal image below depicts a 6-week-old gestational sac. What is the clinical significance of identifying the structure marked with an arrow at this gestational age? 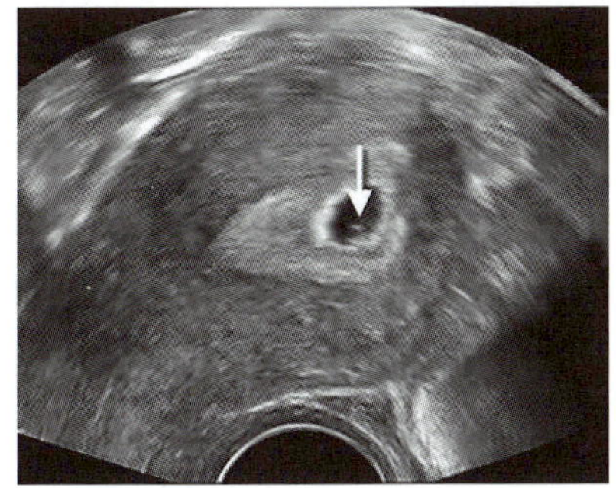 A. It confirms a viable intrauterine pregnancy. B. It indicates an ectopic pregnancy. C. It suggests a molar pregnancy. D. It is a sign of a missed abortion. E. It indicates a blighted ovum.	**Ans: A (It confirms a viable intrauterine pregnancy)** The arrow in the adjacent image shows the presence of yolk sac in the gestational sac at 6 weeks. At 4–5 weeks, before the embryo or yolk sac is visible, a **double-rimmed gestational sac** indicates intrauterine pregnancy **(Fig. 3)**. It results from two echogenic decidual layers (capsularis and parietalis) separated by an anechoic space. 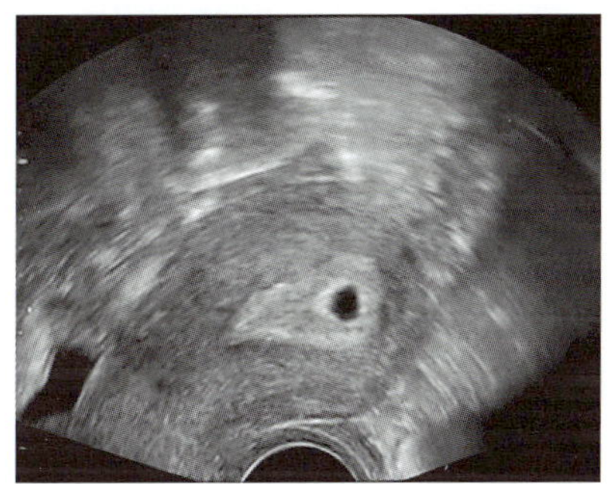 **Fig. 3:** Transvaqinal scan demonstrating an intrauterine pregnancy at 5 weeks of gestation showing a double-rimmed gestational sac.	**Explanation:** In a normal intrauterine pregnancy, the yolk sac normally appears by 5–6 weeks of gestation whereas the embryo appears at about 6 weeks of gestation. The yolk sac appears as a round sonolucent structure surrounded by a bright rim. The presence of a yolk sac helps to confirm that the pregnancy is intrauterine and viable at this early stage. Yolk sac does not increase to a size >6 mm in case of a normal pregnancy. The pregnancy may be abnormal if no yolk sac appears at the gestational sac size of 10 mm or no fetal pole is seen at the gestational sac size of 18 mm. **Potential questions:** There can be questions related to features of normal and abnormal scans encountered during early gestation.

Question	Answer	Comment
Q4. What is the main clinical significance of the red-marked parameter on first-trimester TVS as shown in the image below? 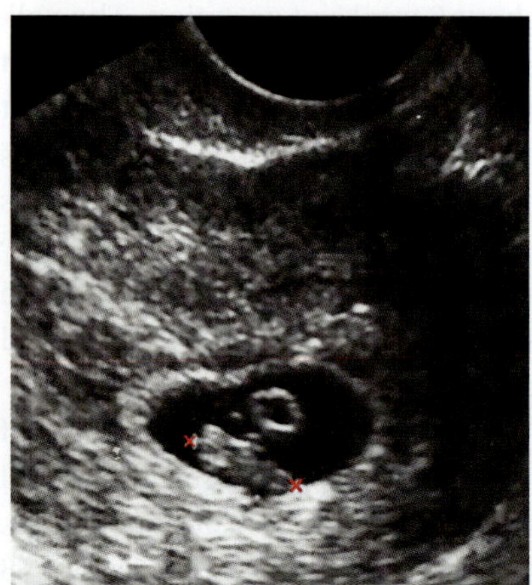 A. Confirm gestational age/EDD B. Assess chromosomal abnormality risk C. Assess miscarriage risk D. Detect structural anomalies E. Diagnose multiple gestations	**Ans: A (Confirm gestational age/ EDD)** The red marks in the adjacent image depict the measurement of crown–rump length (CRL). The CRL is an ultrasonic measurement, which is made earliest in pregnancy, when the gestational age is between 7 to 13 weeks. A diagrammatic representation of CRL is shown in **Figure 4**. 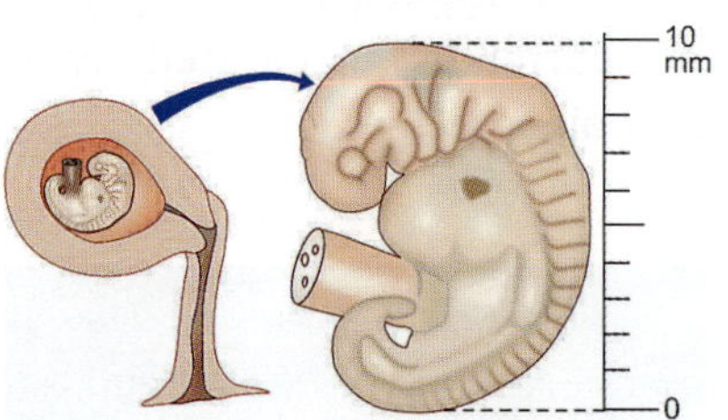 **Fig. 4:** Diagrammatic measurement of the crown–rump length.	**Explanation:** The CRL is the most accurate measurement for determining gestational age in the first trimester. It is the longest length of the fetus excluding the limbs and the yolk sac. It is about 1 mm at 5 weeks and 4 mm at 6 weeks of normal gestation. **Potential questions:** There can be questions related to various important fetal diameters and measurements.

Question	Answer	Comment
Q5. What is the clinical significance of identifying the placental grade as shown in the transvaginal ultrasound image below? 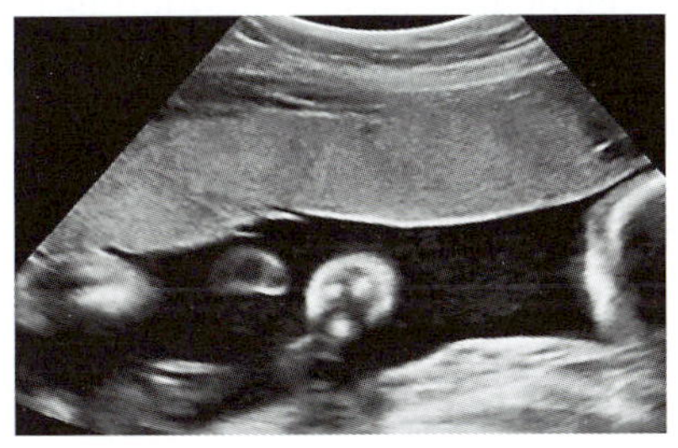 A. It indicates placental abruption B. It suggests a high risk of preterm labor C. It is a normal finding in early pregnancy D. It indicates placenta previa E. It suggests intrauterine growth restriction (IUGR)	**Ans: C (It is a normal finding in early pregnancy)** The adjacent transvaginal ultrasound image shows grade 0 placenta on the ultrasound, placed anteriorly in the fundal region. Placenta is recognized by the presence of chorionic plate. The grading of the placenta is based on its maturity, with Grade 0 being the least mature. As the pregnancy progresses, the placenta matures and its grade increases. Therefore, identifying a Grade 0 placenta in the fundal region on a transvaginal ultrasound can be considered as a normal finding in early pregnancy. **Figure 5** shows grade 2 placenta with deeper coma-like indentations (marked by the whiite arrow), increasing calcifications in the form of hyperechogenic areas and echogenic basal plate. 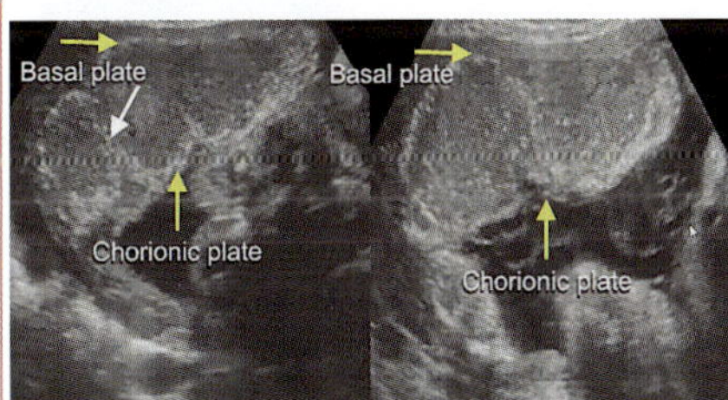 **Fig. 5:** Grade 2 placenta.	**Explanation:** Grading of placenta is as follows: *Grade 0 placenta (first and second trimesters):* It has uniform echogenicity with a smooth chorionic plate without indentations. *Grade I placenta (mid-second trimester to early third trimester):* The chorionic plate shows subtle indentations. There are small diffuse calcifications randomly dispersed throughout the placenta *Grade II placenta (late third trimester):* The indentations throughout the chorionic plate become larger and calcifications also become more prominent. *Grade III placenta (39 weeks to postdated):* Complete indentations of the chorionic plate reaching all the way to the basilar plate are present. This results in the formation of cotyledons with a significant increase in the number of calcifications. **Potential questions:** There can be questions related to features of normal and abnormal scans encountered during early gestation. There can also be questions related to different placental grades.

Question	Answer	Comment
Q6. What is the clinical significance of visualizing the fetal structure as shown in the two-dimensional transvaginal image below? 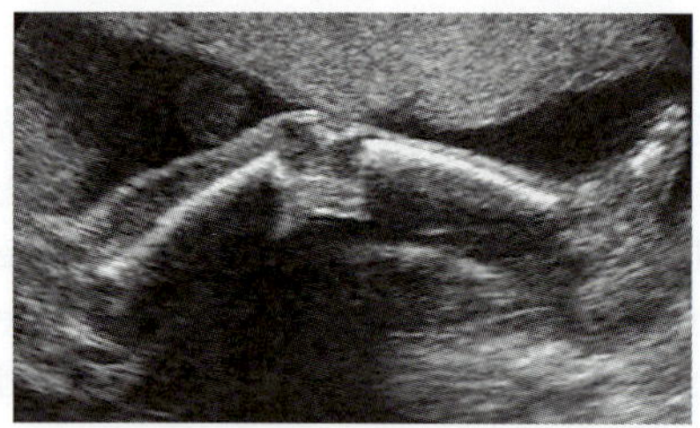 A. It confirms the presence of fetal movement B. It indicates a high risk of limb abnormalities C. It suggests that the fetus is in a breech position D. It is a normal finding in the second trimester E. It indicates oligohydramnios	**Ans: D (It is a normal finding in the second trimester)** The adjacent transvaginal two-dimensional ultrasound scan demonstrates the left lower limb of a 24-week-old fetus with the hip and knee semiextended and feet showing presence of five toes. **Figure 6** shows the three-dimensional ultrasound image of fetal feet. Toes of the feet must be carefully examined for the presence of any abnormalities such as abnormalities in alignment, big toe abnormalities, abnormalities in size and number of toes, etc. 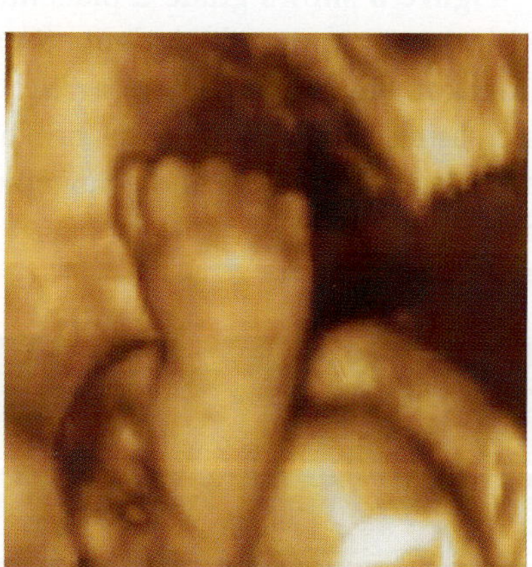 **Fig. 6:** Three-dimensional ultrasound image of fetal feet.	**Explanation:** Visualizing the fetal lower limb on a two-dimensional transvaginal ultrasound is a normal finding, especially in the second trimester when the fetus is more developed and its limbs are more easily seen. This imaging helps in assessing the growth and development of the fetus, including the limbs. It does not necessarily indicate any abnormalities or complications. Regular monitoring through ultrasound helps ensure that the fetus is developing normally and can help detect any potential issues early on. **Potential questions:** There can be questions related to features of normal and abnormal scans encountered during various stages of gestation.

Question	Answer	Comment
Q7. When visualizing a structure on Doppler ultrasound as shown in the image below, which of the following is the most accurate method to ensure a clear and reliable signal related to this structure? 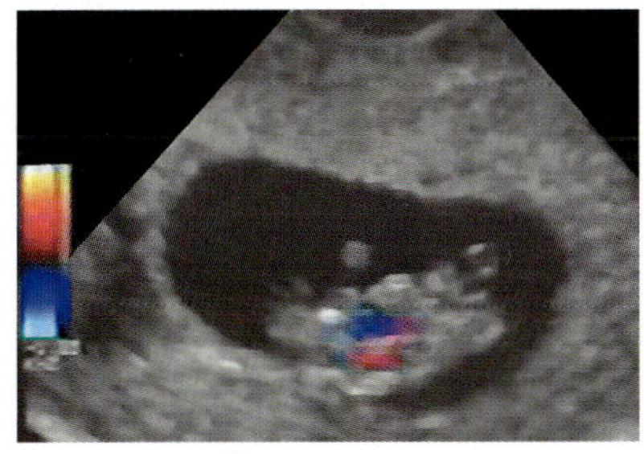 A. Place the transducer at the maternal umbilicus. B. Use a high-frequency transducer. C. Position the transducer over the fetal back. D. Apply minimal pressure with the transducer. E. Use continuous-wave Doppler mode.	**Ans: C (Position the transducer over the fetal back)** The adjacent image shows presence of fetal heart at 8 weeks of gestation as observed on color Doppler examination. Fetal heart can be observed on TVS by 6–7 weeks of gestation. A detailed four-chamber view (with or without Doppler; **Fig. 7**) can help in delineation of various cardiac defects. 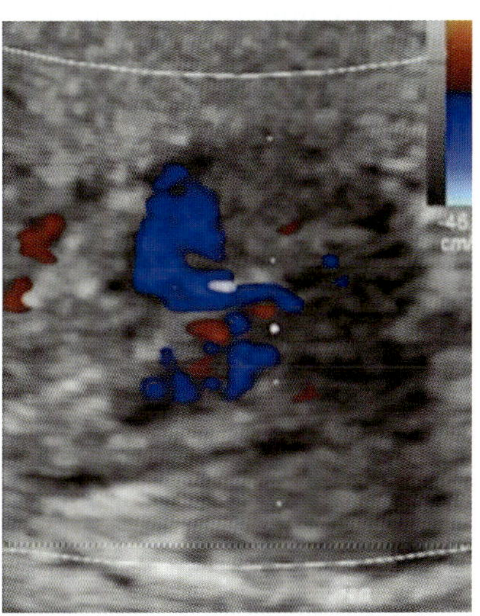 **Fig. 7:** Four-chamber view by color Doppler imaging at 9-week gestation.	**Explanation:** Positioning the transducer over the fetal back is the most accurate method to ensure a clear and reliable signal when detecting the fetal heart using Doppler ultrasound. This is because the fetal back provides a stable and consistent surface that allows for better transmission and reception of the Doppler signals. In the occiput anterior positions of the fetal head especially, the fetal heart is closer to the back, making it easier to detect the heartbeat. In most of the cases, by the time the embryo measures 2 mm, fetal heart activity may be clearly seen and is as high as 85 beats per minute (BPM), which may increase to 100–175 BPM by 5–9 weeks of gestation. If the fetal pole measures 5 mm or more with no heartbeat, diagnosis of miscarriage is usually made. **Potential questions:** There can be different questions related to features of normal and abnormal structures encountered on scans during various stages of gestation.

<table>
<tr><th>Question</th><th>Answer</th><th>Comment</th></tr>
<tr><td>Q8. What is the clinical significance of measuring the parameter as indicated by the arrow in below image?
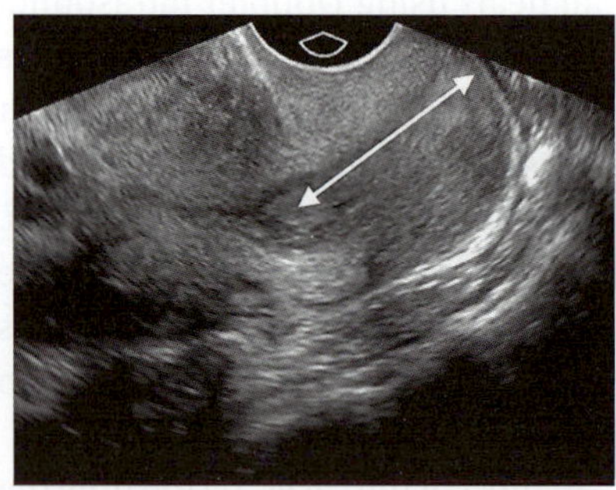
A. It helps diagnose cervical incompetence
B. It indicates the position of the placenta
C. It confirms fetal gender
D. It suggests the presence of gestational diabetes
E. It indicates the presence of multiple pregnancies</td><td>Ans: A (It helps diagnose cervical incompetence)
The arrow in the adjacent image depicts normal cervical length as measured on transvaginal sonography. Measuring cervical length on ultrasound examination is important for assessing the risk of preterm birth. A short cervix (<25 mm) on two occasions at 14–24 weeks of gestation can indicate cervical incompetence, potentially leading to preterm labor or miscarriage. Figure 8 shows normal cervical length as measured on transabdominal sonography (TAS).
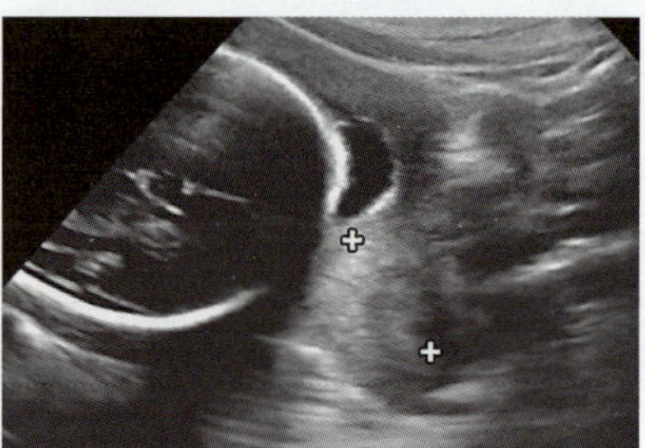
Fig. 8: Normal cervical length as measured on transabdominal sonography.</td><td>Explanation: Regular monitoring of cervical length can help in early identification and management of cervical incompetence, including implementation of interventions like cervical cerclage or progesterone therapy to reduce the risk of preterm birth. This measurement is typically performed during the second trimester and involves measuring the whole length of cervical canal between the external and internal os. Transvaginal sonography (TVS) is more accurate than TAS in measuring the length of cervical canal.
Potential questions: There can be different questions related to features of normal and abnormal structures encountered on scans during various stages of gestation</td></tr>
</table>

NORMAL MID-LATE PREGNANCY SCAN

Question	Answer	Comment
Q9. What is the primary purpose of evaluating the structure shown in the below images during a second-trimester ultrasound? 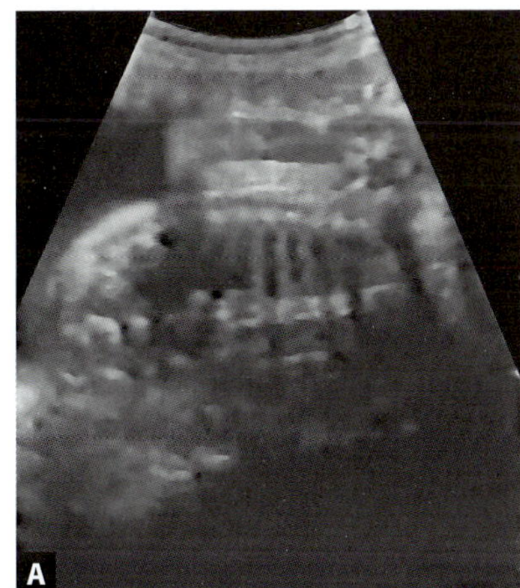 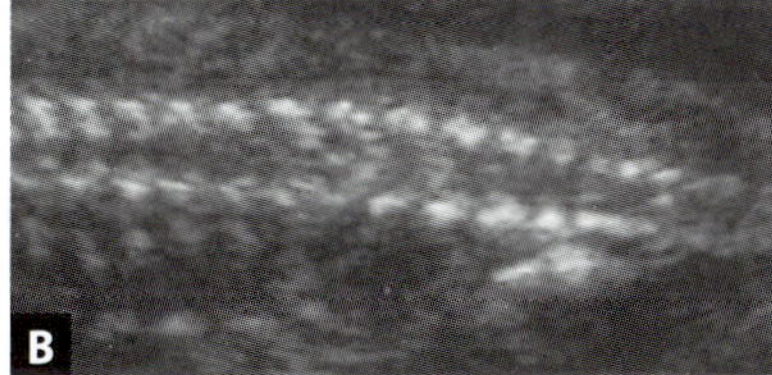 A. To assess fetal heart rate B. To determine fetal position C. To detect neural tube defects D. To measure amniotic fluid volume E. To estimate fetal weight	**Ans: C (To detect neural tube defects)** The adjacent images show fetal spine in longitudinal section (A) and coronal view (B) Evaluating the fetal spine during a second-trimester ultrasound is primarily aimed at detecting neural tube defects, such as spina bifida. This involves examining the alignment and closure of the vertebrae to ensure that there are no gaps or abnormalities. Early detection of these defects is important for planning appropriate medical care and interventions, both during pregnancy and after birth. The optimal time for evaluation of fetal spine is 12–16 weeks of gestation. **Figure 10** shows the three-dimensional ultrasound scan of a 16-week-old fetus. 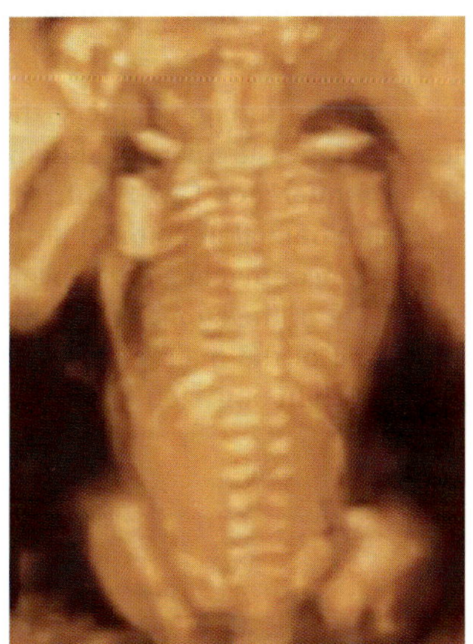 **Fig. 10:** Three-dimensional ultrasound scan of a 16-week-old fetus showing fetal spine.	**Explanation:** Neural tube defects of the central nervous system can be considered as one of the most common congenital malformations. Most scans aimed toward diagnosing the neural congenital anomalies are done around midgestation (at about 20 weeks of pregnancy). Longitudinal section of the fetal spine must be performed because it helps in revealing various spinal malformations such as vertebral anomalies and sacral agenesis. Longitudinal section of the spine (at about 14 weeks) demonstrates three ossification centers (one inside the body and one at the junction between the lamina and pedicle on each side). These appear as three parallel lines depending upon the orientation of ultrasound beams. Attempts must also be made to demonstrate the intactness of the skin overlying the spine. Presence of a mass bulging out must also be observed. **Potential questions:** There can be different questions related to features of normal and abnormal structures encountered on scans during various stages of gestation.

Question	Answer	Comment
Q10. What is the clinical significance of measuring the diameter as depicted by the dotted line on ultrasound examination during pregnancy as shown in the image below? 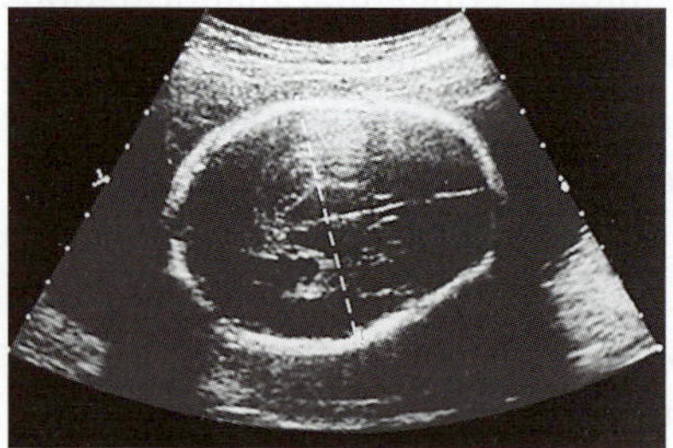 A. Determine the gestational age (GA) B. It indicates the presence of neural tube defects C. It confirms the position of the fetus D. It suggests the presence of polyhydramnios E. It indicates fetal anemia	**Ans: A Determine the GA** The adjacent image shows the measurement of biparietal diameter (BPD). BPD can be measured at level of the plane defined by frontal horns of lateral ventricles and cavum septum pellucidum anteriorly, falx cerebri in the midline, thalami symmetrically positioned on either side of falx in the center, and occipital horns of lateral ventricles, Sylvian fissure, cisterna magna, and insula posteriorly **(Fig. 9)**. 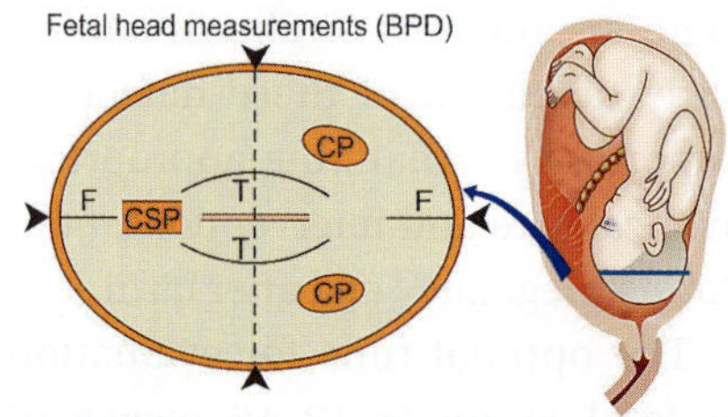 **Fig. 9:** Diagrammatic measurement of fetal biparietal diameter. (CP: choroid plexus; CSP: cavum septum pellucidum; F: falx; T: thalamus)	**Explanation:** Biparietal diameter is the distance between the two sides of the head. Accurate measurement of BPD is crucial for determining the gestational age, monitoring fetal growth, and identifying any potential growth abnormalities. It is one of the key biometric parameters used in prenatal care to ensure that the fetus is developing appropriately. The measurement is taken from the outer table of the proximal skull to the inner table of the distal skull with the cavum septum pellucidum perpendicular to the ultrasound beam. **Potential questions:** There can be questions related to various important fetal diameters and measurements.
Q11. When measuring the fetal circumference on ultrasound as shown in the image below, which of the following steps is important for obtaining an accurate measurement? 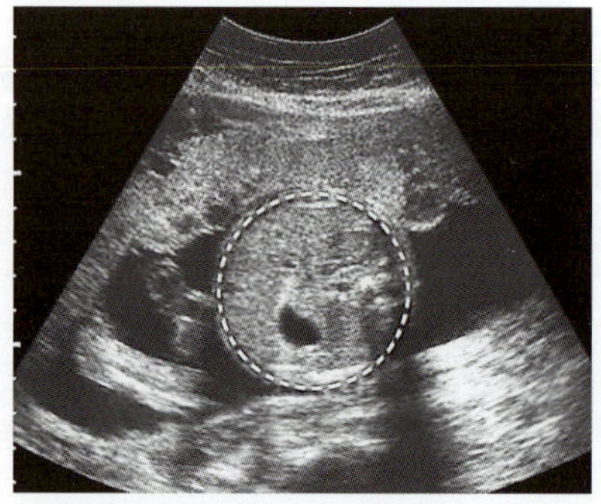 A. Measure the circumference at the level of the fetal kidneys B. Ensure that the image is as round as possible, avoiding an ovoid shape C. Include the limbs D. Use excessive pressure with the transducer to get a clear image E. Measure the circumference at the level of the fetal heart	**Ans: B (Ensure that the image is as round as possible, avoiding an ovoid shape)** The adjacent image depicts the ultrasound measurement of abdominal circumference (AC), which is a measure of fetal abdominal girth. The AC is measured in an axial plane at the level of the stomach and the bifurcation of the main portal vein into the right and left branches **(Fig. 11)**. 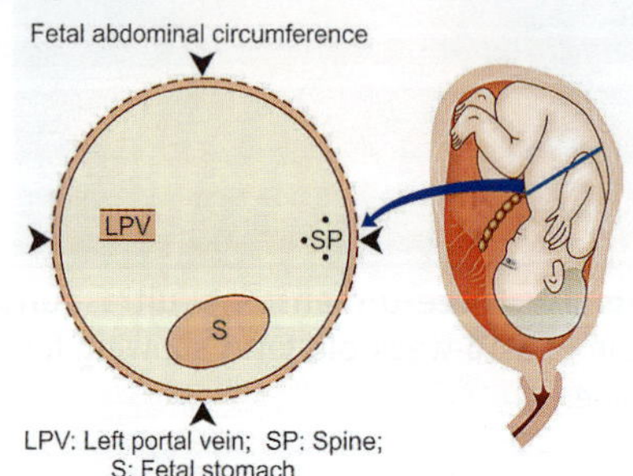 **Fig. 11:** Diagrammatic measurement of fetal abdominal circumference.	**Explanation:** To accurately measure the fetal AC on ultrasound, it is essential to obtain a cross-sectional image of the fetal abdomen that is as round as possible. This ensures that the measurement is taken at the correct anatomical level, typically where the umbilical vein enters the liver and the stomach is visible. Avoiding an ovoid shape helps in reducing measurement errors and provides a more accurate assessment of fetal growth. **Potential questions:** There can be questions related to various important fetal diameters and measurements.

Question	Answer	Comment
Q12. When measuring the measurement on ultrasound as depicted in the image below, which of the following steps is important for obtaining an accurate measurement? 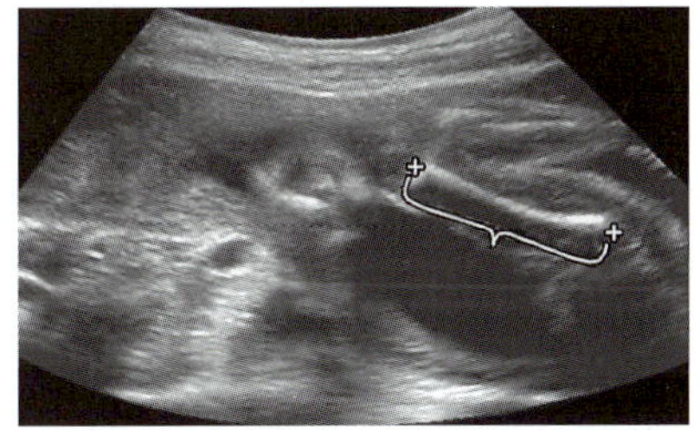 A. Measurement must be done at an oblique angle to the ultrasound beam B. Include the distal femur point in the measurement C. Ensure that both ends of the bone are clearly visualized and measure in a straight line D. Use excessive pressure with the transducer to get a clear image E. Measure at level of fetal kidneys	**Ans: C (Ensure that both ends of the femur are clearly visualized and measure in a straight line)** The adjacent TVS image shows measurement of femur length (FL), which is the length of femoral diaphysis, the longest bone in the body and represents the longitudinal growth of the fetus. Femur appears as an echogenic structure on ultrasound examination. At the time of measuring femur length, the femoral diaphysis should be horizontal showing a homogeneous echogenicity. 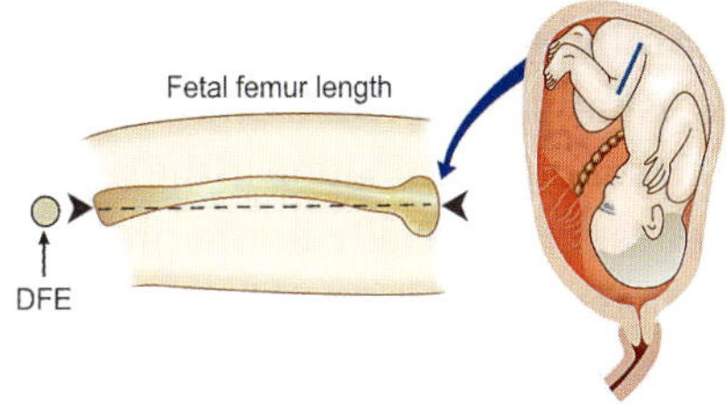 **Fig. 12:** Diagrammatic measurement of the femoral length. (DFE: distal femoral epiphysis)	**Explanation:** To accurately measure the FL on ultrasound, it is essential to visualize both the proximal and distal ends of the femur clearly. The measurement should be taken in a straight line, not following the curvature of the bone **(Fig. 12)**. This ensures that the length is measured accurately, reflecting the true size of the femur. Avoiding oblique angles and excessive pressure with the transducer helps in obtaining a precise measurement. **Potential questions:** There can be questions related to various important fetal diameters and measurements.
Q13. Which step is correct for accurately measuring fetal transverse cerebellar diameter (TCD) on ultrasound as shown? 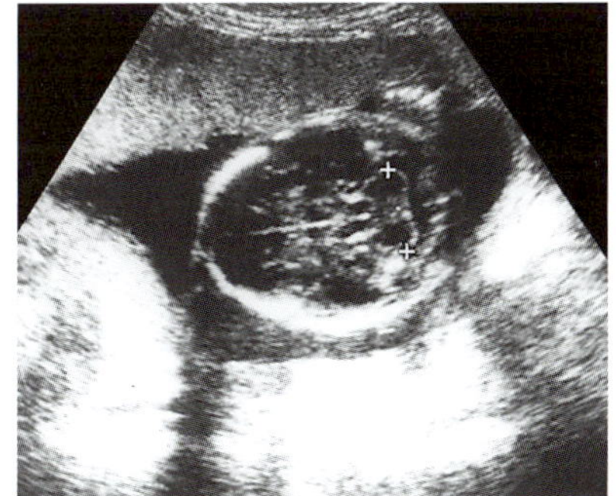 A. Measure at fetal medulla oblongata B. Include thalami and cavum septi pellucidi C. Measure in an oblique plane D. Use excessive transducer pressure E. Visualize cerebellum in axial plane and place calipers at outer margins	**Ans: E (Visualize cerebellum in axial plane and place calipers at outer margins)** The adjacent image demonstrates measurement of TCD, which refers to the widest diameter of cerebellum. The ultrasound appearance of cerebellum seems to progressively change from an eyeglass (grade I, **Fig. 13**) to dumbbell (grade II), and finally to "fan" shape (grade III) with advancing gestational age. 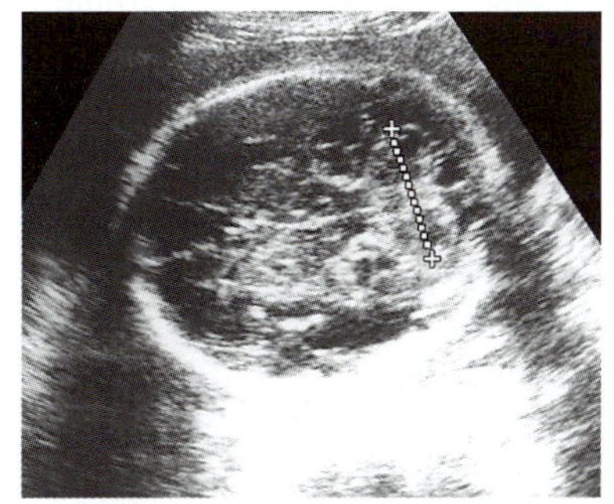 **Fig. 13:** Grade I appearance of cerebellum.	**Explanation:** To accurately measure the TCD on ultrasound, it is essential to obtain an axial view of the fetal head. The cerebellum should appear as a peanut-shaped structure, and the measurement should be taken at the widest diameter across the cerebellar hemispheres. Proper placement of the calipers at the outer margins of the cerebellum ensures an accurate assessment of the TCD. The major advantage of measuring cerebellar diameter is that this parameter allows for the estimation of gestational age that is independent of the shape of the fetal head, throughout the pregnancy. **Potential questions:** There can be questions related to various important fetal diameters and measurements.

Question	Answer	Comment
Q14. When measuring the fetal heart rate (FHR) using M-mode ultrasound as shown in the image below, which of the following steps is important for obtaining an accurate measurement? 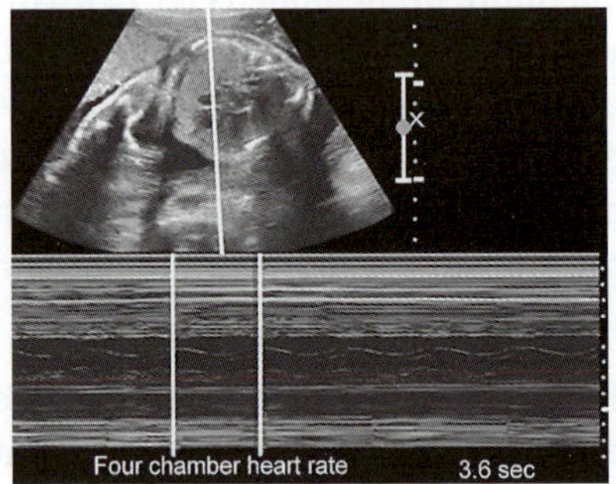 A. Measure the FHR using pulse-wave Doppler B. Place the M-mode cursor over the fetal liver C. Ensure that the M-mode cursor is placed over the beating heart D. Use excessive pressure with the transducer to get a clear image E. Measure the FHR at the level of the fetal bladder	**Ans: C (Ensure that the M-mode cursor is placed over the beating heart)** The adjacent image shows measurement of FHR using M-mode ultrasound, a type of ultrasound which records moving echoes from the heart. The depth of echo-producing interface is displayed along one axis and time is displayed along the second axis. This information is then interpreted in the form of FHR. Besides the measurement of FHR, a detailed assessment of the four chambers of fetal heart **(Fig. 14)** is usually performed routinely on ultrasound examination in the second trimester, especially in the presence of a previous history of heart disease in a parent or sibling or presence of a noncardiac structural defect. 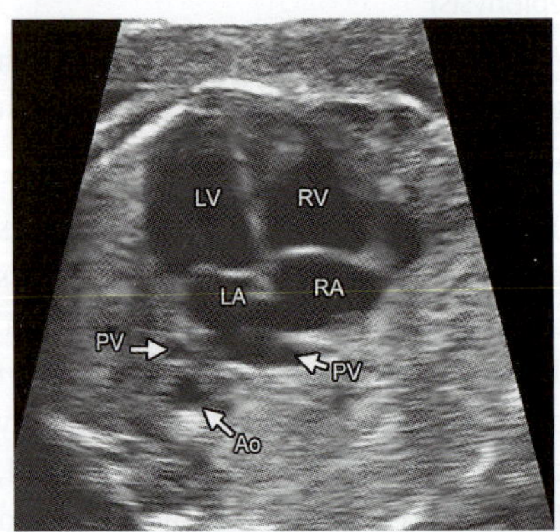 **Fig. 14:** Four-chamber view of fetal heart (Ao: aorta; LA: left atrium; LV: left ventricle; PV: pulmonary vein; RA: right atrium; RV: right ventricle)	**Explanation:** To accurately measure the FHR using M-mode ultrasound, it is essential to place the M-mode cursor over the beating heart. This allows for a real-time representation of the heart's motion, creating a waveform that can be used to measure the heart rate. The measurement is typically taken from peak to peak or valley to valley of the waveform. Using M-mode instead of pulse-wave Doppler is recommended to avoid potential adverse effects on the fetus. The fetal heart rate at term usually varies between 120 to 160 BPM. **Potential questions:** There can be different questions related to features of normal and abnormal structures encountered on scans during various stages of gestation.

DOPPLER ULTRASOUND

Question	Answer	Comment
Q15. In the evaluation of fetal anemia using color Doppler of the vessel as shown in the image below, which parameter is most indicative of severe anemia? 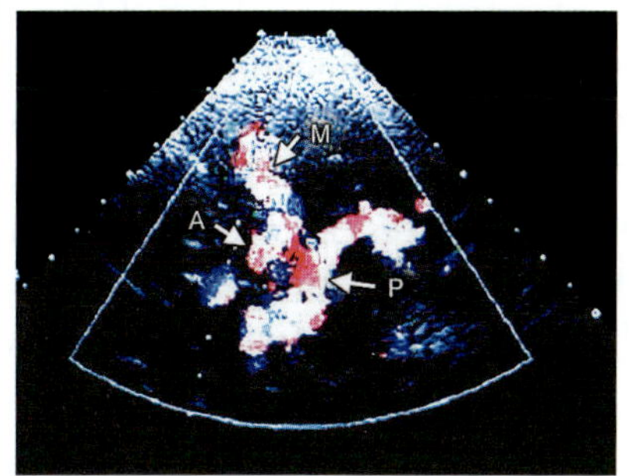 A. MCA pulsatility index (PI) <1.0 B. MCA peak systolic velocity (PSV) >1.5 MoM (multiples of the median) C. MCA systolic/diastolic (S/D) ratio >3.0 D. MCA end-diastolic flow reversal E. MCA cerebroplacental ratio (CPR) <1.0	**Ans: B [MCA peak systolic velocity (PSV) >1.5 MoM (multiples of the median)]** The adjacent color Doppler transvaginal ultrasound image shows evaluation of middle cerebral artery (MCA) showing the circle of Willis. In the adjacent image, A depicts anterior cerebral artery, M depicts MCA, and P depicts posterior cerebral artery. Middle cerebral artery is a major lateral branch of the circle of Willis, which is most accessible to ultrasound imaging and carries nearly 80% of cerebral blood. Peak systolic velocity (PSV) of the MCA is a critical parameter in the assessment of fetal anemia **(Fig. 15)**. 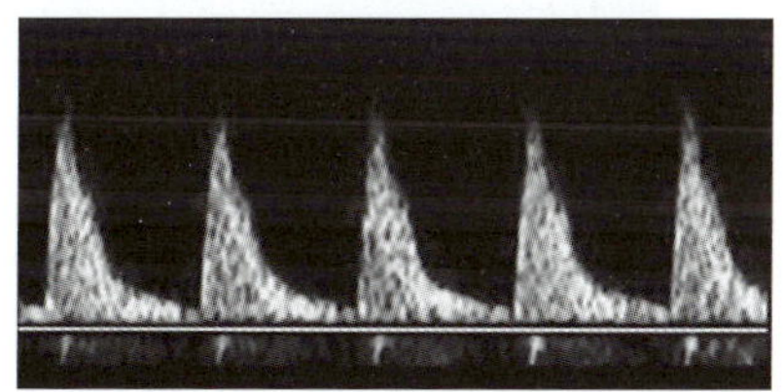 **Fig. 15:** Normal Doppler velocity waveforms in middle cerebral artery (MCA) showing high systolic velocities and minimal diastolic velocities.	**Explanation:** On Doppler imaging, MCA can be seen to be running anterolaterally at the borderline between the anterior and the middle cerebral fossae. An elevated MCA PSV, specifically > 1.5 MoM, is highly indicative of severe fetal anemia. This is because, in anemic fetuses, the blood viscosity decreases, leading to increased blood flow velocity in the MCA. This parameter is widely used due to its high sensitivity and specificity for detecting moderate-to-severe fetal anemia, making it a reliable noninvasive diagnostic tool. **Potential questions:** There can be different questions related to the evaluation of various Doppler waveforms of important fetal vessels.

Question	Answer	Comment
Q16. A Doppler ultrasound of a fetal blood vessel shows a triphasic waveform with forward flow during atrial contraction as shown in the image below. What does this indicate about the fetal circulation? 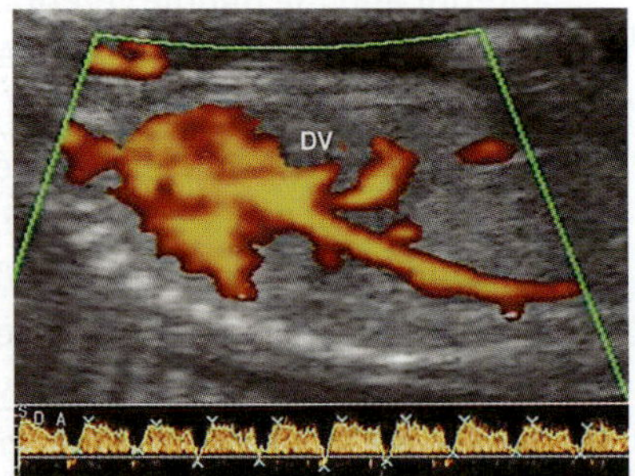 A. Fetal anemia B. Fetal heart failure C. Normal fetal circulation D. Twin-twin transfusion syndrome E. Maternal diabetes	**Ans: C (Normal fetal circulation)** The adjacent image shows normal blood flow in ductus venosus (DV). The typical waveform for the blood flow in DV consists of three phases related to cardiac cycle **(Fig. 16)**. In normal fetuses, the blood flow in the venous system is always in the forward direction throughout the cardiac cycle. Forward blood flow in the venous system is a function of cardiac compliance, contractibility, and afterload. This normal flow pattern ensures that well-oxygenated blood from the placenta is efficiently delivered to the fetal heart and brain, which is essential for healthy fetal development. 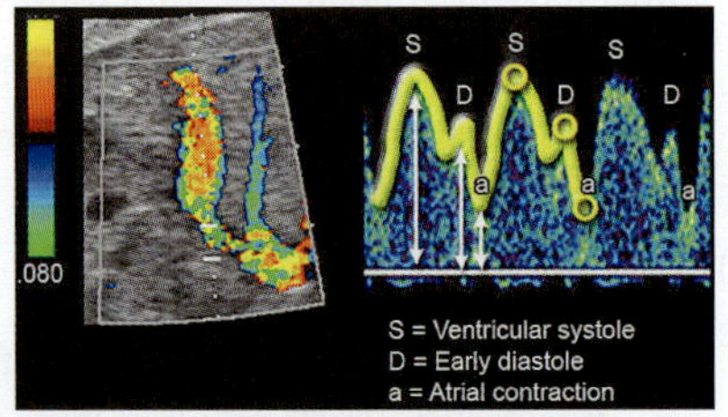 **Fig. 16:** Doppler analysis of ductus venosus waveforms.	**Explanation:** A triphasic waveform with forward flow during atrial contraction in the ductus venosus is indicative of normal fetal circulation. This pattern consists of the S wave (ventricular systolic contraction), D wave (early ventricular diastole), and A wave (atrial contraction), all showing forward flow towards the fetal heart. A decline in forward velocities in venous system results in increased Doppler indices and suggests impaired preload handling. **Potential questions:** There can be different questions related to the evaluation of various normal and abnormal Doppler waveforms of important fetal vessels.
Q17. When assessing blood flow in the ductus venosus on ultrasound as shown in the image below, which of the following findings is most indicative of the abnormality present here? 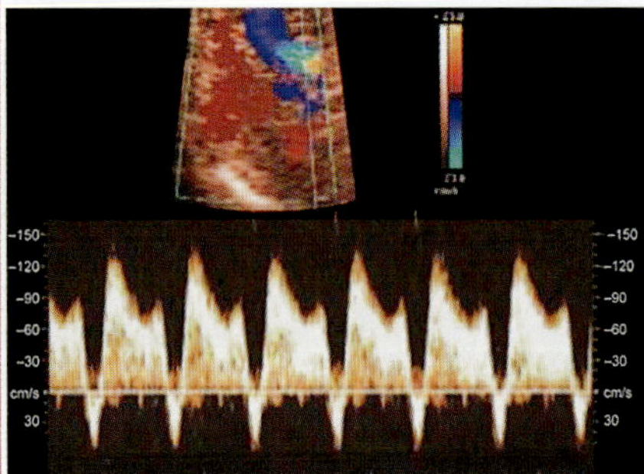 A. Forward flow during the S wave B. Forward flow during the D wave C. Reversed flow during the A wave D. Forward flow during the A wave E. Reversed flow during the S wave	**Ans: C (Reversed flow during the A wave)** The adjacent image depicts reversed blood flow in the DV. Abnormal blood flow in the DV is associated with either absence of A wave or reversal of blood flow in the A wave (as shown in **Figs. 17A and B**). Abnormal DV flow could be indicative of IUGR or cardiac abnormality or underlying Down syndrome. During the periods of fetal hypoxia, a compensatory mechanism occurs, causing transient dilatation of the ductus, which is supposed to increase oxygenated blood flowing through it during these periods of hypoxia or reduced umbilical flow. 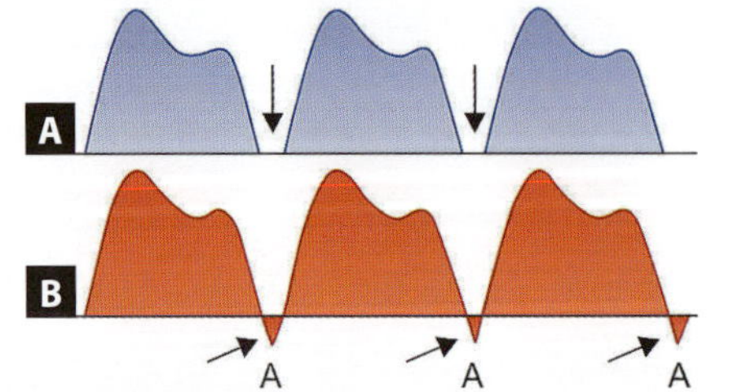 **Figs. 17A and B:** Abnormal waveforms in the ductus venosus: (A) Absent A waves; (B) Reversal of A waves (arrow).	**Explanation:** The DV is a very important part of fetal venous circulation. This vessel acts as a shunt and helps in directly connecting the umbilical vein to the inferior vena cava. The ductus venosus normally exhibits a triphasic waveform on Doppler ultrasound, with forward flow during the S wave (ventricular systole), D wave (early diastole), and A wave (atrial contraction). Reversed flow during the A wave is considered abnormal and can indicate increased cardiac afterload or myocardial dysfunction. **Potential questions:** There can be different questions related to the evaluation of various normal and abnormal Doppler waveforms of important fetal vessels.

<table>
<tr><th>Question</th><th>Answer</th><th>Comment</th></tr>
<tr>
<td>Q18. A 32-year-old woman at 28 weeks of gestation undergoes an umbilical artery Doppler ultrasound, which shows normal blood flow as shown in the image below. What is the significance of this finding?

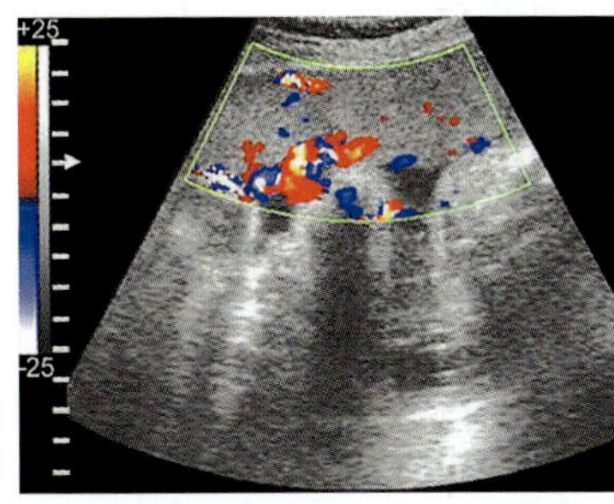

A. No fetal growth restriction
B. Abnormal placental function
C. Increased risk of preeclampsia
D. Normal fetal heart rate
E. Decreased risk of stillbirth</td>
<td>Ans: A (No fetal growth restriction)

The adjacent image shows color Doppler of the umbilical artery, assessing fetoplacental perfusion. Deoxygenated blood from the fetus flows to the placenta via two umbilical arteries, and oxygenated blood returns via the umbilical vein. Normally, vascular resistance decreases with gestation; diastolic flow is absent early but appears later. Characteristic umbilical blood flow has a saw-toothed appearance of pulsatile arterial flow in one direction and continuous umbilical venous blood flow in the other (Fig. 18).

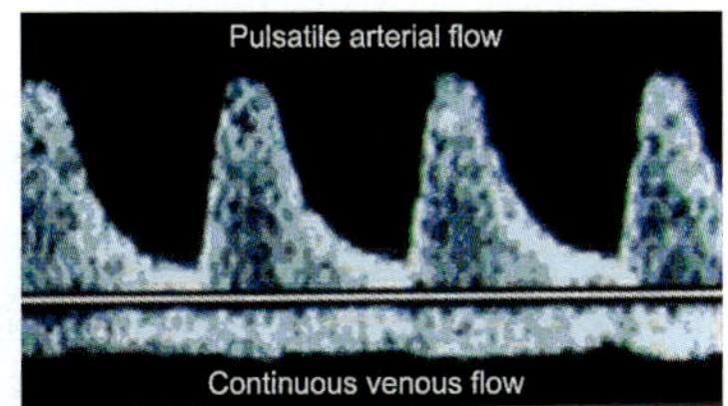

Fig. 18: Umbilical artery Doppler ultrasound waveforms.</td>
<td>Explanation: Normal umbilical artery Doppler flow indicates good placental function and adequate fetal blood supply. Abnormal findings, such as increased S/D ratio or absent/reversed flow, suggest placental insufficiency, commonly linked to IUGR and requires close monitoring or intervention.

Potential questions: There can be different questions related to the evaluation of various normal and abnormal Doppler waveforms of important fetal vessels.</td>
</tr>
</table>

Question	Answer	Comment
Q19. A Doppler ultrasound of the umbilical artery shows a wave pattern as depicted in the image below. What is the most likely cause of this finding? 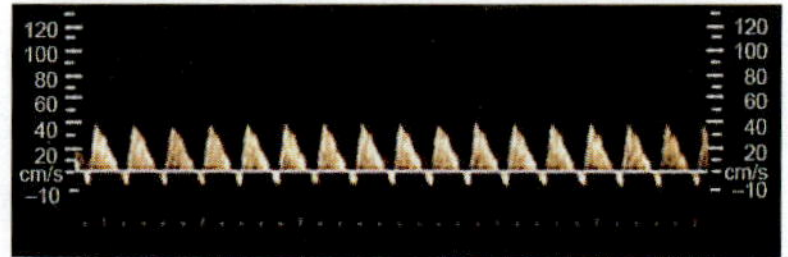 A. Fetal anemia B. Fetal heart failure C. Placental insufficiency D. Twin-twin transfusion syndrome E. Maternal diabetes	**Ans: C (Placental insufficiency)** The Doppler waveforms in the adjacent image show reversed end-diastolic flow. In pregnancies complicated by placental insufficiency such as hypertensive disorders, IUGR, etc., there may be a series of changes occurring in the umbilical blood vessels on Doppler ultrasound. Initially, there may be increased resistance to blood flow in the umbilical artery blood vessels resulting in an increased systolic/diastolic (S/D) ratio and diastolic notching **(Fig. 19A)**, followed by absent blood flow on umbilical artery Doppler **(Fig. 19B)** and eventually reversed blood flow on Doppler ultrasound. 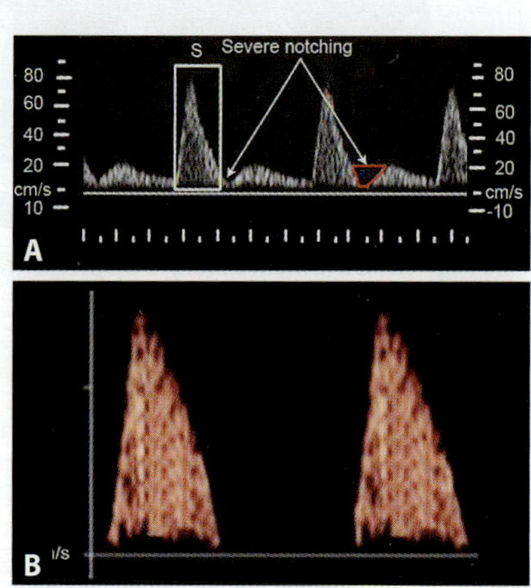 **Figs. 19A and B:** Abnormal umbilical artery blood flow patterns: (A) Diastolic notching in the umbilical blood vessels; (B) Absent blood flow on umbilical artery Doppler.	**Explanation:** Initially in cases of placental insufficiency, the Doppler ultrasound of the umbilical artery shows increased resistance to flow (decreased mean velocity) and reduced diastolic blood flow. This results in an elevated S/D ratio. With further increase in vascular resistance, there occurs an early diastolic notch **(Fig. 19A)**. With yet further worsening of the situation, the blood flow in the diastole stops completely (absent end-diastolic flow) or blood starts flowing in a reverse direction. Absent/reversed end-diastolic flow in the umbilical artery is a significant indicator of placental insufficiency. This abnormal waveform suggests increased resistance in the placental circulation, which can lead to IUGR and other complications. As a result, this finding warrants close monitoring and mandates immediate delivery depending on the clinical situation of the patient. **Potential questions:** There can be different questions related to the evaluation of various normal and abnormal Doppler waveforms of important fetal vessels.

Question	Answer	Comment
Q20. Which Doppler ultrasound waveform in the uterine artery as depicted by an arrow in the below image is most predictive of preeclampsia? 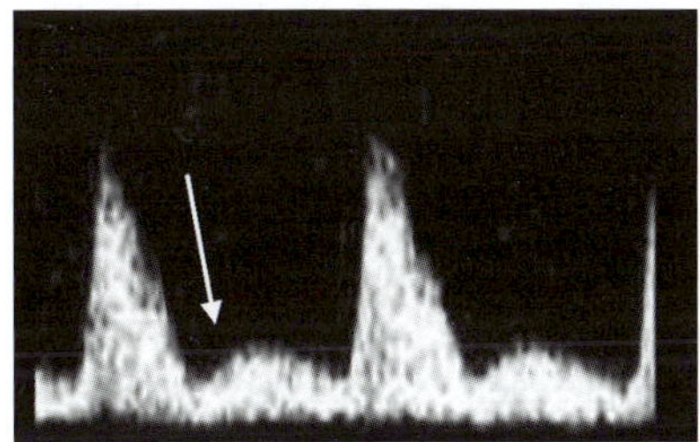 A. Low pulsatility index (PI) B. High resistance index (RI) C. Absent end-diastolic flow D. Presence of early diastolic notch E. Continuous forward flow	**Ans: D (Presence of early diastolic notch)** The arrow in the image shows an early diastolic notch in the uterine artery Doppler waveform, a significant predictor of preeclampsia, indicating increased resistance in the uteroplacental circulation. Normal uterine artery Doppler at 22 weeks is shown in **Figure 20**. 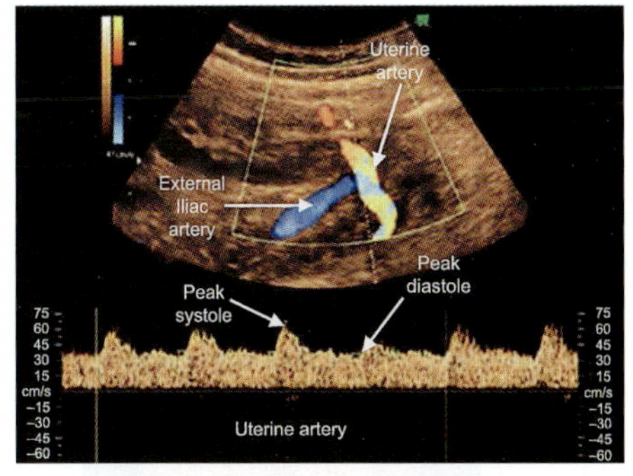 **Fig. 20:** Normal uterine artery Doppler analysis at 22 weeks' gestation.	**Explanation:** Uterine artery Doppler noninvasively assesses uteroplacental perfusion. In normal pregnancies, trophoblastic invasion of spiral vessels increases blood flow and lowers resistance. In preeclampsia or IUGR, inadequate trophoblastic invasion of spiral vessels causes abnormal Doppler waveforms. **Potential questions:** There can be different questions related to the evaluation of various normal and abnormal Doppler waveforms of important fetal vessels.

CONGENITAL ABNORMALITIES

Question	Answer	Comment
Q21. A 12-week pregnant woman undergoes a nuchal translucency (NT) scan. The ultrasound image below shows the findings observed on ultrasound examination. What is the most likely diagnosis associated with this finding? 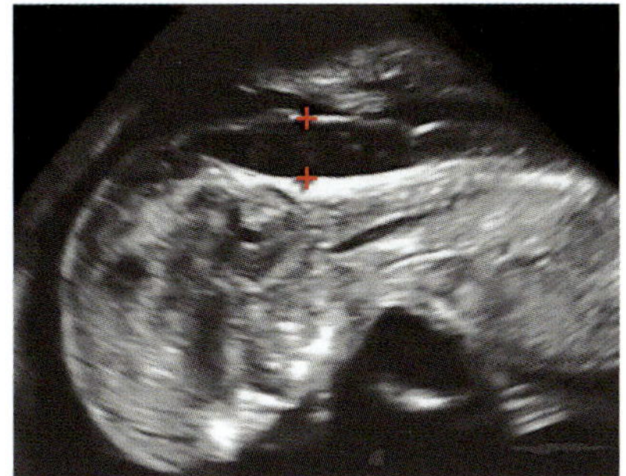 A. Turner syndrome B. Down syndrome C. Patau syndrome D. Edwards syndrome E. Normal variant	**Ans: B (Down syndrome)** The adjacent image shows NT measurement of 6 mm. NT $\geq$3 mm is abnormal, warranting genetic counseling or amniocentesis. The largest of three measurements, taken with calipers perpendicular to the long axis of fetal body, is considered. **Figure 21** shows normal NT. 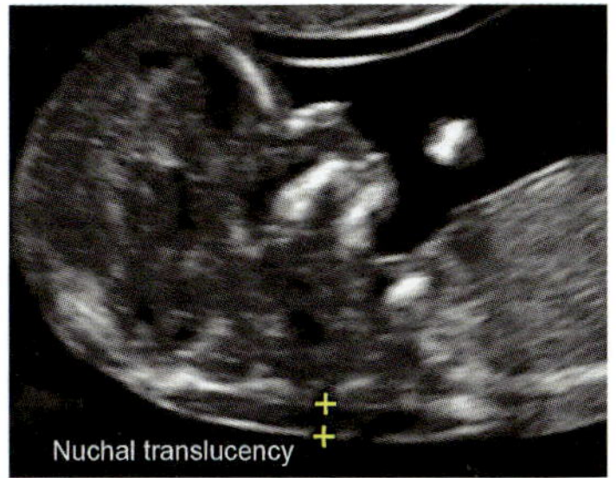 **Fig. 21:** Normal nuchal translucency as observed on the ultrasound examination.	**Explanation:** NT refers to the fluid-filled space at the back of the fetal neck. Increased NT, measured by ultrasound at 11–14 weeks (CRL 45–84 mm), is a key marker for chromosomal abnormalities, especially Down syndrome. Larger NT values indicate higher risk, and may also be associated with other trisomies, Turner syndrome, and congenital heart defects. **Potential questions:** There can be different questions related to various sonographic abnormalities encountered in cases of Down syndrome.

<table>
<tr><th>Question</th><th>Answer</th><th>Comment</th></tr>
<tr><td>

Q22. A 12-week pregnant woman undergoes a first-trimester ultrasound scan. The image reveals an abnormality as shown in the image below. Which additional finding on ultrasound would further increase the suspicion of Down syndrome?

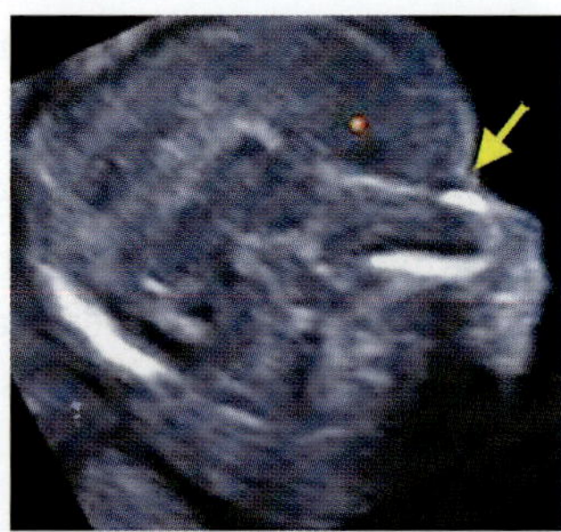

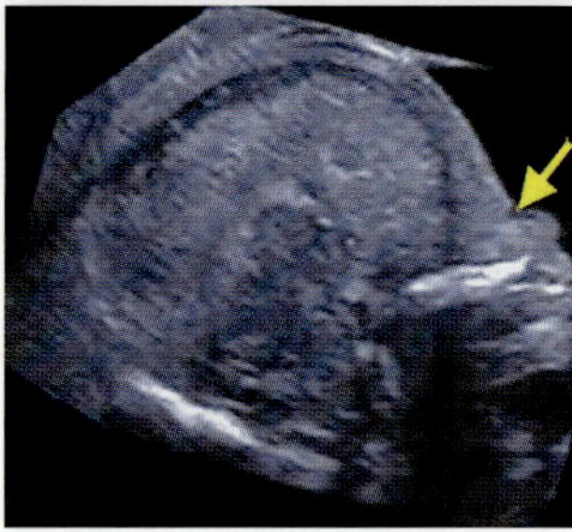

A. Increased nuchal translucency
B. Short femur length
C. Echogenic intracardiac focus
D. Absent nasal bone
E. Choroid plexus cyst

</td><td>

Ans: A (Increased nuchal translucency)

The yellow arrow in the adjacent image depicts the absence of nasal bone. **Figures 22A and B** show the presence of nasal bone in a normal fetus.

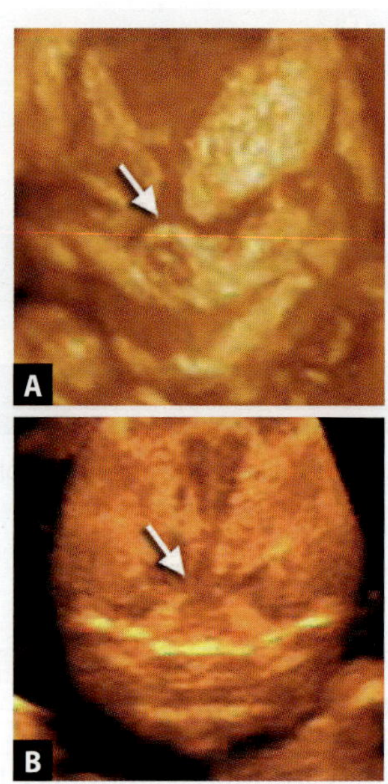

Figs. 22A and B: Presence of nasal bone (as depicted by white arrow).

</td><td>

Explanation: Absence of nasal bone can be considered as a useful ultrasound parameter for identifying fetuses with trisomy 21/Down syndrome because such fetuses may often suffer from hypoplasia or delayed ossification of the nasal bone.

Increased NT is another significant marker for Down syndrome (trisomy 21). When combined with the finding of an absent nasal bone, the presence of increased NT further raises the suspicion of Down syndrome.

However, increased nuchal translucency or absence of nasal bone do not confirm the diagnosis. of Down syndrome. Invasive tests like amniocentesis or CVS may be required to confirm the diagnosis in these cases.

Potential questions: There can be different questions related to various sonographic abnormalities encountered in cases of Down syndrome.

</td></tr>
</table>

Question	Answer	Comment
Q23. A 22-week pregnant woman undergoes a routine ultrasound, which reveals the findings as depicted by an arrow in the image below. What is the most likely cause of this finding? 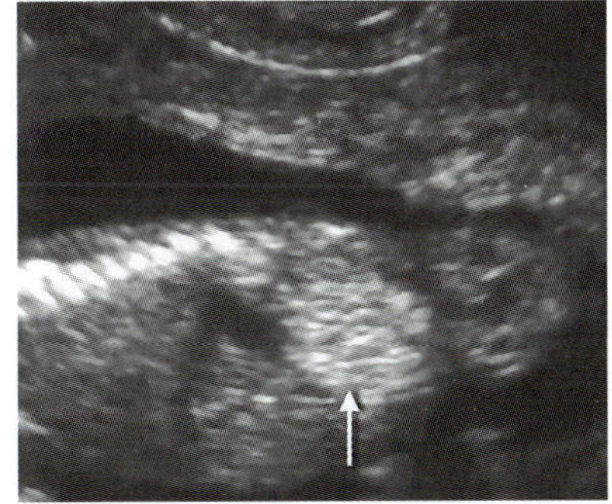 A. Down syndrome (trisomy 21) B. Cystic fibrosis C. Fetal infection (e.g., cytomegalovirus) D. Gastrointestinal obstruction E. Edwards syndrome (trisomy 18)	**Ans: A [Down syndrome (trisomy 21)]** The white arrow in the image points to echogenic bowel, which matches the echogenicity of the adjacent iliac bone. **Figure 23** shows a magnified view of fetal echogenic bowel loops. Slotnick et al. classified bowel echogenicity into three grades: Grade 1 (less than iliac crest), Grade 2 (similar to iliac crest), and Grade 3 (greater than iliac crest). 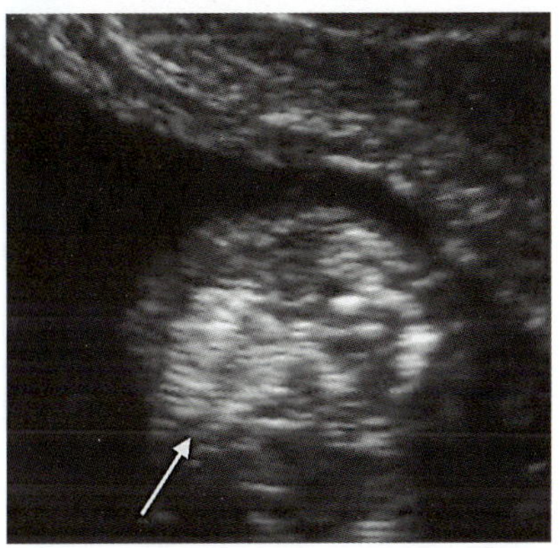 **Fig. 23:** Magnified view showing fetal echogenic bowel loops.	**Explanation:** Echogenic bowel requires detailed ultrasound to check for other anomalies, including renal and cardiac issues. It can be linked to conditions like Down syndrome, cystic fibrosis, fetal infections (e.g., CMV), and gastrointestinal obstructions, or may be a normal variant. The association with Down syndrome and adverse pregnancy outcomes is strongest in cases with moderate-to-severe echogenicity (grades 2 and 3), and amniocentesis may be needed for confirmation. **Potential questions:** There can be different questions related to various sonographic abnormalities encountered in cases of Down syndrome.

Question	Answer	Comment
Q24. A newborn is diagnosed with the abnormality shown in the image below. Which of the following is the most likely associated condition? 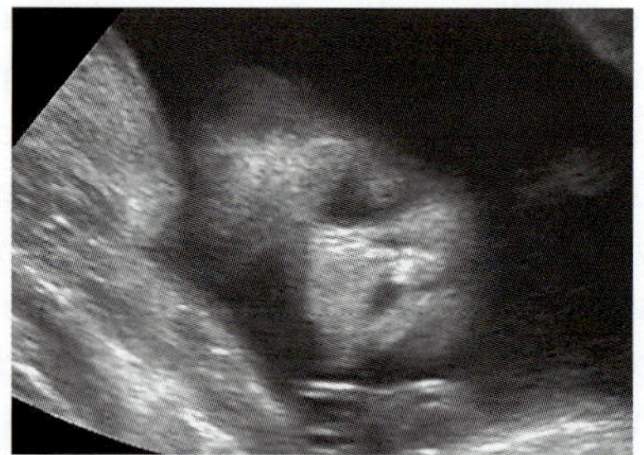 A. Pierre Robin sequence B. Trisomy 13 (Patau syndrome) C. DiGeorge syndrome D. Treacher Collins syndrome E. Down syndrome	**Ans: B [Trisomy 13 (Patau syndrome)]** The adjacent image shows a 2D transvaginal ultrasound of a left unilateral cleft lip. Cleft lip/palate can be diagnosed on a second-trimester 3D scan **(Fig. 24)**, with further evaluation and amniocentesis required for associated anomalies and chromosomal defects. 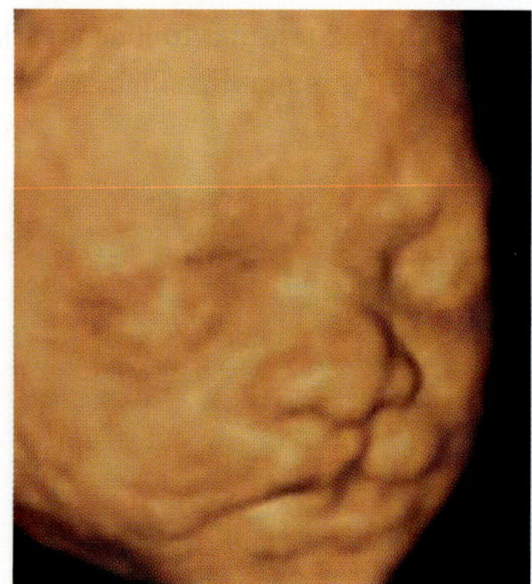 **Fig. 24:** Three-dimensional ultrasound showing cleft lip on the left side.	**Explanation:** Unilateral cleft lip is often linked to genetic syndromes, most commonly Trisomy 13 (Patau syndrome), which involves an extra chromosome 13 and multiple anomalies like cleft lip/palate, polydactyly, and severe intellectual disability. Diagnosis is confirmed by genetic testing, such as karyotyping or chromosomal microarray analysis. Surgical repair is usually done between 1–4 months of age. **Potential questions:** There can be questions related to different abnormalities encountered on ultrasound examination with various syndromes (e.g.. Down syndrome, Edward syndrome, Patau syndrome, etc.).
Q25. Which of the following most appropriate diagnosis can be made from the ultrasound image shown below? 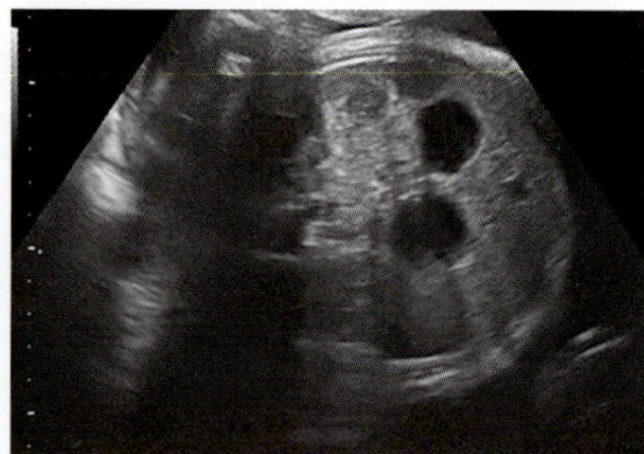 A. Marker for Down syndrome B. Obstructed urethra and bladder C. Dilated kidney D. Obstruction in the bile duct E. Dilatation of intestines	**Ans: A (Marker for Down syndrome)** The ultrasound image shows the "double-bubble sign," indicative of duodenal atresia, with two fluid-filled bubbles in the fetal abdomen representing the dilated stomach and proximal duodenum, caused by a distal obstruction **(Fig. 25)**. 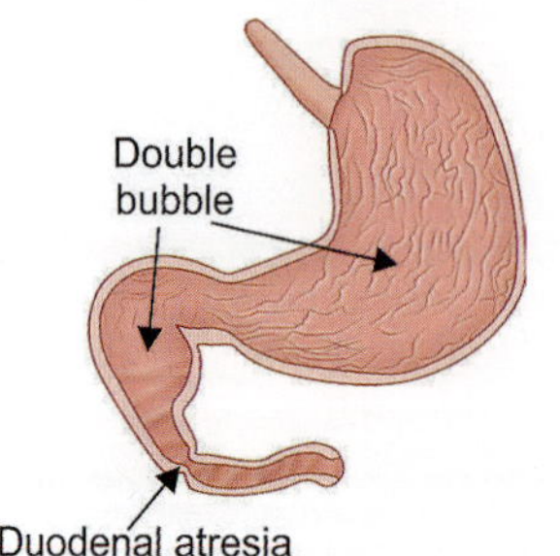 **Fig. 25:** Diagrammatic representation of duodenal atresia.	**Explanation:** The "double-bubble" sign is a classic ultrasound finding indicative of duodenal atresia, a condition frequently associated with Down syndrome (trisomy 21). Typically identified during the anatomy ultrasound performed between 16 to 20 weeks of gestation, the "double-bubble" sign prompts further investigation for chromosomal analysis, such as amniocentesis or chorionic villus sampling. **Potential questions:** There can be different questions related to various sonographic abnormalities encountered in cases of Down syndrome.

Question	Answer	Comment
Q26. A newborn is noted to have an anomaly during three-dimensional ultrasound examination as shown in the image below. Which of the following conditions is most commonly associated with this finding? 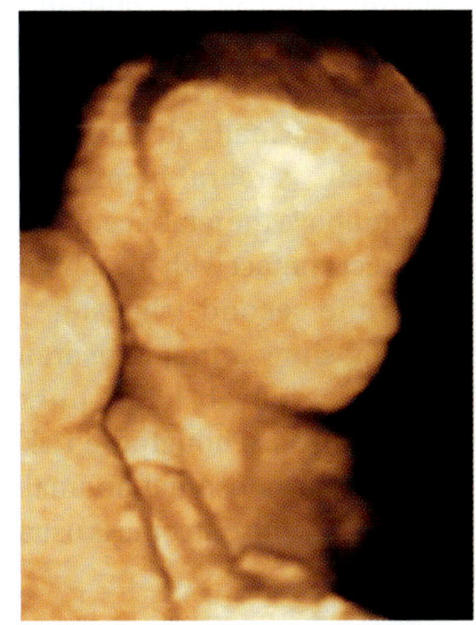 A. Down syndrome (trisomy 21) B. Turner syndrome C. Beckwith-Wiedemann syndrome D. Noonan syndrome E. Fetal alcohol syndrome	**Ans: A [Down syndrome (trisomy 21)]** The adjacent three-dimensional ultrasound image depicts low-set ears and micrognathia at 15 weeks' gestation. Low-set ears and micrognathia (undersized jaws) are commonly associated with anomalies such as aneuploidies (especially Down syndrome). Further evaluation may be required in these cases. **Figure 26** shows the aborted fetus in the same case showing the defect. 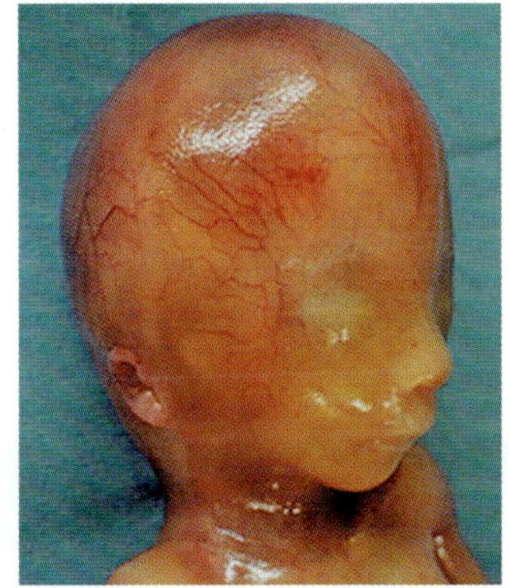 **Fig. 26:** Aborted fetus in the same case showing the defect. The underlying chromosomal anomaly in this patient was detected as trisomy 18. *Courtesy:* Ritsuko K Pooh.	**Explanation:** Three-dimensional ultrasound is able to provide a better description of ear morphology, structure, and position in comparison to two-dimensional ultrasound. By determining the line between the orbits and peak point of auricles, diagnosis of low-set ears can be made. Low-set ears are a clinical feature where the ears are positioned lower on the head than usual. This finding is often associated with various congenital conditions, especially Down syndrome (trisomy 21). In Down syndrome, low-set ears are part of a broader spectrum of dysmorphic features, including a flat facial profile, epicanthal folds, and a single palmar crease. The diagnosis is typically confirmed through genetic testing. **Potential questions:** There can be different questions related to various sonographic/physical abnormalities encountered in cases of Down syndrome.

Question	Answer	Comment
Q27. A prenatal ultrasound at 18 weeks' gestation reveals a fetus with abnormalities of cranial vault and cerebral hemispheres as shown in the images below. What is the most likely diagnosis? 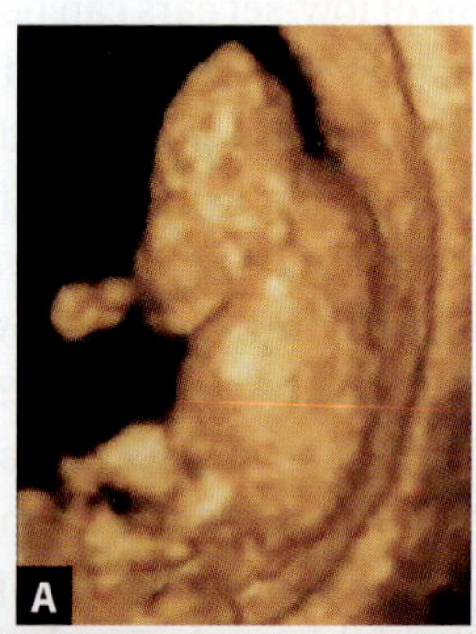 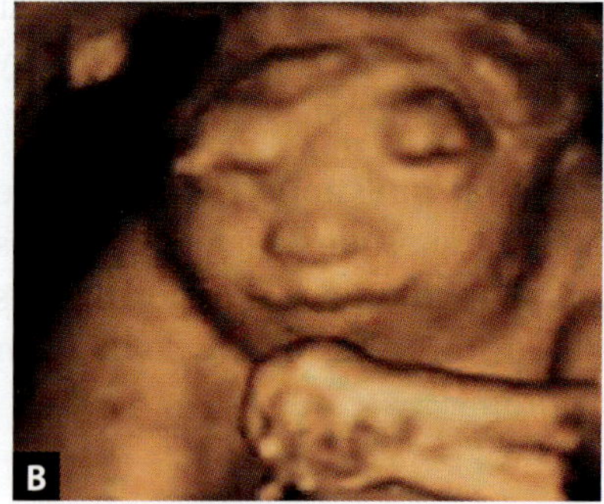 A. Hydrocephalus B. Encephalocele C. Anencephaly D. Holoprosencephaly E. Microcephaly	**Ans: C (Anencephaly)** The adjacent three-dimensional ultrasound image shows an anencephalic fetus. Anencephaly is a severe neural tube defect characterized by absence of a major portion of the brain, skull, and scalp **(Fig. 27)**. It occurs when the upper part of the neural tube fails to close during embryonic development. This condition is typically identified through prenatal ultrasound, which shows an open cranial vault and the absence of cerebral hemispheres. Anencephaly is not compatible with life, and affected infants are either stillborn or die shortly after birth. It is typically detected through prenatal ultrasound and confirmed with maternal blood tests for alpha fetoprotein levels. 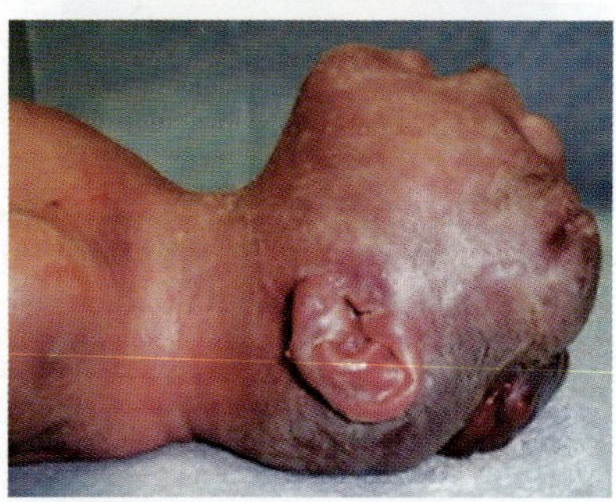 **Fig. 27:** Aborted fetus in the same case at 18 weeks' gestation. *Courtesy:* Ritsuko K Pooh and Kyonghon Pooh.	**Explanation:** Anencephaly refers to the spectrum of various destructive changes in the cranial vault mainly due to its failed development. It occurs due to the deficiency of folic acid. The changes may range from exencephaly (in the first trimester) to frank anencephaly (in the second trimester). There might be exencephaly where the brain hemispheres are intact, though they are abnormally developed. In exencephaly, cerebral hemispheres are visible above the fetal face and they are in direct contact with the amniotic fluid. In the second trimester, the orbits may show a frog appearance with the cerebral hemispheres being destroyed. Though the risk of associated chromosomal anomalies is low (2–11%), the outcome is usually fatal. **Potential questions:** There can be questions related to different abnormalities encountered in various organs on ultrasound examination.

Question	Answer	Comment
Q28. A 20-week gestation ultrasound reveals a fetus with a small defect in the vertebral arch as shown in the ultrasound image below. The overlying skin appears normal. What is the most likely diagnosis? 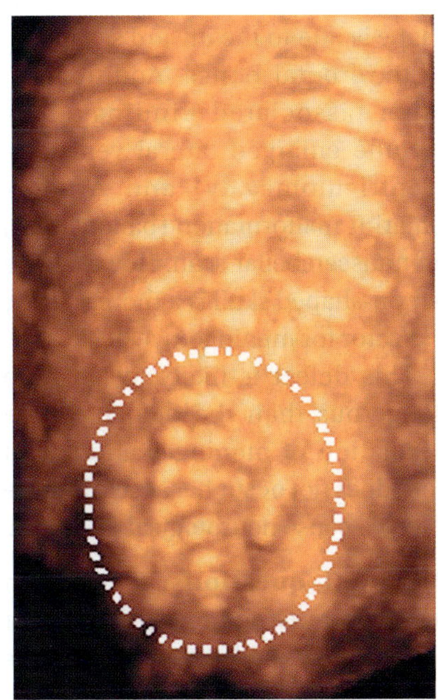 *Courtesy.* Ritsuko K Pooh and Kyonghon Pooh. A. Spina bifida occulta B. Meningocele C. Myelomeningocele D. Encephalocele E. Lipomyelomeningocele	**Ans: A (Spina bifida occulta)** The adjacent three-dimensional ultrasound image shows lumbar spina bifida occulta at 20 weeks' gestation. This defect is characterized by a small gap in one or more of the vertebrae without any protrusion of the spinal cord or meninges **(Fig. 28)**. It is often referred to as "hidden" spina bifida because the defect is covered by skin and typically does not cause any visible abnormalities or symptoms. Spina bifida occulta is the mildest form of spina bifida, resulting due to the failure of posterior vertebral arches to fuse during the early first trimester. 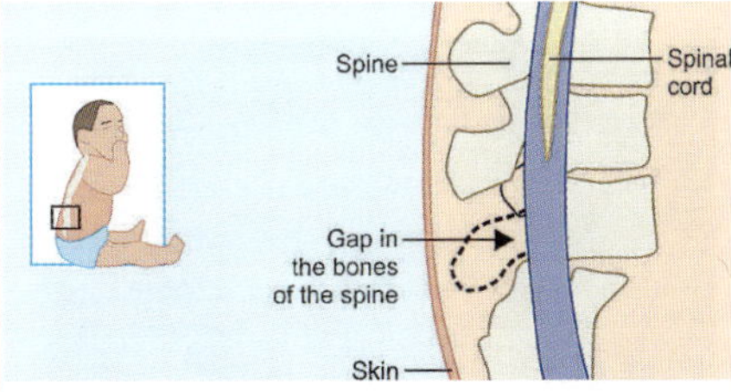 **Fig. 28:** Diagrammatic representation of spina bifida occulta.	**Explanation:** Various types of abnormalities, which may be present in cases of spina bifida are as follows: ▪ *Spina bifida occulta:* This is the mildest type of spina bifida, which is usually asymptomatic and no neural elements are usually involved. The defect in the spine is covered with skin, and spinal cord and meninges remain in place. ▪ *Meningocele:* There is a defect in the spine through which the meninges protrude out, but the spinal cord remains in place. ▪ *Meningomyelocele:* Protrusion of both meninges and spinal cord through the defect in the spine. **Potential questions:** There can be questions related to different abnormalities encountered in various organs on ultrasound examination.

Question	Answer	Comment
Q29. A defect in the spine is observed in a 28-week old abortus as shown in the image below. Which of the following findings is most likely to be observed on the ultrasound in these cases? 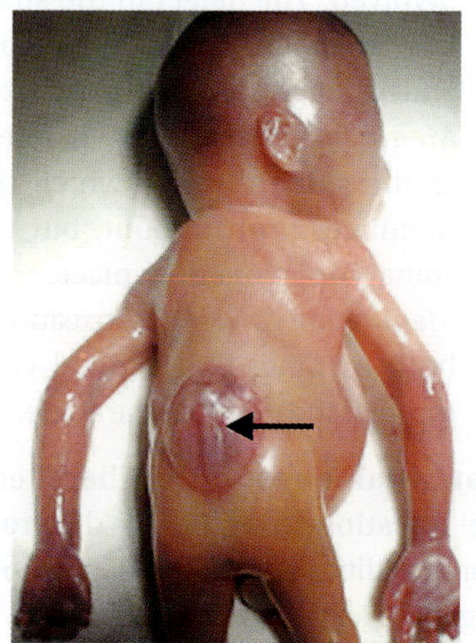 *Courtesy:* Ritsuko K Pooh. A. Enlarged lateral ventricles B. Polyhydramnios C. Lemon-shaped skull D. Clubfoot E. Omphalocele	**Ans: C (Lemon-shaped skull)** The adjacent image shows external appearance of the aborted fetus. There is a defect in the fetal spine through which there is protrusion of meninges and spinal cord. The central canal of the spinal canal has been delineated with a black arrow. This abnormality can be diagnosed as a meningomyelocele, which is a type of spina bifida where the meninges and the spinal cord protrude through a gap in the spine, potentially causing neurological deficits. The three-dimensional ultrasound image in the same patient done at 20 weeks is depicted in **Figure 29**. 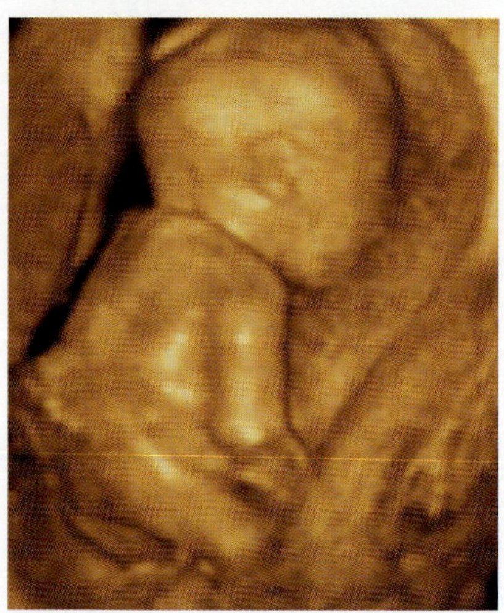 **Fig. 29:** Three-dimensional ultrasound showing a large meningomyelocele at 20 weeks' gestation in the same patient.	**Explanation:** Meningomyelocele, a severe form of spina bifida, is often associated with characteristic cranial findings on ultrasound. One of the hallmark signs is the lemon-shaped skull on transventricular scan, which results from the abnormal development of the neural tube. This shape is due to the inward scalloping of the frontal bones. Additionally, other associated findings may include enlarged lateral ventricles (ventriculomegaly) and Arnold-Chiari II malformation (banana sign) on transcerebellar scan. However, the lemon-shaped skull is a more specific indicator for meningomyelocele. This defect is likely to be more dangerous than the defects where herniation of meninges and spinal cord does not occur because it is more likely to cause neurological disability. **Potential questions:** There can be questions related to different abnormalities encountered in various organs on ultrasound examination.

<table>
<tr><th>Question</th><th>Answer</th><th>Comment</th></tr>
<tr>
<td>Q30. A fetus with 20-week gestational age is diagnosed with clubfoot on antenatal ultrasound as shown in the image below. Which of the following findings is most likely to be observed on the ultrasound?
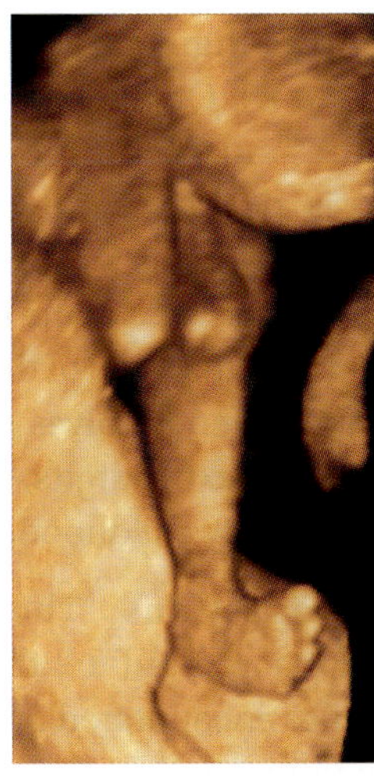
A. Foot positioned downward and inward
B. Foot positioned upward and outward
C. Foot positioned upward and inward
D. Shortened femur
E. Foot positioned downward and outward</td>
<td>Ans: A (Foot positioned downward and inward)
The adjacent three-dimensional ultrasound image shows clubfoot at 15 weeks of gestation, which is a commonly occurring birth defect. The prenatal diagnosis of clubfoot is usually established on ultrasound examination. The appearance of the same fetus when aborted in shown in Figure 30.
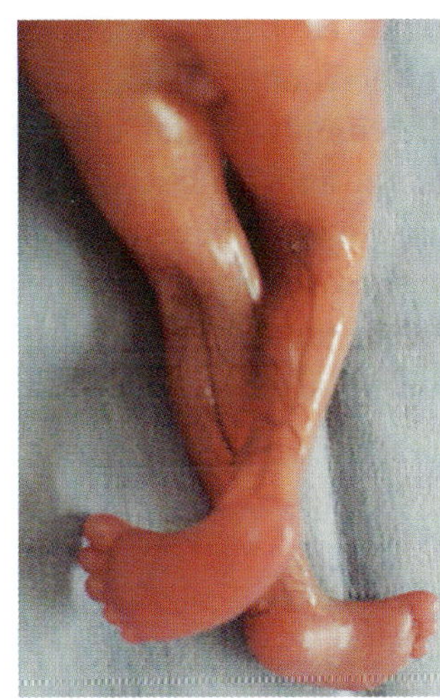
Fig. 30: Aborted fetus of the same case. Karyotype analysis revealed an underlying chromosomal anomaly.
Courtesy: Ritsuko K Pooh.</td>
<td>Explanation: Clubfoot, also known as talipes equinovarus, is a congenital deformity characterized by the foot being excessively plantar flexed, with the forefoot swung medially and the sole facing inward. On antenatal ultrasound, this condition is typically identified by the abnormal positioning of the foot, which appears pointed downward and inward. This distinctive positioning helps in diagnosing clubfoot prenatally.
Management usually involves casting or bracing, often following the Ponseti method, and sometimes surgical intervention.
Potential questions: There can be questions related to different abnormalities encountered in various organs on ultrasound examination.</td>
</tr>
</table>

<table>
<tr><th>Question</th><th>Answer</th><th>Comment</th></tr>
<tr>
<td>

Q31. A 28-year-old pregnant woman undergoes an ultrasound at 20 weeks' gestation. The scan shows abnormality as seen in the image below. What is the most common inheritance pattern associated with the isolated cases of this anomaly?

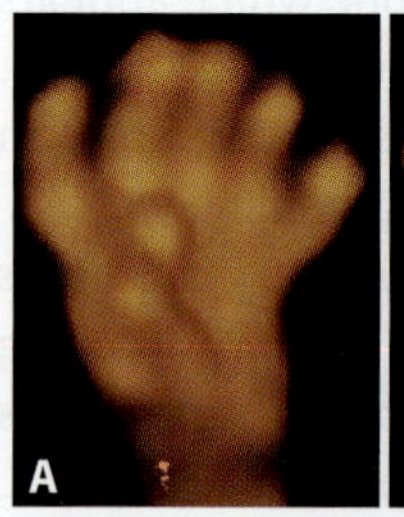

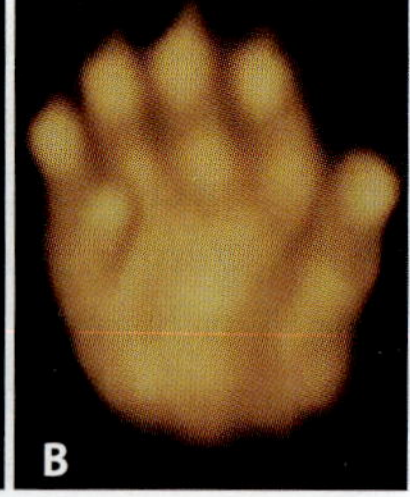

A. Autosomal dominant
B. Autosomal recessive
C. X-linked recessive
D. Mitochondrial inheritance
E. Multifactorial inheritance

</td>
<td>

Ans: A (Autosomal dominant)

The adjacent three-dimensional ultrasound image depicts polydactyly of fetal hands. Polydactyly or an abnormal number of digits, fingers, or toes (6 or more) is the most common abnormality of fetal digits. It may frequently occur as an isolated anomaly or may be associated with an underlying chromosomal abnormality or syndrome (e.g., Laurence-Moon-Biedl syndrome, trisomy 13, etc.). In case of diagnosis of polydactyl on a second-trimester scan, a complete fetal ultrasound evaluation and genetic counseling may be required. Three-dimensional imaging is not mandatory but helps in better delineation of anatomical and morphological details.

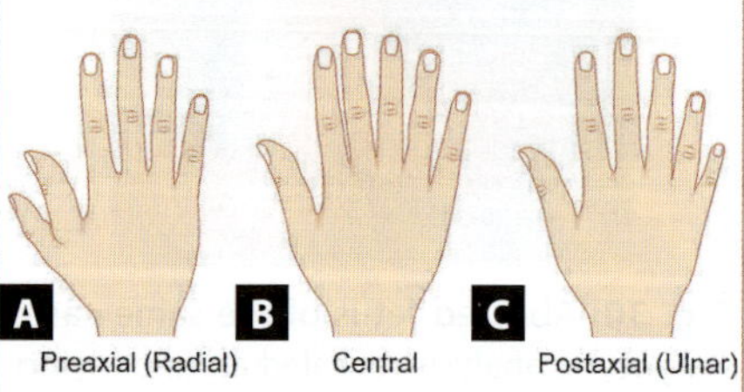

Figs. 31A to C: Types of polydactyly.

</td>
<td>

Explanation: Polydactyly, which refers to the presence of extra fingers or toes, is commonly inherited in an autosomal-dominant pattern when it occurs as an isolated trait. It can be classified as preaxial (affecting the thumbs), postaxial (affecting the little finger), or rarely central (where three central digits are affected) **(Figs. 31A to C)**. On antenatal ultrasound, the most common form observed is postaxial polydactyly, where the extra digit is located on the ulnar (little finger) side of the hand or the fibular (little toe) side of the foot.

Treatment often involves surgical removal of the extra digits, usually performed in early childhood.

Potential questions: There can be questions related to different abnormalities encountered in various organs on ultrasound examination.

</td>
</tr>
</table>

Question	Answer	Comment
Q32. A 28-year-old pregnant woman at 12 weeks' gestation undergoes a three-dimensional ultrasound that shows an abnormality in fetal spine as shown in the image below. What is the most appropriate next step in management? 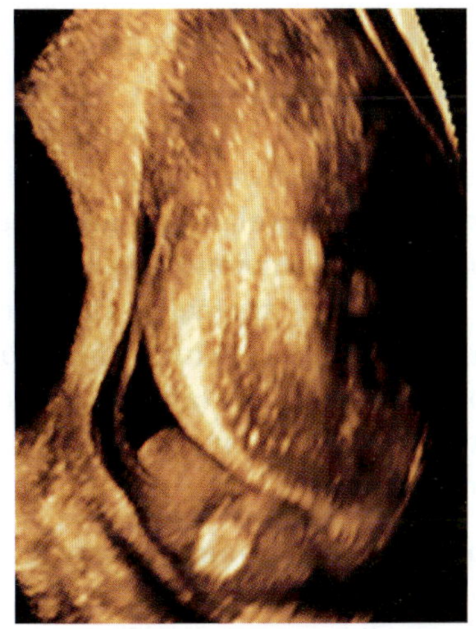 A. Follow-up ultrasound after a week B. Immediate surgical intervention C. MRI of the fetal spine D. Follow-up ultrasound at 20 weeks E. Referral to a pediatric orthopedic specialist	**Ans: D. (Follow-up ultrasound at 20 weeks)** The adjacent three-dimensional ultrasound image shows fetal scoliosis at 12 weeks of gestation. Scoliosis is a spinal deformity associated with both lateral deformity and vertebral rotation. **Figure 32** shows the aborted fetus in the same case showing severe scoliosis. 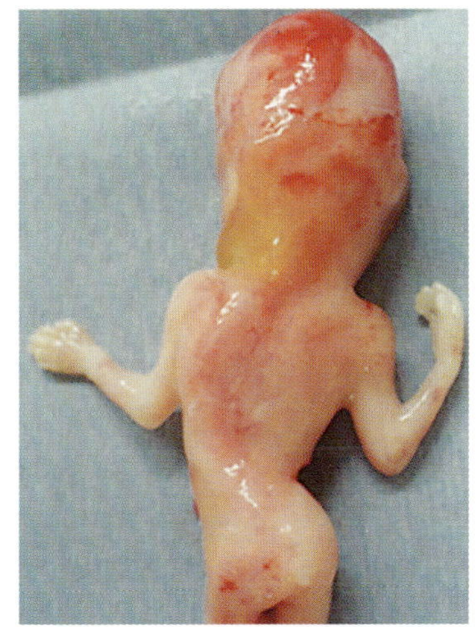 **Fig. 32:** Aborted fetus in the same case showing severe scoliosis. No underlying chromosomal abnormality was detected in this case. *Courtesy:* Ritsuko K Pooh.	**Explanation:** At 12 weeks' gestation, the identification of scoliosis in a fetus primarily warrants close monitoring. A follow-up ultrasound at 20 weeks helps to further assess and confirm the diagnosis and evaluate any progression. Immediate invasive procedures or advanced imaging like MRI are typically not warranted at this early stage. The diagnosis of fetal scoliosis mandates a detailed assessment for other anomalies and genetic counseling regarding the likely fetal outcome. Management can include observation, bracing, or surgery, depending on the severity and progression of the curve. **Potential questions:** There can be questions related to different abnormalities encountered in various organs on ultrasound examination.

Question	Answer	Comment
Q33. A 20-week gestation fetus is diagnosed with an abnormality on antenatal ultrasound as shown in the image below. Which of the following findings is most likely to be observed on the ultrasound? 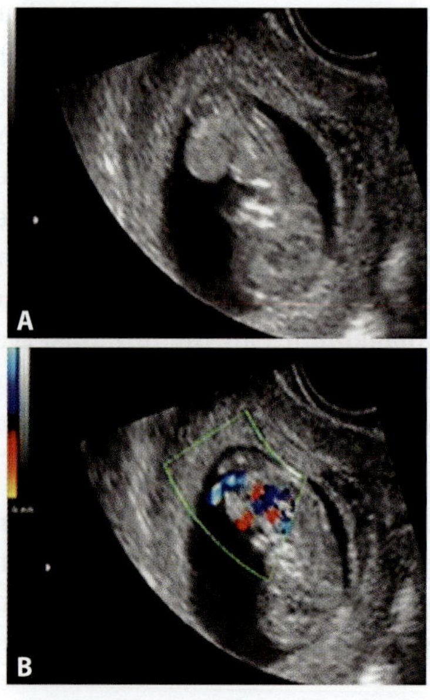 A. Herniation of abdominal contents into a membrane-covered sac B. Free-floating bowel loops in the amniotic fluid C. Enlarged kidneys D. Polyhydramnios E. Shortened femur	**Ans: A (Herniation of abdominal contents into a membrane-covered sac)** The adjacent image A is a two-dimensional ultrasound image showing omphalocele at 12 weeks' gestation. On the other hand, image B is a color Doppler ultrasound image of the same. Omphalocele can be defined as the herniation of intra-abdominal contents into the base of umbilical cord. A membrane almost always covers an omphalocele and the umbilical cord usually inserts onto the membranes in midposition **(Figs. 33A and B)**. 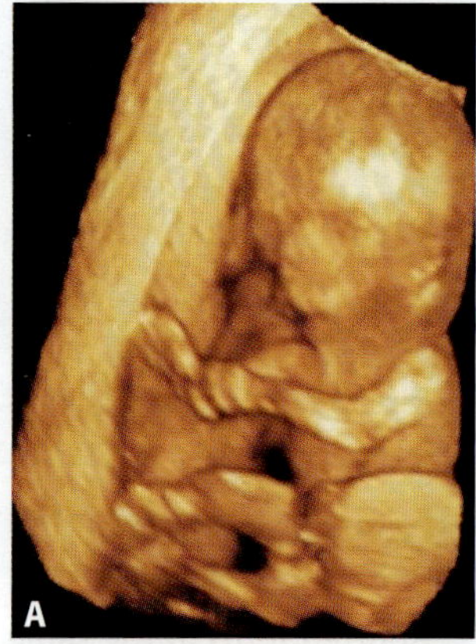 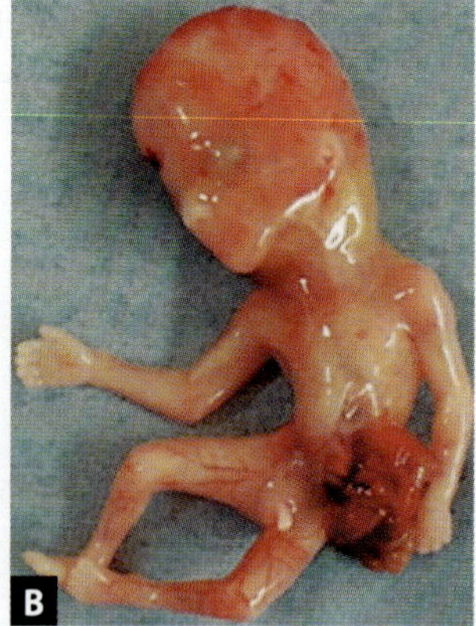 **Figs. 33A and B:** (A) Three-dimensional ultrasound image in the same patient; (B) Aborted fetus showing the ruptured omphalocele sac. No underlying chromosomal anomaly was found in this case. *Courtesy:* Ritsuko K Pooh.	**Explanation:** Omphalocele is a congenital defect characterized by the herniation of abdominal contents through the base of the umbilical cord, covered by a membrane consisting of amnion, Wharton's jelly, and peritoneum. On antenatal ultrasound, this condition is identified by the presence of abdominal organs, such as the liver and intestines, within a membrane-covered sac outside the fetal abdomen. This differentiates omphalocele from gastroschisis, where the bowel loops are free-floating in the amniotic fluid. Treatment typically involves surgical repair, which may be done immediately after birth or later, depending on the size of the omphalocele. **Potential questions:** There can be questions related to different abnormalities encountered in various organs on ultrasound examination.

<table>
<tr><th>Question</th><th>Answer</th><th>Comment</th></tr>
<tr>
<td>Q34. A 34-year-old G3P2L2 with 14 completed weeks of gestation presented to the gynecological emergency with complaints of reduced fetal movements since the last 3–4 days. An ultrasound examination was performed in the patient, which revealed the findings as shown in the image below. What is the likely diagnosis in this case?
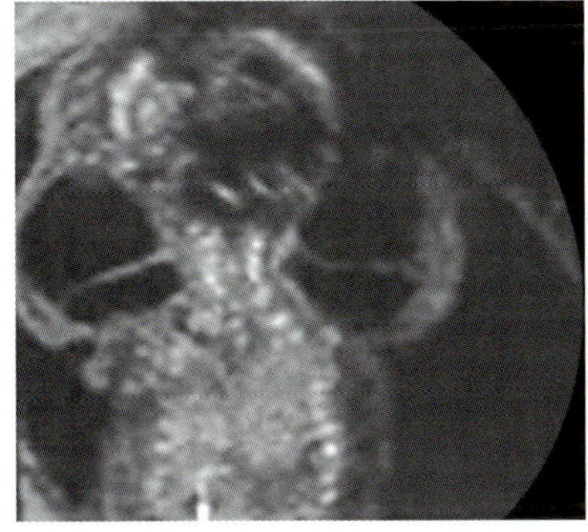
A. Single, solid mass in the neck
B. Multiloculated cystic mass in the neck
C. Hyperechoic mass in the neck
D. Simple cyst in the liver
E. Echogenic bowel</td>
<td>Ans: B (Multiloculated cystic mass in the neck)
The adjacent two-dimensional ultrasound image demonstrates presence of multiple, discreet, and circumscribed cystic areas in the neck region. Fetal heart rate was found to be absent. A tentative diagnosis of cystic hygroma was made.
Three-dimensional ultrasound examination was performed to further confirm the diagnosis (Fig. 34A). In lieu of dead baby in this case, the labor was induced. Aborted fetus demonstrated the presence of cystic hygroma (Fig. 34B).
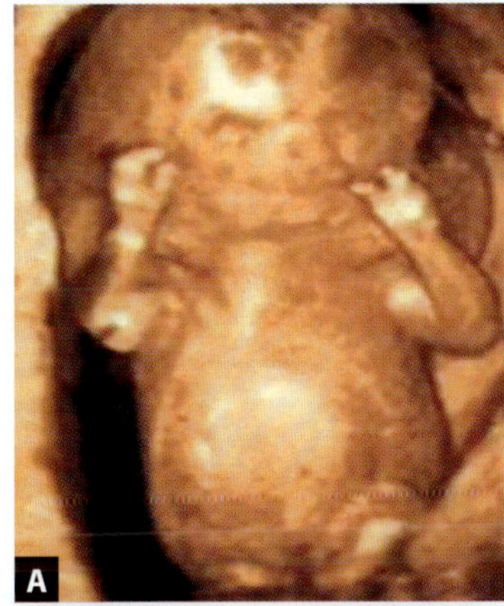
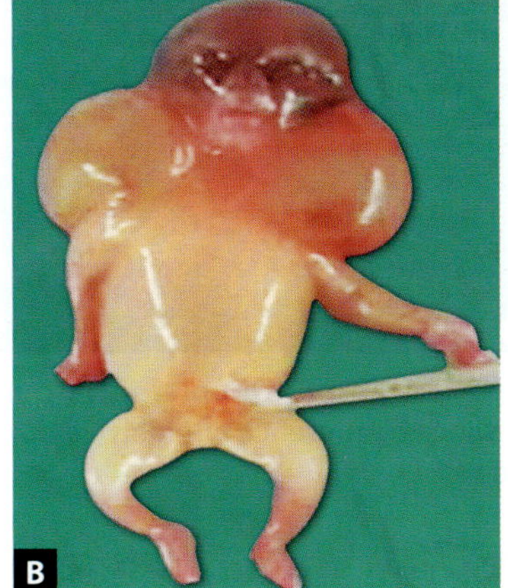
Figs. 34A and B: (A) Three-dimensional image in the same patient as the adjacent image; (B) Aborted fetus in the same patient. Fetal karyotype was found to be 45X.
Courtesy: Ritsuko K Pooh.</td>
<td>Explanation: Also known as cystic lymphangioma, cystic hygroma is characterized by cystic dilation of the lymphatic tissue in the neck region. A cystic hygroma is characterized by a multiloculated cystic mass typically found in the neck region on ultrasound. These masses are due to lymphatic malformations and can appear as fluid-filled spaces with septations. They are often associated with chromosomal abnormalities such as Turner syndrome and Down syndrome.
Management can include observation, drainage, or surgical removal, depending on the size and location of the cystic hygroma.
Potential questions: There can be questions related to different abnormalities encountered in various organs on ultrasound examination.</td>
</tr>
</table>

OBSTETRIC, GYNECOLOGICAL AND GENERAL ABNORMALITIES

Question	Answer	Comment
Q35. A 20-year-old primigravida patient presented with bleeding at 9 weeks of gestation. A transvaginal ultrasound was done which revealed findings as shown in the image below. What is the likely characteristic finding of this pathology on color Doppler ultrasound? 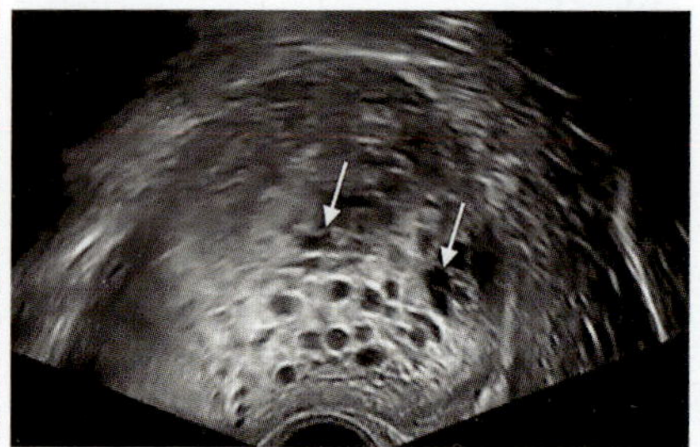 A. High-velocity, low-impedance flow B. Low-velocity, high-impedance flow C. Absence of blood flow D. Uniform echogenic mass without vascularity E. High-resistance, low-velocity flow	**Ans: A (High-velocity, low-impedance flow)** The white arrows in the adjacent image point toward a cluster of grape-like appearance on TVS. There was presence of numerous anechoic cysts with intervening hyperechoic material. A diagnosis of hydatidiform mole was made. Doppler ultrasound examination showed presence of highly vascularized tissues with low-resistance blood flow **(Figs. 35A and B)**. 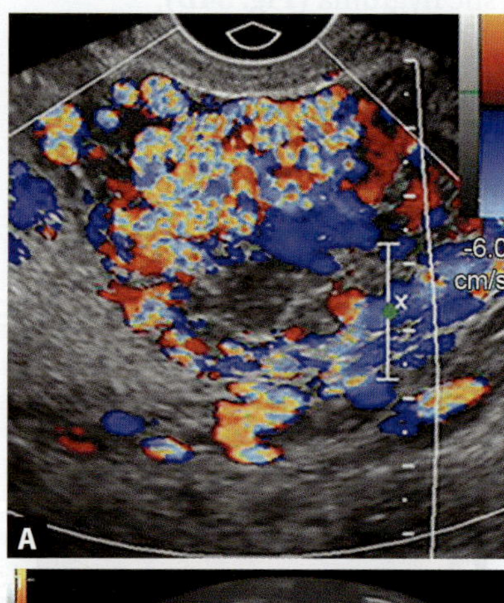 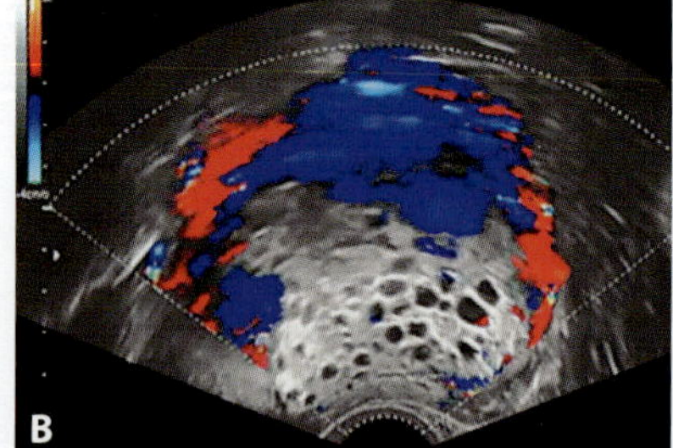 **Figs. 35A and B:** Doppler ultrasound showing the presence of highly vascularized tissues.	**Explanation:** On color Doppler ultrasound, a hydatidiform mole typically shows high-velocity, low-impedance flow. This is due to the increased vascularity of the trophoblastic tissue, which is a hallmark of molar pregnancies. This finding helps differentiate a hydatidiform mole from other conditions such as missed abortion, which would not exhibit such vascular patterns. **Potential questions:** There can be questions related to etiology, diagnosis, and management of the cases of hydatidiform mole.

Question	Answer	Comment
Q36. During the routine antenatal ultrasound of a 32-year-old gravida 2, para 1 woman, at 30 weeks of gestation, the sonographer observes a typical sign as shown in the image below. Which of the following is the primary pathological process associated with this sign? 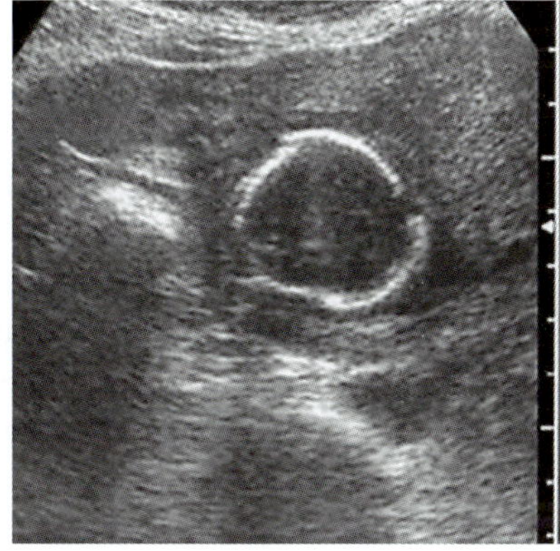 A. Polyhydramnios B. Maternal coagulopathy C. Uterine rupture D. Placental insufficiency E. Fetal maceration	**Ans: E (Fetal maceration)** The adjacent image shows overlapping bones of the fetal skull. This is depicted by an arrow in **Figure 36**. This sign is indicative of intrauterine fetal death, which can be defined as the diagnosis of the stillborn infant (with the period of gestation being > 24 weeks and fetal weight > 500 g). Definitive diagnosis of intrauterine death is made by observing the lack of fetal cardiac motion during a 10-minute period of careful examination with real-time ultrasound. 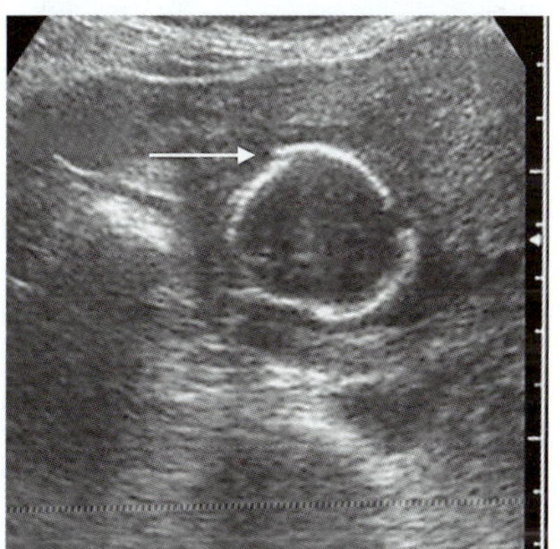 **Fig. 36:** Spalding sign, showing overlapping of the fetal skull bones (indicated by arrow).	**Explanation:** Spalding sign is an indicator of fetal demise and is characterized by the overlapping of fetal skull bones on ultrasound. This occurs due to the loss of alignment and overriding of the bones of the cranial vault, which occurs due to maceration, a pathological process where the fetus undergoes autolysis and soft tissue breakdown in utero. This sign typically appears several days after fetal demise and is a crucial diagnostic feature in confirming intrauterine fetal death. Other signs of fetal death may include hyperflexion of the spine, crowding of ribs, and appearance of gas shadows in the heart and great vessels (Robert's sign). **Potential questions:** There can be questions related to different abnormalities encountered in various organ-structures on ultrasound examination.

<table>
<tr><th>Question</th><th>Answer</th><th>Comment</th></tr>
<tr>
<td>Q37. A 25-year-old woman presents with right-sided pelvic pain for more than 1 year. An ultrasound scan is arranged which shows a 5-cm well-defined cystic lesion in the right adnexa with mixed echoes as shown in the image below. There is no fluid in the cul-de-sac with the following sonographic image. What is the most likely diagnosis for this?
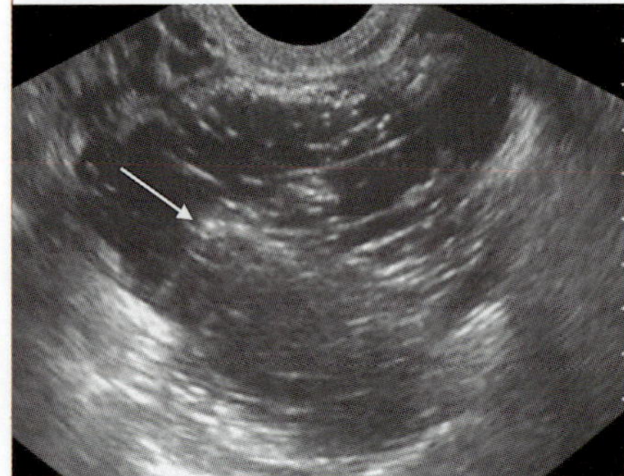
A. Benign cystic teratoma
B. Endodermal sinus tumor
C. Endometrioma
D. Mucinous cystadenoma
E. Serous cystadenoma</td>
<td>Ans: A (Benign cystic teratoma)
The arrow in the adjacent image refers to a mass with heterogeneous echogenicity. This is suggestive of a benign cystic teratoma.
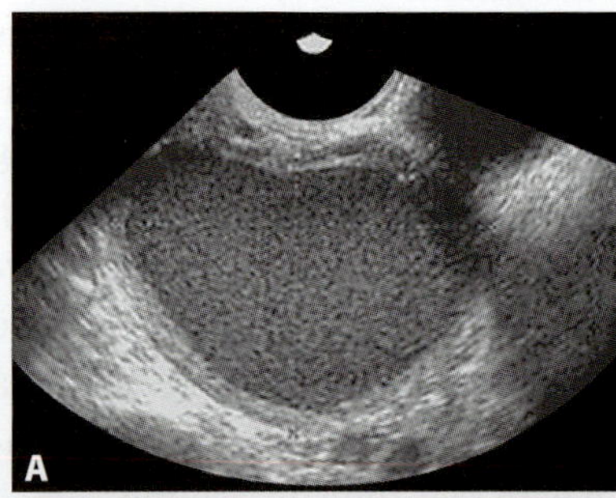

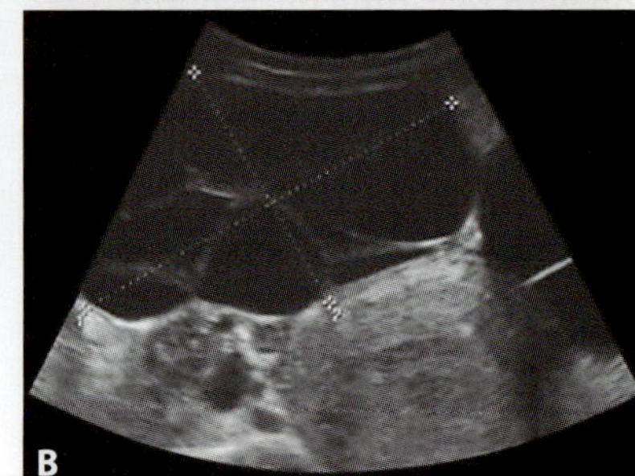

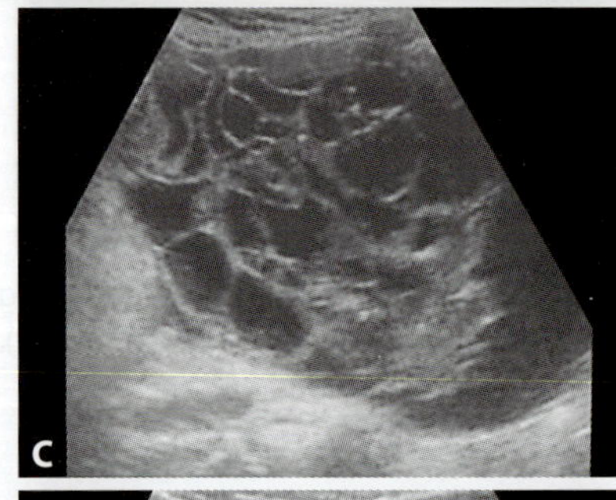

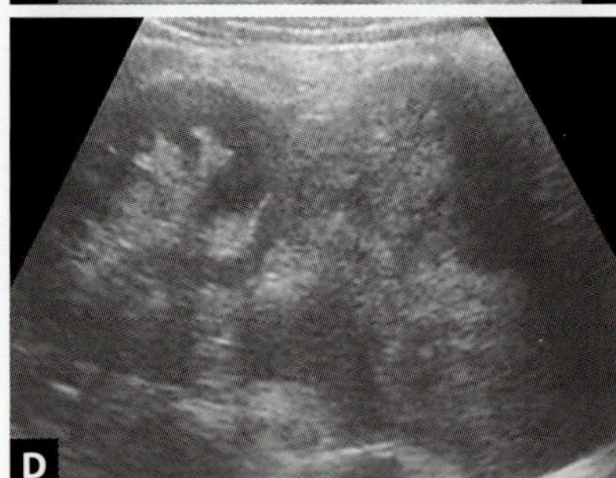

Figs. 37A to D: (A) Endometrioma showing ground-glass appearance; (B) Serous cystadenoma; (C) Mucinous cystadenoma; (D) Endodermal sinus tumor.</td>
<td>Explanation: Presence of other types of tumors can be ruled out as follows:
Endometrioma (Fig. 37A) shows a homogenous, grainy or ground-glass appearance. The most commonly occurring appearance of an endometrioma is the presence of a unilocular cyst showing acoustic enhancement with diffuse homogeneous ground-glass echoes, which can be observed in this case.
Serous cystadenoma presents as a smooth, thin-walled, anechoic, fluid-filled structure (Fig. 37B). Mucinous cystadenoma (Fig. 37C) appears as a large cystic adnexal mass. Multiple loculi may be present separated by thin septae. Loculations may present with varied levels of echogenicity based on different levels of mucin content in various loculi. Endodermal sinus tumor presents as a multiloculated solid mass (Fig. 37D).
Potential questions: There can be questions related to different tumors of the ovaries and adnexa on ultrasound examination.</td>
</tr>
</table>

Question	Answer	Comment
Q38. A 33-year-old woman with known stage III cervical cancer post hysterectomy presents to the A & E department with lower abdominal and unilateral flank pain. CT scan contrast urogram was done and is shown below. From the below-mentioned options, what is the likely diagnosis? 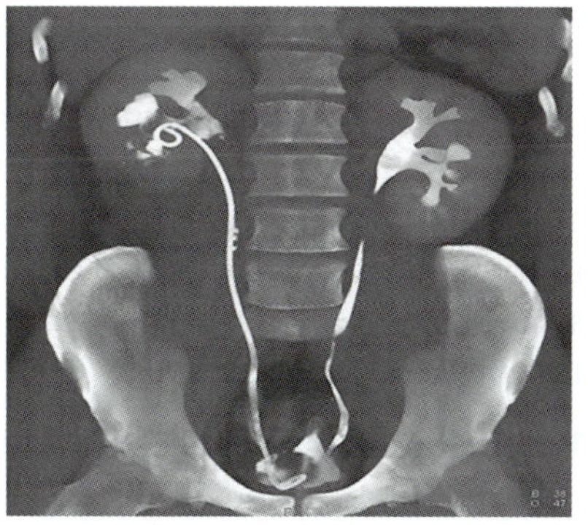 A. Renal stones B. Ischemia secondary to uterine artery obstruction C. Urinary tract infection D. Urethral obstruction E. Ureteric obstruction	**Ans: E (Ureteric obstruction)** The adjacent CT scan image shows interruption of the dye flow, approximately 1 cm below the pelvis–ureteral junction. The area of interruption has been depicted with the help of an arrow in **Figure 38**. 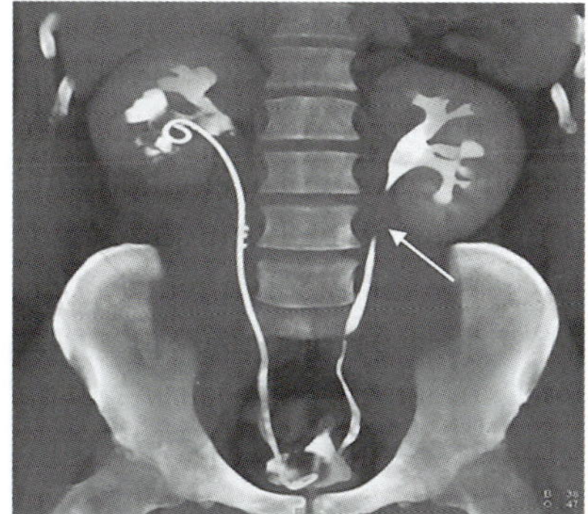 **Fig. 38:** Arrow showing interruption of the flow of dye on CT contrast urogram.	**Explanation:** The ureteric obstruction is related to stage III cervical cancer in this case. This can lead to a blockage in the kidneys known as hydronephrosis. Hydronephrosis is associated with worse outcomes in cervical cancer patients. Treatment options in these cases include ureteral stenting, percutaneous nephrostomy, chemoradiotherapy, etc. If left untreated, ureteric obstruction can lead to chronic kidney disease or acute kidney injury, necessitating urgent interventions like dialysis. **Potential questions:** There can be questions related to different complications associated with various gynecologic malignancies.
Q39. The below image was obtained after imaging a 35-year-old woman complaining of heavy menstrual bleeding. What investigation was done in this case? 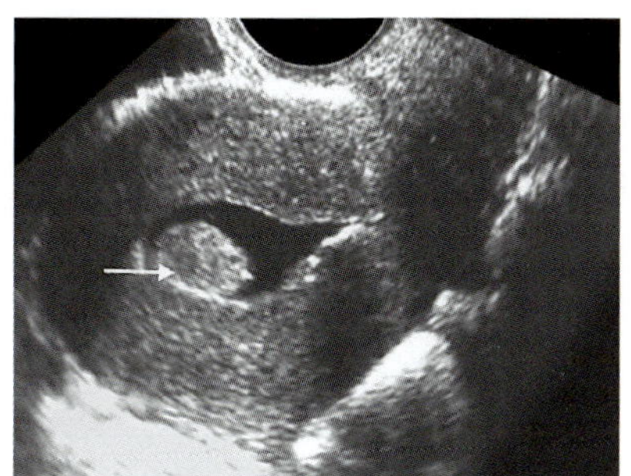 A. Transabdominal sonography B. Transvaginal sonography C. Saline infusion sonography D. Magnetic resonance imaging E. Computed tomography	**Ans: C (Saline infusion sonography)** The figure in the adjacent question shows distension of the uterine cavity with saline, revealing presence of a solitary endometrial polyp (indicated by an arrow). This polyp is probably responsible for causing heavy menstrual bleeding in this patient. **Figure 39** shows the diagrammatic representation of the procedure of saline infusion sonography. 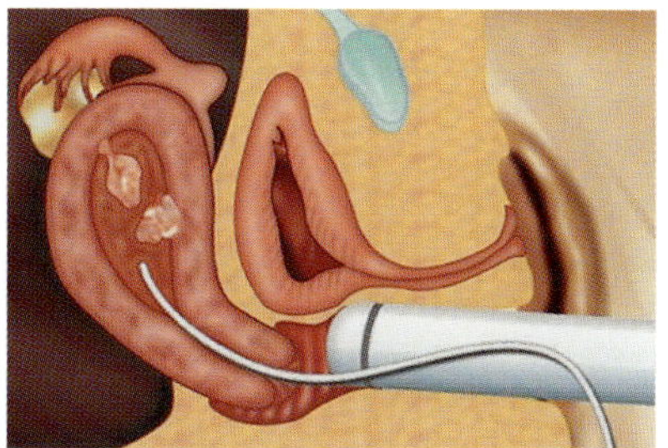 **Fig. 39:** Diagrammatic representation of the procedure of saline infusion sonography.	**Explanation:** A newer technique, called saline infusion sonography or sonohysterography, uses saline infusion into the endometrial cavity to enhance the detection of submucosal fibroids and polyps at the time of transvaginal sonography. Though transvaginal ultrasonography is associated with higher resolution in comparison to transabdominal sonography, it may not always be useful in distinguishing between a submucosal fibroid, endometrial polyp, and adenomyosis. **Potential questions:** There can be questions related to the diagnosis of different endometrial pathologies.

Question	Answer	Comment
Q40. A 35-year-old patient post abortion came in with difficulty of breathing and hemoptysis. Her β-hCG levels are raised. Chest X-ray was done, which revealed findings as shown in the image below. With the following findings, what is the tumor marker that is possibly elevated? 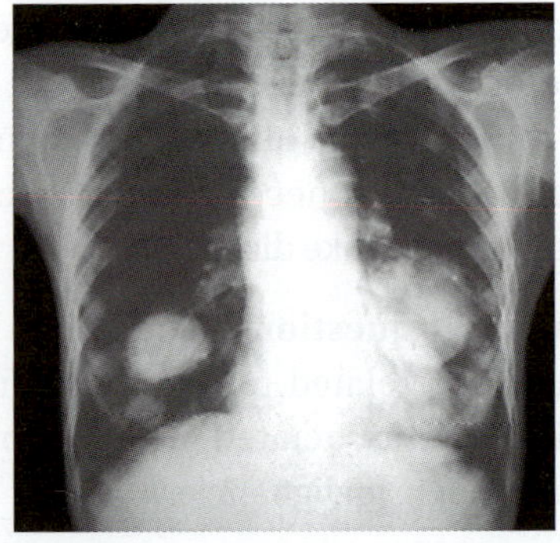 A. AFP (alpha-fetoprotein) B. CEA (carcinoembryonic antigen) C. hCG D. CA-125 E. LDH (lactate dehydrogenase)	**Ans: C (hCG)** The chest X-ray in the adjacent figure shows a cannon ball appearance, in which there are multiple, well-defined, pulmonary nodules of varied sizes suggestive of pulmonary metastasis. **Figure 40** shows the primary tumor in this case. There is a presence of focal intramural tumor with high vascularity. This is highly suggestive of a choriocarcinoma in the presence of raised hCG levels. 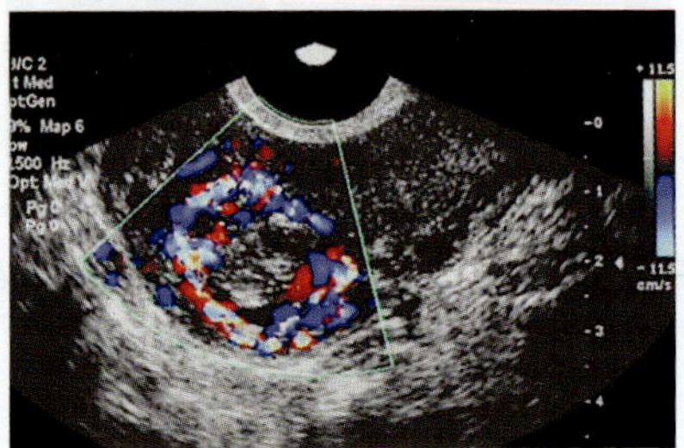 **Fig. 40:** Color doppler ultrasound showing choriocarcinoma.	**Explanation:** Presence of pulmonary metastasis appears to be most likely associated with choriocarcinoma, which has caused elevated levels of β-hCG in the blood. Treatment is mainly by chemotherapy. Stage I is treated with a single-agent therapy comprising methotrexate. Stages II to IV are treated with multiagent chemotherapy comprising methotrexate, actinomycin D, and etoposide. Monitoring must be continued with serial hCG levels every week until normal for 3 consecutive weeks. This is followed by monthly hCG levels for 1 year. **Potential questions:** There can be questions related to diagnosis, management and complications of hydatidiform mole.

Question	Answer	Comment
Q41. A 22-year-old presented to the accident and emergency department with history of severe abdominal pain and nausea. She had undergone surgery in lieu of severe endometriosis and was discharged two days back from the hospital. The X-ray abdomen shown in the image below revealed multiple air-fluid levels. Which of the following is not correct regarding the symptoms of associated pathology? 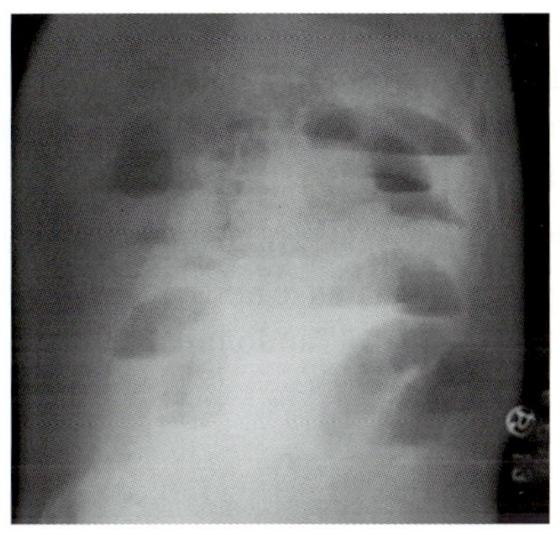 A. Constipation B. Crampy pain due to intermittent vigorous peristalsis C. Distension due to fluid and gas proximal to the obstruction D. Hypotension E. Vomiting which is more severe with low than with high bowel obstruction	**Ans: E (Vomiting which is more severe with low than with high bowel obstruction)** The adjacent image shows an erect abdominal X-ray with multiple air-fluid levels, which are suggestive of intestinal obstruction. The abdominal X-ray is likely to show dilated loops of small bowel proximal to the site of obstruction. Air fluid levels can be observed especially in cases of erect films The red arrows in **Figure 41** indicate air-fluid levels. 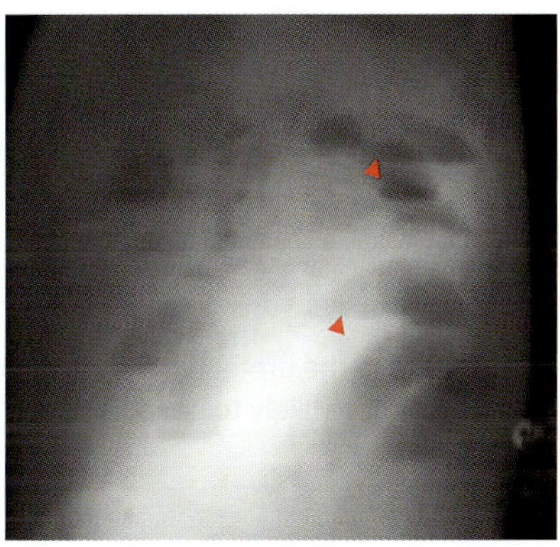 **Fig. 41:** Presence of multiple air-fluid levels in erect X-ray films, indicating intestinal obstruction.	**Explanation:** Obstruction of intestines is likely to cause a buildup of food, fluid, gastric acid, and gas behind the site of blockage. It may result in signs and symptoms such as colicky abdominal pain, nausea and vomiting, abdominal distension or bloating, constipation and inability to pass stool, gas, or flatus. Loss of body fluids can result in the development of hypotension. Vomiting is likely to be more severe in high bowel obstructions because the blockage occurs closer to the stomach (duodenum/proximal jejunum), causing rapid accumulation of gastric and bilious contents with limited absorption capacity. In low bowel obstructions, the distal location (ileum/colon) allows some absorption and storage of intestinal contents, reducing the immediacy and intensity of vomiting. **Potential questions:** There can be questions related to diagnosis and management of various postoperative complications.

Question	Answer	Comment
Q42. A 52-year-old menopausal patient comes with a complaint of groin pain. An X-ray shows the finding as depicted by the arrow in the below image. 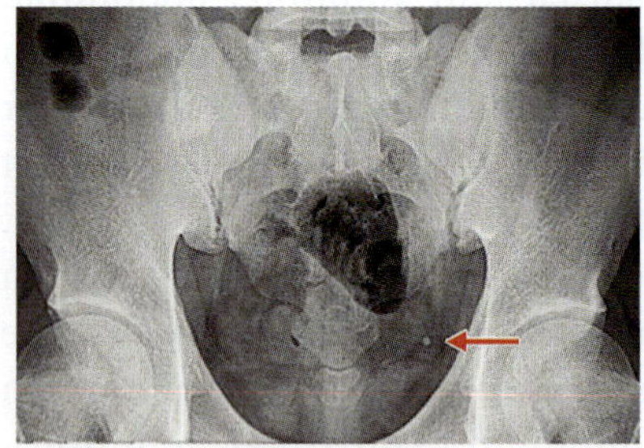 At what level are you expected to see this pathology? A. Iliac crest B. Paravertebral C. Pelvic brim D. Mid-clavicular line E. Mid-axillary line	**Ans: C (Pelvic brim)** The red arrow in the adjacent image points toward a calcification in the course of ureter, suggestive of a ureteric stone. There are three narrow areas of the ureter, where the ureteric stone is most likely to lodge **(Fig. 42)**. 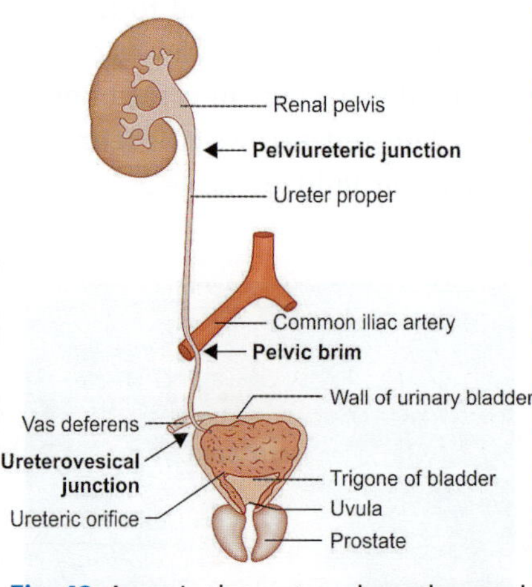 **Fig. 42:** Areas in the ureter where the renal stone is more likely to be located.	**Explanation:** Areas of the ureter, where the ureteric stone is most likely to lodge, include the following: ▪ *Ureteropelvic junction:* Stone lodged at the ureteropelvic junction results in mild-to-severe deep pain in the flank, which does not get radiated to the groin. ▪ Pelvic brim ▪ Ureterovesical junction Stones at the pelvic brim or ureterovesical junction may result in abrupt, severe, colicky pain in the flank and ipsilateral lower abdomen. This pain may radiate to the groin or testicle in men or to the groin or labia majora in women. **Potential questions:** There can be questions related to nongynecological causes of pelvic/abdominal pain.

CHAPTER 14

Data Interpretation

FETAL MONITORING USING CARDIOTOCOGRAPHY

Question	Answer	Comment
Q1. When using the process of fetal monitoring as shown in the image below, which of the following is the most effective way to ensure accurate and continuous monitoring? 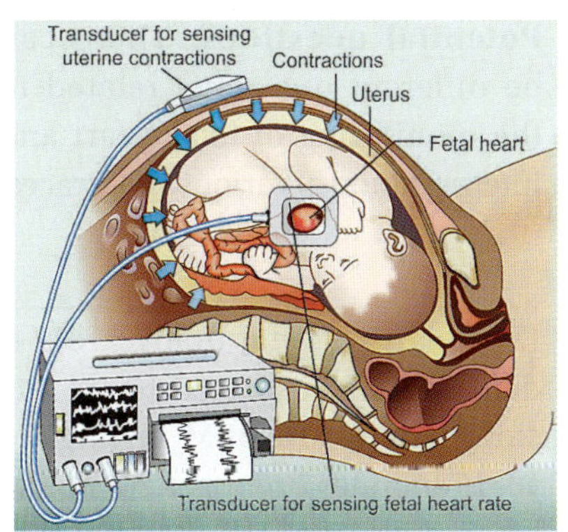 A. Place the transducer at the maternal umbilicus B. Use a high-frequency transducer. C. Position the transducer over the fetal back D. Apply minimal pressure with the transducer E. Ensure that the mother is in semi-Fowler's position	**Ans: C (Position the transducer over the fetal back)** The adjacent image depicts electronic external fetal heart rate monitoring (EFM) using cardiotocograph (CTG). EFM has been defined by both American College of Obstetricians and Gynecologists (ACOG) and Royal College of Obstetricians and Gynaecologists (RCOG) as monitoring the baby's heart rate for indicators of stress, usually during labor and birth using electronic fetal heart rate monitoring device. Based on the types of transducers used (external or internal), electronic fetal monitoring can be of two types: External or internal cardiac monitoring. **Figure 1** shows an obstetrician taking a cardiotocographic trace of a patient in labor. 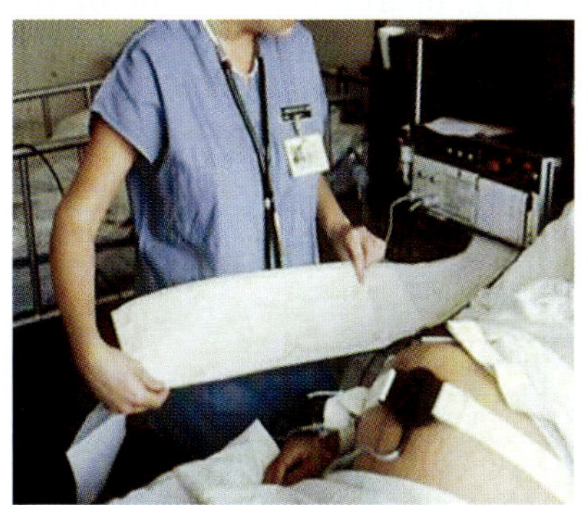 **Fig. 1:** An obstetrician taking a cardiotocographic trace of a patient in labor.	**Explanation:** External fetal heart monitoring as shown in the adjacent figure is performed by attaching the cardiotocograph machine through external transducers to the mother's abdomen with elastic straps. Positioning the transducer over the fetal back is the most effective way to ensure accurate and continuous monitoring of the fetal heart rate using electronic EFM. The fetal back provides a stable and consistent surface that allows for better transmission and reception of the heart rate signals. This positioning helps in obtaining a clearer and more reliable signal. Though routine use of EFM in every pregnancy is not recommended, it is widely used in the assessment of fetal health, particularly in high-risk pregnancies and unbooked patients with low-risk pregnancy, presenting for the first time late in labor. **Potential questions:** There can be different questions related to the monitoring of fetal heart and interpretation of various CTG traces.

Question	Answer	Comment
Q2. Which of the following fetal heart rate (FHR) patterns indicated by the arrow in the below image is considered reassuring? 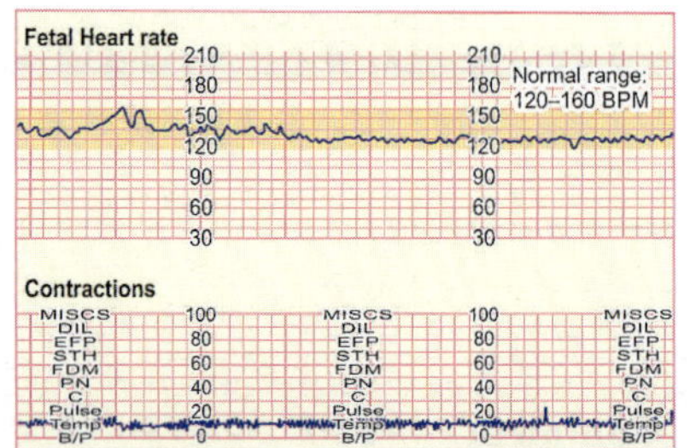 A. Late decelerations B. Variable decelerations C. Early decelerations D. Sinusoidal pattern E. Presence of acceleration	**Ans: E (Presence of acceleration)** The arrow in the adjacent image points toward the presence of accelerations. Reassuring FHR pattern can be defined as a baseline FHR of 120–160 BPM, having preserved beat-to-beat variability along with the presence of accelerations. Presence of accelerations is a reassuring sign that the fetus is adequately responsive and an indicator that the integrity of mechanisms controlling the fetal heart is intact. **Figure 2** illustrates reassuring heart rate pattern on FHR trace. 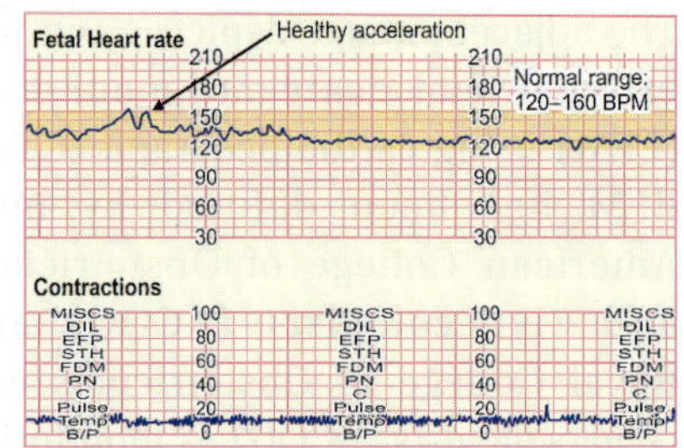 **Fig. 2:** Reassuring fetal heart rate patterns.	**Explanation:** Fetal heart tracing should be interpreted using a systematic approach, which involves evaluation of four main parameters, such as baseline heart rate, variability, absence of decelerations, and presence of accelerations. Accelerations are transient increases in the FHR, typically defined as an increase of more than 15 BPM lasting for at least 15 seconds. These accelerations are often associated with fetal movements. In the normal mature fetus, accelerations can be triggered by fetal body movements, sounds, and other stimuli. **Potential questions:** There can be different questions related to the monitoring of fetal heart and interpretation of various CTG traces.
Q3. What kind of fetal heart rate (FHR) pattern is indicated by the image below? 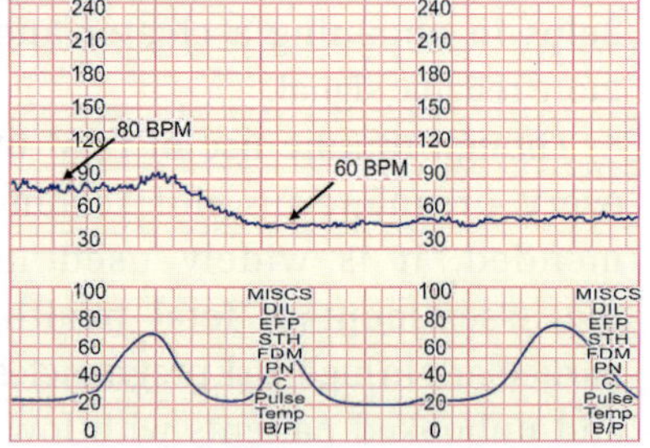 A. Baseline heart rate of 160 BPM B. Baseline heart rate of 110 BPM C. Baseline heart rate of less than 110 BPM D. Baseline heart rate of 130 BPM E. Baseline heart rate of 150 BPM	**Ans: C (Baseline heart rate of less than 110 BPM)** The adjacent image shows fetal heart rate pattern between 60 to 80 BPM. This is suggestive of fetal bradycardia. In contrast, baseline heart rates between 110 to 160 BPM are generally considered normal and reassuring. Fetal heart rate above 160 BPM for a period of 10 minutes or more is defined as tachycardia **(Fig. 3)**. 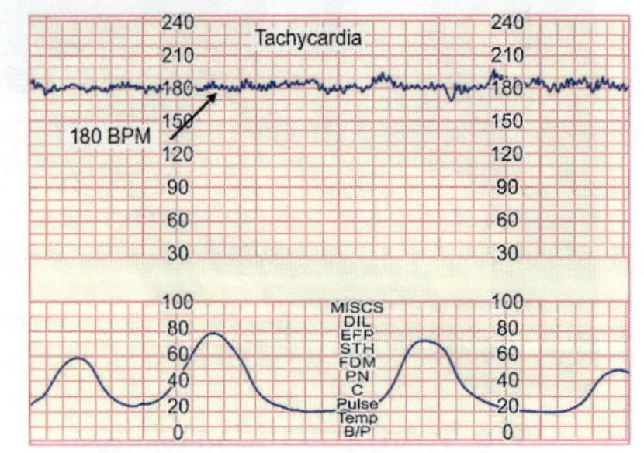 **Fig. 3:** Fetal heart tracing showing tachycardia.	**Explanation:** Fetal bradycardia is defined as a sustained heart rate slower than 110 BPM lasting for 10–15 minutes or longer. Moderate bradycardia is an FHR of 80–100 BPM and severe bradycardia is 80 BPM or less lasting for 3 minutes or longer. Monitoring and further evaluation are necessary to determine the cause and appropriate management of fetal bradycardia. Bradycardia is a late sign of fetal hypoxia (a continued lack of oxygen supply to fetus). Mild bradycardia can also sometimes result from compression of the umbilical cord. Since fetal bradycardia may be an emergency, seeking immediate assistance becomes mandatory. **Potential questions:** There can be questions related to the interpretation and significance of various FHR patterns on CTG traces.

Question	Answer	Comment
Q4. Which of the following descriptions best describes the FHR variability depicted in the image below? 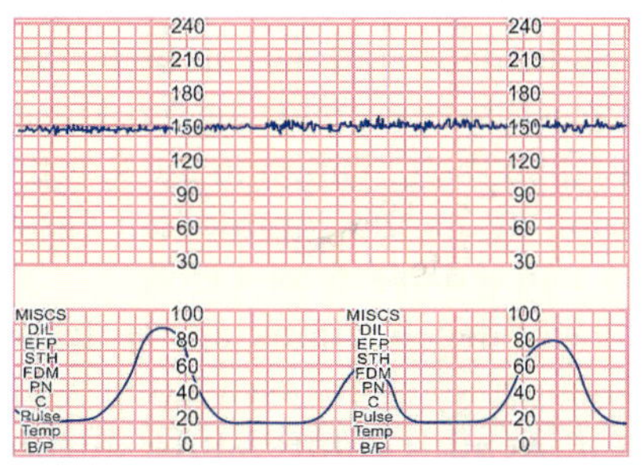 A. Amplitude range undetectable B. Amplitude range less than 5 beats per minute C. Amplitude range 6–25 beats per minute D. Amplitude range greater than 25 beats per minute E. No variability with a sinusoidal pattern	**Ans: C (Amplitude range 6–25 beats per minute)** The adjacent figure illustrates normal short-term variability. Baseline variability implies that the FHR is under constant variation from the baseline. A normal, healthy fetus should exhibit average to moderate variability varying between 5 to 25 BPM every 10–20 seconds, i.e., at the frequency of three to six cycles per minute. Variability can normally be both short term and long term **(Fig. 4)**. Long-term variability denotes the fluctuations or oscillatory changes that occur during the course of 1 minute in the fetal heart tracing relative to its baseline rate. 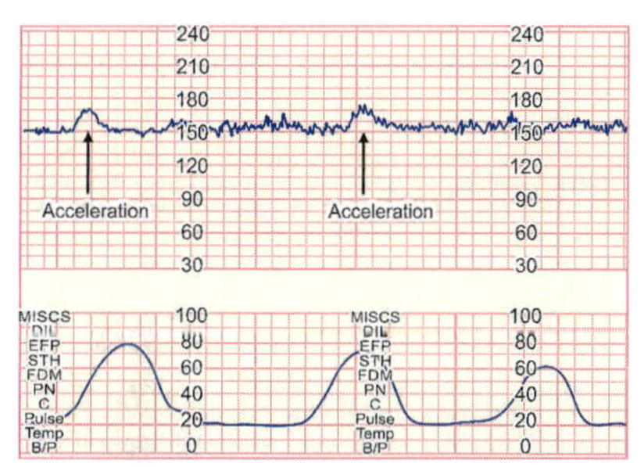 **Fig. 4:** Long-term variability.	**Explanation:** Beat-to-beat or short-term variability is the minute irregularity that occurs from one beat to the other on the CTG trace line, responsible for giving it a saw-toothed appearance. Moderate FHR variability, defined as an amplitude range of 5–25 BPM, is considered reassuring and indicates a well-oxygenated fetus with an intact central nervous system. Normal beat-to-beat variability indicates the ability of the fetal heart to respond to external stimuli through well-balanced sympathetic and parasympathetic nervous systems. Minimal variability (<5 BPM) or marked variability (>25 BPM) can be concerning and may indicate fetal distress or compromise. **Potential questions:** There can be different questions related to the interpretation and significance of FHR pattern on various types of CTG traces, including long-term and short-term variability.

Question

Q5. Which of the following characteristics best describes the type of deceleration in FHR as depicted by arrows in the image below?

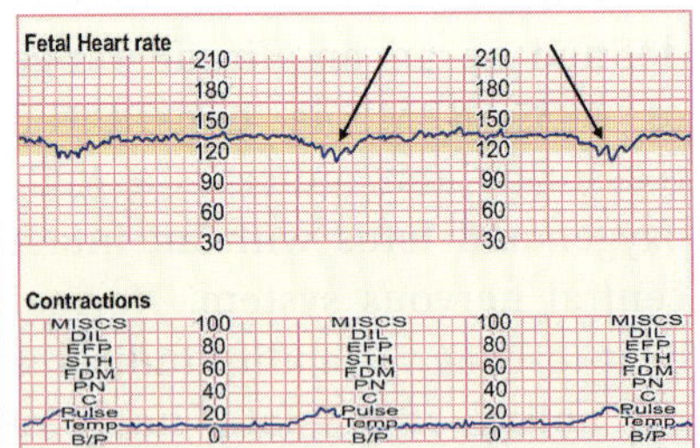

A. Gradual decrease in fetal heart rate with the nadir occurring after the peak of a contraction
B. Abrupt decrease in fetal heart rate with the nadir occurring after the peak of a contraction
C. Gradual decrease in fetal heart rate with the nadir occurring at the same time as the peak of a contraction
D. Abrupt decrease in fetal heart rate with the nadir occurring at the same time as the peak of a contraction
E. Gradual decrease in fetal heart rate with the nadir occurring before the peak of a contraction

Answer

Ans: C (Gradual decrease in fetal heart rate with the nadir occurring at the same time as the peak of a contraction)

The adjacent image shows the pattern of early deceleration. The onset and return of the deceleration typically coincide with the start and end of the contraction, respectively (**Fig. 5**). These decelerations are characterized by a gradual decrease and return to baseline of the FHR, with the nadir (lowest point) occurring simultaneously with the peak of a uterine contraction. These decelerations recover fully by the end of the uterine contraction.

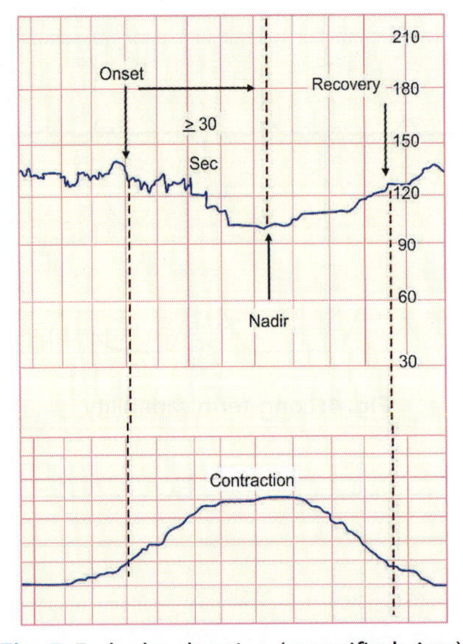

Fig. 5: Early deceleration (magnified view).

Comment

Explanation: A sudden decrease in FHR by more than 15 BPM lasting for more than 15 seconds but less than 2 minutes from the baseline is considered as a deceleration and can be either periodic or episodic. Periodic decelerations can be further subclassified into following three types based on their relation to the specific period of uterine contraction: Early, late, and variable decelerations.

Early decelerations are typically benign and often associated with fetal head compression during contractions, which is a normal part of labor. Unlike late decelerations, which occur after the peak of a contraction and can indicate fetal distress, early decelerations are usually not a cause for concern. Uncomplicated early deceleration does not signify hypoxia or acidosis; hence, immediate intervention is usually not necessary.

Potential questions: There can be different questions related to the interpretation and significance of FHR pattern on various types of CTG traces, including the presence of various types of decelerations (early, variable, and late).

Question	Answer	Comment
Q6. Which of the following interventions is most appropriate for managing the decelerations caused by umbilical cord compression as shown in the image below? 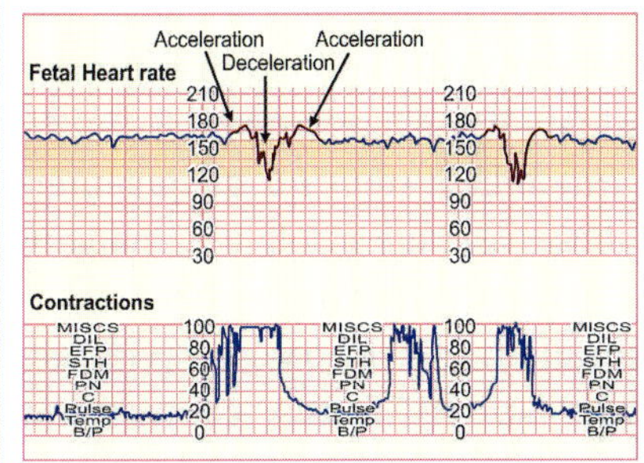 A. Administering oxygen to the mother B. Increasing intravenous fluid administration C. Changing the mother's position D. Performing an immediate cesarean section E. Administering tocolytics to stop contractions	**Ans: C (Changing the mother's position)** The adjacent image depicts variable decelerations, which are named so as they can occur at any time during a contraction. These decelerations are often variable in duration, intensity, and timing **(Fig. 6)**. These decelerations can occur at any time in relation to uterine contractions and are often caused by umbilical cord compression. However, severe atypical (associated with loss of variability) variable decelerations are commonly associated with fetal acidosis and low APGAR scores. 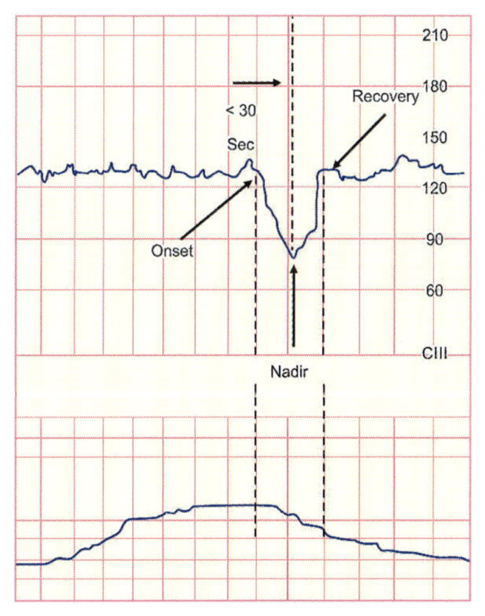 **Fig. 6:** Variable decelerations (magnified view).	**Explanation:** Variable decelerations are characterized by the presence of a frequently short acceleration pattern followed by a rapid deceleration for some seconds. This is again followed by a rapid rise and a short acceleration before returning to baseline. This results in acceleration "shoulders" before and after a deceleration and is responsible for their V or W-shape. Management of variable decelerations is as follows: ▪ Changing the maternal position ▪ If the patient is on oxytocin, it should be discontinued. ▪ Performing a vaginal examination to rule out cord prolapse. Changing the mother's position is often the first and most appropriate intervention for managing variable decelerations caused by umbilical cord compression. This can help relieve the pressure on the umbilical cord and improve fetal blood flow. **Potential questions:** There can be different questions related to the interpretation and significance of fetal heart rate pattern on various types of CTG traces, including the presence of various types of decelerations (early, variable, and late).

Question	Answer	Comment
Q7. Which of the following fetal heart rate patterns is most concerning when observed alongside the decelerations shown in the image below? 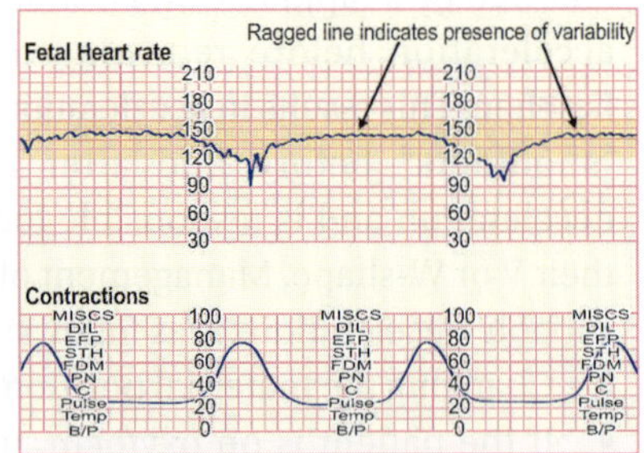 A. Moderate variability B. Early decelerations C. Accelerations D. Minimal variability E. Sinusoidal pattern	**Ans: D (Minimal variability)** The adjacent image shows late decelerations with preserved baseline variability. The onset of late decelerations occurs after the beginning of the contraction, and the nadir of the deceleration occurs after the peak of the contraction **(Fig. 7)**. Since deceleration starts late during the contraction, it is known as late deceleration. These decelerations may be associated with reduced placental perfusion resulting in uteroplacental insufficiency, which can result in development of hypoxia and metabolic abnormalities in the baby. 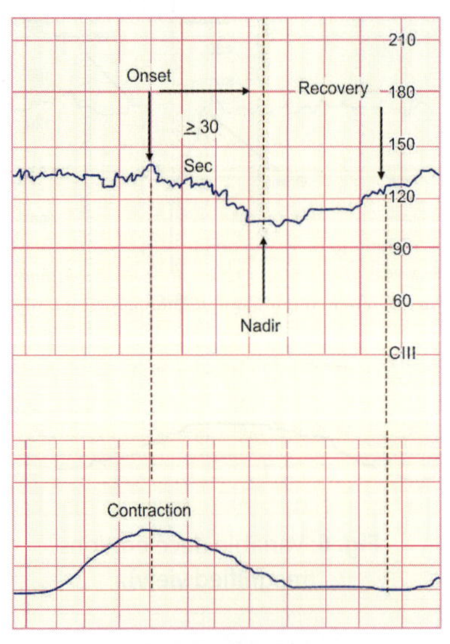 **Fig. 7:** Late deceleration (magnified view).	**Explanation:** Late decelerations are the most ominous fetal heart rate pattern. Persistent late decelerations with decreased variability (<5 BPM) or absent variability is associated with an even worse prognosis. This combination indicates a higher risk of fetal hypoxia and requires prompt evaluation and intervention. Immediate steps for management in these cases are as follows: Changing the patient position to left lateral, administration of oxygen (via face mask) and IV fluids, cessation of oxytocin if being administered, administration of subcutaneous terbutaline in case of uterine hyperstimulation, etc. If despite the above-mentioned steps, maternal decelerations persist for more than 30 minutes, measurement of fetal scalp pH may be done based on physician's discretion. As per the latest NICE guidelines (2022), no recommendation has been made about fetal blood sampling due to lack of suitable evidence. Fetal scalp stimulation may be considered in these cases. If the CTG trace still remains pathological, the overall clinical condition must be evaluated, and the obstetrician must consider expediting baby's delivery. **Potential questions:** There can be different questions related to the interpretation and significance of fetal heart rate pattern on various types of CTG traces, including the presence of various types of decelerations (early, variable, and late).

Question	Answer	Comment
Q8. Which of the following characteristics best describes the fetal heart rate pattern as observed in the image below? 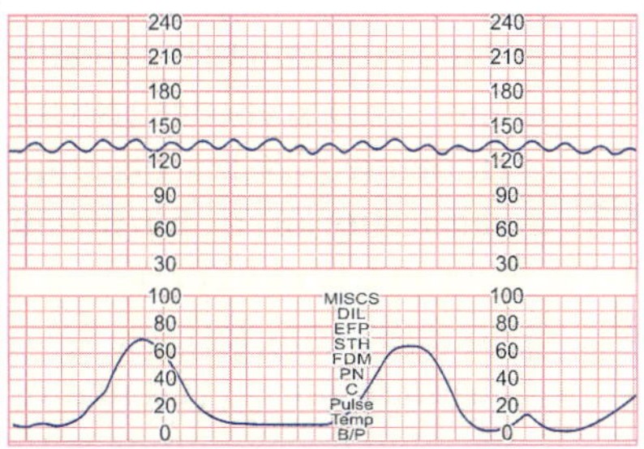 A. Pseudosinusoidal pattern B. Saltatory pattern C. Sinusoidal pattern D. Persistent late decelerations E. Absent variability	**Ans: C (Sinusoidal pattern)** The adjacent image shows a sinusoidal pattern, in which the amplitude of oscillations and period of short term (beat-to-beat variability) remain more or less constant. This gives the fetal heart trace a smooth, undulating, regular wavy appearance. The fetal heart pattern is labeled as sinusoidal, if this pattern lasts for at least 10 minutes. Fetal activity may be minimal or absent, and FHR accelerations are usually lacking. Sinusoidal pattern is known as the pseudosinusoidal pattern **(Fig. 8)**, when in the in- between period, the baseline variability is preserved. It is not flattened as in the true sinusoidal pattern. 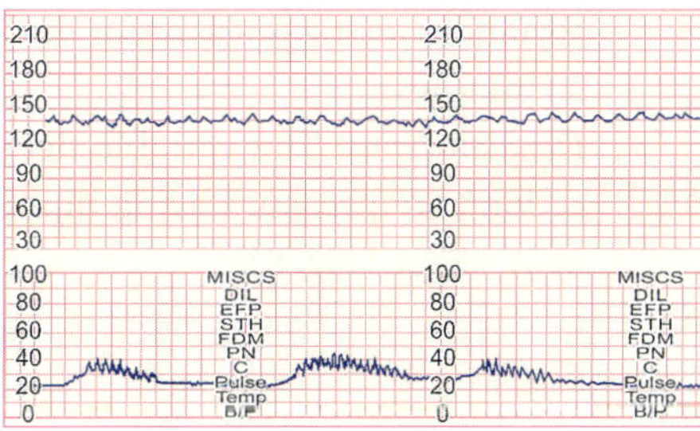 **Fig. 8:** Pseudosinusoidal pattern.	**Explanation:** A true sinusoidal pattern in FHR is characterized by a regular, smooth, wave-like pattern with a cycle frequency of 3–5 per minute and no variability. This pattern is concerning and often indicates severe fetal anemia or hypoxia, which is likely to be associated with a high rate of fetal morbidity and mortality. This pattern may be associated with conditions, such as Rh alloimmunization, severe anemia, asphyxiation (occasionally), and maternal administration of some sedative and analgesic drugs like meperidine, pethidine, butorphanol, etc. It is distinct from other patterns due to its regularity and lack of variability, which can be a sign of significant fetal compromise. Immediate evaluation and intervention are typically required when a true sinusoidal pattern is observed. **Potential questions:** There can be different questions related to the interpretation and significance of FHR pattern on various types of CTG traces, including the presence of sinusoidal, pseudosinusoidal, and saltatory patterns.

Question	Answer	Comment
Q9. A midwife asks the obstetric registrar to review a primigravida in labor who has progressed to 6 cm dilatation with an abnormal CTG. The CTG has been normal up to 30 minutes previously. The registrar reviews the patient and confirms that the CTG has a baseline heart rate of 150 BPM with a baseline variability of 4 for the last 30 minutes. There were no accelerations, but variable decelerations were present. What would be the appropriate management with these CTG findings? 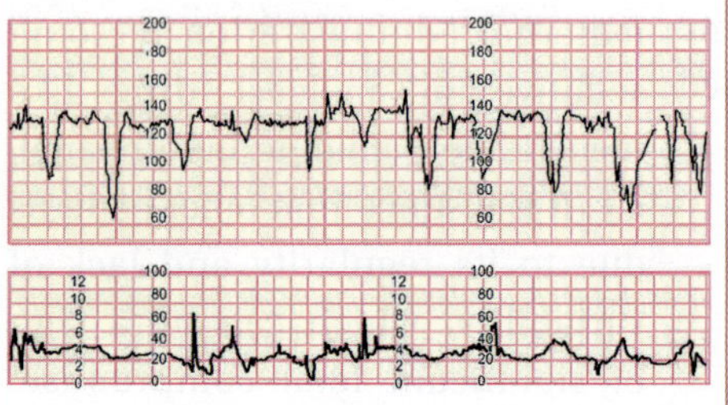 A. This is a normal CTG and no intervention is required B. This is a suspicious CTG and requires continued obstetric review C. This is a pathological CTG and fetal scalp stimulation is required D. This is a pathological CTG and urgent delivery is required (category 1 caesarean section) E. This is a suspicious CTG and fetal blood sampling is required	**Ans: C (This is a pathological CTG and fetal scalp stimulation is required)** The CTG can be interpreted following the mnemonic DR C BRaVADO, according to which the parameters assessed in this CTG are as follows: ▪ *Define risk:* Based on the clinical history, the patient is not at risk. ▪ *Contractions:* The rate of maternal contractions is within normal limits. ▪ *Baseline heart rate:* A heart rate of 150 BPM in this case can be considered as a reassuring feature as it lies within the normal range (110–160 BPM). ▪ *Variability:* Normal baseline variability can be considered to be between 5 and 25 BPM between contractions. In this case, baseline variability of 4 is present for the last 30 minutes. ▪ *Decelerations:* The variable decelerations are present having biphasic or W-shape **(Fig. 9)**. 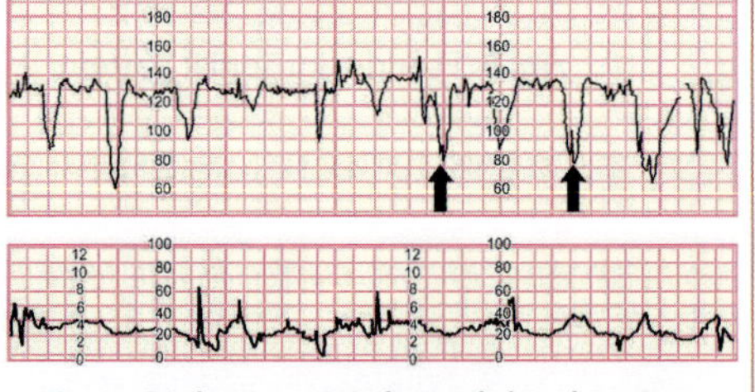 **Fig. 9:** Biphasic or W-shaped decelerations (indicated by arrows).	**Explanation:** The overall impression of the adjacent CTG trace is the presence of two features in the amber category. These include the following: ▪ *Variability:* According to National Institute for Health and Care Excellence (NICE) guidelines (2022), baseline variability of <5 for 30–50 minutes is considered as a nonreassuring feature. ▪ *Decelerations:* Presence of variable decelerations with any concerning characteristics in up to 50% of contractions for 30 minutes or more is the second feature in the amber category present in this case. Due to the presence of two features in the amber category, this CTG can be classified as pathological. Therefore, a fetal scalp stimulation must be performed in this case. **Potential questions:** There can be questions related to the interpretation of various parameters as well as their significance in various types of CTG traces.

Question	Answer	Comment
Q10. A 39-year-old female presented with spontaneous rupture of membrane. Below image is the CTG of the patient. Maternal heart rate is 80 BPM and fetal heart rate is 120 BPM, and the liquor is clear. After 2 hours, she is 4 cm dilated and CTG shows FHR 120 BPM with clear liquor. Maternal uterine contractions are reduced. What is the management option? 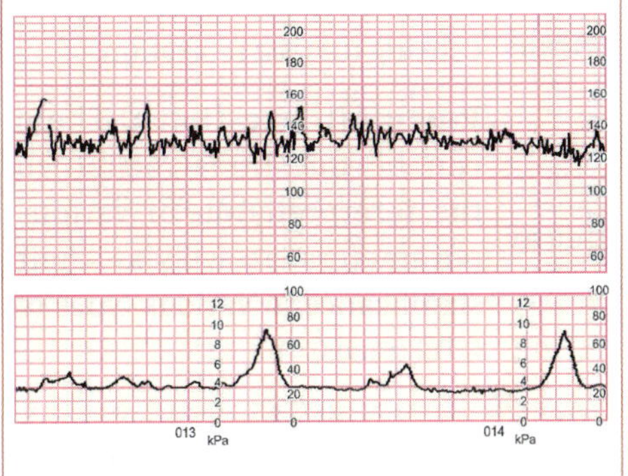 A. Category 1 cesarean B. Category 2 cesarean C. Category 3 cesarean D. Observe E. Fetal blood sampling	**Ans: D (Observe)** Following the mnemonic, DR C BRaVADO, the parameters assessed in this CTG are as follows: ▪ *Define risk:* The patient is not at high risk because the meconium is clear. ▪ *Contractions:* There are 1–2 contractions occurring every 5–6 minutes **(Fig. 10)**. ▪ *Baseline FHR:* It is within normal limits. ▪ *Variability:* Baseline variability is also normal. ▪ *Decelerations:* No decelerations can be observed. 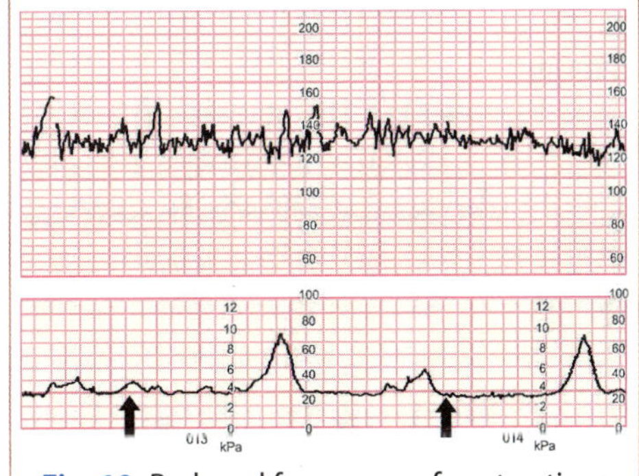 **Fig. 10:** Reduced frequency of contractions (indicated by the arrows).	**Explanation:** During the active stage of labor, normal uterine contractions occur every 2–3 minutes. In the adjacent case study, the overall impression is that the frequency of uterine contractions is reduced. Therefore, the patient just needs to be observed for some time to assess if the frequency of uterine contractions improves on its own. Stimulation with oxytocic may be required if contractions do not improve on their own. **Potential questions:** There can be questions related to the interpretation of various parameters as well as their significance in various types of CTG traces.

Question	Answer	Comment
Q11. The CTG of a multiparous patient with 40 weeks of gestation, who was induced with misoprostol pessary, is shown below. The pessary was removed after 20 minutes. The cervix is dilated to about 4 cm. What should be the next step of action in this patient? 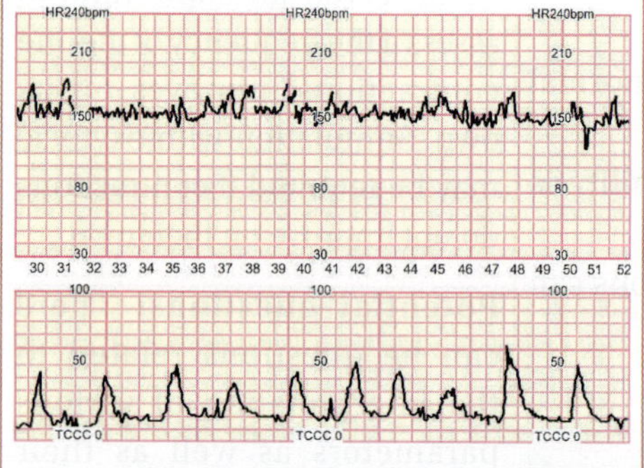 A. Administration of terbutaline 20 mg subcutaneously B. Category 1 cesarean section C. Category 2 cesarean section D. Reassurance and observation E. Performing fetal blood sampling	**Ans: A (Administration of terbutaline 20 mg subcutaneously)** Following the mnemonic, DR C BRaVADO, the parameters assessed in this CTG are as follows: ▪ *Define risk:* The patient does not appear to be at high risk. ▪ *Contractions:* There are 3–4 contractions every 1–2 minutes, which appear to be unusually high during this stage of labor **(Fig. 11)**. ▪ *Baseline FHR:* It is within normal limits. ▪ *Variability:* Baseline variability is also normal. ▪ *Decelerations:* No significant decelerations can be observed. 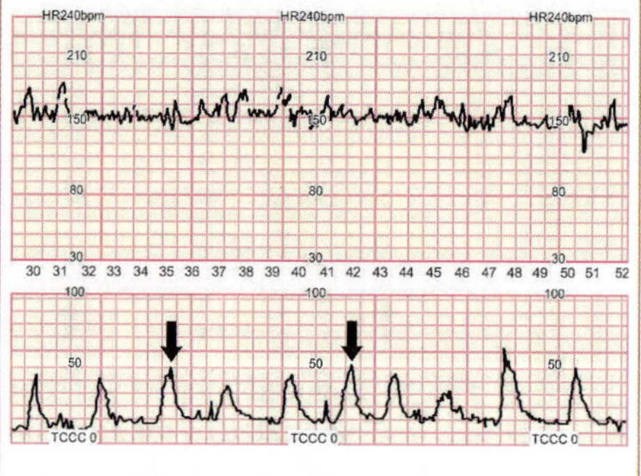 **Fig. 11:** Increased frequency of contractions (indicated by the arrows).	**Explanation:** The overall impression of the adjacent CTG trace is that the uterine contractions are increased. During the active stage of labor, normal contractions occur every 2–3 minutes. This frequency is greatly increased. This appears to be a case of uterine hyperstimulation. Therefore, the patient must be administered tocolytic drugs for causing uterine relaxation. **Potential questions:** There can be questions related to the interpretation of various parameters as well as their significance in various types of CTG traces.

Question	Answer	Comment
Q12. A 28-year-old primigravida patient, whose antenatal period had been largely uneventful, developed obstetric cholestasis with raised bile acids at 37 weeks' gestation. Growth of the baby was observed to be within normal limits on ultrasound scan. At 38 weeks, labor was induced with Prostin, followed by infusion of oxytocics. CTG revealed the trace shown in the image below. What should be the next step of management in this patient? 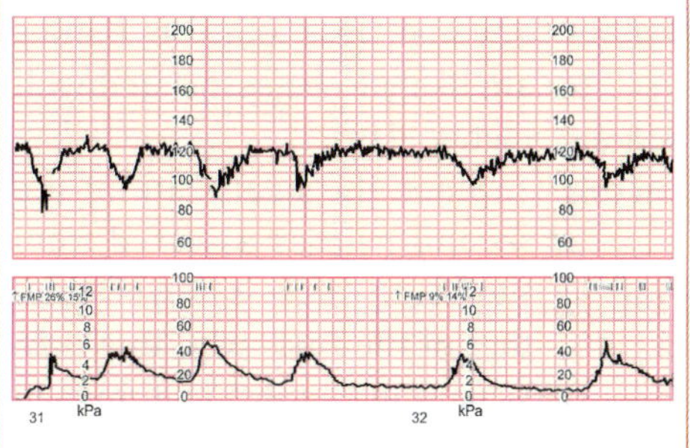 A. Encourage woman to be mobile or move to left lateral to ease head compression B. Fetal scalp pH C. Instrumental delivery in the labor ward D. Instrumental delivery in the operation theatre E. Category 1 caesarean delivery	**Ans. A (Encourage woman to be mobile or move to left lateral to ease head compression)** Following the mnemonic DR C BRaVADO, the parameters assessed in the adjacent CTG trace are as follows: ▪ *Define risk:* The patient is at high risk in view of obstetric cholestasis ▪ *Contractions:* 1–2 contractions every 2–3 minutes, which is normal during this stage of labor. ▪ *Baseline FHR:* Baseline heart rate is within normal limits. ▪ *Variability:* Baseline variability is also normal. ▪ *Decelerations:* Early decelerations can be observed **(Fig. 12)**. 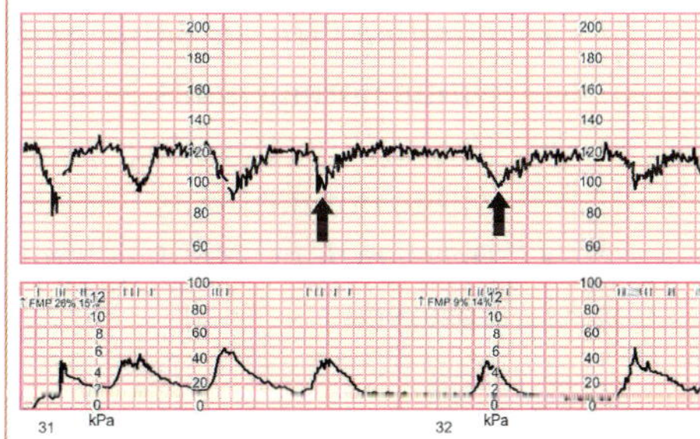 **Fig. 12:** Presence of early deceleration (indicated by the arrow).	**Explanation:** The overall impression of the adjacent CTG trace is the presence of early decelerations. These decelerations commence with the beginning of the uterine contraction and end with the end of the uterine contraction. The nadir of deceleration coincides with the peak of contraction. These decelerations are probably related to the compression of the fetal head. Therefore, the woman must be asked to be mobile and adopt a left lateral position while lying down to ease the fetal head compression. **Potential questions:** There can be questions related to the interpretation of various parameters as well as their significance in various types of CTG traces.

Question	Answer	Comment
Q13. A 27-year-old woman with pregnancy of 28 weeks attends the obstetrics and gynecology department following rupture of membranes. CTG was done to assess fetal heart rate. What can be the likely diagnosis after observing such fetal heart traces shown in the figure below? 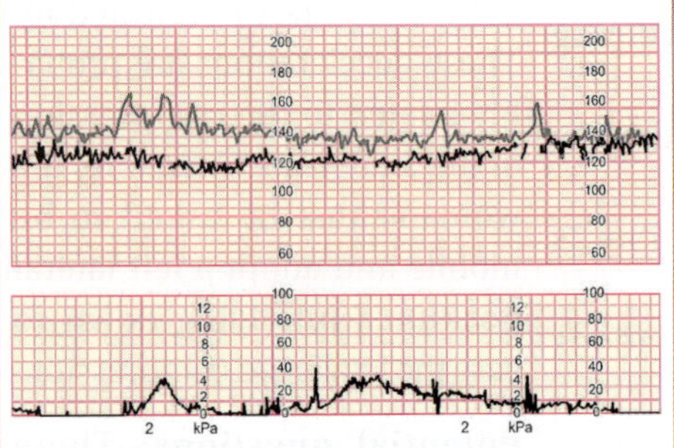 A. Nonreassuring fetal trace B. Abnormal fetal trace C. Reassuring fetal heart rate patterns D. Normal twin gestation E. Compromised twins	**Ans: D (Normal twin gestation)** In the adjacent figure, two fetal heart traces can be seen, which is suggestive of twin gestation. Following the mnemonic, DR C BRaVADO, the parameters assessed in this CTG for both the twins are as follows **(Fig. 13)**: Twin 1 (lighter trace on CTG, indicated by the red arrow): Twin 2 (darker trace, indicated by the black arrow): ▪ *Define risk:* The patient does not have any other risk factor besides twin gestation. ▪ *Contractions:* Uterine contractions are not adequately monitored in this case. ▪ *Baseline FHR:* Baseline heart rate is within normal limits. ▪ *Variability:* Baseline variability is within normal limits. ▪ *Decelerations:* No decelerations are observed. 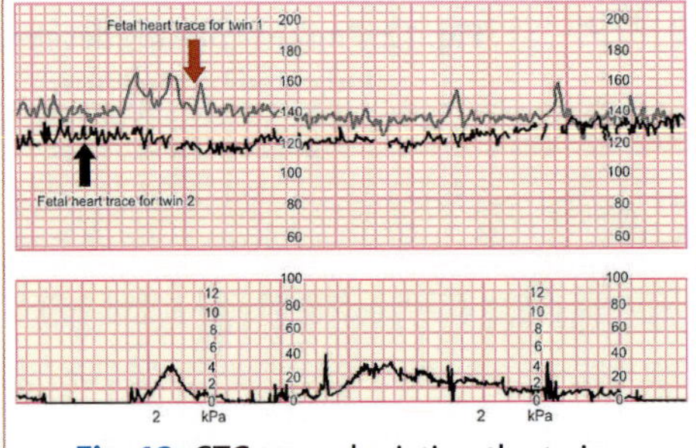 **Fig. 13:** CTG trace depicting the twins.	**Explanation:** In the adjacent figure, two fetal heart traces can be seen, which is suggestive of twin gestation. The overall impression given by the CTG trace of both first twin (lighter trace) and second twin (darker trace) is that all the parameters appear to be within normal limits. Since the heart rate of the first twin as assessed from the CTG trace is higher than that of the second twin, this twin is likely to be less mature because less mature babies are likely to be associated with higher FHRs. Since the heart rate of the second twin as assessed from the CTG trace is lower than that of the first twin, this twin is likely to be more mature than the second twin because more mature babies are likely to be associated with a lower FHR. **Potential questions:** There can be questions related to the interpretation of various parameters as well as their significance in various types of CTG traces.

Question	Answer	Comment
Q14. A 40-year-old woman at 33 weeks' gestation presents with a 2-hour history of heavy vaginal bleeding and lower abdominal pain. The placenta is not low-lying, and she is rhesus D positive. Examination shows a firm, tender abdomen and moderate active bleeding from closed cervical os. CTG monitoring shows an atypical fetal heart rate pattern for 30 minutes with no accelerations as shown in the image below. What is the most appropriate management? 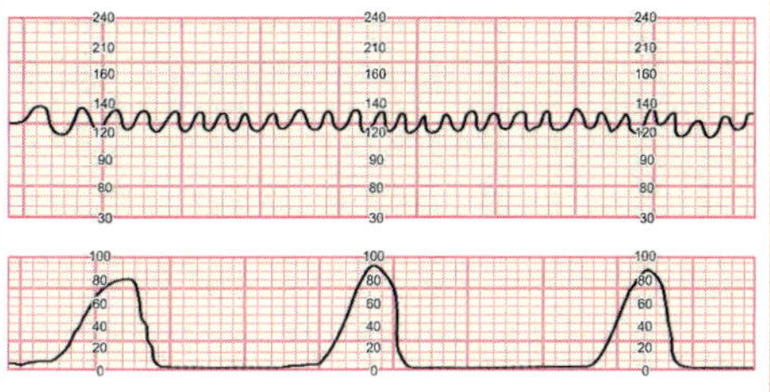 A. Induce labor with prostaglandin B. Steroids—two doses, 24 hours apart C. Steroids—two doses, 24 hours apart with tocolytics D. Tocolysis E. Urgent cesarean delivery	**Ans: E (Urgent cesarean delivery)** The CTG trace shown in the adjacent figure is suggestive of a sinusoidal heart rate pattern. The fetal heart pattern is labeled as sinusoidal, because it follows a sine-wave pattern **(Fig. 14)**. In this pattern, the amplitude of oscillations usually varies between 5 and 15 BPM with a fixed period of 3–5 cycles per minute. This gives the fetal heart trace a smooth, undulating, regular wavy appearance. Fetal activity may be minimal or absent, and FHR accelerations are usually lacking. 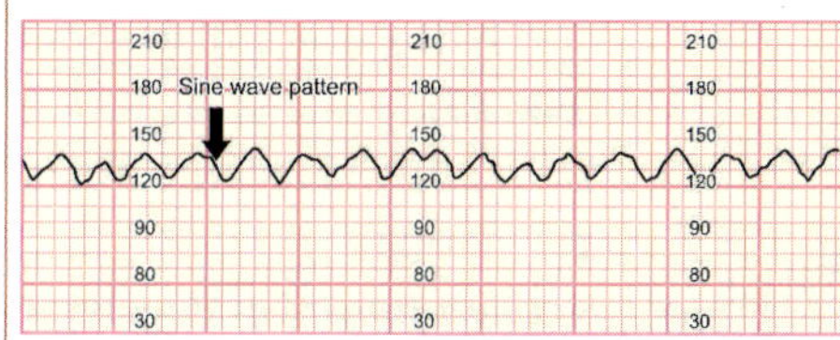 **Fig. 14:** Magnified view showing a sinusoidal heart rate pattern.	**Explanation:** In the sinusoidal type of heart rate pattern, the amplitude of oscillations and period of short-term (beat-to-beat) variability remain more or less constant. This type of FHR pattern may be associated with conditions such as fetomaternal hemorrhage (e.g., due to Rh alloimmunization) resulting in fetal anemia, hydrops fetalis, etc. A true sinusoidal pattern is rare but ominous and is associated with a high rate of fetal morbidity and mortality. Therefore, emergency delivery (by any route) becomes mandatory in these cases. Since the patient's cervical os is closed in this case, delivery through cesarean section appears to be the best option. **Potential questions:** There can be questions related to the interpretation of various parameters as well as their significance in various types of CTG traces.

Question	Answer	Comment
Q15. A woman with a previous cesarean section is in labor at 39 weeks of gestation. She is 2 cm dilated. The image below is the CTG trace, initially classified as normal. You have now been asked to review the situation because the fetal heart rate has acutely dropped from 140 to 70 BPM for 9 minutes, in spite of left lateral position. What is the most appropriate course of action? 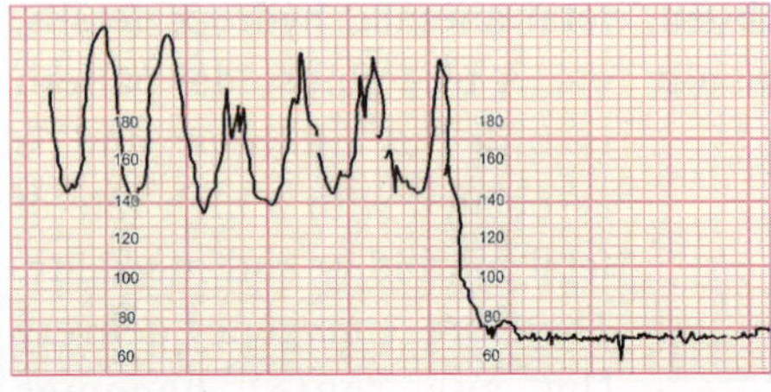 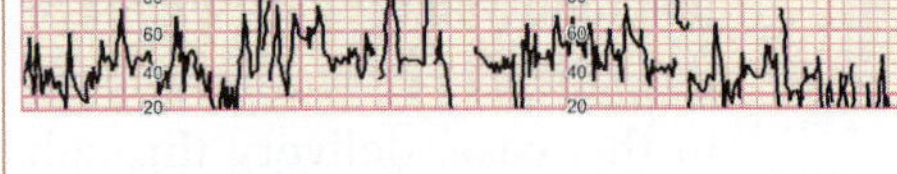 A. Doppler assessment of the umbilical artery blood flow B. Fetal blood sampling C. Oxygen therapy D. Prepare for a cesarean section E. Prepare for a ventouse delivery	**Ans: D (Prepare for a cesarean section)** Following the mnemonic DR C BRaVADO, the parameters assessed in this CTG are as follows: ▪ *Define risk:* The patient is at high risk in view of her previous cesarean delivery. ▪ *Contractions:* Uterine contractions cannot be adequately assessed in this case. ▪ *Baseline FHR:* Baseline heart rate is within normal limits (140–150 BPM) initially, on the left-hand side of the graph. However, somewhere in the middle, there occurs an acute dip in the FHR to an extent to about 70 BPM **(Fig. 15)**. ▪ *Variability:* Baseline variability is also normal. ▪ *Decelerations:* No decelerations are present. 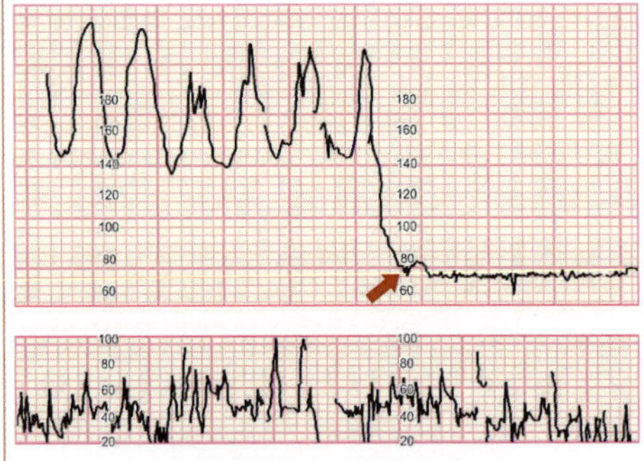 **Fig. 15:** Acute dip in the fetal heart rate (indicated by the arrow).	**Explanation:** The overall impression of the adjacent CTG trace is the presence of acute bradycardia. This is an indication for urgent delivery, by whichever route possible. Since the woman in adjacent case study is only 2 cm dilated, cesarean section appears to be the fastest route for delivery. **Potential questions:** There can be questions related to the interpretation of various parameters as well as their significance in different types of CTG traces.

Question	Answer	Comment
Q16. A primigravida is in labor at 38 weeks of gestation. The midwife has called you as the mother is exhausted. The CTG in the image below is showing late decelerations, a baseline of 140 BPM, and adequate variability. On examination, none of the presenting part is palpable per abdomen. The cervix is fully dilated, vertex is at +1 station, and position is occipitoposterior. What is the most appropriate management? 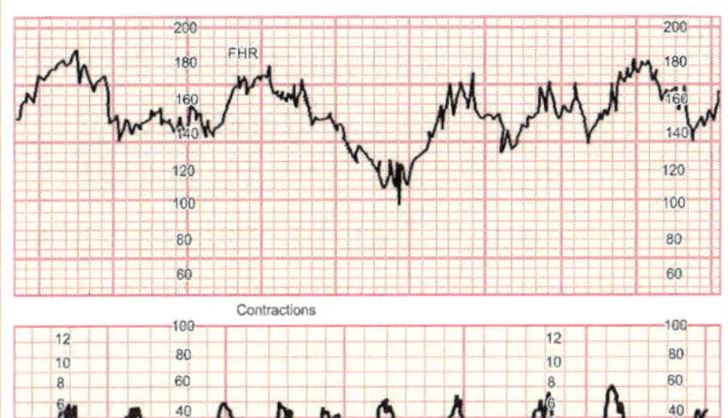 A. Wait for spontaneous vaginal delivery. B. Perform fetal blood sample. C. Instrumental delivery in the labor ward D. Instrumental delivery in the operation theater E. Emergency cesarean section	**Ans: D (Instrumental delivery in the operation theater)** Following the mnemonic DR C BRaVADO, the parameters assessed in this CTG are as follows: ▪ *Define risk:* The patient is at a high risk in view of her occipitoposterior position. ▪ *Contractions:* Uterine contractions in this case are occurring at the rate of 1–2 contractions per 1–2 minute, which is within normal limits during the second stage of labor. ▪ *Baseline FHR*: Baseline heart rate is within normal limits. ▪ *Variability*: Baseline variability is also normal. ▪ *Decelerations:* Several late decelerations can be observed. However, there is one late deceleration in the center of the CTG trace, which is prolonged for more than 3 minutes **(Fig. 16)**. 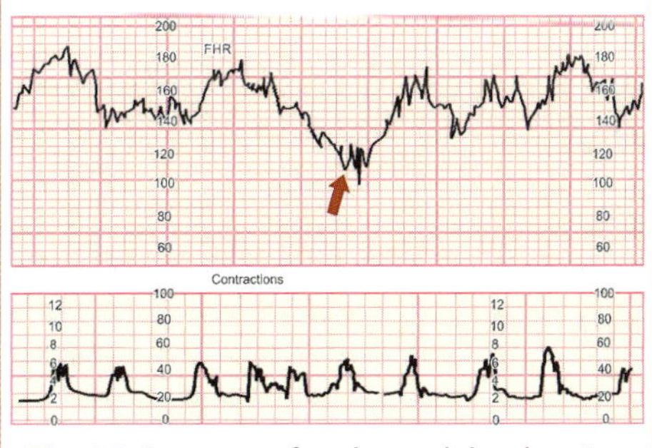 **Fig. 16:** Presence of prolonged deceleration in CTG (indicated by an arrow).	**Explanation:** The overall impression of the adjacent CTG is the presence of a single prolonged deceleration (>3 minutes). This is an indication for urgent delivery, which in this case appears to be possible with the help of instrumental delivery. Instrumental delivery is possible in this case because the cervix is fully dilated; the fetal head is engaged and has descended to +1 station. Instrumental delivery in this case needs to be conducted in the operation theater and not in the labor ward because the fetal head is in occipitoposterior position. Therefore, anesthesia may be required before application of Kielland forceps for rotating the fetal head or before manual rotation of the fetal head. **Potential questions:** There can be questions related to the interpretation of various parameters as well as their significance in various types of CTG traces.

ECG CHANGES

Question	Answer	Comment
Q17. A 67-year-old woman attends the gynecology ward for a preoperative assessment. She has been taking bendroflumethiazide for several years for hypertension. Her ECG trace has been shown in the image below. What is the most likely electrolyte imbalance in this case? 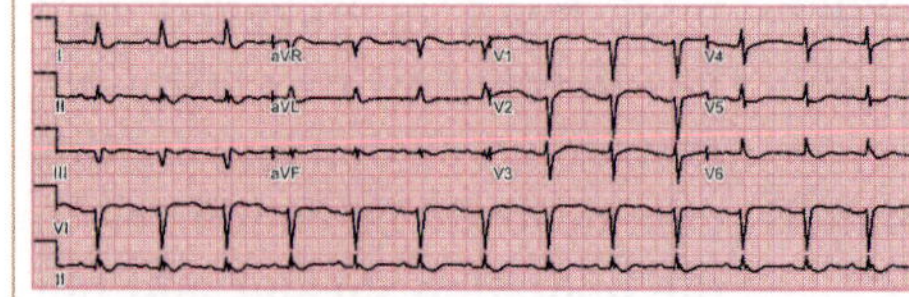 A. Hypokalemia B. Hyperkalemia C. Hypercalcemia D. Hypocalcemia E. Hypernatremia	**Ans: A (Hypokalemia)** The ECG changes in the adjacent image are suggestive of hypokalemia (serum potassium level of <3.5 mEq/L) and include the following **(Fig. 17)**: ▪ *Mild hypokalemia:* Reduced amplitude of the T wave ▪ *Moderate hypokalemia:* Flattened T wave with prominent U wave ▪ *Severe hypokalemia:* ST- segment sagging, only U waves; absent T waves 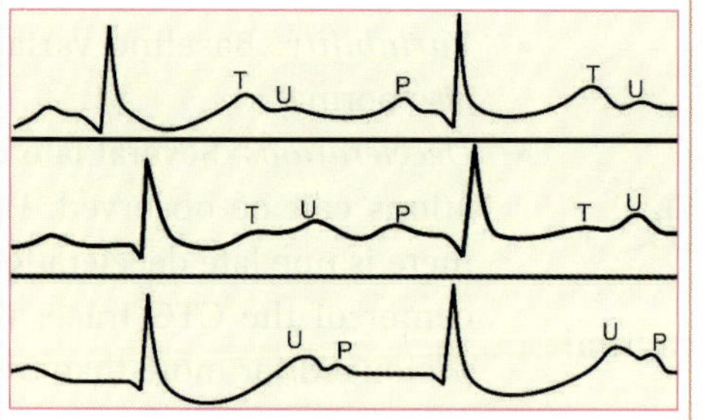 **Fig. 17:** ECG features suggestive of progressive hypokalemia.	**Explanation:** Diuretics can be considered as the most commonly used drugs responsible for causing hypokalemia. Potassium-wasting diuretics which block sodium reabsorption proximal to the distal nephron include diuretics such as thiazides, loop diuretics, osmotic diuretics, etc. These can cause hypokalemia. In this case, the woman is on thiazide diuretics, bendroflumethiazide, which is likely to result in hypokalemia. The adjacent ECG image also shows the features of hypokalemia such as presence of prominent U waves, absent T waves, and ST segment depression. **Potential questions:** There can be questions related to interpretation of common ECG changes, especially myocardial infraction and different electrolyte abnormalities, especially in the MRCOG part 1 exam.

Question	Answer	Comment
Q18. A 46-year-old woman has persistent hypertension during a workup for gynecology operation. Her laboratory investigations revealed a diagnosis of pheochromocytoma. The ECG trace obtained in this woman is depicted in the image below. Which biochemical change is most likely observed in this patient? 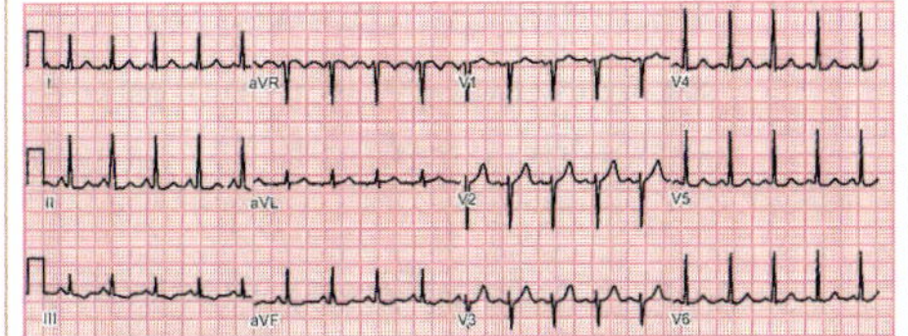 A. Hypokalemia B. Hyperglycemia C. Hyperkalemia D. Hypocalcemia E. Reduced urinary catecholamines	**Ans: B (Hyperglycemia)** The ECG figure of the given question is suggestive of sinus tachycardia which may be sometimes observed in the cases of pheochromocytomas. Sinus tachycardia is characterized by heart rate between 100 to 160 BPM **(Figs. 18A to C)**. The atrial rate indicated by P waves and ventricular rate indicated by QRS complex are > 100 BPM in this case. Since the P wave conducts through the atrioventricular node to the ventricles, the ratio of P waves to QRS complex is 1:1. The sinus rhythm remains regular with a normal P wave before each QRS complex. The heart rate in the given ECG graph varies between 120 to 150 BPM and the sinus rhythm remains regular. Heart rate in an ECG can be calculated by dividing 300 by number of large squares between the two R waves, which in this case is 2-2.5. 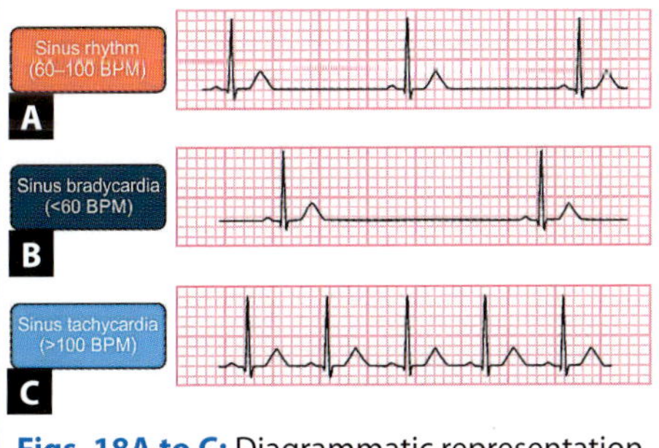 **Figs. 18A to C:** Diagrammatic representation of sinus tachycardia.	**Explanation:** Pheochromocytomas is caused by tumor of chromophil cells in adrenal medulla and is characterized by hypersecretion of catecholamines. Excessive secretion of catecholamines is likely to result in a triad of clinical presentation including headache, palpitations, and diaphoresis. The most important clinical signs associated with the cardiovascular system include sinus tachycardia and labile hypertension. Catecholamines have been shown to directly suppress insulin secretion from the pancreas and induce glycogenolysis in the liver via alpha-adrenergic receptor stimulation, resulting in hyperglycemia. Though pheochromocytomas usually do not cause any electrolyte abnormality, they can rarely cause hypokalemia. **Potential questions:** There can be questions related to interpretation of common ECG changes, especially myocardial infraction and different electrolyte abnormalities, particularly in the MRCOG part 1 exam.

Question	Answer	Comment
Q19. A 38-year-old pregnant woman with the diagnosis of acute renal failure was admitted into the critical care unit. The ECG trace of this patient is shown in the image below. What is the likely electrolyte abnormality in this case? 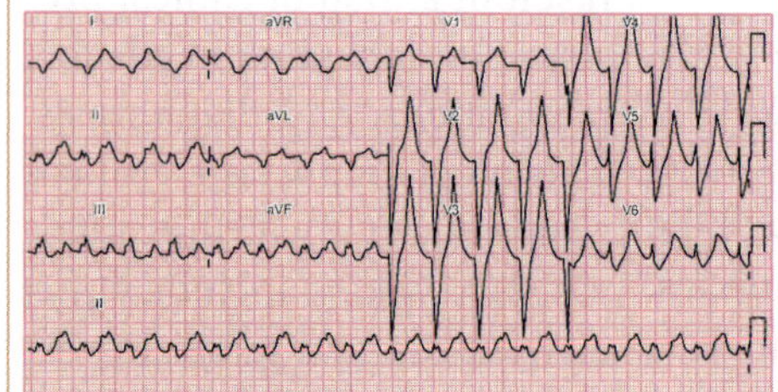 A. Hypokalemia B. Hyperkalemia C. Hypercalcemia D. Hypocalcemia E. Hypernatremia	**Ans: B (Hyperkalemia)** The adjacent image shows ECG findings suggestive of hyperkalemia. Hyperkalemia can be defined as the serum potassium concentration >5.0–5.5 mEq/L. ECG features suggestive of hyperkalemia include the following **(Fig. 19)**: ▪ Bizarre and wide QRS complex ▪ Tall, peaked T waves ▪ Short QT interval ▪ Flat P waves 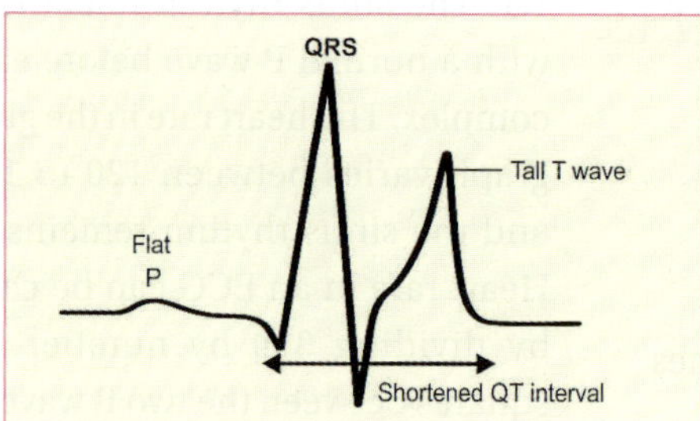 **Fig. 19:** ECG features suggestive of hyperkalemia.	**Explanation:** Findings in this ECG graph are as follows: Broad, bizarre QRS complexes—these merge with both the preceding P wave and subsequent T wave. Also, T waves are typically peaked. This is suggestive of hyperkalemia. Acute renal failure may be associated with hyperkalemia in this case. **Potential questions:** There can be questions related to interpretation of common ECG changes especially myocardial infarction and different electrolyte abnormalities, especially in the MRCOG part 1 exam.

Question	Answer	Comment
Q20. A 34-year-old woman of Pakistani origin was admitted in the accident and emergency department with a history of generalized tetany. She gives a history of wearing hijab all the time, whenever she is not at home. The image below illustrates the ECG findings in this case. What is the likely electrolyte abnormality in this case 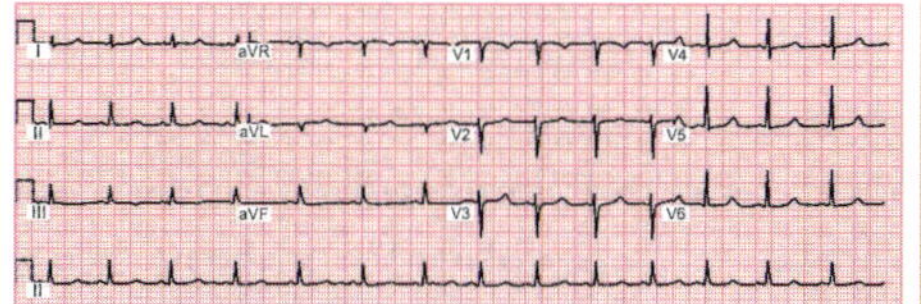 A. Hypokalemia B. Hypocalcemia C. Hypernatremia D. Hyponatremia E. Hyperkalemia	**Ans: B (Hypocalcemia)** The adjacent image in this case shows prolonged QT interval which is suggestive of hypocalcemia. Hypocalcemia can be defined as low serum calcium (Ca^{2+}) levels, less than the normal calcium levels of 2.1–2.6 mmol/L. Electrocardiography findings suggestive of hypocalcemia are as follows **(Figs. 20A and B)**: ▪ True prolongation of the QT interval without any alteration of the ST segment or T wave ▪ Dysrhythmias are uncommon ▪ Torsades de pointes may occur 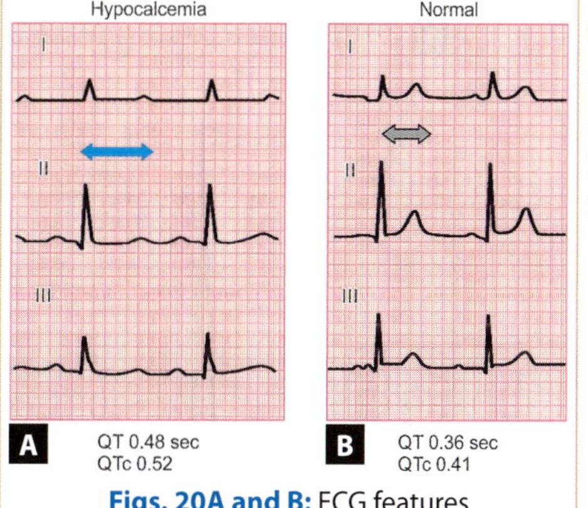 **Figs. 20A and B:** ECG features (A) Hypocalcemia; (B) Normal.	**Explanation:** The clinical scenario in this case is suggestive of reduced exposure to sunlight, resulting in vitamin D deficiency which can cause hypocalcemia. The adjacent image in this case shows prolonged QT interval which is suggestive of hypocalcemia. Some common causes of hypocalcemia include, hypoparathyroidism, vitamin D deficiency, acute pancreatitis, hyperphosphatemia, hypomagnesaemia, diuretics (furosemide), pseudohypoparathyroidism, etc. **Potential questions:** There can be questions related to interpretation of common ECG changes, especially myocardial infraction and different electrolyte abnormalities, particularly in the MRCOG part 1 exam.

Question	Answer	Comment
Q21. A 70-year-old woman with history of lung cancer, operated 2 months back, presented with worsening polyurea and has depression. Her parathyroid hormone (PTH) levels were raised. Her ECG trace is shown in the image below. What is the most likely electrolyte imbalance in this patient? 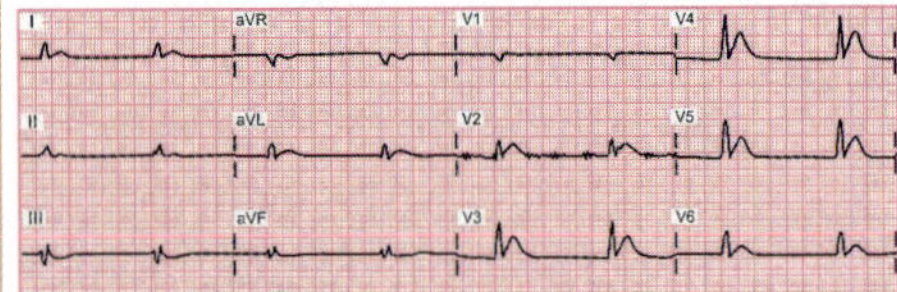 A. Hypokalemia B. Hypercalcemia C. Hypernatremia D. Hyponatremia E. Hyperkalemia	**Ans: B (Hypercalcemia)** The ECG findings in the adjacent image are suggestive of hypercalcemia, which can be defined as high calcium (Ca^{2+}) levels in the blood/serum, which is more than the normal calcium levels of 2.1–2.6 mmol/L. **Figures 21A and B** illustrate ECG features suggestive of hypercalcemia. 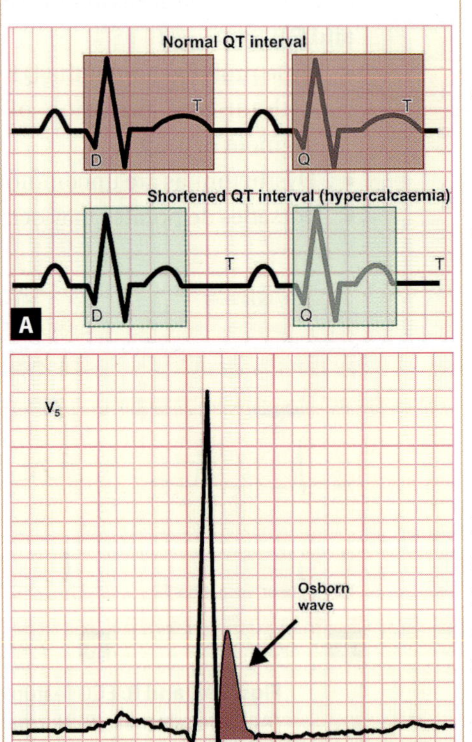 **Figs. 21A and B:** ECG features suggestive of hypercalcemia: (A) Shortening of the QT interval; (B) Osborn waves (J waves).	**Explanation:** Elevated PTH levels are likely to cause hypercalcemia. The ECG figure in this case shows reduced QT interval, which is suggestive of hypercalcemia. Electrocardiography changes in hypercalcemia are as follows **(Figs. 21A and B):** ▪ Shortening of the QT interval; no changes in the morphology of the QRS deflection or of the P and T waves ▪ ST segment may be completely absent and replaced by inverted small T wave directly after R wave ▪ In severe hypercalcemia, Osborn waves (J waves) may be seen. Osborn waves can be described as the waves occurring at the J point, which is the point of junction between the QRS complex and ST segment. **Potential questions:** There can be questions related to interpretation of common ECG changes, especially myocardial infarction and different electrolyte abnormalities, particularly in the MRCOG part 1 exam.

URODYNAMICS

Question	Answer	Comment
Q22. What does the bladder urodynamic graph shown in the image below describe? 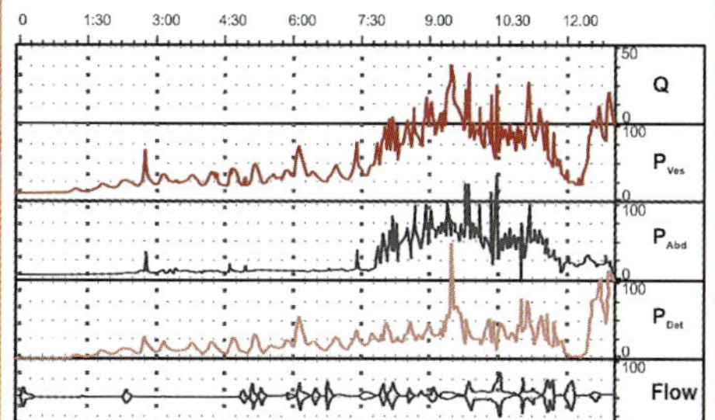 A. Detrusor muscle overactivity B. Detrusor muscle instability C. Stress incontinence D. Urge incontinence E. Urinary tract infection	**Ans: A (Detrusor muscle overactivity)** The adjacent urodynamic curve demonstrates detrusor muscle overactivity. This has been demonstrated with the help of arrows in **Figure 22**. The left-hand side of the adjacent urodynamic graph represents the filling phase, whereas the right side represents the voiding phase. The uppermost curve represents intravesical pressure. The second curve from the top represents intra-abdominal pressure. 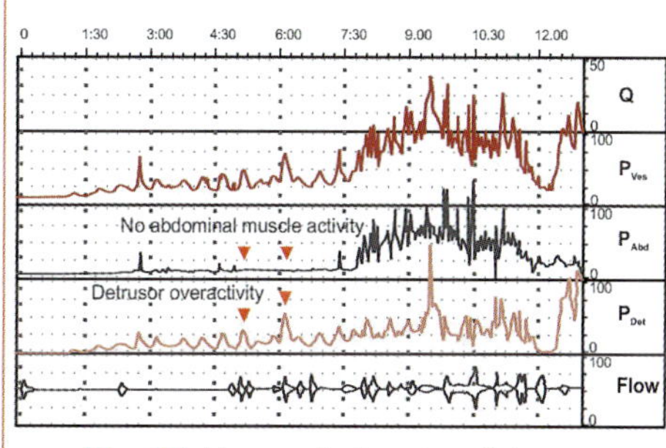 **Fig. 22:** Urograph showing detrusor hyperactivity with the help of arrows.	**Explanation:** The adjacent image shows that intravesical and intra-abdominal pressures remain stable during the filling phase. The detrusor pressure, calculated by subtracting abdominal pressure from intravesical pressure, displays hyperactivity during this phase, with isolated detrusor contractions indicated by arrows. There is no simultaneous rise in intra-abdominal pressure, suggesting detrusor muscle overactivity. **Potential questions:** There can be questions pertaining to the interpretation of urodynamic graphs in cases of both urge and stress incontinence.

<table>
<tr><th>Question</th><th>Answer</th><th>Comment</th></tr>
<tr>
<td>

Q23. What does the bladder urodynamic graph shown in the image below describe?

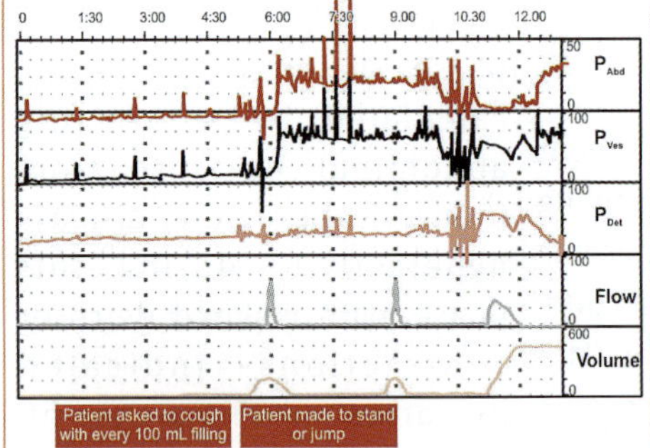

A. Detrusor muscle overactivity
B. Detrusor muscle instability
C. Stress incontinence
D. Urge incontinence
E. Urinary tract infection

</td>
<td>

Ans: C (Stress incontinence)

The adjacent urograph shows leakage during coughing and other maneuvers, indicating stress incontinence. The detrusor pressure remains low, and the leakage occurs without detrusor contraction. Coughing and other maneuvers cause a sharp rise and fall in pressure, equally affecting the bladder and abdominal channels **(Figure 23)**.

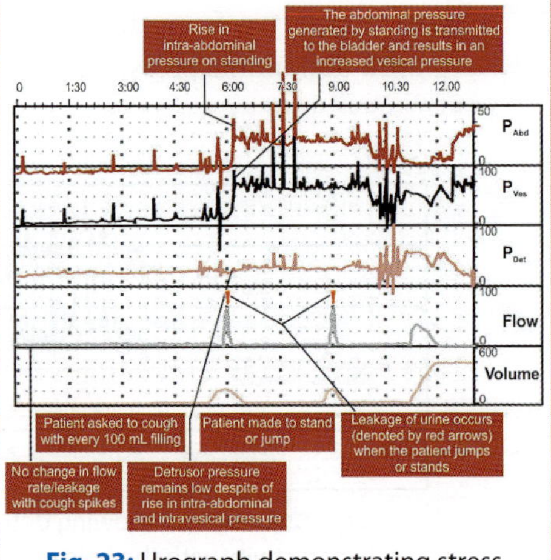

Fig. 23: Urograph demonstrating stress incontinence in the same patient.

</td>
<td>

Explanation: Figure 23 shows that the cough causes similar spikes in PVes and PAbd, but no rise in detrusor pressure or urine leakage. However, when the patient stands, urine leakage occurs with a rise in intra-abdominal pressure, without a concurrent rise in detrusor pressure or involuntary detrusor contractions, indicating stress incontinence.

Potential questions: There can be questions pertaining to the interpretation of urodynamic graphs in cases of both urge and stress incontinence.

</td>
</tr>
</table>

Index

Page numbers followed by *f* refer to figure.

D

E

F

G